Physicochemical Principles of Pharmacy

In Manufacture, Formulation and Clinical Use

SIXTH EDITION

Alexander T Florence CBE, DSc, FRSE, FRSC, FRPharmS
UCL School of Pharmacy, University College London, UK

David Attwood PhD, DSc, CChem, FRSC
Manchester Pharmacy School
University of Manchester, UK

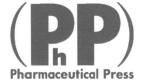

Pharmaceutical Press

Published by Pharmaceutical Press

66–68 East Smithfield, London E1W 1AW

© Royal Pharmaceutical Society 2016

(**PP**) is a trade mark of Pharmaceutical Press

Pharmaceutical Press is the publishing division of the
Royal Pharmaceutical Society

First, second and third editions published by
Palgrave (formerly Macmillan Press Ltd) 1981, 1988, 1998
Third edition reprinted 2004, 2005
Fourth edition 2006
Fourth edition reprinted 2007, 2009
Fifth edition 2011
Sixth edition 2016
Sixth edition reprinted 2022, 2023

Typeset by Data Standards Ltd, Frome, Somerset, UK
Printed in Great Britain by TJ Books Limited, Padstow, Cornwall

ISBN: 978 0 85711 174 6 (print)
ISBN: 978 0 85711 258 3 (ePDF)
ISBN: 978 0 85711 259 0 (ePub)
ISBN: 978 0 85711 260 6 (mobi)

A catalogue record for this book is available from the British Library.

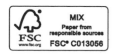

Physicochemical Principles of Pharmacy

In Manufacture, Formulation and Clinical Use

To our wives
Florence and Renee
for their long-standing patience and understanding.

Contents

Preface

Physicochemical Principles of Pharmacy emerged first in 1981, partly as a result of our frustration when teaching physical pharmacy to undergraduate pharmacy students that there was no European text that covered the subject using pharmaceutical examples to illustrate the topics. Having been brought up ourselves on a diet of physical chemistry of little obvious pharmaceutical relevance, we decided we should write a book that illustrated pharmaceutical themes with pharmaceutical examples. We also argued that if a particular concept had never been used in a published pharmacy or pharmaceutical science paper, then it perhaps could be ignored. We have felt that the book served as an important component of the sciences of pharmacy, complementing and recognising pharmaceutical and medicinal chemistry and pharmacology.

The first edition was well received and a second and third followed, all published by the Macmillan Press. It was encouraging that the text was used widely throughout the world. Charles Fry in a previous existence with Macmillan Press encouraged us to publish the book. His career took him to the Pharmaceutical Press where he negotiated the rights of the book and reapplied gentle pressure for us to complete the fourth edition. The fifth edition and now this, the sixth edition, are the result of considerable revision, to capture the basics from production of dosage forms to clinical pharmaceutics.

There have of course been changes in pharmacy education since the first edition appeared. We have tried wherever possible to make links with real situations that occur with medicines or that might be important in pharmacy today or in the future. Some of the examples we have used are those in the original editions, because they have now become classics. New material has been added, remembering that this is not a monograph on the latest advances, but a textbook of the physicochemical principles of pharmacy for undergraduates and postgraduates. All the editions of the book have made reference to clinical issues, but in this edition we have combined parts of the text from *An Introduction to Clinical Pharmaceutics* to give a more overt practice base.

We strongly believe that all pharmacy including clinical pharmacy practice must be based firmly in quantitative pharmaceutical science, otherwise it will not be distinguishable from other forms of clinical input practised by physicians and nurses and related staff. Another natural extension has been to add sections on the formulation and manufacture of solid-dose forms, as it is essential that pharmacy retains and indeed expands its role in industry and elsewhere in manufacture and design of delivery systems, not least with the challenging medicines now emerging. Not only that, but a true understanding of dosage form design will aid pharmacy practitioners to advise patients expertly on the optimum use of medicines.

We hope that the book will continue to be used in undergraduate and postgraduate pharmacy courses in many parts of the world, and by students of pharmaceutical science and the increasing number of students of cognate disciplines interested in pharmaceutical formulation and the properties of medicines.

We thank especially Erasmis Kidd for her encouragement and Linda Paulus for her valuable assistance during the production of this new and expanded edition.

Alexander T Florence
Dundee
David Attwood
Manchester
October 2015

About the authors

Alexander Florence was Dean of The School of Pharmacy, University of London from 1989 to 2006 and is Professor Emeritus at University College London. He was previously James P Todd Professor of Pharmaceutics at the University of Strathclyde. His interests are in drug delivery and targeting and nanotechnology. He is the author of *An Introduction to Clinical Pharmaceutics*, 2010, published by the Pharmaceutical Press.

David Attwood is Emeritus Professor of Pharmacy at the University of Manchester; he previously lectured at the University of Strathclyde. His research interests are in the physicochemical properties of drugs and surfactants, and in polymeric drug delivery systems. He has many years' experience in the teaching of physical pharmacy.

They co-authored *Surfactant Systems: Their Chemistry, Pharmacy and Biology* (Chapman and Hall, 1983) and *FASTtrack Physical Pharmacy* (Pharmaceutical Press, 2008, 2012).

Introduction

Pharmacy has several component disciplines, all interlinked. Pharmaceutics or physical pharmacy or the physicochemical principles of pharmacy, as in the title of this book, is one of these. It comprises the study of drug formulations and their design, manufacture and delivery to the body. In brief, pharmaceutics is about the conversion of drug substances into medicines suitable for administration by or to patients. It is not a static discipline: the definition of pharmaceutics extends now into the targeting of drugs and delivery systems to specific sites in the body and the fabrication of nanoparticles and delivery devices, as well as monitoring the behaviour of dose forms in the body.

There are other vital component disciplines in pharmacy. The way drugs act in and on the body is the domain of pharmacology; the science of drug design and analysis belongs to medicinal and pharmaceutical chemistry. One cannot design formulations without a comprehensive knowledge of the chemistry of the drug substance, nor study how medicines behave in the laboratory or in patients without good analytical skills. An understanding of the pharmacology of a drug is crucial not only with respect to the optimal design of a delivery system, but also to the wider practice of pharmacy.

There is certainly no dividing line in the sciences underlying these subjects: the physical chemistry that operates in the formulation laboratory is the same that holds within the human body. The forces acting between suspension particles and the walls of a container are the same as those acting on bacteria adsorbed on to a catheter or intestinal cell wall. The boundary conditions and the degree of complexity might differ, but the principles are the same. An understanding of the rules that govern what keeps drugs in solution in an infusion fluid allows us also to predict the extent to which a drug might precipitate in the renal tubules or in the blood after injection.

Studying the solid-state properties of drugs should not only provide vital information for formulators but might also help us to understand the formation of crystals in joints or in the kidneys, and how to dissolve them or prevent their formation. You will find many such examples in this book. We use 'memory diagrams' to assist in thinking about links between topics, dissect medicines that are used in the clinic and bring examples of the clinical aspects as well as newer concepts in the physical arena.

Physical chemistry and pharmacy

Undergraduates beginning their study of pharmacy are often surprised at the amount of physical chemistry they are expected to absorb, when they had expected perhaps a more biological flavour to their diet. Physical pharmacy is sometimes still thought of as a subject only for those who will become formulators and industrial pharmacists, but this view neglects the fact that pharmacy is, as it were, the 'guardian' of this subject. How can a practitioner advise physicians, nurses or patients on medicines without a sure knowledge of their composition and nature? The biological processes in the body do not operate and exist in some special non-physical world, although it is true that they are usually more complex than the processes we control in the test tube. So in this book we not only try to give the physicochemical basis for understanding pharmaceutical formulation and drug delivery but we also stray into related areas, frequently referring of course to chemical structures and biological and clinical issues. It is important that the underpinning sciences are used intelligently by pharmacy graduates, and not separated into compartments or silos.

Although in this edition of the book we have selected key equations that illustrate key points, we do not derive all of them from first principles. The value in appreciating the way in which an equation is derived lies with the fact that one can better understand the limitations of the equation. Equations often apply only in certain conditions, for example in extremely dilute solution, so the caveats in the derivations of equations must be heeded. Sometimes it is useful to be able to derive an equation from first principles. It would be sad if modern pharmacists were to become empiricists at a time when the science of drug development and drug therapy is becoming much more quantitative and predictable.

We have to admit that it is not always possible to apply precisely the equations in this book in the complex world of multicomponent medicines, especially after their administration, but rigorous physical chemistry is the starting point for a better understanding of these limits. As an example, the knowledge of the way in which the solubility of a drug increases or decreases with change in the acidity of the stomach or the intestine is an essential starting point in the understanding of the complex process of drug absorption and of the stability of drugs in solution. We also introduce in this edition some discussion of processes which have elements of randomness, such as the interaction between nanoparticles and receptors, or their escape from the blood circulation into target tissues. Static equations sometimes give the impression of certainty, when in real situations in complex environments these stochastic processes play their part in outcomes. Diffusion of molecules and particles results from stochastic interactions, as we will see.

This book is not of course a complete survey of all the physical chemistry underlying pharmacy, but we have selected what we feel is the most important in pharmaceutics and biopharmaceutics, without dealing with pharmacokinetics *per se* or with many aspects of pharmaceutical processes or pharmaceutical microbiology, which are covered in specialised textbooks.

The clinical relevance of physical pharmacy: clinical pharmaceutics

To some it seems a long extrapolation from physical pharmacy to patient care. There are those who argue that, with the increased emphasis on a clinical role for pharmacy, the importance of pharmaceutics diminishes. We certainly do not hold to this view. First we need products of high quality that are consistent and that work under a variety of circumstances. We need to understand the material in this book before embarking on a career in which medicines are central. But clinical pharmaceutics is more than biopharmaceutics: it is about applying knowledge of physical processes and phenomena, such as surface activity, rheology, precipitation and crystallisation and diffusion, to events in patients. We have not introduced a special chapter to deal with these issues, but rather each chapter provides selected examples where the physical chemistry assists in the understanding of adverse events, action of agents, and so on. We have used many examples and text from A T Florence, *An Introduction to Clinical Pharmaceutics*, Pharmaceutical Press, London, 2010.

Pharmacists must be comfortable with the properties of dosage forms, conventional and otherwise; they must understand how they work, what features can cause problems and which formulation might be better suited to one patient rather than another. More than that, we need practitioners who can predict trends in medication, drug delivery and targeting, personalised medicines, special formulations for paediatric and geriatric patients and the growing use of biologicals. Graduates should be able to evaluate critically what pharmaceutical manufacturers say about their products: the 'skeptical' pharmacist (following Robert Boyle's 17th-century *Skeptical Chymist*) is needed more and more in today's health care environment.

Adjuvants or excipients

It is forgotten by many, patients and other health care professionals included, that medicines contain much more than the drug, the active substance. Medicines contain so-called inactive materials, that is, *excipients* or *adjuvants*. In any medicine, the drug is of course central, whether we are dealing with its formulation, its delivery, its analysis or its activity. The formulation itself might simply be a means of delivering the dose in a convenient form to the patient, or it might have an influence on the site of delivery or the time over which the drug exerts its action, as with controlled-release products. Rational formulation requires a firm understanding of the physical mode of action of excipients in formulations. It is therefore vital that we understand the physical chemistry of materials used in formulations to control the rate of release or to solubilise insoluble molecules, to stabilise or to suspend drugs or to form microspheres and nanoparticles. These so-called adjuvants or excipients are generally regarded as inert, but few substances are totally inert and some, such as a number of surfactants, dyes and stabilisers, may be biologically active and indeed harmful if used inappropriately.

Arrangement of the book

In the first few chapters we examine the properties of drugs and excipients in the solid state and in solution. A new feature of the text is that we incorporate the physical aspects of manufacture of tablets and related products in Chapter 1. Formulation is discussed throughout the text. Gases are considered because of their importance in the design and use of therapeutic pressurised aerosols and implanted pumps. Special classes of materials and systems are also considered in separate chapters. Colloidal systems (which are those comprising particulates generally below 1 μm in diameter), including many suspensions and emulsions, have experienced a renaissance because of the use of microparticles and nanoparticles in drug targeting and controlled drug delivery. Polymers and macromolecules, used widely in pharmaceutical formulations as excipients in many forms as hydrogels, lipogels, viscous solutions and solid matrices or membranes, are treated in one chapter. Proteins, peptides and monoclonal antibodies have a chapter devoted to the pharmaceutical challenges they pose because of their size, lability and physical properties.

Surface activity is a phenomenon that has widespread consequences. Surface-active substances are those that adsorb at surfaces and lower surface tension; these so-called surfactant materials have a wide applicability in pharmacy. In micellar form they can solubilise water-insoluble drugs and many at low concentrations can increase membrane permeability and aid the transport of drugs across biological barriers. Many drugs have surface-active properties and this might have consequences for their activity and behaviour. The topic is summarised in a chapter on surface activity and surfactants.

Crucial to the whole subject is the process of drug absorption and how the physical properties of drugs and their formulation can influence the rate and extent (and sometimes site) of absorption. The basics of drug absorption and the oral route are discussed in one chapter, while the many alternative (parenteral) routes to achieving systemic levels of drugs are reviewed in a separate chapter. The emphasis is on the way in which the physiology of the route influences the design of formulations and the behaviour of drugs and dose forms.

Drugs are frequently given together and some interact, with clinically important consequences. Often these interactions are pharmacological, but some have a basis in physical chemistry. Incompatibilities might arise from electrostatic interactions between oppositely charged drugs, or from complexation between drugs and ions or drugs and polymers; these and a variety of other interactions are discussed in the book. There are special needs for some patients, those at the beginning of their lives, from neonates to 12-year-olds, and those who have matured to be 'geriatric', a term which covers many decades, as we discuss in a chapter on the topic. This discusses the need for more personalised medicines, attuned to the search for drugs with more predictable actions in individuals rather than cohorts. It is not always possible to predict the behaviour of drugs and formulations in the complicated environments in which they find themselves *in vivo*, but this should not deter us from at least attempting to rationalise events once they have become known. In this way our predictive powers will be honed and will allow us to prevent adverse events in the future. Some unwanted effects are due to the degradation of drugs and drug formulations; the examination of stability is an important part of assessing the suitability of formulations. This requires a good understanding of the chemistry of the drug substance and reaction kinetics. This, too, is the subject of a chapter.

Pharmaceutical nanotechnology is discussed because of the growing importance of this field and the increasing number of formulations and systems in the nanoscale. Many drug targeting systems are nanoparticles; some liposomes have diameters below 200 nm and dendrimers can be as small as 5–6 nm in diameter. Issues of particle size, flocculation and aggregation are important when size can determine the fate in the body. With many biological agents one must also think of molecular size as a factor in restricting the diffusion and translocation of the molecules in question. Many of the properties of systems, such as flowing suspensions, diffusion, surface activity and stability (either in storage or in patients) have wider implications. This is an aspect we try to convey.

One abiding object of pharmaceutical science is the production of high-quality medicinal products from high-quality drugs. One of the assurances for quality can be measured by *in vitro* experimentation, a field that is growing because of the new techniques now available to assess the physical and chemical nature of products. One chapter is devoted to discussing a selection of these as examples of what can be done, even with quite simple instruments. Nothing can replace studies in patients, but *in vitro* testing can predict the robust nature of products and their consistency in performance.

The book ends with a discussion of the issue of generic medicines of great importance in the economics of health care and the affordability of medication. Evaluation of the pharmacokinetics of products that are essentially interchangeable has to be assessed within certain limits, which must be understood against the background of the clinical relevance of peak plasma levels and times to maximum concentrations. These are more critical in some disease states than in others. The difficulty in creating generic proteins is also discussed in the chapter, which explains why in this domain the biological products are called biosimilars.

Nowhere do we claim that the physicochemical principles of pharmacy operate in isolation: the alliance between chemistry, biology, pharmacology and physics in determining outcomes of medicinal therapy is acknowledged. What we do argue is that understanding the physicochemical principles assists us in having a more quantitative and predictive view of the use of medicinal products by each route of administration.

Objectives

If one wishes to understand at more than a superficial level what makes modern delivery systems work, physical chemistry forms one important part. Examination of just one such delivery system (Fig. I.1), a simple

transdermal patch, brings into focus the diversity of physical phenomena that are involved in the design, use and action of delivery systems. One could list these in just this one example as:

- adsorption
- the stability of suspensions
- molecular transport through polymeric membranes
- adhesion
- the interaction of drugs with polymers
- the physicochemical properties of the skin
- the diffusional characteristics of drugs in the subsections of the skin, including crossing the capillary membrane into the blood.

'Reading' structures and formulae

Throughout this book you will come across two types of formulae: structural chemical formulae and physicochemical equations. 'Reading' and understanding formulae – of both kinds – is in a way like learning a language. We often equate reading chemical formulae to reading Chinese characters. To a person without any knowledge of the components of Chinese pictograms, the beautiful shapes mean nothing: 化学结构. A physical equation, similarly, is possibly more akin to the first sight of Arabic: a jumble of unfamiliar letters to the unversed: المعادلات الرياضية. Before we delve into the book proper, we can rehearse how to see the important features of chemical structures and equations.

Chemical structures

It is not necessary always to understand at this stage how a drug is synthesised, but it is important to know about the chemistry of a drug, as this determines so many features important in its formulation: its solubility in water, solubility in lipid phases, stability, interaction with excipients and, of course, absorption, not to mention the ultimate metabolism of the active.

There are of course classes of drugs with the same central 'core' to which are added substituents. It is important that we have a feel for the properties of the 'core' and the substituent groups, that is, whether they are ionised or non-ionised, polar or non-polar, water-soluble (hydrophilic) or hydrophobic. A hydrophobic

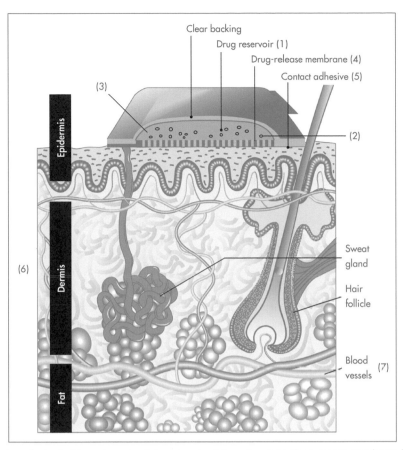

Figure I.1 A drawing of a typical transdermal patch system to deliver drug into the systemic circulation by way of the skin. Drawn here is the system with (1) a reservoir containing the drug adsorbed to (2) lactose particles in (3) an oil; (4) the rate-controlling membrane, a copolymer whose thickness and composition are altered to achieve the desired rate of transport of the drug; and (5) the adhesive layer, also a polymer, although liquid, which attaches the patch to the skin. The basic structure of the skin (6) illustrates the routes of penetration of the drug through this barrier layer into the systemic circulation via the capillary blood supply (7).

aromatic ring can have substituents that make the molecule water-soluble. Much of this is discussed in the text itself. This section simply asks that you look at the drug molecule (or an excipient or an additive molecule) in a certain way. Two drugs, meperidine (pethidine) (**I**) and procainamide (**II**) are shown below. Meperidine possesses an aromatic hydrocarbon ring and a piperidine ring and it is a carboxylic acid ester. The nitrogen is a tertiary amine and will be protonated at low pH; the ester is neutral. So one can predict something about the way the molecule will behave in solution and its relative hydrophobicity once the influence of substituent groups is realised. Also, a drug's name will often reveal something of its structure, hence the piperidine clue in meperidine. So too with procainamide (**II**), which is an amide with a primary amine

group and a tertiary alkylamine as well. This drug will have two pK_a values (or pK_b values) and this will have consequences for its solubility and absorption.

Structure I Meperidine

Structure II   Procainamide

It is not so simple with larger drugs such as docetaxel (**III**) and paclitaxel (**IV**), but the relationships between drugs in a class can be identified at least.

Structure III   Docetaxel

Structure IV   Paclitaxel

With proteins and peptides structural formulae are complex. Proteins have not only chemical structures, as we discuss, but have different conformations and three- and four-dimensional structures, which can be appreciated at a different level.

Physical equations

One equation often used in pharmaceutical development is the Noyes–Whitney equation, which relates the surface area of a solid drug to its rate of solution. Some equations are phenomenological (that is, they are derived as a result of experiment and observation) and do not necessarily have a deep theoretical base, so there is no need to be apprehensive of them. These are often intuitive equations, quite logical, as this one is:

$$\frac{\mathrm{d}w}{\mathrm{d}t} = \frac{DA}{\delta}(c_s - c)$$

where $\mathrm{d}w$ is the increase of the mass of material going into solution with increase of time $\mathrm{d}t$; D is the diffusion coefficient of the molecules escaping from the crystal surface; A is the surface area of the powder or of the crystal (if it is a single crystal); δ is the diffusion layer thickness; c_s is the saturation solubility of the drug; and c is the concentration of drug at any time point, t.

It is quite logical that the rate of solution should increase as the available surface area for dissolution increases, so you would expect $\mathrm{d}w/\mathrm{d}t$ to be directly proportional to A. D is a property of the drug molecule diffusing in concentrated drug solution. As the diffusion coefficient increases, one would expect the rate to increase. Diffusion takes place through a concentrated layer – the diffusion layer – and the thicker this is (i.e. the larger δ is), the further the drug has to diffuse to reach the bulk of the solution, hence $\mathrm{d}w/\mathrm{d}t$ is proportional to $1/\delta$. Stirring reduces the thickness of the stationary layer, hence aids dissolution. The more soluble a compound is (i.e. the higher c_s is), the higher the rate of solution; it is clear that if $c_s = c$, then the dissolution stops.

So, by thinking of a process logically, one can almost formulate the equation. Noyes and Whitney did this for us, and precisely, although as with all equations, this is robust only under certain conditions. Nevertheless, from the Noyes–Whitney equation one can predict accurately what the effect on dissolution will be if the solubility of the drug in the medium is increased, for example, by a change in pH. There are other equations for calculating the effect of pH on the equilibrium solubility, so this helps us get a more quantitative view of the complex world of medicines *in vitro* and *in vivo*.

1

Solids

The physical properties of the solid state seen in crystals and powders of both drugs and pharmaceutical excipients are of interest because they can affect both the production of dosage forms and the performance of the finished product. Powders, as Pilpel[1] reminded us, 'can float like a gas or flow like a liquid', but when compressed can support a weight. Fine powders dispersed as suspensions in liquids are used in injections and aerosol formulations. Both liquid and dry-powder aerosols are available and are discussed in Chapter 9.

In this chapter we will discuss:

- the form and particle size of crystalline and amorphous drugs and the effect these characteristics have on drug behaviour, especially on drug dissolution and bioavailability
- the properties of several subphases of crystalline solids, such as polymorphs, which are different crystalline forms (at different free-energy states) of the same molecule or molecules; and solvates, hydrates and cocrystals, which consist of more than one type of molecule, one of which is the drug, while the other can be either an organic solvent (to form a solvate) or water (to form a hydrate), or another crystalline solid (to form cocrystals)
- the wetting of powders, which influences, for example, their dispersion as suspensions and their spreading on tablet cores during spray coating; their flow and compaction properties, which are important during many of the unit operations involved in the tableting process; and the process of sublimation, which forms the basis of the technique of freeze drying
- the many physicochemical factors which come into play during the formulation and production of tablets and capsules, including: the cohesive and adhesive forces between particles that influence the flow and mixing properties; particle–particle interactions in both wet and dry granulation processes; and the mechanisms of compression and film coating of tablets

● the formulation and properties of solid dispersions and their potential for increasing the solubility of poorly water-soluble drugs.

The objectives of this chapter are to demonstrate how the nature of the crystalline form of a drug substance may affect its stability in the solid state, its solution properties, its absorption and its formulation as a solid-dosage form. It is with this topic that we start, to consider later other properties of the solid state that are important in production and formulation, for example, the production of nanocrystals of poorly soluble drugs to improve their dissolution and absorption.

1.1 Classification of solids

The solid phase can be classified into two major categories based on the order of molecular packing. The most common type of state is the crystalline state, in which there is both short-range and long-range order; that is, there is a regular structure that extends throughout the crystal. This contrasts with amorphous solids, in which the regularity of structure is limited to the immediate neighbours of any particular molecule within the solid. Crystalline solids can be further subdivided, as shown in Fig. 1.1, into polymorphs, which result from different crystalline forms of the same molecule, and multicomponent crystals such as hydrates, solvates and cocrystals, which consist of more than one type of molecule.

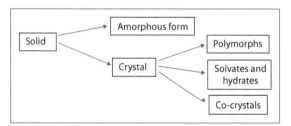

Figure 1.1 Classification of solids.

1.2 Crystalline solids: structure and properties

1.2.1 Crystal structure

Crystals contain highly ordered arrays of molecules and atoms held together by non-covalent interactions. We can consider as a simple example the unit cell of an inorganic salt, sodium chloride. Figure 1.2 shows the ordered arrangement of Cl^- ions and Na^+ ions that make up the sodium chloride crystal structure. We can draw a square on one side connecting the chloride ions.

Similar squares could be drawn on all the sides to form a cubic repeating unit, which we call the *unit cell*. Within a specific crystal, each unit cell is the same size and contains the same number of molecules or ions arranged in the same way. It is usually most convenient to think of the atoms or molecules as points and the crystal as a three-dimensional array of these points, or a *crystal lattice*.

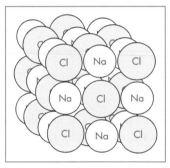

Figure 1.2 Space lattice of the sodium chloride crystal. Each sodium ion is octahedrally surrounded by six chloride ions and each chloride ion is octahedrally surrounded by six sodium ions.

For all possible crystals there are seven basic or primitive unit cells, which are shown in Fig. 1.3. We will represent the lengths of the sides as *a*, *b* and *c* and the angles as

α (between sides *b* and *c*)
β (between sides *a* and *c*)
γ (between sides *a* and *b*)

Figure 1.3 shows the characteristic side lengths and angles for these 'primitive' unit cells. The structures in Fig. 1.3 have atoms or molecules only at each corner of the unit cell. It is possible to find unit cells with atoms or molecules also at the centre of the top or bottom faces (*end-centred*), at the centre of every face (*face-centred*) or with a single atom in the centre of the cell (*body-centred*), as in Fig. 1.4.

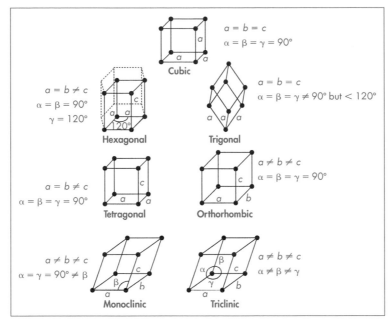

Figure 1.3 The seven possible primitive unit cells with atoms or molecules only at each corner of the unit cell. Drug molecules will typically form triclinic, monoclinic and orthorhombic unit cells.

Note that these variations do not occur with every type of unit cell: we find

- end-centred monoclinic and orthorhombic
- face-centred cubic and orthorhombic
- body-centred, cubic, tetragonal and orthorhombic.

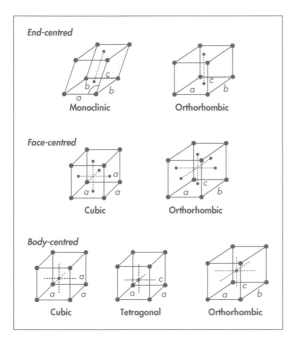

Figure 1.4 Variations on primitive cells.

Altogether there are 14 possible types of unit cell and we call these the *Bravais lattices*. For drugs there are three common types of unit cell: triclinic, monoclinic and orthorhombic.

Key points

- The crystal lattice is constructed from repeating units called unit cells; all unit cells in a specific crystal are the same size and contain the same number of molecules or ions arranged in the same way.
- There are seven primitive unit cells – cubic, trigonal, orthorhombic, triclinic, hexagonal, tetragonal and monoclinic – which have molecules or ions arranged at each corner.
- In addition, monoclinic and orthorhombic unit cells may be end-centred; cubic and orthorhombic unit cells may be face-centred; and cubic, tetragonal and orthorhombic unit cells may be body-centred.
- There are therefore only 14 possible types – the Bravais lattices.
- Drug molecules usually have triclinic, monoclinic or orthorhombic unit cells.

Miller indices

We can identify the various planes of a crystal using the system of *Miller indices*. To understand how this system is used, let us consider the plane drawn through the cubic crystal shown in Fig. 1.5a. The plane cuts the *a* axis at one unit length and also the *c* axis at one unit length. It does not, however, cut the *b* axis, and hence the intercept to this axis is infinity. One way we could label planes is to denote each set by the distances along the axes to the point where the plane crosses the axis. So, for example, the planes marked in Fig. 1.5a would have intercept lengths of $a = 1$, $b = \infty$, $c = 1$. This system of labelling the faces is inconvenient because of the appearance of ∞. A way around this problem is to take the reciprocals of the numbers (since the reciprocal of $\infty = 0$). The plane shown then becomes 1/1, 1/∞, 1/1 for the *a*, *b* and *c* axes, i.e. 1, 0, 1. The Miller indices for this plane are then written as (101).

A second example is illustrated in Fig. 1.5b. This plane does not cut the *a* axis: it cuts the *b* axis at a unit cell length of ½, and does not cut the *c* axis. The intercept lengths are therefore $a = \infty$, $b = 1/2$, $c = \infty$,

which on taking reciprocals become 0, 2, 0. A second rule of Miller indices is now applied, that is, to reduce the numbers to the lowest terms – in this case by dividing them all by 2. The Miller indices for this plane are therefore (010).

Other rules for applying Miller indices are shown by the following examples, which for ease of illustration are shown using a two-dimensional array (the *c* axis can be imagined to be at right angles to the page). None of the sets of planes we will consider crosses the *c* axis, i.e. we consider them to intersect it at ∞. The plane X in Fig. 1.6 has *a*, *b* and *c* intercepts of 3, 2 and ∞, giving reciprocals of ⅓, ½ and 0. The procedure is now to clear the fractions, in this case by multiplying each term by 6, giving 2, 3 and 0. It is not possible to reduce these further, and the Miller indices are therefore (230). The plane Y in Fig. 1.6 shows an example of a negative intercept where the *a* axis is crossed. The reciprocals of the *a*, *b* and *c* intercepts are -1, 1 and 0. The procedure that is now used is to write the negative number using a bar above it, giving Miller indices for this plane of ($\bar{1}$10). We should notice that the smaller the number in the Miller index for a particular axis, the more parallel is the plane to that axis – a zero value indicates a plane exactly parallel to that axis. The larger a Miller index, the more nearly perpendicular a plane is to that axis.

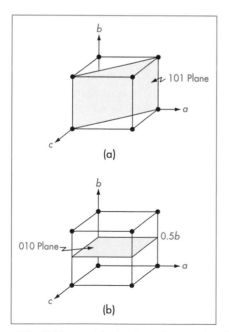

Figure 1.5 Cubic crystal showing planes with Miller indices of (a) (101) and (b) (010).

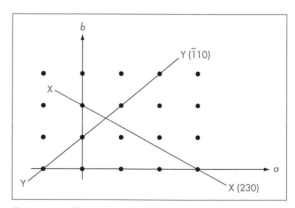

Figure 1.6 Planes in a two-dimensional array.

Key points

The general rules for expressing planes using the system of Miller indices:

- Determine the intercepts of the plane on the *a*, *b* and *c* axes in terms of unit cell lengths.
- Take the reciprocals of the intercepts.
- Clear the fractions by multiplying by the lowest common denominator.
- Reduce the numbers to the lowest terms.
- Indicate negative numbers with a bar above the number.

Example 1.1 Use of Miller indices

Draw a two-dimensional lattice array and indicate the planes with the following Miller indices:

(i) (100); (ii) (010); (iii) (110); (iv) (120); (v) (230); and (vi) (410).

Answer

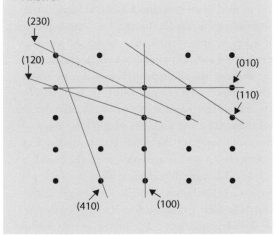

1.2.2 Crystal form

The solid state is important for a variety of reasons, summarised in Fig. 1.7: morphology, particle size, polymorphism, solvation or hydration can affect filtration, flow, tableting, dissolution and bioavailability. These are described below. In addition, crystallisation can sometimes occur *in vivo*, often, as in the case of gout and urinary stones (see below), with painful consequences.

The crystals of a given substance may vary in size, the relative development of the given faces and the number and kind of the faces (or forms) present; that is, they may have different crystal *habits*. The habit describes the overall shape of the crystal in rather general terms and includes, for example, acicular (needle-like), prismatic, pyramidal, tabular, equant, columnar and lamellar types. Figure 1.8 shows the crystal habits of a hexagonal crystal.

Although there may not be significant differences in the bioavailability of drugs with different crystal habits, the crystal habit is of importance from a technological point of view. The ability to inject a suspension containing a drug in crystal form will be influenced by the habit: plate-like crystals are easier to inject through a fine needle than are needle-like crystals. The crystal habit can also influence the ease of compression of a powder and the flow properties of the drug in the solid state. The plate-like crystals of tolbutamide, for example, cause powder bridging in the hopper of the tablet machine and also capping problems during tableting. Neither of these problems occurs with tolbutamide in other crystal habits. The habits acquired depend on the conditions of crystallisation, such as the solvent used, the temperature, the concentration and presence of impurities. Ibuprofen crystallises from hexane as elongated needle-like crystals, which have been found to have poor flow properties; crystallisation from methanol produces equidimensional crystals with better flow properties and compaction characteristics, making them more suitable for tableting. The crystal morphology of the excipients (such as powdered cellulose) included in tablet formulations can also have a significant influence on the strength and disintegration time of tablets.

Crystallisation and factors affecting crystal form[2]

Crystallisation from solution can be considered to be the result of three successive processes:

1. supersaturation of the solution
2. formation of crystal nuclei
3. crystal growth round the nuclei.

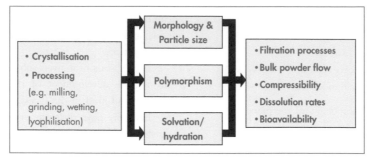

Figure 1.7 The solid state in pharmaceutical science: potential causes and effects of structural change (after AJ Florence).

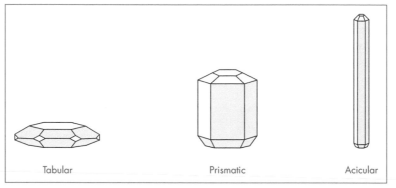

Figure 1.8 Crystal habits of a hexagonal crystal.

 Clinical point **Painful examples of crystallisation: gout and kidney stones**

Gout usually manifests itself as a sudden excruciating pain in the big toe (usually of men), although other joints such as the ankle, heel, instep, knee, wrist, elbow, fingers or spine may be affected. It is a consequence of the precipitation of needle-like crystals of uric acid, in the form of monosodium urate, on the articular cartilage of joints when the levels of uric acid in blood serum exceed a critical solubility level (approximately 6.7 mg dL^{-1}); the crystals inside the joint cause intense pain whenever the affected area is moved. Uric acid is a normal component of blood serum and is a product of the metabolism of purines, which are generated by the body via breakdown of cells in normal cellular turnover, and also are ingested as part of a normal diet in foods such as liver, sardines, anchovies and dried peas and beans. The uric acid is normally filtered out of the blood by the kidneys and excreted in the urine. Sometimes, however, too much uric acid is produced by the body or the kidneys are not sufficiently efficient at removing it and it accumulates in the blood, a condition known as hyperuricaemia. Precipitation of uric acid is also markedly enhanced when the blood pH is low (acidosis), a consequence of reduced solubility under such conditions. Patients with long-standing hyperuricaemia can have uric acid crystal deposits called tophi in other tissues, such as the helix of the ear.

Urinary stone formation (urolithiasis) is a common disorder affecting 1–5% of the population in industrialised countries. Although it is a consequence of complex physicochemical processes, the major driving force behind the formation of many stones is the state of saturation of urine with crystal-forming substances such as oxalic or uric acid. For example, urinary uric acid solubility is limited to 9.6 mg dL^{-1}. Since uric acid excretion in humans generally exceeds 600 mg day^{-1}, this poses a great risk for its precipitation. Uric acid is a weak acid (pK_a of 5.35 at 37°C) with a solubility of 158 mg dL^{-1} at pH 7.0. Reducing the urinary pH to 5.0 decreases the solubility of uric acid to less than 8.0 mg dL^{-1}, leading to supersaturation of the urine and precipitation of sparingly soluble uric acid in the kidney or bladder in the form of stones.

Supersaturation can be achieved by cooling, by evaporation, by the addition of a precipitant or by a chemical reaction that changes the nature of the solute. Supersaturation itself is insufficient to cause crystals to form; the crystal embryos must form by collision of molecules of solute in the solution, or sometimes by the addition of seed crystals, or dust particles, or even particles from container walls. Deliberate seeding is often carried out in industrial processes; seed crystals do not necessarily have to be of the substance concerned but may be isomorphous substances (i.e. of the same morphology). As soon as stable nuclei are formed, they begin to grow into visible crystals.

Crystal growth can be considered to be a reverse dissolution process and the diffusion theories of Noyes and Whitney, and of Nernst, consider that matter is deposited continuously on a crystal face at a rate proportional to the difference of concentration between the surface and the bulk solution. Thus an equation for crystallisation can be proposed in the form:

$$\frac{dm}{dt} = Ak_m(c_{ss} - c_s) \tag{1.1}$$

where m is the mass of solid deposited in time t, A is the surface area of the crystal, c_s is the solute concentration at saturation and c_{ss} is the solute concentration at supersaturation. As $k_m = D/\delta$ (D being the diffusion coefficient of the solute and δ the diffusion layer thickness; see Fig. 1.19), the degree of agitation of the system, which affects δ, also influences crystal growth. Crystals generally dissolve faster than they grow, so growth is not simply the reverse of dissolution. It has been suggested that there are two steps involved in growth in addition to those mentioned earlier, namely, transport of the molecules to the surface and their arrangement in an ordered fashion in the lattice. Equation (1.1) turns out to be better written in a modified form:

$$\frac{dm}{dt} = Ak_g(c_{ss} - c_s)^n \tag{1.2}$$

k_g being the overall crystal growth coefficient and n the 'order' of the crystal growth process. For more details, reference 2 should be consulted.

Precipitation

Precipitation may be induced by altering the pH of the solution so that the saturation solubility is exceeded. Precipitation may be made to occur from a homoge-neous solution by slowly generating the precipitating agent by means of a chemical reaction, a process likely to occur, for example, in intravenous infusion fluids and liquid pharmaceuticals. Precipitation by direct mixing of two reacting solutions sometimes does not bring about immediate nucleation and, as a result, the mixing stage may be followed by an appreciable lag time. The rate of precipitation is an important factor in determining habit, as might be imagined with a dynamic process such as crystallisation, involving nucleation and subsequent crystal growth. The form of phenylsalicylate, for example, depends on rate of crystal growth. Transition to an acicular shape occurs when the rate of growth increases. At low rates of growth, crystals of a more regular shape are obtained. In studies of the effect of solvents on habit it is generally found that less viscous media favour the growth of coarse and more equidimensional crystal forms.

Habit modification

Crystal habit can be modified by adding impurities or 'poisons'; for example, sulfonic acid dyes alter the crystal habit of ammonium, sodium and potassium nitrates.

Surfactants in the solvent medium used for crystal growth (or, for example, in stabilisation or wetting of suspensions) can alter crystal form by adsorbing on to growing faces during crystal growth. This is best illustrated by the effect of anionic and cationic surfactants on the habit of adipic acid crystals.[3] X-ray analysis showed that the linear six-carbon dicarboxylic acid molecules were aligned end to end in a parallel array in the crystal, with their long axis parallel to the (010) faces, so that the (001) face is made up entirely of −COOH groups while the (010) and (110) faces contain both −COOH and hydrocarbon (HC) portions of the molecule (Fig. 1.9). The cationic surfactant trimethyldodecylammonium chloride is twice as effective in hindering the growth of the (001) face as that of the (110) and (010) faces. In high concentrations it causes the formation of very thin plates or flakes. Conversely, the anionic surfactant sodium dodecylbenzene sulfonate at 55 parts per million (ppm) is three times as effective in reducing the growth rates of the (110) and (010) faces as of the (001) face. Higher levels of sodium dodecylbenzene sulfonate cause extreme habit modification, producing not hexagonal plates but long, thin

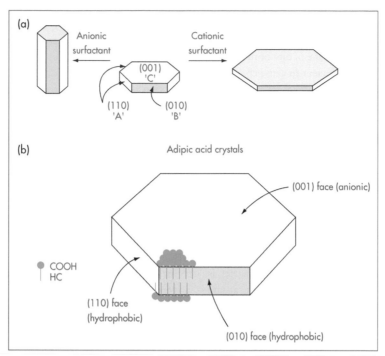

Figure 1.9 (a) Effect of anionic and cationic surfactants on the habit of adipic acid crystals. (b) A diagrammatic (not to scale) representation of the arrangement of molecules at the crystal surface.

rods or needles. The crystallographic faces whose growth rates are depressed most are those upon which surfactant adsorption is the greatest. Cationic additives adsorb on the face composed of carboxylic groups (001), and anionic additives on the (110) and (010) faces, which are hydrophobic. A coulombic interaction of the cationic head groups and the $-COO^-$ groups on the (001) faces has been suggested. The adsorption of the anionic surfactant, repelled from the anionic (001) faces, takes place amphipathically on the hydrophobic (110) faces and (010) faces (Fig. 1.9).

1.2.3 Polymorphism[4]

As we have seen, compounds can crystallise out of solution in a variety of different habits depending on the conditions of crystallisation. These crystal habits usually have the same internal structure and so have the same X-ray diffraction patterns. A more fundamental difference in properties may be found when the compounds crystallise as different *polymorphs*. When *polymorphism* occurs, the molecules arrange themselves in two or more different ways in the crystal: either they may be packed differently in the crystal lattice or there may be differences in the orientation or conformation of the molecules at the lattice sites. These variations cause differences in the X-ray diffraction patterns of the polymorphs and this technique is one of the main methods of detecting the existence of

Key points

- The crystal habit describes the external appearance of a crystal, i.e. its overall shape and the number and kind of faces. Common types of habit include acicular, prismatic, pyramidal, tabular, equant, columnar and lamellar.
- The crystal habit depends on the conditions of crystallisation and may affect the syringeability of suspensions of the drug, its ease of compression into tablets and its flow properties.
- The crystal habit can be modified by adding impurities (called poisons) or surfactants to the solvent used for crystallisation.

polymorphs. The polymorphs have different physical and chemical properties; for example, they may have different melting points and solubilities and they also usually exist in different habits.

We will consider two drugs that exhibit this phenomenon. Spironolactone (I), which is a diuretic steroidal aldosterone agonist, crystallises as two polymorphic forms and also as four solvated crystalline forms depending on the solvents and methods used for crystallisation.[5] We will consider the occurrence of solvated forms in section 1.2.4; at the moment we will concentrate on the two polymorphs only. Form 1 is produced when spironolactone powder is dissolved in acetone at a temperature very close to the boiling point and the solution is then cooled within a few hours down to 0°C. Form 2 is produced when the powder is dissolved in acetone, dioxane or chloroform at room temperature and the solvent is allowed to evaporate spontaneously over a period of several weeks. In both polymorphs the steroid nuclei (A, B, C and D rings) are almost planar and perpendicular to the E ring and to the 7α-acetothio side-chain. The packing of the molecules in the two polymorphs is compared in Fig. 1.10. Both unit cells are orthorhombic but they differ in their dimensions. The *a*, *b* and *c* axes of Form 1 were found to be 0.998, 3.557 and 0.623 nm, respectively, compared with equivalent lengths for Form 2 of 1.058, 1.900 and 1.101 nm. There are also differences in the crystal habits: Form 1 crystals are needle-like, while those of Form 2 are prisms (Fig. 1.11). The melting points are slightly different: Form 1 melts at 205°C whereas Form 2 has a melting point of 210°C.

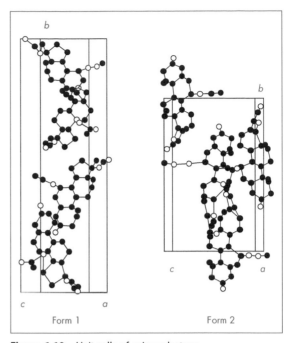

Figure 1.10 Unit cells of spironolactone.

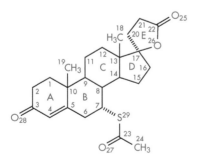

Structure I Spironolactone

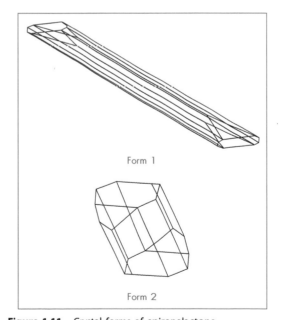

Figure 1.11 Crystal forms of spironolactone.

Our second example of a drug exhibiting polymorphism is paracetamol (**II**). This drug is known to exist in two polymorphic forms, monoclinic (Form 1) and orthorhombic (Form 2), of which Form 1 is the more thermodynamically stable at room temperature and is the commercially used form.[6] However, this form is not suitable for direct compression into tablets and has to be mixed with binding agents before tableting, a procedure that is both costly and time consuming. In contrast, Form 2 can readily undergo plastic deformation upon compaction and it has been suggested that this form may have distinct processing advantages over the monoclinic form. Monoclinic paracetamol is readily produced by crystallisation from aqueous solution and many other solvents; production of the orthorhombic form has proved more difficult but may be achieved, at least on a laboratory scale, by nucleating a supersaturated solution of paracetamol with seeds of Form 2 (from melt-crystallised paracetamol). Figure 1.12 shows scanning electron micrographs of the two polymorphic forms when crystallised from industrial methylated spirit. Form 1 is described as having a prismatic to plate-like habit that is elongated in the direction of the *c*-axis, while Form 2 crystallises as prisms that are elongated along the *c*-axis.

Structure II Paracetamol

Polymorphism is common with pharmaceutical compounds. Although we do not yet understand the process sufficiently well to predict which drugs are likely to exhibit this phenomenon, it is clear that certain classes of drug are particularly susceptible. Eight crystal modifications of phenobarbital have been isolated, but 11 have been identified, with melting points ranging from 112 to 176°C. Of the barbiturates used medicinally, about 70% exhibit polymorphism. The steroids frequently possess polymorphic modifications, testosterone having four: these are cases of true polymorphism and not pseudopolymorphism, in which solvent is the cause (see section 1.2.4). Of the commercial sulfonamides, about 65% are found to exist in several polymorphic forms. Examples of the differing solubilities and melting points of polymorphic sulfonamides and steroids are given in Table 1.1.

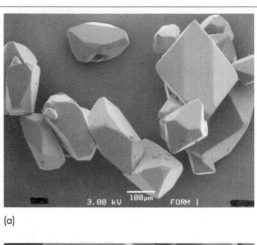

(a)

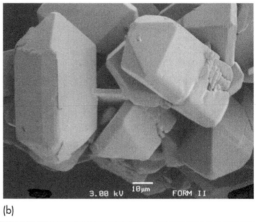

(b)

Figure 1.12 Scanning electron micrographs showing the crystal habit of (a) Form 1 and (b) Form 2 of paracetamol grown from supersaturated industrial methylated spirit. Note different scales.

Reproduced from Nichols G, Frampton CS. Physicochemical characterization of the orthorhombic polymorph of paracetamol crystallized from solution. *J Pharm Sci* 1998;87:684–693. Copyright Wiley-VCH Verlag GmbH & Co. KGaA. Reproduced with permission.

Predictability of the phenomenon is difficult except by reference to past experience. Its pharmaceutical importance depends very much on the stability and solubility of the forms concerned. It is difficult, therefore, to generalise, except to say that where polymorphs of insoluble compounds occur there are likely to be biopharmaceutical implications. Table 1.2 is a partial listing of the drugs for which polymorphic and pseudopolymorphic states have been identified or for which an amorphous state has been reported.

Table 1.1 Melting points of some polymorphic forms of steroids, sulfonamides and riboflavin

Compound	Form and/or melting point (°C)			
Polymorphic steroids	(I)	(II)	(III)	(IV)
Corticosterone	180–186	175–179	163–168	155–160
β-Estradiol	178	169		
Estradiol	225	223		
Testosterone	155	148	144	143
Methylprednisolone	I (205, aqueous solubility 0.075 mg cm^{-3}) II (230, aqueous solubility 0.16 mg cm^{-3})			
Polymorphic sulfonamides				
Sulfafurazole	190–195	131–133		
Acetazolamide	258–260	248–250		
Tolbutamide	127	117	106	
Others				
Riboflavin	I (291, aqueous solubility 60 mg cm^{-3}) II (278, aqueous solubility 80 mg cm^{-3}) III (183, aqueous solubility 1200 mg cm^{-3})			

Reproduced with permission from Kuhnert-Brandstatter M. *Thermomicroscopy in the Analysis of Pharmaceuticals.* New York: Pergamon Press, 1971.

Pharmaceutical implications of polymorphism

We have already considered the problems in tableting and injection that may result from differences in crystal habit (see section 1.2.2). Since polymorphs frequently have different habits, they too will be subject to these same problems. However, polymorphs also have different crystal lattices and consequently their energy contents may be sufficiently different to influence their stability and biopharmaceutical behaviour.

As the different polymorphs arise through different arrangement of the molecules or ions in the lattice, they will have different interaction energies in the solid state. Under a given set of conditions the polymorphic form with the lowest free energy will be the most stable, and other polymorphs will tend to transform into it. The rate of conversion is variable and is determined by the magnitude of the energy barrier between the two polymorphs – the higher the energy barrier and the lower the storage temperature, the slower is the conversion rate. Occasionally, the most stable polymorph appears only several years after the

Table 1.2 Polymorphic and pseudopolymorphic drugs

Compound	Number of forms		
	Polymorphs	Amorphous	Pseudopolymorphs
Ampicillin	1	–	1
Beclometasone dipropionate	–	–	2
Betamethasone	1	1	–
Betamethasone 21-acetate	1	1	–
Betamethasone 17-valerate	1	1	–
Caffeine	1	–	1
Cefaloridine	4	–	2
Chloramphenicol palmitate	3	1	–
Chlordiazepoxide HCl	2	–	1
Chlorthalidone	2	–	–
Dehydropregnenolone	1	–	7
Dexamethasone acetate	3	–	1
Dexamethasone pivalate	4	–	7
Digoxin	–	1	–

Table 1.2 *(continued)*

Compound	Number of forms		
	Polymorphs	**Amorphous**	**Pseudopolymorphs**
Erythromycin	2	–	–
Fludrocortisone acetate	3	1	–
Fluprednisolone	3	–	2
Glutethimide	1	–	1
Hydrocortisone TBA	1	–	3
Indometacin	3		
Mefenamic acid	2	–	–
Meprobamate	2	–	–
Methyl *p*-hydroxybenzoate	6	–	–
Methylprednisolone	2	–	–
Novobiocin	1	1	–
Prednisolone	2	–	–
Prednisolone TBA	2	–	2
Prednisolone TMA	3	–	–
Prednisolone acetate	2	–	–
Prednisone	1	–	1
Progesterone	2	–	–
Sorbitol	3	–	–
Testosterone	4	–	–
Theophylline	1	–	1
Triamcinolone	2	–	–

Modified with permission from Bouché R, Draguet-Brughmans M. [Recent developments of thermal analysis.] *J Pharm Belg* 1977;32:347, with additions.
HCl, hydrochloride; TBA, tertiary butyl acetate (tebutate); TMA, trimethyl acetate.

compound was first marketed. We can determine which of two polymorphs is the more stable by a simple experiment in which the polymorphs are placed in a drop of saturated solution under the microscope. The crystals of the less stable form will dissolve and those of the more stable form will grow until only this form remains. Figure 1.13 shows this process occurring with the two polymorphs of paracetamol, discussed earlier. Figure 1.13a shows the presence of both forms of paracetamol at room temperature in saturated benzyl alcohol. Over a time interval of 30 minutes the less stable of the two forms, the orthorhombic Form 2, has completely converted to the more stable monoclinic

Form 1 (Fig. 1.13b). For drugs with more than two polymorphs we need to carry out this experiment on successive pairs of the polymorphs of the drug until we eventually arrive at their rank order of stability.

Transformations

The transformation between polymorphic forms can lead to formulation problems. Phase transformations can cause changes in crystal size in suspensions and their eventual caking. Crystal growth in creams as a result of phase transformation can cause the cream to become gritty. Similarly, changes in polymorphic forms of vehicles, such as theobroma oil used to make

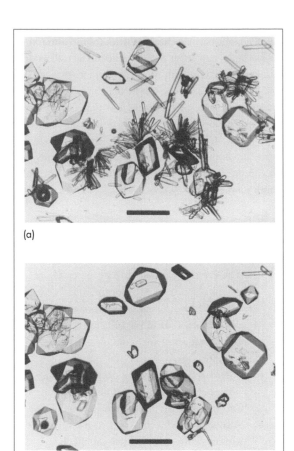

(a)

(b)

Figure 1.13 Photomicrographs showing the solution-phase polymorphic conversion of orthorhombic paracetamol (needles) to monoclinic paracetamol (prisms and plates). Micrograph (a) was taken at $t = 0$ and (b) was taken at $t = 30$ minutes. Scale bars = 250 μm.

Reproduced from Nichols G, Frampton CS. Physicochemical characterization of the orthorhombic polymorph of paracetamol crystallized from solution. *J Pharm Sci* 1998;87:684–693. Copyright Wiley-VCH Verlag GmbH & Co. KGaA. Reproduced with permission.

suppositories, could cause products with different and unacceptable melting characteristics.

Analytical issues

For analytical work it is sometimes necessary to establish conditions whereby different forms of a substance, where they exist, might be converted to a single form to eliminate differences in the solid-state infrared spectra that result from the different internal structures of the crystal forms. As different crystal forms arise through different arrangements of the molecules or ions in a three-dimensional array, this implies different interaction energies in the solid state. Hence, one would expect different melting points and different solubilities (and of course different infrared spectra). Changes in infrared spectra of steroids due to grinding with potassium bromide have been reported; changes in the spectra of some substances have been ascribed to conversion of a crystalline form into an amorphous form (as in the case of digoxin), or into a second crystal form. Changes in crystal form can also be induced by solvent extraction methods used for isolation of drugs from formulations prior to examination by infrared spectroscopy. Difficulties in identification arise when samples that are thought to be the same substance give different spectra in the solid state; this can happen, for example, with cortisone acetate, which exists in at least seven forms, or dexamethasone acetate, which exists in four. Therefore, where there is a likelihood of polymorphism it is best where possible to record solution spectra if chemical identification only is required. The normal way to overcome the effects of polymorphism is to convert both samples into the same form by recrystallisation from the same solvent, although obviously this technique should not be used to hide the presence of polymorphs.

Consequences

The most important consequence of polymorphism is the possible difference in the bioavailability of different polymorphic forms of a drug, particularly when the drug is poorly soluble. The rate of absorption of such a drug is often dependent upon its rate of dissolution. The most stable polymorph usually has the lowest solubility and slowest dissolution rate and consequently often a lower bioavailability than the metastable polymorph. Fortunately, the difference in bioavailability of different polymorphic forms of a drug is usually insignificant. It has been proposed that when the free energy differences between the polymorphs are small there may be no significant differences in their biopharmaceutical behaviour as measured by the blood levels they achieve. Only when the differences are large may they affect the extent of absorption. For example, $\Delta G_{B \to A}$ for the transition of chloramphenicol palmitate Form B to Form A is -3.24 kJ mol^{-1}; ΔH is -27.32 kJ mol^{-1}. For mefenamic acid $\Delta G_{II \to I}$ is -1.05 kJ mol^{-1} and ΔH is -4.18 kJ mol^{-1}. Whereas differences in biological activity are shown by the palmitate polymorphs, no such differences are observed with the mefenamic acid polymorphs. When little energy is required to convert one polymorph into another, it is likely that the forms will interconvert *in vivo* and that the administration of one form in place of the other will be clinically unimportant.

Particle size reduction may lead to fundamental changes in the properties of the solid. Grinding of crystalline substances such as digoxin can lead to the formation of amorphous material (see section 1.3) that has an intrinsically higher rate of solution and therefore apparently greater activity. Such is the importance of the polymorphic form of poorly soluble drugs that it has to be controlled. For instance, there is a limit on the inactive polymorph of chloramphenicol palmitate. Of the three polymorphic forms of chloramphenicol palmitate, Form A has a low biological activity because it is so slowly hydrolysed *in vivo* to free chloramphenicol.[7] We can see from Fig. 1.14 that the maximum blood levels attained with 100% Form B polymorph are about seven times greater than with 100% Form A polymorph, and that with mixtures of A and B the blood levels vary in proportion to the percentage of B in the suspension.[8]

During formulation development it is vital that sufficient care is taken to determine polymorphic tendencies of poorly soluble drugs. This is so that formulations can be designed to release drug at the correct rate and so that intelligent guesses can be made before clinical trial about possible influences of food and concomitant therapy on drug absorption. As will be seen later, particle characteristics (of nitrofurantoin, for example) can affect drug interaction as well as drug absorption. Above all, it is important that during toxicity studies care is given to the characterisation of the physical state of the drug, and that during development the optimal dosage form is attained. It is insufficient that drug is 'available' from the dosage form; on both economic and biological grounds, the maximum response must be achieved with the minimum amount of drug substance.

Key points

- The crystals of some drugs can crystallise in more than one polymorphic form characterised by differences in packing in the crystal lattice or in the orientation or conformation of the molecules at the lattice sites.
- Polymorphs of the same drug may have different melting points and solubilities and usually exist in different habits.
- Although polymorphism is common with pharmaceutical compounds, its likely occurrence cannot be predicted with confidence.
- The polymorphic form with the lowest free energy will be the most stable and other polymorphs will tend to transform into it over time.
- Polymorphism may cause problems in the formulation, analysis and bioavailability of drugs.

1.2.4 Multicomponent crystals

Crystal hydrates and solvates

When some compounds crystallise they may entrap solvent in the crystal. Crystals that contain solvent of crystallisation are called crystal *solvates*, or crystal *hydrates* when water is the solvent of crystallisation. Crystals that contain no water of crystallisation are termed *anhydrates*.

Crystal solvates exhibit a wide range of behaviour depending on the interaction between the solvent and the crystal structure. With some solvates the solvent

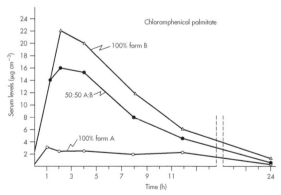

Figure 1.14 Comparison of serum levels ($\mu g\ cm^{-3}$) obtained with suspensions of chloramphenicol palmitate after oral administration of a dose equivalent to 1.5 g of chloramphenicol.

Redrawn from Aiguiar AJ, Zelmer JE. Dissolution behaviour of polymorphs of chloramphenicol palmitate and mefanamic acid. *J Pharm Sci* 1969;58:983–987. Copyright Wiley-VCH Verlag GmbH & Co. KGaA. Reproduced with permission.

plays a key role in holding the crystal together; for example, it may be part of a hydrogen-bonded network within the crystal structure. These solvates are very stable and are difficult to desolvate. When these crystals lose their solvent they collapse and recrystallise in a new crystal form. We can think of these as *polymorphic solvates*. In other solvates, the solvent is not part of the crystal bonding and merely occupies voids in the crystal. These solvates lose their solvent more readily and desolvation does not destroy the crystal lattice. This type of solvate has been called a *pseudopolymorphic solvate*.

By way of illustration of this phenomenon, we return to the case of spironolactone which we considered earlier. As well as the two polymorphs, this compound also possesses four solvates, depending on whether it is crystallised from acetonitrile, ethanol, ethyl acetate or methanol. Each of these solvates is transformed to the polymorphic Form 2 on heating, indicating that the solvent is involved in the bonding of the crystal lattice.

The stoichiometry of some of the solvates is unusual. Fluordrocortisone pentanol solvate, for example, contains 1.1 molecules of pentanol for each steroid molecule, and its ethyl acetate solvate contains 0.5 molecules of ethyl acetate per steroid molecule. A succinylsulfathiazole solvate appears to have 0.9 moles of pentanol per mole of drug. Beclometasone dipropionate forms solvates with chlorofluorocarbon propellants.

Infrared measurements show that cefaloridine exists in α, β, δ, ε, ζ and μ forms (that is, six forms after recrystallisation from different solvents).[9] Proton magnetic resonance spectroscopy showed that, although the μ form contained about 1 mole of methanol and the ε form about 1 mole of dimethyl sulfoxide, ethylene glycol or diethylene glycol (depending on the solvent), the α, β, anhydrous δ and ε forms contained less than 0.1 mole, that is, non-stoichiometric amounts of solvent. The α form is characterised by containing about 0.05 mole of N,N-dimethylacetamide. This small amount of 'impurity', which cannot be removed by prolonged treatment under vacuum at 10^{-5}–10^{-6} Torr, is apparently able to 'lock' the cefaloridine molecule in a particular crystal lattice.

Pharmaceutical consequences of solvate formation

Modification of the solvent of crystallisation may result in different solvated forms. This is of particular relevance because the hydrated and anhydrous forms of a drug can have melting points and solubilities sufficiently different to affect pharmaceutical behaviour. For example, glutethimide exists in both an anhydrous form (m.p. 83°C, solubility 0.042% at 25°C) and a hydrated form (m.p. 68°C, solubility 0.026% at 25°C). Other anhydrous forms show similar higher solubilities than the hydrated materials and, as expected, the anhydrous forms of caffeine, theophylline, glutethimide and cholesterol show correspondingly higher dissolution rates than their hydrates.

One can assume that, as the hydrate has already interacted intimately with water (the solvent), then the energy released for crystal break-up, on interaction of the hydrate with solvent, is less than for the anhydrous material. The non-aqueous solvates, on the other hand, tend to be more soluble in water than the non-solvates. The *n*-amyl alcohol solvate of fludrocortisone acetate is at least five times as soluble as the parent compound, while the ethyl acetate solvate is twice as soluble.

The equilibrium solubility of the non-solvated form of a crystalline organic compound that does not dissociate in the solvent (for example, water) can be represented as:

$$A_{(c)} \xrightleftharpoons{K_s} A_{(aq)}$$

where K_s is the equilibrium constant. This equilibrium will of course be influenced by the crystal form, as we have seen, as well as by temperature and pressure. For a hydrate $A \cdot xH_2O$, we can write:

$$A \cdot xH_2O_{(c)} \xrightleftharpoons{K_{sh}} A_{(aq)} + xH_2O$$

K_{sh} is then the solubility of the hydrate. The process of hydration of an anhydrous crystal in water is represented by an equation of the type:

$$\underset{\text{(anhydrate)}}{A_{(c)} + xH_2O_{liquid}} \xrightleftharpoons[K_{sh}]{K_s} \underset{\text{(hydrate)}}{A \cdot xH_2O_{(c)}}$$

and the free energy of the process is written:

$$\Delta G_{trans} = RT \ln \frac{K_{sh}}{K_s} \tag{1.3}$$

ΔG_{trans} can be obtained from the solubility data of the two forms at a particular temperature, as for theophylline and glutethimide in Table 1.3.

Table 1.3 Solubility of theophylline and glutethimide forms at various temperatures

		Solubility	
	Temperature (°C)	Hydrate (mg cm^{-3})	Anhydrate (mg cm^{-3})
Theophylline	25	6.25	12.5
	35	10.4	18.5
	45	17.6	27.0
	55	30	38
Glutethimide		(%w/v)	(%w/v)
	25	0.0263	0.042
	32	0.0421	0.0604
	40	0.07	0.094

Reproduced with permission from Eriksen SP. *Am J Pharm Educ* 1964;28:47.

The dissolution rates of solvates can vary considerably. Table 1.4 shows the range of intrinsic dissolution rates reported for solvates of oxyphenbutazone into a dissolution medium containing a surface-active agent (to avoid wetting problems). The superior dissolution rates of the benzene and cyclohexane solvates (B and C respectively) are apparent but, of course, the possible use of these solvates is prohibited because of their likely toxicity.

Differences in solubility and dissolution rate between solvates can lead to measurable differences in their bioavailabilities. You can see in Table 1.5 the differences in *in vivo* absorption rates of solvates of prednisolone *t*-butyl acetate and hydrocortisone *t*-butyl acetate after implantation of pellets of these compounds. Note, for example, that the monoethanol solvate of prednisolone has an absorption rate *in vivo* that is nearly five times greater than that of the anhydrous *t*-butyl acetate. Differences in the absorption of ampicillin and its trihydrate can be observed (Fig. 1.15), but the extent of the difference is of doubtful clinical significance. The more soluble anhydrous form appears at a faster rate in the serum and produces higher peak serum levels.

Cocrystals

Cocrystals are an important class of pharmaceutical materials that have the potential to enhance solubility, dissolution and consequent bioavailability of poorly water-soluble drugs. A pharmaceutical cocrystal is a multicomponent crystal comprising two or more com-

Table 1.4 Intrinsic dissolution rates of the crystal forms of oxyphenbutazone

Sample	Intrinsic dissolution rate[a] (μg min^{-1} cm^{-2})
Solvate C	21.05 ± 0.02
Solvate B	18.54 ± 0.47
Anhydrate	14.91 ± 0.47
Hemihydrate	17.01 ± 0.78
Monohydrate	9.13 ± 0.23

Reproduced with permission from Stoltz M, Lotter AP, van der Walt JG. Physical characterization of two oxyphenbutazone pseudopolymorphs. *J Pharm Sci* 1988;77:1047.
[a]Mean ± range of uncertainty of two determinations.

Table 1.5 Absorption rate of hydrocortisone tertiary butyl acetate and prednisolone tertiary butyl acetate (mg h^{-1} cm^{-2})

Compound	Absorption rate (mg h^{-1} cm^{-2})
Prednisolone tertiary butyl acetate	
Anhydrous	1.84 x 10^{-3}
Monoethanol solvate	8.7 x 10^{-3}
Hemiacetone solvate	2.2 x 10^{-1}
Hydrocortisone tertiary butyl acetate	
Anhydrous	4.74 x 10^{-3}
Monoethanol solvate	1.83 x 10^{-3}
Hemichloroform solvate	7.40 x 10^{-1}

Modified with permission from Ballard BE, Biles J. Effect of crystallizing solvent on absorption rates of steroid implants. *Steroids* 1964;4:273.

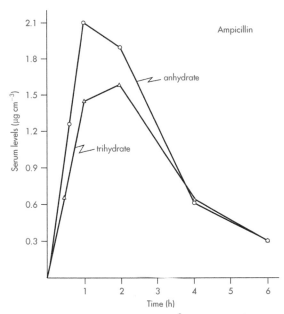

Figure 1.15 Serum levels (μg cm^{-3}) obtained after oral administration of a suspension containing 250 mg ampicillin as the anhydrate and as the trihydrate.

Reproduced with permission from Poole JW *et al.* Physicochemical factors influencing the absorption of the anhydrous and trihydrate forms of ampicillin. *Curr Ther Res* 1968;10:292.

pounds (at least one of which is a drug molecule) that are solids under ambient conditions, present in a stoichiometric ratio and interact by non-covalent interactions such as hydrogen bonding. They are similar to crystal solvates in that the crystal is composed of the drug and another molecule; in cocrystals, however, the other molecule (the coformer) is a pharmaceutically acceptable compound that is a solid under ambient conditions rather than a liquid as in crystal solvates. An important advantage of cocrystals compared to solvates and hydrates is that it is easier to control the ratio of components (i.e. the stoichiometry) and therefore the physicochemical properties of the cocrystal.

Cocrystals differ from solid dispersions (section 1.9), which are *physical* mixtures of drug and a highly water-soluble carrier molecule in microcrystalline or molecular form. The aim with each of these solid-state dosage forms is nevertheless the same – to alter the physicochemical properties of the drug, for example, to increase solubility or reduce hygroscopicity. In this respect cocrystallisation provides a means of presenting very different physicochemical properties compared to the parent drug without covalent modification of its molecular structure, whereas it is only possible to achieve marginal changes in solubility with solvates,

hydrates and polymorphs. The potential for improvement of solubility and dissolution profile is similar to that which can be achieved by forming more soluble salts of the drug. Cocrystal development is, however, particularly attractive when salt formation is not feasible or when existing salts fail to exhibit suitable properties for use in a drug product. In addition, cocrystals of pharmaceutical salts, namely ionic cocrystals, can also be prepared and evaluated. These potentially offer more scope for solubility enhancement since both the counterion and the coformer can be varied to achieve optimum solubility.

In selecting a suitable molecule to cocrystallise with the drug, consideration is made of the potential for hydrogen bonding between the two molecules. Figure 1.16 shows the molecular packing within the 1 : 1 cocrystals of carbamazepine and saccharin. The carbamazepine molecules hydrogen bond to each other to form a dimer and saccharin molecules form double hydrogen bonds to both N—H donor and O acceptor atoms on this dimer. Other drugs forming cocrystals include caffeine and theophylline, both of which form cocrystals with a range of dicarboxylic acids that have improved stability to high humidity.

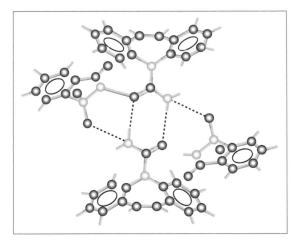

Figure 1.16 Packing of molecules in cocrystals of carbamazepine and saccharin. The dashed lines indicate hydrogen bonding of carbamazepine molecules to each other to form a dimer and the formation of double hydrogen bonds between saccharin and N—H donor and O acceptor atoms on the dimer.

Reprinted with permission from Fleischman SG *et al.* Crystal engineering of the composition of pharmaceutical phases: multi-component crystalline solids involving carbamazepine. *Cryst Growth Des* 2003;3:909. Copyright 2003, American Chemical Society.

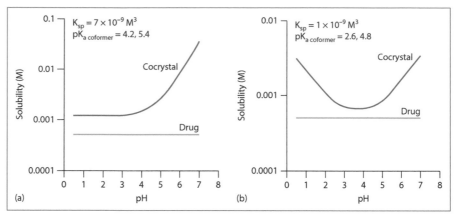

Figure 1.17 Manipulation of the pH-solubility profile of carbamazepine by forming cocrystals with (a) succinic acid and (b) 4-aminobenzoic acid hydrate.

Reproduced with permission from Thakuria R *et al.* Pharmaceutical cocrystals and poorly soluble drugs. *Int J Pharm* 2013;453:101. Copyright Elsevier 2013.

It is interesting to note that not only is cocrystal formation a means of increasing the intrinsic solubility of a poorly soluble drug, but it also provides an opportunity to alter its pH-solubility profile through the choice of a suitable ionisable coformer. Figure 1.17 shows that cocrystals of a non-ionisable drug (carbamazepine) can exhibit very different pH-solubility profiles depending on the coformer ionisation properties. A diprotic coformer such as succinic acid leads to an increase of solubility with pH; an amphoteric coformer such as 4-aminobenzoic acid will, however, result in a U-shaped curve with a solubility minimum in a pH range between the two pK_a values.

Despite the successful application of cocrystallisation in manipulation of the physical properties of a drug, there are currently no marketed products utilising cocrystals. One of the difficulties encountered in the design of possible cocrystals for a particular drug is that, although cocrystal solubility often correlates strongly with coformer solubility, there are insufficient data to predict the solubility enhancement with certainty. A more important concern, however, is that these metastable crystal forms may change their form during storage. However, a recent review[10] discusses potential developments in cocrystal technology and concludes that 'the systematic commercialisation of cocrystal drug substances into drug products is likely just a matter of time'.

Key points

- Some drugs can entrap solvent in their crystals during crystallisation, forming crystal solvates (or hydrates when the solvent is water).
- In *polymorphic* solvates the solvent plays an important role in the crystal structure; these solvates are very stable and difficult to desolvate. This type of solvate collapses when it loses its solvent of crystallisation and recrystallises in a different crystal form.
- In *pseudopolymorphic* solvates the solvent is not part of the crystal bonding and simply occupies voids in the crystal. This type of solvate loses its solvent more readily and desolvation does not destroy the crystal lattice.
- The anhydrous form has a higher aqueous solubility than the hydrated form of the same drug, whereas the non-aqueous solvates tend to be more water soluble than the non-solvates.
- There is often a wide variation in the dissolution rates of different solvates of the same drug.
- Differences in solubility and dissolution rates of solvates can cause measurable differences in their bioavailabilities.

- Cocrystals are combinations of the drug and another crystalline solid (coformer) to which it is hydrogen bonded; for example, combinations of carbamazepine and saccharin. They are designed to have a higher solubility and often lower hygroscopicity than the crystals of the drug itself.

1.3 Amorphous solids

Solids in which there is no long-range ordering of the molecules are said to be *amorphous*. These disordered systems differ in solubility, stability, dissolution properties and compression characteristics from the more traditionally used crystalline counterparts and provide attractive alternatives to them in drug delivery formulations. In principle, most classes of material can be prepared in the amorphous state if the rate at which they are solidified is faster than that at which their molecules can align themselves into a crystal lattice with three-dimensional order. It is also possible to convert crystalline material to amorphous inadvertently when supplying mechanical or thermal energy, for example, during grinding, compression and milling the solid or during drying processes. Some materials, notably polymers such as poly(lactic acid), polyvinylpyrrolidone and polyethylene glycol, are inherently amorphous. Even at slow solidification rates, large molecules such as these are often unable to form perfect crystals because of the difficulty in arranging the chains of these flexible molecules in an ordered manner; such materials are frequently *semicrystalline*, with areas of a crystalline nature surrounded by amorphous regions, as shown in Fig. 1.18.

Unlike crystals, amorphous or semicrystalline materials do not have sharp melting points, but instead there is a change in the properties of the material at a characteristic temperature, called the *glass transition temperature, T_g*. Below T_g, the material is said to be in its glassy state and is brittle; as the temperature is increased above T_g, the molecules become more mobile and the material is said to become rubbery. The transition temperature may be lowered by the addition of plasticisers, which are generally small molecules that are able to fit between the glassy molecules, so increasing their mobility. Water, for example, is used as a plasticiser for a wide range of polymers used in film coating.

Amorphous solids, because they exhibit a higher energy state than crystalline solids, are inherently less stable and have the potential for converting to the thermodynamically more stable crystalline form over time. In addition, because of their higher molecular mobility, they often show stronger chemical reactivity and hence a faster rate of chemical degradation. Nevertheless, the amorphous form of a drug often has a higher solubility than its crystalline form and the use of the amorphous form of a drug may provide an opportunity to enhance its bioavailability in the case of poorly water-soluble drugs.

1.4 Dissolution of solid drugs

Whether the solution process takes place in the laboratory or *in vivo*, there is one law that defines the rate of solution of solids when the process is diffusion controlled and involves no chemical reaction. This is the *Noyes–Whitney equation*, which may be written:

$$\frac{dw}{dt} = kA(c_s - c) \tag{1.4}$$

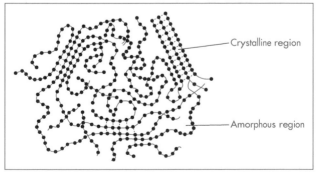

Figure 1.18 Diagrammatic representation of a solid polymer showing regions of crystallinity and regions that are amorphous.

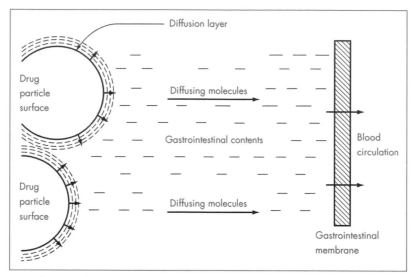

Figure 1.19 Schematic diagram of dissolution from a solid surface.

where $k = D/\delta$. The equation is the analogue of equation (1.1), discussed previously. Figure 1.19 shows the model on which this equation is based. The terms of the equation are: dw/dt, the rate of increase of the amount of material in solution dissolving from a solid; k, the rate constant of dissolution; c_s, the saturation solubility of the drug in solution in the diffusion layer; and c, the concentration of the drug in the bulk solution. A is the area of the solvate particles exposed to the solvent, δ is the thickness of the diffusion layer and D is the diffusion coefficient of the dissolved solute. The relevance of polymorphism and solid-state properties to this equation lies in the fact that A is determined by particle size. Particle size reduction, if it leads to a change in polymorph, results in a change in c_s, and if dissolution is the rate-limiting step in absorption, then bioavailability is affected. In more general terms, one can use the equation to predict the effect of solvent change or other parameters on the dissolution rate of solid drugs. These factors are listed in Table 1.6.

1.5 Biopharmaceutical importance of particle size

As discussed in Chapter 9, control of particle size is important in pulmonary delivery because only very fine particles are able to penetrate the alveolar regions of the respiratory tract. But there is an optimum. Indeed,

Table 1.6 How the parameters of the dissolution equation can be changed to increase (+) or decrease (−) the rate of solution

Equation parameter	Comments	Effect on rate of solution
D (diffusion coefficient of drug)	May be decreased in presence of substances which increase viscosity of the medium	(−)
A (area exposed to solvent)	Increased by micronisation and in 'amorphous' drugs	(+)
δ (thickness of diffusion layer)	Decreased by increased agitation in gut or flask	(+)
c_s (solubility in diffusion layer)	That of weak electrolytes altered by change in pH, by use of appropriate drug salt or buffer ingredient	(−)(+)
c (concentration in bulk)	Decreased by intake of fluid in stomach, by removal of drug by partition or absorption	(+)

if the particle size is reduced too far, particles may be exhaled and not deposited. The vital influence (for mainly aerodynamic reasons) of particle size and density in the activity of inhaled drug particles is discussed in Chapter 9, section 9.8.1. In this section

Example 1.2 Use of Noyes–Whitney equation

A preparation of drug granules weighing 5.5 g and having a total surface area of 2.8×10^3 cm^2 dissolves in 500 mL of water at 25°C. The quantity of drug dissolved after the first minute is 0.76 g. The saturated solubility of the drug is 15 mg mL^{-1} and the diffusion layer thickness is 5×10^{-3} cm. Calculate: (a) the dissolution rate constant; (b) the diffusion coefficient; and (c) the effect on the dissolution rate of an increase of surface area to 5×10^3 cm^2.

Answer

(a) Converting the mass of drug dissolved into mg gives the rate of dissolution at $t = 60$ s as:

$$dw/dt = 0.76 \times 1000/60 = 12.67 \text{ mg s}^{-1}$$

The concentration of the drug in the bulk solution is

$$c = 0.76 \times 1000/500 = 1.52 \text{ mg cm}^{-3}$$
$$c_s - c = 15 - 1.52 = 13.48 \text{ mg cm}^{-3}$$

Therefore, from equation (1.4),

$$k = (12.67/2.8 \times 10^3) \times (1/13.48) = 3.36 \times 10^{-4} \text{ cm s}^{-1}$$

(b) The diffusion coefficient D can be calculated from:

$$D = k\delta = 3.36 \times 10^{-4} \times 5 \times 10^{-3} = 1.68 \times 10^{-6} \text{ cm}^2 \text{ s}^{-1}$$

(c) When the surface area is increased to 5×10^3 cm^2,

$$dw/dt = 3.36 \times 10^{-4} \times 5 \times 10^3 \times 13.48 = 22.65 \text{ mg s}^{-1}$$

i.e. the increase in surface area has caused an increase of the rate of dissolution from 12.67 to 22.65 mg s^{-1}.

Note the importance of ensuring that the parameters are converted to the appropriate units when substituting in equation (1.4) or indeed in any equation. If you are in doubt about units then it is easy to carry out a check to ensure that the units balance on both sides of the equation. In the particular example of equation (1.4) we have:

$$\text{mg s}^{-1} = \text{cm s}^{-1} \times \text{cm}^2 \times \text{mg cm}^{-3} = \text{mg s}^{-1}$$

we will consider the influence of particle size on the dissolution and absorption of drugs.

It has generally been believed that only substances in the molecularly dispersed form (that is, in solution) are transported across the intestinal wall and absorbed into the systemic circulation. This is the premise on which much thinking on bioavailability from pharmaceutical dosage forms is based. Although this is generally true, it has been shown that very small particles in the nanometre size range can also be transported through enterocytes by way of pinocytosis, and that solid particles of starch, for example, in the micrometre size range enter by a mechanism involving passage of particles between the enterocytes.[11] Sub-micrometre particulate uptake by the M cells of the gut-associated lymphoid tissue is a phenomenon of increasing importance.[12] Because of the much greater absorptive area available to molecules, however, the opportunity for molecules to penetrate the cell membrane is obviously higher than that for particles.

The rate of absorption of many slightly soluble drugs from the gastrointestinal tract and other sites is limited by the rate of dissolution of the drug. The particle size of a drug is therefore of importance if the substance in question has a low solubility. In some cases, notably that of griseofulvin, there is pharmacopoeial control of particle size; the *British Pharmacopoeia* (2010) specifies for this drug 'a microfine powder, the particles of which generally have a maximum dimension of up to 5 μm, although larger particles that may exceed 30 μm may occasionally be present'. The control exercised over the particle size is due to its very low solubility; the experience is that if the solubility of a drug substance is about 0.3% or less then the dissolution rate *in vivo* may be the rate-controlling step in absorption.

The Noyes–Whitney equation demonstrates that solubility is one of the main factors determining rate of solution. When the rate of solution is less than the rate of absorption, the solution process becomes rate limiting. Generally speaking, it should become so only when the drug is of low solubility at the pH of the stomach and intestinal contents. The rate of absorption, the speed of onset of effect and the duration of therapeutic response can all be determined by particle size for most routes of administration. Figure 1.20 shows the effect of particle size of phenobarbital suspensions on the drug's bioavailability after intramuscular injection compared with a solution of the drug, which probably precipitates in fine crystal form at the site of injection. The rate of solution of the drug crystals controls the extent of absorption from the intramuscular site.

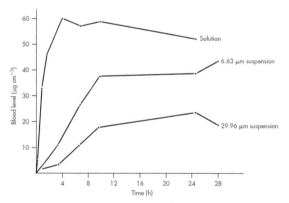

Figure 1.20 Blood levels (μg cm^{-3}) of phenobarbital versus time after intramuscular injection of three formulations.
Redrawn from Miller LG, Fincher JH. Influence of drug particle size after intramuscular dosage of phenobarbital to dogs. *J Pharm Sci* 1971;60:1733, with permission from Wiley.

We have seen in the previous section that particle size has an important influence on dissolution rate, the larger surface exposed to the solvent increasing significantly the dissolution rate of smaller particles. The effect of particle size reduction on dissolution rate is one of exposure of increasing amounts of surface of

the drug to the solvent. It is only when comminution reduces particle size below 0.1 μm that there is an effect on the intrinsic solubility of the substance (see Chapter 4), and thus on its intrinsic dissolution rate. Very small particles have a very high surface/bulk ratio. If the surface layer has a higher energy than the bulk, as is the case with these small particles, they will interact more readily with solvent to produce higher degrees of solubility.

It was with the action of phenothiazine that the importance of particle size was first recognised, in 1939, in relation to its toxicity to codling moth larvae, and in 1940 in relation to its anthelmintic effect, in both of which it was shown that reduction in particle size increased activity. The improvement in biological response to griseofulvin on micronisation is well known; similar blood levels of the drug were obtained with half the dose of micronised drug compared with those of non-micronised griseofulvin.[13] The influence of particle size on the bioavailability of digoxin[14] and dicoumarol (bishydroxycoumarin)[15] has also been investigated. In both cases, plasma levels of drug are of high significance in clinical and toxic responses.

In the case of digoxin there is evidence that milling to reduce particle size can produce an amorphous modification of the drug with enhanced solubility and hence increased bioavailability. The possibility of changing the crystal structure during processing is therefore important: comminution, recrystallisation and drying can all affect crystal properties.

During the pharmacological and toxicological testing of drugs before formal formulation exercises have been carried out, insoluble drugs are frequently administered in suspension form, often routinely in a vehicle containing gum arabic or methylcellulose. Without adequate control of particle size or adequate monitoring, the results of these tests must sometimes be in doubt, as both pharmacological activities and toxicity generally result from absorption of the drug. In a few cases particle size influences side-effects such as gastric bleeding or nausea. Gastric bleeding may in part be the direct result of contact of acidic particles of aspirin or non-steroidal anti-inflammatory agents with the mucosal wall. The influence of drug form on the LD$_{50}$ of pentobarbital in mice is shown in Table 1.7. A twofold range of LD$_{50}$ values is obtained by the use of different, simple formulations of the barbiturate. Even in solution form, sodium carboxymethylcellulose affects

Table 1.7 Influence of formulation on the potency ratios of pentobarbital in the form of the sodium salt and the free acid

Pentobarbital form	Dosage form	Vehicle	Particle size (μm)	LD$_{50}$	Potency ratio[a]
Sodium salt	Solution	Water	–	132	1
Sodium salt	Solution	1% NaCMC	–	170	0.78
Free acid	Suspension	1% NaCMC		189	0.70
Free acid	Suspension	1% NaCMC	297–420	288	0.46

Reproduced with permission from Ritschel WA *et al.* Biopharmaceutical factors influencing LD$_{50}$. Part II: Particle size. *Arzneim Forsch* 1975;25:853.
[a] Relative to aqueous solution of the sodium salt.
NaCMC, Aqueous solution of sodium carboxymethylcellulose.

the LD$_{50}$ by mechanisms that are not confirmed. Adsorption of the polymer at the intestinal surface may retard absorption, or some of the drug may be adsorbed on to the polymer.

The deliberate manipulation of particle size leads to a measure of control of activity and side-effects. Rapid solution of nitrofurantoin from tablets of fine particulate material led to a high incidence of nausea in patients, as local high concentrations of the drug produce a centrally mediated nausea. Development of macrocrystalline nitrofurantoin (as in Macrodantin) has led to the introduction of a form of therapy in which the incidence of nausea is reduced. Capsules are used to avoid compression of the large crystals during manufacture. Although the urinary levels of the anti-bacterial are also lowered by the use of a more slowly dissolving form of the drug, levels are still adequate to produce efficient antibacterial effects.[16]

Key points

The size of drug particles has important effects on:

- the dissolution rate, because the rate at which the drug dissolves is proportional to the surface area exposed to the solvent (see the Noyes–Whitney equation), which increases as the particle size is reduced
- the uniformity of dosage of very potent drugs formulated as a solid-dosage form; this is greater with smaller particles because of the larger number of particles constituting the dose
- pulmonary delivery of drugs, because only very fine particles are able to remain dispersed and thus penetrate to and deposit in the alveolar regions of the respiratory tract
- the rate of absorption, the speed of onset of effect and the duration of therapeutic response of slightly soluble drugs, because of its effect on their rate of dissolution.

1.6 Wetting of powders

Penetration of water into tablets or into granules precedes dissolution. The wettability of the powders, as measured by the contact angle (θ) of the substance with water (Fig. 1.21), therefore determines the contact of solvent with the particulate mass. The measurement of the contact angle gives an indication of the nature of the surface. The behaviour of crystalline materials can be related to the chemical structure of the materials concerned, as is shown by the results in Table 1.8 on a series of substituted barbiturates. The more hydrophobic the individual barbiturate molecules, the more hydrophobic the crystal that forms, although this would not be necessarily a universal finding but one dependent on the orientation of the drug molecules in the crystal and the composition of the faces, as we have already seen with adipic acid. Thus, hydrophobic drugs have dual problems: they are not readily wetted, and even when wetted they have low solubility. On the other hand, because they are lipophilic, absorption across lipid membranes is facilitated.

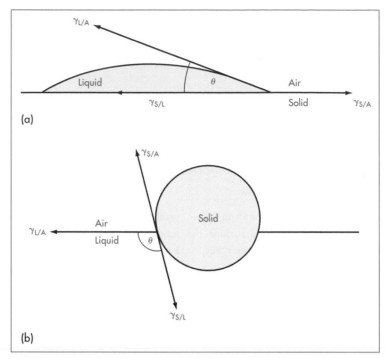

Figure 1.21 Equilibrium between forces acting on (a) a drop of liquid on a solid surface, and (b) a partially immersed solid.

Table 1.8 Relationship between chemical structure of barbiturates and contact angle (θ) with water

R^1	R^2	θ (deg)
Et	Et	70
Et	Bu	78
Et	CH$_2$CH$_2$CH(CH$_3$)$_2$	102
—CH—CH$_3$ CH$_3$	CH$_2$—CH=CH$_2$	75
—CH$_2$—CHCH$_3$ CH$_3$	CH$_2$—CH=CH$_2$	87

Reproduced with permission from Lerk CF *et al.* Contact angles of pharmaceutical powders. *J Pharm Sci* 1977;66:1480.

1.6.1 Contact angle and wettability of solid surfaces

There are many situations in which the wetting of surfaces is important, not only in the action of surfactants in aqueous media wetting hydrophobic drugs discussed above, but also in the case of polymer solution droplets spreading on tablet cores during spray coating (see Chapter 7). Tear fluids wet the cornea, and dewetting results in dry-eye syndrome (see Chapter 9). A representation of the several forces acting on a drop of liquid placed on a flat, solid surface is shown in Fig. 1.21a. The surface tension of the solid, $\gamma_{S/A}$, will favour spreading of the liquid, but this is opposed by the solid–liquid interfacial tension, $\gamma_{S/L}$, and the horizontal component of the surface tension of the liquid $\gamma_{L/A}$ in the plane of the solid surface, that is, $\gamma_{L/A} \cos \theta$. Equating these forces gives:

$$\gamma_{S/A} = \gamma_{S/L} + \gamma_{L/A} \cos \theta \qquad (1.5)$$

Equation (1.5) is generally referred to as *Young's equation*. The angle θ is termed the *contact angle*. The condition for complete wetting of a solid surface is that the contact angle should be zero. This condition is fulfilled when the forces of attraction between the liquid and solid are equal to or greater than those between liquid and liquid.

The type of wetting in which a liquid spreads over the surface of the solid is referred to as *spreading wetting*. The tendency for spreading may be quantified in terms of the spreading coefficient S, where $S = \gamma_{S/A} - (\gamma_{S/L} + \gamma_{L/A})$. The surface tension at the solid–air interface is not a readily measured parameter, but this term may be replaced by substitution from equation (1.5), giving:

$$S = \gamma_{L/A}(\cos \theta - 1) \qquad (1.6)$$

If the contact angle is larger than 0°, the term ($\cos \theta - 1$) will be negative, as will the value of S. The condition for complete, spontaneous wetting is thus a *zero* value for the contact angle.

A useful indicator of the wettability of a solid surface is its *critical surface tension for spreading*, γ_c. This parameter is determined from measurements of the contact angle θ of drops of a series of liquids of known surface tension when placed on a flat non-porous surface of the chosen solid. Extrapolation of a plot of $\cos \theta$ against surface tension (a Zisman plot) to a value of $\cos \theta = 1$ (i.e. to $\theta = 0$) (Fig. 1.22) provides a value of γ_c.

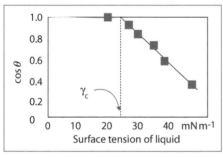

Figure 1.22 Determination of critical surface tension for wetting, γ_c, from a plot of the cosine of the contact angle against surface tension.

Only those liquids or solutions having a surface tension less than γ_c will wet the surface. γ_c is a characteristic property of a solid and is determined by the polarity; solid hydrocarbons and waxes have a low critical surface tension and will be wetted only by solutions of low surface tension; more polar solids such as those of nylon and cellulose have higher γ_c values and consequently are more easily wetted. Human skin has a γ_c of between 22 and 30 mN m^{-1} and it is usual to add surfactants to lotions for

application to the skin to ensure adequate wetting. Similarly, insecticide sprays have to be formulated to wet the surfaces of leaves.

The measurement of γ_c values for tablet surfaces can provide useful information for use in developing an adequate film coating for the tablets. For example, pure acetylsalicylic acid tablets present a surface with a γ_c value of about 31 mN m^{-1}. The addition of a lubricant such as magnesium stearate decreases the γ_c value because the surface is richer in $-CH_3$ and $-CH_2$ groups, whereas the inclusion in the tablet of excipients such as starch, cellulose and talc results in surface richer in $=O$ and $-OH$, causing an increase in γ_c value. Increased γ_c values result in increased wetting by the coating solution and an increased bonding force between the tablet surface and the polymer film coating after the solvent has evaporated.

1.6.2 Wettability of powders

When a solid is immersed in a liquid, the initial wetting process is referred to as *immersional wetting*. The effectiveness of immersional wetting may be related to the contact angle that the solid makes with the liquid–air interface (Fig. 1.21b). The condition for complete immersion of the solid in the liquid is that there should be a decrease in surface free energy as a result of the immersion process. Once the solid is submerged in the liquid, the process of spreading wetting (see the previous section) becomes important.

Table 1.9 gives the contact angles of a series of pharmaceutical powders. These values were determined using compacts of the powder (produced by compressing the powder in a large-diameter tablet die) and a saturated aqueous solution of each compound as the test liquid. Many of the powders are slightly hydrophobic (for example, indometacin and stearic acid), or even strongly hydrophobic (for example, magnesium stearate, phenylbutazone and chloramphenicol palmitate). Formulation of these drugs as suspensions (for example, Chloramphenicol Palmitate Oral Suspension USP) presents wetting problems. Table 1.9 shows that θ can be affected by the crystallographic structure, as for chloramphenicol palmitate. Surface modification or changes in crystal structure are clearly not routine methods of lowering the contact angle and the normal method of improving wettability is by the inclusion of surfactants in the formulation.

Table 1.9 Contact angles of some pharmaceutical powders

Material	Contact angle θ (deg)
Acetylsalicylic acid (aspirin)	74
Aluminium stearate	120
Aminophylline	47
Ampicillin (anhydrous)	35
Ampicillin (trihydrate)	21
Caffeine	43
Calcium carbonate	58
Calcium stearate	115
Chloramphenicol	59
Chloramphenicol palmitate (α form)	122
Chloramphenicol palmitate (β form)	108
Diazepam	83
Digoxin	49
Indometacin	90
Isoniazid	49
Lactose	30
Magnesium stearate	121
Nitrofurantoin	69
Phenylbutazone	109
Prednisolone	43
Prednisone	63
Salicyclic acid	103
Stearic acid	98
Succinylsulfathiazole	64
Sulfadiazine	71
Sulfamethazine	48
Sulfathiazole	53
Theophylline	48
Tolbutamide	72

Selected values from Lerk CF *et al. J Pharm Sci* 1976;65:843; *J Pharm Sci* 1977;66:1481.

The surfactants not only reduce $\gamma_{L/A}$ but also adsorb on to the surface of the powder, thus reducing $\gamma_{S/L}$. Both of these effects reduce the contact angle and improve the dispersibility of the powder.

Key points

- The type of wetting that occurs when a liquid spreads over a solid surface is referred to as spreading wetting. The tendency for spreading is described by the spreading coefficient, which for spontaneous spreading should be positive or zero. The value of the spreading coefficient depends on the contact angle; complete wetting occurs when the contact angle is zero.
- Solid surfaces may be characterised by their critical surface tension for wetting, γ_c; low γ_c values indicate poor wetting properties.
- The process of initial wetting when a powder is immersed in a liquid is referred to as immersional wetting. Wetting problems occur when the contact angle is greater than 90°; several pharmaceutical powders have been identified that, because of their high contact angle, present wetting problems.
- Wettability may be improved by the inclusion of surfactants in the formulation.

1.7 Freeze drying

Sublimation, i.e. the direct transition from the solid to the vapour phase, forms the basis of the widely used technique of *freeze drying* (lyophilisation), for the drying of heat-sensitive materials such as proteins and blood products. The process may be understood by reference to the phase diagram for water (Fig. 1.23), which shows the changes in the melting point of ice and the boiling point of water as the external pressure above the water is decreased from atmospheric pressure. Also shown is the equilibrium between ice and vapour when the external pressure has been reduced below the *triple point*, when all the liquid water has

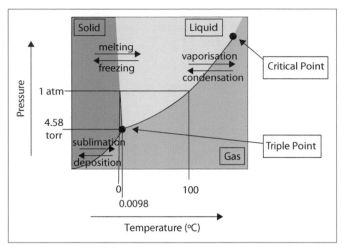

Figure 1.23 Phase diagram of water (not to scale) showing the boundaries between liquid, solid and vapour phases.

been solidified. The triple point is the unique point at which all three phases coexist. In the process of freeze drying, an aqueous solution of the heat-sensitive material is frozen and its pressure is reduced to below the triple point; a small amount of heat is then supplied to increase the temperature to the sublimation curve, at which the ice changes directly to vapour without passing through the liquid phase. The pressure is prevented from increasing above the triple point during the freeze-drying process by removing the vapour as it is formed. Removal of water, i.e. drying, is therefore achieved at temperatures well below room temperature, so preventing decomposition of the thermolabile product.

The handling and storage of some drugs in their solid state can pose problems arising from the sublimation of the drug. Evidence for a transition from solid to vapour is seen from the haze developed on the inner walls of the glass vials containing solid ibuprofen when these are stored at 40°C.[17] The Clausius–Clapeyron equation describes the variation of vapour pressure with temperature (Derivation Box 1A). Over the temperature range 23–64°C ibuprofen vapour pressure–temperature data obey a generalised form of the Clausius–Clapeyron equation:

$$\log P = \frac{-\Delta H_{vap}}{2.303RT} + \text{constant} \tag{1.7}$$

where P is the vapour pressure, R is the gas constant, T is temperature and ΔH_{vap} is the molar enthalpy of vaporisation of ibuprofen (121 kJ mol^{-1}). Figure 1.24 shows that, although the vapour pressure exerted at 25°C is negligible (9×10^{-6} Torr), the value increases

by several orders of magnitude as the temperature is increased and as a result the rate of loss of ibuprofen becomes significant at higher temperatures. For example, the measured weight loss at 55°C is 4.15 mg day^{-1}. Weight losses of this magnitude are significant during drying and coating processes and during accelerated stability-testing procedures.

Two factors – the vapour pressure of the drug and the particle size – are influential in determining the rate of evaporation of the drug in powdered form. Table 1.10 shows the significantly higher evaporation times calculated for several widely used antineoplastic agents when the mean particle size is 1 μm compared with those of 100 μm particles[18] and emphasises the greatly increased risks involved when handling fine powder.

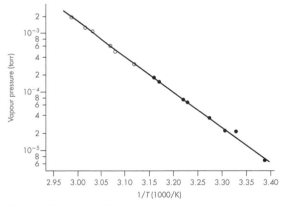

Figure 1.24 Ibuprofen vapour pressure data plotted according to the Clausius–Clapeyron equation.

Reproduced from Ertel KD *et al.* Determination of ibuprofen vapor pressure at temperatures of pharmautical interest. *J Pharm Sci* 1990;79:552. Copyright Wiley-VCH Verlag GmbH & Co. KGaA. Reproduced with permission.

Table 1.10 Vapour pressure and evaporation time for drug particles of diameter, *d*

Compound	Measured vapour pressure (Pa)		Calculated evaporation time (s)	
	20°C	**40°C**	**d = 1 μm**	**d = 100 μm**
Carmustine	0.019	0.530	12	1.2×10^5
Cisplatin	0.0018	0.0031	110	11.0×10^5
Cyclophosphamide	0.0033	0.0090	44	4.4×10^5
Etoposide	0.0026	0.0038	51	5.1×10^5
Fluorouracil	0.0014	0.0039	210	21.0×10^5

Reproduced with permission from Kiffmeyer TK *et al*. Vapour pressures, evaporation behaviour and airborne concentrations of hazardous drugs: implications for occupational safety. *Pharm J* 2002;268:331–337.

Clinical point

There are risks associated with the handling of hazardous drugs, particularly by personnel who are potentially exposed to cytostatic agents routinely used for cancer chemotherapy, which occur because of spillage, inhalation of aerosolised liquid (which can occur, for example, when a needle is withdrawn from a drug vial) or direct contact with contaminated material such as gloves. Some powders do not pour easily or are readily carried away by air currents, making them very difficult to work with directly in a fume hood; others may be subject to electrostatic charge effects, making it difficult to transfer them even if there is no air flow. There is, however, also evidence that cytotoxic agents evaporate and form a vapour during normal handling, which presents a risk to personnel from inhalation of this vapour.[18]

The influence of temperature on the vapour pressure of these drugs is plotted according to equation (1.7) in Fig. 1.25. The vapour above the drugs behaves as an ideal gas because of the low quantity of drug transferred to the gaseous phase and the Clausius–Clapeyron equation is obeyed in all cases. The vapour pressure of carmustine is about 10–100 times greater than that of the other antineoplastic agents and approaches that of mercury (1.0 Pa at 40°C) at elevated temperature, with implications for occupational safety when handling this drug.

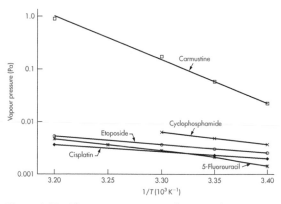

Figure 1.25 The vapour pressures of antineoplastic agents plotted according to the Clausius–Clapeyron equation.
Redrawn with permission from Kiffmeyer TK *et al*. Vapour pressures, evaporation behaviour and airborne concentrations of hazardous drugs: implications for occupational safety. *Pharm J* 2002;268:331–337.

1.8 Solid-dosage forms: formulation and manufacture

As oral dosage forms are the predominant means of administering medication it is necessary to address some of the factors in their composition and manufacture, since Chapter 8 is largely devoted to their performance once administered. By far the most common solid-dosage forms for oral administration are tablets and the emphasis of this section will be on their formulation and manufacture, although many of the processes discussed are common to other solid-dosage forms, particularly capsules, which may be filled with powders, granules and tablets. It is important that pharmacists, even if they are not engaged in the formulation and production of dosage forms, understand the basis of the most common forms of medica-

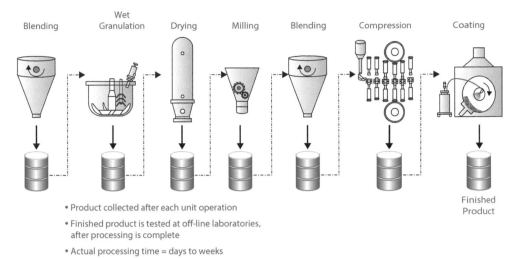

Blending Wet Granulation Drying Milling Blending Compression Coating

Finished Product

- Product collected after each unit operation
- Finished product is tested at off-line laboratories, after processing is complete
- Actual processing time = days to weeks

Figure 1.26 An overview of a typical tableting process.

tion and the differences that might lead to adverse events or generic inequivalence. There are many textbooks completely devoted to the pharmaceutical production of dosage forms, thus our intention here is to discuss the many physicochemical factors which come into play during the formulation and production of tablets and capsules, in line with the objectives of this book. Although this is not a technology manual, it is useful to an understanding of the issues involved in the large-scale production of both tablets and capsules to review briefly the various unit operations involved. Figure 1.26 shows schematically some of the stages that may be involved in the formulation, manufacture and coating of tablets, although, as we will see, there are many possible variations on this simplified depiction of the overall process. Most tablets are manufactured by compression of granules prepared from the powder mix, although an alternative method, in which the powder mix itself is directly compressed into tablets, may be preferable when it is necessary to avoid contact with water or other solvents.

In addition to the active drug(s), the powder mix used in the manufacture of tablets and the powder fills of capsules contains a variety of excipients designed to aid the manufacture of the dosage form, ensure its quality and control its biopharmaceutical properties. In this section we will discuss the choice of excipients to be included in the formulation, examine some of the properties of powders which are important to the smooth functioning of the industrial manufacturing processes involved in the production of tablets and capsules, and discuss some of the relevant physicochemical phenomena involved in the unit operations employed in these processes.

1.8.1 Excipients

In addition to the active therapeutic agent, several other ingredients are generally included in the formulation of the powder mix which is compressed to form the tablet or filled into the shells of hard capsules. These include:

- fillers to add bulk to low-dose tablets
- binders, which, as the name suggests, enhance the cohesion of particles of drug and excipients to form granules suitable for compression
- disintegrants to aid the break-up of tablets in contact with aqueous media
- lubricants to reduce friction between particles during compression and between the compressed tablet and the die walls to aid ejection of the tablet core
- glidants to enhance the flow of powders
- buffering agents to engineer the pH of tablets to aid stability or dissolution of the drug
- wetting agents such as surfactants to aid ingress of water and wetting of hydrophobic drug particles to optimise release.

Filler/diluent

To achieve an appropriate and convenient size of tablet which might contain very low doses of active ingredient, it is usual to include fillers or diluents as part of the formulation to increase the bulk volume of the powder. These are inert, inexpensive materials with an acceptable taste. When added to tablet formulations they should also have good compression properties.

The most commonly used filler for tablets is *lactose*. In its anhydrous crystalline form it is commonly used as a diluent when wet and dry granulation processes are employed and is available in a range of particle sizes depending on crystallisation and subsequent milling conditions. When direct compaction methods of tableting (i.e. those not involving a granulation process) are employed, an amorphous form of lactose produced by spray drying a lactose solution may be used, which dissolves more rapidly than crystalline lactose and has better compaction properties; it is, however, hygroscopic and care must be taken with drugs susceptible to degradation in the solid state. Other sugars, particularly *mannitol*, are used as fillers in chewable tablets because of their sweet taste.

Microcrystalline cellulose is prepared by the controlled acid hydrolysis of cellulose and is available in several grades with different degrees of crystallinity and physicochemical properties. In addition to its use as a filler, it may function as a binder and disintegrating agent (see below).

A commonly used inorganic filler is *dicalcium phosphate*, which, although water-insoluble, is easily wetted by water. In its fine particulate form it is suited to granulation, whereas in an aggregated form it has excellent flow and compression properties and is used when tablets are produced by direct compression. Because of its basic nature it may be incompatible with drugs sensitive to alkaline conditions.

Disintegrants

Disintegrants are included in tablet formulations to ensure that the tablet breaks down into smaller fragments when in contact with liquids, thereby increasing the effective surface area and promoting rapid dissolution of the drug. The first stage of disintegration is wetting the tablet surface; this is a particularly important step when the tablet has been manufactured using a high compression force or has a hydrophobic surface. Without the inclusion of a disintegrant aiding the wetting of the surface, the release rate from such tablets would be unacceptably low. Once the liquid has penetrated the pores of the tablet matrix, the tablets disintegrate into granules which subsequently deaggregate into the primary drug particles. There are two main mechanisms of action of the disintegrant: it may increase the porosity and wettability of the tablet, allowing liquid to penetrate the matrix readily and cause its breakdown, an obvious candidate being a surface-active agent; or it may swell in the presence of liquid, so increasing the pressure within the matrix, resulting in its disintegration. The most widely used excipients acting via a swelling mechanism are starch (at concentrations up to 10%), or modified starches such as sodium starch glycolate or pregelatinised starch (at concentrations between 2 and 5%). Modified celluloses such as crosslinked sodium carboxymethylcellulose (0.5–5.0%) and crosslinked polyvinylpyrrolidone (2–5%) are also commonly used as swelling agents. The disintegration of effervescent tablets occurs by a different mechanism: here the disintegrant functions by producing a gas when exposed to water which causes the rapid disruption of the tablet matrix. The disintegrant is usually a bicarbonate or carbonate salt which liberates carbon dioxide in an acidic aqueous environment.

Binders

The function of binders is to increase the mechanical strength of the tablet. They can act in several ways: they may be added as a dry powder to the powder mix and subsequently dissolve when liquid is added during the granulation process; they may be added as a solution during granulation (*solution binders*); or they may be mixed as a dry powder with the other excipients before compaction (*dry binders*). Solution binders are usually polymers such as polyvinylpyrrolidone and hydroxypropylcellulose; dry binders include microcrystalline cellulose and crosslinked polyvinylpyrrolidone.

Lubricants

Lubricants are added to almost all tablet formulations and act by reducing the friction between the tablet surface and the face of the die during the ejection of the tablet from the die at the end of the extremely rapid cycles of modern tablet presses. Without adequate lubrication, capping may occur or tablets having pitted or scratched surfaces may be produced, leading to rejection of the batch. The most common lubricants (often referred to as boundary lubricants) are fine particulate solids, in particular stearic acid or stearic acid salts such as magnesium stearate. It is important when using this type of insoluble lubricant to avoid mixing it with the disintegrant as this leads to the formation of a film of lubricant on the surface of the disintegrant, reducing its wettability and hence having a deleterious effect on the disintegration time of the tablets. Other factors that may lead to poor tablet disintegration include the use of too high a concentration of lubricant, and excessive mixing time. These problems may be addressed by the use of soluble lubricants such as polyethylene glycols or sodium lauryl sulfate, although their efficiency is generally lower than that of their insoluble counterparts.

Glidants

During the large-scale manufacture of tablets the powders or granules are loaded into hoppers from which they flow into the tablet dies to be compressed into tablets. Glidants are included in the formulation to improve the flow of the powder in the hopper when direct compression is used, and even when a granulation stage is employed they are often added to the granules to ensure sufficiently high flow rates for high-speed tablet production. To reduce the friction between the powder and hopper surface and also between the particles themselves the glidant particles need to be hydrophobic and sufficiently small to locate at the surface of the particles or granules. Talc (hydrated magnesium silicate, $Mg_6(SiO_2)_4(OH)_4$) has traditionally been used as a glidant but is now usually replaced by colloidal silicon dioxide which typically has a particle size of <15 nm.

Flavouring agents and colourants

Flavouring and sweetening agents are added to the formulation to give the tablet a more pleasant taste, particularly when the tablet contains a bitter-tasting drug or when the tablet is a chewable tablet. Typical sweetening agents include sorbitol, glycerol, sucrose and aspartame. Tablets are coloured as a means of identification and/or to improve their appearance, particularly if the drug itself is coloured, giving an otherwise speckled appearance to the tablet. The required

colour can be incorporated into the film coating or can be included in the formulation prior to compaction.

Some examples of excipients are given in Fig. 1.27. Chapters 10 and 12 treat some aspects of the use of excipients, in particular the reactions that some patients have to certain materials used in formulation.

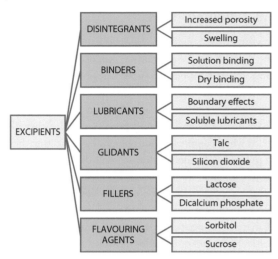

Figure 1.27 Some excipients used in tablet formulation and their functions.

 Key points

- Tablet formulations typically contain several ingredients to optimise their manufacture and disintegration, including: fillers to add bulk to low-dose tablets; binders to enhance the cohesion of particles of the powder mix during granulation and compression; disintegrants to aid the break-up of tablets in contact with aqueous media; lubricants to reduce friction between particles during compression; glidants to enhance the flow of powders; buffering agents to control pH of tablets; and surfactants to aid wetting of hydrophobic drug particles to optimise release from the tablets.

- The unit operations involved in the manufacture of tablets can include: mixing of ingredients, granulation, milling, compression and coating. The manufacture of most tablets involves the granulation of the tablet formulation and compression of the granules; an alternative method of direct compression of the powder mix is used when it is necessary to avoid contact of the powder mix with water or other solvents.

1.8.2 Powder flow

Powders have remarkable properties – they can float like a gas, flow like a liquid or support a weight in the same way as hard-packed snow. They behave rather like gases when in the form of smoke or dust in the atmosphere, rather like liquids when poured or conveyed during manufacturing processes and rather like solids when compressed into blocks by subjecting them to pressure.[1] In this section we will discuss their flow properties and in particular examine the important influence of particle size on the flow of a powder during manufacturing processing when large quantities of material are handled. It is important that pharmaceutical powders or granules are able to flow freely into storage containers or hoppers of tablet- and capsule-filling equipment so that a uniform packing of the particles and hence a uniform tablet or capsule weight is achieved. It is important to remember that in the manufacturing process the die into which the powder flows to be compressed to form the tablet does not weigh the material and hence the tablet or capsule weight is regulated by the flow properties. The possibility of particle jamming, illustrated in Figure 1.28, is relevant to any process where particles compete for a single route of escape (as in particle escape from the hopper).

Uneven particle flow can also cause excessive entrapment of air within the powders, which may promote capping of tablets. Particle size influences the flow properties of powders mainly through its effect on the *cohesivity* of the particles and the *adhesivity* of the particles to a surface in contact with the powder. Cohesion and adhesion are recurrent themes in pharmaceutical science: cohesion between particles or bacteria, adhesion of particles or bacteria to surfaces, flow of particles in processing, flow of particles in inhalation devices and in the blood circulation. The importance of avoiding cohesion (e.g. in colloidal systems) is another issue, discussed in Chapter 6. Cohesive and adhesive forces between particles arise from short-range van der Waals forces,

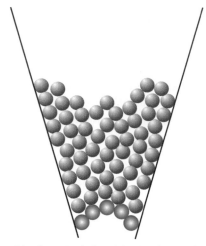

Figure 1.28 'Jamming' of particles in a hopper by particle bridge formation. The size distribution, shape and cohesivity of the particles influence flow, which is complicated by the presence of two or more materials with different characteristics (as shown in Fig. 1.33).

electrostatic forces from frictional charging during handling or surface tensional forces between adsorbed liquid layers on the particle surface. These are all related to the surface area of the particle and increase as the particle size decreases. Particles larger than about 250 µm are usually relatively free flowing but flow problems are likely to be observed when the size falls below 100 µm because of cohesion. Very fine particles (below 10 µm) are usually extremely cohesive and have a high resistance to flow. We should, however, note when making these generalisations that particle shape also influences flow properties and particles of similar sizes but different shapes can have markedly different flow properties because of differences in interparticulate contact areas. Spherical particles, for example, have minimum area of contact with each other compared to more irregular particles and as a consequence have better flow properties. The extent of cohesion of particles or the adhesion of particles to a substrate can be determined by a variety of experimental methods, including indirect methods such as the measurement of the angle of repose, the shear strength and the bulk density, and more direct measurements of flow through an orifice. The principles underlying these methods are outlined below.

The simplest method is measurement of the *angle of repose* assumed by a cone-like pile of the powder formed on a horizontal surface when the powder is allowed to fall under gravity from a nozzle (Fig. 1.29). Particles in the pile will start to slide when the angle of inclination of the pile becomes large enough to overcome the frictional forces. The particles continue to slide over each other until the gravitational forces balance the interparticulate forces; the angle between the sides of the pile and the horizontal surface at equilibrium is called the angle of repose and is a measure of the internal friction or cohesion of the particles of the powder. The angle of repose (α) may be calculated from the height (H) and radius of the cone (R) using $\tan \alpha = H/R$. An angle of about 25° is indicative of a powder that should have suitable flow properties for use in manufacturing processes; angles exceeding 50° indicate poor flow properties and will necessitate the inclusion of a glidant to reduce the interparticulate cohesion.

Shear strength is a measure of the resistance to flow of a powder bed caused by cohesional or adhesional forces and can be determined using a simple shear cell. A typical type of shear cell (the Jenike shear cell) is shown in Figure 1.30. Powder is packed into the two halves of the cell and a vertical (normal) force is applied to the lid of the assembled cell by the application of weights. A horizontal force is applied by the slow, steady movement of the upper half, the drive mechanism of which is connected to a force transducer which measures the applied shear force; the shear stress is determined by dividing the shear force by the cross-sectional area of the powder bed. Measurements are repeated using a range of applied normal forces and the measured shear stress is plotted against the applied normal stress. Extrapolation back to zero normal force gives a value for the cohesion of the powder; the higher the intercept, the higher is the cohesion: a graph for a completely non-cohesive powder would pass through the origin.

The bulk density of a powder is related to particle flow via the relationship between particle flow and packing characteristics; the more tightly a powder is able to pack, the more resistant it will be to flow. The principles of methods devised to measure bulk density are relatively simple: the powder is placed into a measuring cylinder and mechanically tapped by means of a constant-velocity rotating cam. During this process the packing volume decreases from an initial value, V_0, as the void space decreases (the process of consolidation), eventually reaching a stable

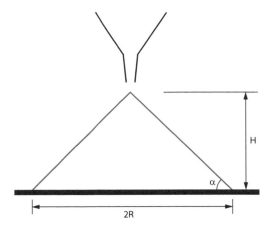

Figure 1.29 Measurement of the angle of repose. Powder is allowed to fall under gravity from the funnel until equilibrium is reached. The angle of repose (α) is calculated from the height (H) and radius of the cone (R) using $\tan \alpha = H/R$.

final volume, V_f. The initial bulk density (also referred to as the fluff density), $\rho_{Bmin} = m/V_0$, and final bulk density (also called the tapped density), $\rho_{Bmax} = m/V_f$, can then be calculated from the mass, m, of the powder. The cohesivity of the powder may be derived from these measurements using the Hausner ratio or the Carr's index.

$$\text{Hausner ratio} = \rho_{Bmax}/\rho_{Bmin} \times 100 \qquad (1.8)$$

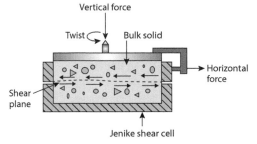

Figure 1.30 The Jenike cell for measurement of the shear strength of a powder. A vertical (normal) force is applied to the lid of the assembled cell by the application of weights and a shear force is applied by the slow, steady movement of the upper half of the cell.

Hausner showed that this ratio was predictive of particle flow characteristics; ratios of less than 1.25 are indicative of low cohesive forces, whereas values greater than 1.5 are obtained when the powder has poorer flow characteristics. Carr's index or % compressibility is also derived from bulk densities and is calculated from:

$$\% \text{ compressibility} = \frac{\rho_{Bmax} - \rho_{Bmin}}{\rho_{Bmax}} \times 100 \qquad (1.9)$$

The lower the value of percentage compressibility, the better the flow properties; values above about 25 are indicative of poor flow characteristics. It should be noted that neither the Hausner ratio nor the Carr's index gives an indication of the ease or speed at which consolidation occurs. Some powders may have quite a high index, suggesting poor flow, and yet may be able to consolidate rapidly. Such powders may be useful in providing uniform die filling since they may be able to flow into the tablet die close to their minimum density and then quickly consolidate to maximum density prior to compression.

Measurement of the powder *flow through an orifice* is the most direct method of assessing flow rate. The orifice of the hopper is sealed with a shutter and the hopper filled with the powder. Complete emptying of the hopper after shutter removal is timed and the mass flow rate is calculated by dividing the mass of discharged powder by this time. The rate of flow through the orifice of the hopper will depend on several factors, including the orifice diameter, so the flow rates obtained are not absolute values; nevertheless they are useful in comparing different powders using the same hopper.

 Key points

- Particle size has an important influence on the flow properties of powders and granules; uneven flow can cause non-uniform tablet weight, jamming in tablet hoppers and entrapment of air, causing tablet capping.
- Particles larger than about 250 μm are usually relatively free flowing but flow problems are likely to be observed when the size falls below 100 μm because of cohesion. Very fine particles (below 10 μm) are usually extremely cohesive and have a high resistance to flow.
- The extent of cohesion of particles or the adhesion of particles to a substrate can be determined by a variety of experimental methods, including indirect methods such as the measurement of the angle of repose, the shear strength and the bulk density, and more direct measurements of flow through an orifice.
- The cohesivity of the powder may be expressed using the Hausner ratio or the Carr's index (percentage compressibility). Hausner ratios of less than 1.25 are indicative of low cohesive forces, whereas values greater than 1.5 are obtained when the powder has poorer flow characteristics; the lower the value of percentage compressibility, the better the flow properties; values above about 25 are indicative of poor flow characteristics.

1.8.3 Particle size reduction

Particle size and size distribution influence many aspects of the production of solid-dosage forms. Of particular importance in tablet manufacture are the flow properties of the powder mix. Powders with different particle sizes have different flow and packing properties and, as explained in section 1.8.1, this affects the mass of drug filled into the tablet or capsule and the uniformity of the dosage. It is unlikely, for example, that raw material will be of a suitable particle size specification for use as an excipient in tablet manufacture, and milling of the material is usually required.

Particle size reduction (comminution) of crystalline material results from fracture at cleavage planes where there are weaknesses in the crystal lattice; in non-crystalline material fracture is more random. Localised stresses are set up within the material which produce strains in the particles and the propagation of the crack through regions of the material that have the most flaws and discontinuities. This is a cascade effect; crack propagation is such a rapid process that the excess energy released during strain relaxation is dissipated throughout the material and concentrates at other discontinuities, setting up new cracks, so spreading the cracking process and causing almost instantaneous fracture of the material.

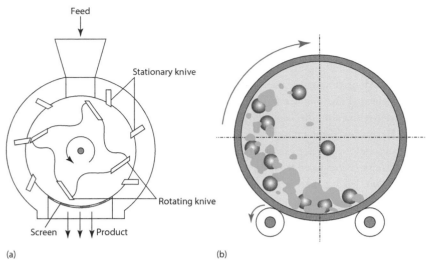

Figure 1.31 Schematic representation of (a) cutter mill and (b) ball mill.

Comminution is a most inefficient process with only a very small percentage (possibly as low as 2%) of the energy input actually involved in process of size reduction; the remainder is lost through elastic deformation of the particles, friction between particles themselves and between particles and the walls of the equipment, and the usual energy losses associated with machine processes – e.g. heat, vibration and sound.

A variety of industrial equipment is available for particle size reduction, the selection largely depending on the initial particle size and the degree of size reduction required:

- *Cutting methods* are suitable when coarse particles are involved, for example, in reducing the size of granules prior to tableting. In cutter mills, size reduction is achieved by a series of rotating knives which act against stationary knives in the metal casing of the mill at a clearance of a few millimetres, so fracturing the particles (Fig. 1.31a).
- A similar degree of size reduction may be achieved by *compression methods*, for example, in roller mills. Here the particles are compressed between two horizontal rollers which can rotate about their long axes. One of the rollers is driven directly; the other rotates by friction as the powder is passed through the narrow gap between them.
- In cases where finer particles of narrower size distributions are required, *impact methods* are considered more suitable. Several designs of mill cause size reduction by impact, including hammer

mills and vibration mills. The impact in hammer mills comes from a series of hammers hinged on a central rotating shaft enclosed in a metal casing. The swinging hammers generate a high impact force which causes brittle fracture of the particles enclosed in the casing, which when sufficiently small are forced out through a fine screen (sieve) of suitable aperture. In vibration mills, the metal casing of the mill is filled to about 80% with stainless-steel or porcelain balls. Vibration of the milling balls causes repeated impact, with the particles contained within the mill causing a reduction in their particle size. When sufficiently fine, the particles fall through a screen at the base of the mill.

- To achieve the finest particles, methods which use a combination of *impact and attrition* forces are generally used. The two main types of mill are the ball mill and the fluid energy mill. In the ball mill, the balls have many different diameters and occupy between 30 and 50% of the drum volume. As the mill rotates, a cascading motion is imparted to the balls as they are lifted up the sides of the drum and fall back to the base across the diameter of the mill (Fig. 1.31b). Collision of the balls with the particles contained within the drum chamber as they fall from the highest part on the wall imparts impact forces sufficient to fragment the larger particles. The particles are also subjected to shear forces (attrition forces) as they move between the cascading balls which are travelling at different velocities, and this causes a further reduction in particle size. A typical fluid energy mill consists of a hollow toroid in which the material is suspended and conveyed at high velocity by compressed air through a region of high turbulence. Repeated high-momentum collisions of the particles with each other and with the walls of the mill in this turbulent zone causes size reduction by impact and, to a lesser extent, attrition. Finer particles may be removed from the mill by a centrifugal action, leaving the coarser particles to undergo further size reduction.

1.8.4 Powder mixing and demixing

The process of mixing the powdered excipients and drug(s) is a complex process involving three main mechanisms: convective, shear and diffusive mixing. *Convective* mixing refers to the movement of groups of particles from one region to another rather than the movement of individual particles within the mix; *shear* mixing occurs when layers of material moving at different speeds flow over each other and mix at the layer interface; in *diffusive* mixing there is movement of individual particles through voids created as a consequence of expansion of the powder bed during some types of mixing. Since the mixing process involves the movement of particles within the powder mix it is not surprising that the efficiency of mixing is influenced by the flow characteristics of the particles and their relative sizes – ideally the particles should all be of similar size, although this is frequently not the case in practice. It is also influenced to a considerable degree by the type of mixer and the processing conditions. It is instructive to consider briefly the principal types of industrial mixer since the contribution of each of the three mechanisms of mixing varies with the design of the mixer.

In planetary bowl mixers (Fig. 1.32), the powders are mixed in a bowl by a rotating blade attached to a rotating shaft, which is offset rather than centrally placed so that the blade rotates around the circumference of the bowl as well as on its own axis. The main mixing mechanism is convective.

In tumbling drum mixers (Fig. 1.32), the drum containing the powders is attached to a drive shaft and rotated by the action of a motor. As a consequence of the tumbling action a velocity gradient through the powder bed is produced, layers nearest the surface move with the greatest velocity and the velocity decreases with distance from the surface. Shear mixing occurs as these layers move relative to each other. In addition, the powder bed expands or dilates as it tumbles, allowing particles to move downwards under gravity, and diffusive mixing occurs.

High-speed mixers have excellent powder-mixing properties and have the added advantage that the mixing process can be followed by wet granulation in the same equipment if required. The powders are contained in a mixing bowl on the bottom of which is an impeller capable of high-speed rotation. During the mixing process the material is thrown towards the wall of the bowl by centrifugal force and then forced upwards before finally falling down to the centre of the mixer. Expansion of the powder bed during this highly efficient mixing process allows diffusive mixing to occur.

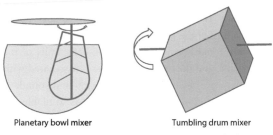

Planetary bowl mixer   Tumbling drum mixer

Figure 1.32 Diagrammatic representations of planetary bowl and tumbling drum mixers.

With each type of mixer, the processing variables, particularly the mixer load and the speed and time of mixing, are carefully controlled to ensure that a homogeneous mixture is produced, that is, one in which the concentration of each component in each region of the mixture is identical.

Having achieved homogeneity of mixing, it is important to ensure that there is no separation of the components of the mixture during handling processes. This process of separation is often referred to as *segregation* or *demixing*. It usually arises because of large differences in the characteristics of the components of the mixture, particularly variations in the size, shape, density and surface properties of the particles. Figure 1.33 shows how, in a rotating device, granules with different radii, density and surface properties may separate. Such events can cause variability in the drug dose between individual dosage units.

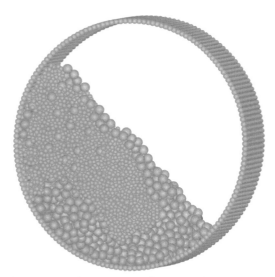

Figure 1.33 The separation of two granule types due to differences in density and size. Such separation could cause problems in the accurate dosing of tablets when the system feeds into the tabletting device.

The two main types of demixing are *trajectory segregation*, in which particles with similar characteristics congregate together, and *percolation segregation*, in which smaller particles fall through voids created when the powder bed dilates on being disturbed by, for example, vibration or pouring. Demixing may be avoided or at least minimised in several ways. Since the problem arises mainly as a consequence of differences in particle size and density, attempts may be made to achieve a narrower size range of ingredients, for example, by sieving the ingredients to remove clumps or fines, by milling components to reduce their size range or by controlled crystallisation of the ingredients to give components of similar size range. It is interesting to note that a mixture containing both very small and very much larger particles, contrary to expectations, does not readily segregate. This is because the very small particles tend to adsorb on to the larger particles, which act as 'carrier particles', resulting in minimal segregation and good flow properties. The phenomenon, referred to as *ordered mixing*, is utilised, for example, in the production of dry-powder inhalations for delivery to the lungs. Here the drug needs to be in a micronised form to reach its site of action and is usually formulated in combination with lactose as the carrier particle to which it becomes adsorbed.

Key points

- The process of mixing the powdered excipients and drug(s) is a complex process involving three main mechanisms: convective, shear and diffusive mixing.
- Convective mixing refers to the movement of groups of particles from one region to another and is the predominant type of mixing in planetary bowl mixers.
- Shear mixing occurs when layers of material moving at different speeds flow over each other and mix at the layer interface; it occurs in tumbling drum mixers.
- Diffusive mixing involves the movement of individual particles through voids created as a consequence of expansion of the powder bed and occurs in high-speed mixers and to some extent in tumbling drum mixers.
- Segregation or demixing usually arises because of large differences in the size, shape, density and surface properties of the components of the mixture.
- The two main types of demixing are trajectory segregation, in which particles with similar characteristics congregate together, and percolation segregation, in which smaller particles fall through voids created when the powder bed dilates on being disturbed by, for example, vibration or pouring.
- Demixing may be minimised by sieving the ingredients to remove clumps or fines; by milling components to reduce their size range; or by controlled crystallisation of the ingredients to give components of similar size range.

1.8.5 Granulation

Granulation is the process whereby the dry-powder mix of active ingredient and suitable excipients (excluding the lubricant) are aggregated into larger particles either by mixing with a suitable fluid (*wet granulation*) or by the application of high stresses without solvent addition (*dry granulation*). The granules may constitute a dosage form in their own right, in which case they are usually produced with a size range of between 1 and 4 mm, but more usually they are an intermediate stage in the production of tablets or capsules and are between 0.2 and 0.5 mm in size.

There are several reasons for the use of granules in the production of tablets:

- to prevent segregation of the constituents of the powder mix. The process of segregation (or demixing) is discussed in section 1.8.4 and arises mainly as a consequence of differences in the size and density of each of the components of the mix. Compression of the segregated powder into tablets would result in an unacceptable variation of composition within a batch of tablets. Ideally, each granule formed in the granulation process will contain the same proportion of each ingredient and provided the size range of the granules is sufficiently narrow to avoid any significant segregation, tablets of a uniform composition will be produced.
- to enhance the flow properties of the mix. As we have seen in section 1.8.2, poor powder flow will occur when particles are below a minimum size and/or have irregular shape. The consequences of this were discussed in this section; unless the powder can flow freely from the hopper into the tablet die there is a possibility that the tablets will not contain a uniform mix of ingredients and also that 'jamming' may occur in the hopper outlet. The formation of granules obviates these problems by improving powder flow characteristics.
- to improve the compaction properties. In general, granules are more easily compacted than powder mixes mainly because of the presence of binder on the granule surface, which improves the adhesion between granules and leads to a stronger tablet of compression.
- to minimise dust production during handling. This is of particular importance when toxic materials are being processed and is greatly reduced when the material is present as granules rather than as a powder mix.

Key points

- Granulation is the process whereby the dry-powder mix is aggregated into larger particles. It is carried out to prevent segregation of the constituents of the powder mix, to enhance the flow properties of the mix, to improve the compaction properties and to minimise dust production during handling.
- There are two types of granulation: wet granulation, in which a solvent is added to the powder mix to aggregate the particles, and dry granulation, in which a high stress is applied to form granules without adding solvent.

Wet granulation

The essential stages in the wet granulation process are as follows:

1. A suitable liquid, usually water, ethanol or isopropanol (or mixtures of these solvents), is added to the powder mixture. To ensure efficient binding of the granules, a binder is either included in the powder mix or dissolved in the granulating fluid. The wet mass is forced through a sieve, producing granules.
2. The wet granules are dried, milled to break down large agglomerates, screened to remove fine material and finally mixed with the lubricant in readiness for the compression process.

Stage 1: Granule formation

In most modern industrial processes the powder-mixing and wet granulation stages are carried out in a single operation using a *high-speed mixer/granulator*. This equipment is based on the planetary bowl mixer shown diagrammatically in Figure 1.32. After mixing the dry ingredients, the granulating fluid is added and mixed with the impeller blades to form a wet mass, which is then broken up into granules by the action of a rotating chopper located in the mixer bowl. Once granules of a suitable size have been produced, they are passed through a wire mesh (screen) to break down any large agglomerates and transferred to the drying equipment.

An alternative technique employs a *fluidised-bed granulator*. The process is shown diagrammatically in Figure 1.34.

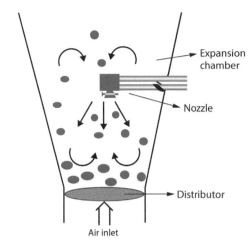

Figure 1.34 Diagrammatic representation of a fluidised-bed granulator. The dry powders are suspended (fluidised) by a vertical stream of warm air entering the base of the equipment and the granulating fluid sprayed through a nozzle located near the top on to the dispersed particles. When granules of the required size have been formed, the spraying process is terminated but the air flow is continued to dry the suspended granules.

Extrusion/spheronisation techniques

For certain applications, particularly where it is required to control the release rate, the drug is incorporated into spherical particles of uniform size (pellets), which can either be filled into hard gelatin capsule shells or compacted into tablets. Controlled release may be achieved by filling the capsule with several batches of pellet in each batch with a coating designed to release drug after different time intervals. The manufacturing process by which such uniformly sized pellets are produced is *extrusion* or *spheronisation*. In the extrusion technique the required quantity of granulation fluid is added to the mix of drug and excipients using similar equipment to that described above, but then transferred to extrusion equipment designed to produce rod-shaped particles of uniform diameter. There are several types of extruders which differ in the mechanism by which the wet mass is forced through the perforated plate (the die). The extrudate particles which emerge break at similar lengths under their own weight into the rod-shaped particles of uniform size. If spherical particles are required, the rods are transferred to a spheroniser which consists of

a bowl having a rapidly rotating bottom plate which rounds off the particles by frictional forces as they collide with each other.

Bonding mechanisms in wet granulation

Several bonding mechanisms operate during the various stages, from the initial cohesion of the particles to the final formation of granules, as follows:

- adhesion and cohesion forces in the stationary films between particles. The presence of the thin stationary liquid film around and between the powder particles brings them closer together and increases the area of contact between them. Because, as discussed in section 6.2.1 in Chapter 6, van der Waals forces of attraction between particles are inversely proportional to the sixth power of the distance between them, there will be increased particle cohesion as a result of this interparticle film and small agglomerates are formed.

- interfacial forces in mobile liquid films within the granules. The quantity of granulating fluid added to the dry-powder mix is usually more than that required to coat the powder particles and the excess forms mobile films between the particles within the granules. The forces acting between particles are dependent on the amount of water present in the mix. When insufficient fluid has been added to displace all of the air originally present, the particles within the granules are held together by surface tension forces at the air/liquid interface of liquid bridges formed between the particles; this is referred to as the pendular state (Fig. 1.35a). In the presence of larger amounts of fluid, the liquid bridges become thicker (the funicular state: Fig. 1.35b) and finally the capillary state (Fig. 1.35c) is reached when the amount of water is sufficient to displace all of the entrapped air or this has been removed by an extended mixing process. The particles are now held together by capillary forces at the liquid/air inter-

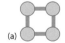   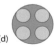

(a)   (b)   (c)   (d)

Figure 1.35 Diagrammatic representation of interfacial forces between granules during granulation showing: (a) pendular; (b) funicular; (c) capillary; and (d) overwetted states.

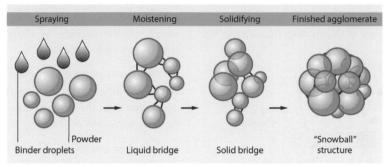

| Spraying | Moistening | Solidifying | Finished agglomerate |

Binder droplets / Powder — Liquid bridge — Solid bridge — "Snowball" structure

Figure 1.36 Processes occurring in wet granulation, using a liquid binder that forms liquid bridges between the particles, which then solidify on drying to provide a quasi-spherical granule suitable for processing.

face, which now exists only at the granule surface. These small agglomerates grow to form larger granules either by addition of single particles via pendular bridges or by combining together to form larger units, which become reshaped during the mixing process. The quantity of added granulating fluid is critical for the formation of granules of the required size and properties. Overwetting (Fig. 1.35d) and continued agitation can produce large granules that are unsuitable for pharmaceutical use, mainly because individual granules are not produced on drying, but also because of problems of tablet disintegration and dissolution due to an excessive amount of binder. Insufficient quantities of granulating fluid, on the other hand, can lead to disintegration of the granules during subsequent processing and, as a consequence, tablets of poor mechanical strength are produced.

● formation of solid bridges between particles. A binder is usually dissolved in the granulating fluid which, during the drying process, solidifies the liquid bridges, so binding the particles together to form a granule with suitable mechanical strength for processing into tablets or capsules (Fig. 1.36). As discussed in section 1.8.1, binders are usually polymeric (e.g. polyvinylpyrrolidone and hydroxypropylcellulose) and the solid bridges resemble a polymeric network holding the particles together in the granule. In some instances, the solvent used for granulation may partially dissolve one of the powdered excipients, which then crystallises out during drying and acts as a hardening agent.

Stage 2: Drying and milling

The objective of these two unit operations is to produce dried granules of a size suitable for processing

into tablets by compression or for filling into hard gelatin capsules.

There is a variety of equipment available for *drying* the wet granules; the choice of method depends on factors, including the stability of the material to heat, the nature of the liquid to be removed and the physical characteristics of the material. In *shelf or tray driers* heat transfer is mainly by conduction; the wet granules are placed on a series of horizontal shelves, hot air is passed across the surface of the granules and moisture is removed through an outlet. Greater efficiency is achieved if drying is carried out using a specially designed oven connected via a condenser (to remove the moisture released) to a vacuum pump. The use of vacuum ovens is mainly restricted to the drying of thermolabile materials, since much lower drying temperatures can be used, or those subject to oxidation, since little air is present. When granulation is carried out in a fluidised-bed granulator the granules are usually dried as part of the process using a current of warm air as described above; efficient convective drying is achieved because of the excellent transfer of heat to the suspended granules and removal of moisture released. Because of the efficiency of the process drying times are generally short, which is not only an economic advantage but also minimises the exposure of thermolabile material to high temperatures.

One of the problems associated with granule drying is that of *solvent migration*. The movement of solvent either through individual granules (intragranular migration) or from granule to granule (intergranular migration) during the drying process carries with it any dissolved solutes to the surface of the granule or the granule bed where they are deposited when the solvent evaporates. As a consequence, there may be variability in the concentration of both drugs and excipients, leading to an unacceptable variation of drug content in the finished tablets. Intergranular migration is a particular problem when drying is carried out in static beds, as in tray driers, and leads to a deposit of solute on the top surface of the bed. Contact between granules is minimised in fluidised-bed driers and hence intergranular migration is less of a problem, although intragranular migration may still occur.

The main reason for *milling* the granules is to achieve the particle size required for smooth flow of the dried granules into the tablet die, which, as we have seen, is an important factor affecting the uniformity of weight of the tablet. The size of the granules is determined by the size of the tablet; smaller tablets require proportionally smaller granules for efficient filling of the smaller dies used for their manufacture. Particle size reduction may be achieved by, for example, a cutter mill, as described in section 1.8.3.

Before final compaction into tablets, the granules are dry-mixed with lubricant, which, as discussed above, reduces the friction between the tablet surface and the face of the die during the ejection of the tablet from the die. Other excipients, such as glidants, and disintegrants may be added at this stage.

Key points

- Wet granulation may be performed using a high-speed mixer/granulator or a fluidised-bed granulator. When high-speed mixers/granulators are used, a suitable solvent is added to the powder mix together with a binder and the wet mass is forced through a sieve to produce the granules, which are then dried using, for example, a shelf or tray drier. In fluidised-bed granulators the dry powders are suspended (fluidised) by a vertical stream of warm air and sprayed with the granulating fluid to produce granules, which are then dried in the same equipment by the current of warm air. Granules produced by both of these techniques are milled to produce granules of the size required for tableting.
- For certain applications, for example, when it is required to control the release rate, uniformly sized pellets are produced using extrusion or spheronisation techniques.
- Several bonding mechanisms operate during the various stages of wet granulation from the initial cohesion of the particles to the final formation of granules; these include adhesion and cohesion forces in the stationary films between particles; interfacial forces in mobile liquid films within the granules; and formation of solid bridges between particles.

Dry granulation

In the process of dry granulation the powder mix is converted to granules by the application of high pressure. Unlike wet granulation, no solvent is added to the powder, so avoiding issues with chemical degradation or solubility of drug in the granulation fluid, and consequently heating to remove solvent is not necessary, which is an advantage if the active ingredients are thermolabile. Despite these potential advantages, dry granulation is not as widely used as wet granulation and has, to some extent, been superseded by direct compression methods, as discussed in the following section.

There are two stages involved in dry granulation: the first involves compression of the powder into a compact; the second involves milling to produce the granules. The compression step may be carried out either by slugging or by roller compaction. In the slugging technique large tablets (usually about 25 mm diameter) are produced in a tableting press capable of applying a high stress. In roller compaction the powder is fed via a hopper on to a moving belt to pass between two rollers rotating in opposite directions, which compress the powder into a thin sheet. In the second stage, conventional milling equipment is employed to break down the tablet or compressed sheet into granules of the required size, and these are then mixed with lubricant ready for compression into tablets.

Bonding mechanisms in dry granulation

Three types of particle–particle interaction are involved in the dry granulation process.

1. The high stresses applied in this method force the particles of the powder mix into close contact and hence increase the van der Waals interactions between them, making this a major contributor to the overall particle–particle attraction.
2. Electrostatic forces between powder particles contribute to the initial cohesion of the particles.
3. There may be partial melting of those excipients of the powder mix which have low melting points because of the high shear stresses involved in compression. Solidification on cooling may increase the interaction between particles.

 Key points

- There are two stages involved in dry granulation: the first involves either compression of the powder into large tablets by slugging under high stress, or compression of the powder into thin films by roller compaction. The second stage involves milling the tablets or films to produce granules of the required size which are then mixed with lubricant ready for compression into tablets.
- Cohesion of the particles of the powder mix in the dry granulation process is mainly due to van der Waals interactions and electrostatic forces, but increased interaction may arise from the partial melting and subsequent solidification of low-melting-point excipients.

1.8.6 Tablet manufacture

In this section we will examine the various unit operations involved as the granules (or powder mix) are compressed to form tablets and some of the techniques used in the coating of these tablets. For each process we will discuss the physicochemical factors involved.

Compression and compaction of powders

The most commonly used manufacturing process employed in the manufacture of tablets involves the formation of granules, either by wet or dry techniques, and it is these granules that are fed into the die of the tablet press and compressed into tablets. An alternative

method, termed *direct compression*, avoids the time-consuming process of granulation and instead the powder mix itself is fed directly into the die of the tablet press. This is a seemingly attractive option since fewer steps are involved, making this a less expensive process, and in addition, no water or other solvents are used, which is an advantage when the excipients or drugs are susceptible to hydrolysis (or solvolysis). However, there are many potential problems associated with the direct compression method:

- The excipients have usually to be specially processed and care has to be taken to ensure that their physical properties, such as morphology, particle size and density, are similar to avoid demixing (as discussed in section 1.8.4).
- The tablets produced by this method tend to be softer than those formed by compression of granules and are consequently more difficult to film coat (see below).
- Although it is possible to manipulate the properties of the excipients to be suitable for successful direct compression, this is often not the case with the drug itself; this may cause problems if the drug is present in amounts exceeding about 10% of the final formulation.
- Direct compression is not usually suitable for the manufacture of coloured tablets because of the mottled appearance of the resulting tablet.

The two alternative processes used for tablet manufacture are shown diagrammatically in Figure 1.37.

The compression process

The three phases of basic tablet formation are, in essence:

1. die filling
2. compaction by the punch
3. ejection from the die.

The process of compression of the powder into tablets takes place in the die of the tablet press, which is filled from a hopper (Fig. 1.38). Flow from the hopper into the die is by gravity and it is essential that the flow properties of the powders or granules are carefully controlled to ensure smooth flow at a controlled rate. Tablets are formed by the action of two punches: the lower punch seals the bottom of the die, allowing a measured amount of powder to be filled into the die

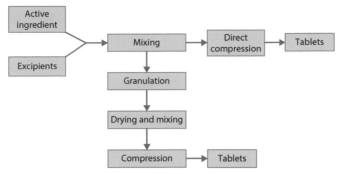

Figure 1.37 Unit operations involved in tablet manufacture by direct compression and by an intermediate granulation process.

cavity from a hopper shoe which moves backwards and forwards over the top of the die, and the upper punch descends to compact the granules (or powder) under high pressure. The tablet so formed is then ejected as the lower punch is pushed upwards and is pushed away by the hopper shoe, which then refills the die to repeat the operation. High-speed tablet manufacture is achieved using rotary presses operating with a number of dies and sets of punches, but the required properties of the powder for optimum tablet production remain essentially the same.

Clearly the particles of drug and excipients are subject to changing forces, often at high speed during the manufacturing process. The particles rearrange during this process, and there is friction between the particles and, dependent on the elasticity of the material, recovery of form after compression.

Mechanisms of compression

The events that occur in the process of compression depend on whether the tableting process involves a granulation stage (as is usually the case) or is by direct compression of the powder mix; we will examine the differences between the two processes for each of the following stages involved in the compression process:

1. *Transitional repacking.* After application of the initial stress as the upper punch descends into the die, there is a small movement of the granules as they rearrange within the space between the two punches. In the direct compression process the extent of the rearrangement is usually greater and depends on the size of the particles and the frictional forces between them.

2. *Deformation under the applied stress.* At a certain load, the granules can no longer continue to rearrange because of reduced space and an increase of interparticulate friction. Reduction of the volume of the die contents is now associated with changes in the shape of the particles, initially by *elastic* deformation and then by *plastic* deformation. Elastic deformation is a reversible effect, i.e. the particles can regain their shape when the loading is removed; plastic deformation results in a permanent change of particle shape. The loading applied in tablet manufacture is generally greater than that required for elastic deformation to avoid the possibility of tablet failure associated with

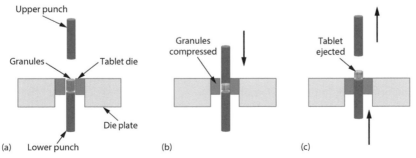

Figure 1.38 Events occurring in the manufacture of tablets in a tablet press: (a) measured amount of granules/powder filled into tablet die from shoe; (b) granules compressed into tablet as upper punch descends; and (c) tablet ejected as lower punch is pushed upwards.

low stress levels. Successful achievement of plastic deformation necessitates the inclusion of excipients that can themselves undergo plastic deformation, otherwise the quality of the compressed tablet will be adversely affected. Following plastic deformation, the granules retain their structure, but the applied stress causes changes in both granule shape and porosity because of the movement of individual particles within the granule. When tablets are produced by the direct compression method, an additional type of deformation, termed *particle fragmentation*, also occurs. In this, the intraparticle bonds are broken and the particle is fractured into a number of smaller discrete particles, which repack to reduce the volume of the powder bed further. These smaller particles may then undergo further deformation with increase of the applied stress. The two main mechanisms of deformation during compression of powder mixes are plastic deformation and fragmentation.

3. *Bonding.* The compressional forces involved in the production of the tablet are sufficient to overcome repulsive forces between adjacent particles and these are forced together into close proximity, causing the formation of intergranule or interparticle bonds which are responsible for the mechanical strength of the tablet. The two main mechanisms involved in tablets produced by both granulation and direct compression techniques are bonding by intermolecular forces (or *adsorption bonding*) and the formation of solid bridges (or *diffusion bonding*). In adsorption bonding, the particles or granules are held together by van der Waals forces between component molecules at the surface. In diffusion bonding the interaction forces are a consequence of the temporary increased mobility of molecules at the particle surface due to melting of components or induced rubbery properties under compression; as a consequence there is the possibility of molecular diffusion and mixing at the surfaces of adjacent particles to form a continuous solid phase (bridge) which bonds them together. Granules formed by the wet granulation process usually include a binder which plays an important role in the cohesion of the tablet through the formation of binder bridges between adjacent granules.

4. *Stress relaxation.* After the release of the compaction forces on ejection of tablets from the tablet press, there may be a continuing viscous deformation of particles, referred to as stress relaxation, which

occurs for a limited time following compaction and leads to a significant increase of tablet strength without any noticeable changes in the physical appearance. It should be noted, however, that such increases of mechanical strength are reliant on careful control of the conditions, particularly relative humidity and temperature, under which tablets are stored. For example, the condensation of water in the pores of the tablet under conditions of high relative humidity can drastically reduce the tablet strength, eventually leading to the collapse of the tablet.

A common problem that occurs during ejection of the tablets is the mechanical splitting of the tablets. This is referred to as *capping,* when the top of the tablet is fractured, and *lamination,* when fracture occurs in the body of the tablet (Fig. 1.39). This defect can be a consequence of the application of excessive stress during compression or an intricate punch geometry.

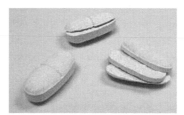

Figure 1.39 Tablet defects: capping in which the top is fractured, and lamination where fracture occurs in the body of the tablet.

 Key points

- Tablets are usually manufactured by compression of the granulated powder mix. In an alternative method (direct compression) the granulation stage is omitted and the powder mix itself is compressed; this method is advantageous when the ingredients are susceptible to hydrolysis but is less frequently used because of the potential problems associated with it.
- The process of compression takes place in the die of the tablet press and involves three steps: filling of the die from the hopper, compression by the upper punch, and ejection of the tablet as the lower punch is pushed upwards.

- The events that occur in the process of compression include: transitional repacking of the granules after application of the initial stress; deformation under the applied stress; formation of intergranule or interparticle bonds during compaction; and stress relaxation after the release of the compaction forces on ejection of tablets.

Tablet coating

Coatings are applied to tablets and capsules for a variety of decorative, protective and functional purposes, including:

- to improve the aesthetic appearance of the product and aid identification by health care professionals and patients
- to enhance the chemical stability of a drug by protecting it from the environment, particularly light, oxygen and moisture
- to mask the bitter taste or unpleasant odour of certain drugs
- to modify drug-release profiles, for example to provide controlled release of drug throughout the gastrointestinal tract or target release of drug at a specific site
- to protect the drug from degradation in the stomach (enteric coating).

Essentially, the coating process involves the application of a layer of coating material to the outer surface of the solid-dosage form, and in this section we will examine the variety of materials used and the methods by which the coat is applied.

The earliest compound applied to tablets was sucrose, which was traditionally used for coating confectionery products, but this has now been mostly replaced by polymeric materials, which, as discussed in section 7.6.1 in Chapter 7, are able to form rate-controlling barriers to drug release. The traditional technique for sugar-coating tablets involved a pan-coating process in which the sucrose solution was manually ladled on to the tablets as they tumbled in a rotating sugar-coating pan. Conventional technologies for the application of film coatings now usually involve the atomisation of the polymeric material dispersed as a solution or suspension, which is then sprayed on to a rotating or fluidised mass of tablets. Subsequent drying to remove the solvent leaves a thin deposit of the coating material on the tablet surface. Several alternative techniques have been developed in order to reduce the use of water or organic solvents which involve the compaction of dry material around the tablet cores, a process referred to as dry or compression coating. We will briefly review both film-coating and dry-coating techniques, indicating their advantages and limitations.

Film coating

Most solid-dosage forms are coated using either a pan (drum) coating or fluidised-bed technique. Although these methods are quite different (see below), the underlying principle of the film-coating process is the same in both. Mechanisms of polymeric film coating have been reviewed by Felton.[19,20] Conceptually, the process involves the repeated exposure of the tablets to a spray containing the polymeric coating material dissolved or suspended in a suitable solvent. As the tablet moves through the spray zone, it receives a partial coating which is then solidified by heating to evaporate the solvent. This cycle of spraying and drying is repeated until the desired coating mass and uniformity are achieved (Fig. 1.40).

The mechanism by which films are formed is dependent on whether the polymer is dissolved or dispersed in the spray liquid. When the polymer is in the *dissolved state* the process of film formation is relatively straightforward. The droplets of the atomised spray spread over the surface of the tablets to form a film of liquid, which becomes a gel when the polymer concentration increases during evaporation of the solvent and the polymer chains interact to form a three-dimensional network (see section 7.3.2 in Chapter 7). Finally, a film is formed when more solvent is lost during the drying process. Adhesion between the polymer chains and the tablet surface, which increases with polymer chain length, secures the film to the surface.

The mechanism of film formation from *aqueous-based polymeric dispersions* is more complex. The major steps involved in this process are shown in Figure 1.41. The atomised droplets initially remain as discrete droplets on the surface rather than spreading over it. Before a film can form, these droplets must first coalesce; this occurs as the water is evaporated. The

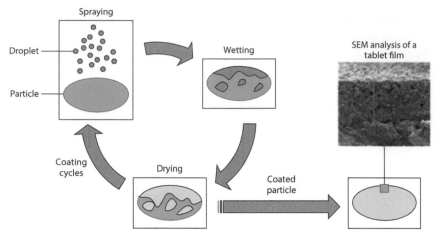

Figure 1.40 General principles of a film-coating process showing repeated spraying and drying cycles. SEM, scanning electron microscopy.

Reproduced with permission from Suzzi D *et al.* Local analysis of the tablet coating process: impact of operation conditions on film quality. *Chem Eng Sci* 2010;65:5699–5715. Copyright Elsevier 2010.

polymer spheres first deform to fill the void spaces left by the evaporating water and eventually, with continued drying, they coalesce to form the film. These

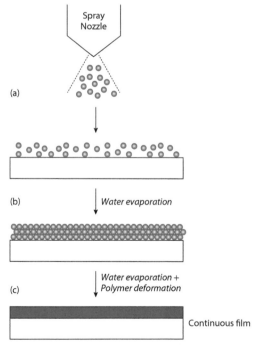

Figure 1.41 Major steps in film formation from an aqueous polymeric dispersion. (a) Atomisation of fine droplets and impingement on to substrate surface; (b) water evaporation causes close packing of polymer spheres; (c) further water evaporation causes polymer deformation and coalescence to form film.

Reproduced with permission from Felton LA. Mechanisms of polymeric film formation. *Int J Pharm* 2013;457:423–427. Copyright Elsevier 2013.

differences in mechanisms of film formation when the polymer is dissolved in an organic solvent and when it is dispersed as a suspension in an aqueous solvent affect the formulation of the spray liquid and the operational conditions under which the film is formed.

Several operational parameters are important in ensuring efficient film formation when the polymer is *dissolved* in the spray liquid. The droplet size of the atomised spray and the rate of solvent evaporation are critical: large droplets caused by inadequate atomisation of the spray liquid or a slow solvent evaporation rate may overwet the tablet surface, possibly causing dissolution of the surface materials, whereas fine droplets, arising when the solvent evaporates too rapidly, may dry before reaching the tablet or spreading over its surface, resulting in rougher surfaces and high loss of material. Similarly, there are specific requirements for the formulated spray solution. The process by which the polymer solution wets the tablet surface and spreads over it to form a liquid film is an example of the phenomenon of spreading wetting, discussed in section 1.6. The ability of the sprayed polymer solution to wet the surface, in the initial stages of the coating process (but not when the surface is already covered by a film), is related to the nature of the solid surface, particularly its hydrophobicity, and the surface tension of the polymer solution. As discussed in section 1.6.1, a measure of the wettability of the surface is the contact angle formed between the solution and the surface, which for perfect wetting should be zero.

Improvement of the wetting capabilities of the polymer solutions can be achieved by reduction of the surface tension of the spray formulation by the inclusion of an appropriate surfactant. The viscosity of the formulation is also important in coating operations involving solutions. The viscosity generally increases with chain length of the polymer and the concentration of its solution. Higher solution viscosities require more energy to atomise the solution and this is a limiting factor restricting the concentration of polymer that can be used. Viscosity also influences the spreading of the droplets; more viscous solutions do not readily spread across the tablet surface and spreading will become increasingly difficult due to an increase of viscosity as the concentration increases during drying.

The processing variables such as spray rate and temperature required for efficient film formation by polymers *dispersed in an aqueous solvent* have to be adjusted to allow for the higher latent heat of water compared to organic solvents. In addition, unlike films formed from solutions, it is often necessary to store the film-coated tablets in an oven at a controlled temperature and humidity to ensure complete coalescence of the polymer spheres, a procedure often referred to as curing. There are also different requirements for the formulated spray solutions compared to those when the polymer is in solution. Although the viscosity of the spray formulation is important in determining the ease of atomisation, it does not influence the spreading since the polymer is present as discrete droplets rather than a solution. Consequently, it is possible to use higher polymer concentrations in the coating process.

An important variable in the coating process is the temperature, which influences the ability of the polymer spheres to deform and fuse together to form a continuous film. For each system there is a minimum film-forming temperature (MFFT) below which the polymeric dispersion will form an opaque discontinuous material upon solvent evaporation rather than the desired clear continuous film. In contrast, there is no MFFT for polymer solutions, which will form films at room temperature. The inclusion of plasticisers in the formulation affects the MFFT, as they soften the polymer spheres (lower the T_g), allowing coalescence at lower temperatures.

Film-coating formulations

The spray liquid typically comprises a polymer, a solvent, a plasticiser, a surfactant, and a colourant or opacifier.

Solvent

Although the use of volatile organic solvents, for example, methanol/dichloromethane combinations, to dissolve the polymer in the spray liquid generally provides a more rapid process, the use of aqueous solutions or dispersions remains the preferred manufacturing approach due to the absence of solvent toxicity, increased process safety and lower manufacturing costs. There are several cases, however, where aqueous systems are inappropriate and organic solvent coatings may be necessary, for example, when the active ingredient is sensitive to water. As discussed above, film formation is more complicated when the polymer is dispersed in an aqueous medium, as the dispersed polymer spheres must also coalesce to form a uniform film. This generally necessitates postcoating storage at elevated temperatures.

Polymer

The choice of film-forming polymer is determined primarily by the proposed use of the dosage form: rapidly dissolving polymers are required when immediate release of active ingredient is intended, whereas film coatings for sustained or controlled-release products should have limited or no solubility in aqueous media. The latter polymers are usually applied in organic solvents or as aqueous dispersions. In addition to this important solubility requirement, polymers are selected for their influence on the physical properties of the film-coating liquid. As we have discussed above, this liquid should have low viscosity to aid atomisation to form the spray, its surface tension should facilitate spreading of the film to cover the tablet surface, the polymer should have good adhesive properties and should be able to pack within the film to provide the desired permeability of the coating. Some examples of the types of polymer used in film coating are given in section 7.6.1 in Chapter 7.

Plasticiser

Plasticisers are generally non-volatile substances that exhibit little or no tendency for evaporation or volatilisation. Commonly used plasticisers include polyols (e.g. polyethylene glycols and propylene glycol), oils (e.g. fractionated coconut oil), citrate esters (e.g. triethyl citrate) and phthalate esters (e.g. diethyl phthalate). The plasticiser molecules increase the flexibility of the film by intercalating between the polymer molecules, allowing increased motion within the film; this reduces problems as the film shrinks and tends to become brittle during the drying process. Plasticisers also facilitate coalescence of the discrete polymer spheres of aqueous-based dispersed systems in the film formation process. The plasticiser must be miscible with the polymer and, for aqueous-based disperse systems, must also partition into the polymer phase. Water-soluble polymer plasticisers partition into the polymer quite rapidly, whereas longer mixing times are required for uptake of the water-insoluble plasticisers. A commonly used method of evaluating the effectiveness of a plasticiser is to determine changes in the glass transition temperature (T_g) of the polymer as the concentration of added plasticiser is increased. As discussed in section 1.3, the T_g is the temperature at which amorphous material changes from a glassy, brittle state to become more mobile and elastic with temperature increase. A more effective plasticiser will cause a greater decrease in T_g of the film. The T_g of a Eudragit polymer is shown in Table 1.11; the most effective plasticiser of those examined was triethyl citrate, which caused the greatest lowering of T_g. Note also that, for all of the compounds examined, an increase of plasticiser concentration resulted in a greater lowering of T_g.

Table 1.11 Influence of plasticiser type and concentration on the T_g of Eudragit RS 30D polymeric films

	Tg of Eudragit RS 30D[a]	
Plasticiser	10% plasticiser	20% plasticiser
Triethyl citrate	34.3°C	12.8°C
Acetyl triethyl citrate	37.0°C	17.5°C
Tributyl citrate	38.2°C	20.5°C
Acetyl tributyl citrate	38.2°C	22.2°C
Triacetin	42.2°C	27.4°C

[a] Unplasticised film is 55.0°C.

Reproduced with permission from Felton LA. Mechanisms of polymeric film formation. *Int J Pharm* 2013;457:423–427.

Colourant

Although water-soluble dyes may be used as colourants, it is more usual to select water-insoluble pigments such as titanium dioxide and the iron oxides, which tend to be more stable to light and also do not readily migrate within the film as do some water-soluble dyes – a process that produces mottled tablets. Pigments can significantly affect the mechanical and permeability properties of the film. For example, large pigment particles are thought to disrupt the interfacial bonding between the polymer and the tablet surface, and the extent of polymer–pigment interaction may influence the elastic modulus of polymer films. The maximum pigment concentration that can be incorporated into a film without compromising film properties is denoted by the critical pigment volume concentration. When this concentration is exceeded there will be insufficient polymer to surround all the insoluble particles and there will be a consequent deterioration in the mechanical and permeability characteristics of the film.

Surfactant

Surfactants may be included in the film-coating formulation in low concentration to emulsify water-insoluble plasticisers, to stabilise suspensions (when the polymer is dispersed in the formulation), to improve the wettability of the tablet surface and to facilitate spreading of the sprayed droplets over the tablet surface.

Film-coating techniques

The most commonly used processes for film coating are pan (or drum) coating and fluidised-bed coating. Differences between these two methods primarily relate to the way particles move between the spray and drying zones and the method used to remove the solvent.

Drum or pan coating

In the usual pan-coating method the tablet cores are placed in a round drum that rotates on an inclined axis (Fig. 1.42). The tablets cascade down the top of the bed, some passing through the atomised spray from one or more nozzles mounted at the top of the drum.

Fluidised-bed coating

This technique is commonly used for multiparticulates rather than larger particles such as tablets. In this method particles are suspended and circulated within a

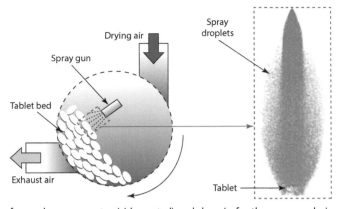

Figure 1.42 Schematic of a modern pan coater (side-vented) and domain for the spray analysis.

Reproduced with permission from Suzzi D *et al*. Local analysis of the tablet coating process: impact of operation conditions on film quality. *Chem Eng Sci* 2010;65:5699–5715. Copyright Elsevier 2010.

cylinder by heated air introduced from below. The air flow mixes and dries the particles which are constantly recirculated, making multiple passes through the spray zone. The high level of air flow makes this coating method more efficient at water removal than the pan-coating technique. The coating liquid is sprayed on to the particles from a nozzle located above or, as shown in Fig. 1.43, below the fluidised bed. The top spray method tends to produce less uniform film coats and is used mainly for taste- and odour-masking purposes.

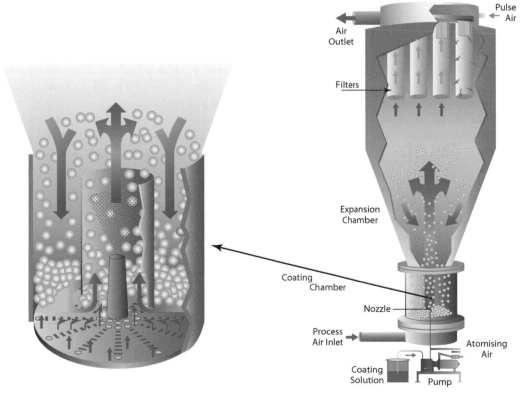

Figure 1.43 Schematic representation of a fluidised-bed film coater in which particles are suspended and circulated in a cylinder by heated air introduced from below. The air flow mixes and dries the particles, which are constantly recirculated, making multiple passes through the spray zone. The coating liquid is sprayed on to the particles from a nozzle located in this case below the fluidised bed.

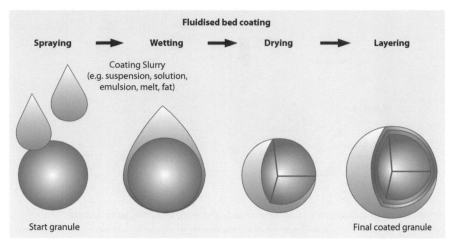

Figure 1.44 Processes involved in the production of a coated granule by film coating using the fluidised-bed technique: spraying, wetting, drying and layering of the coating material.

Figure 1.44 depicts the processes leading to the production of a multilayered granule using the fluidised-bed film-coating technique.

Dry coating

Although film coating using dispersions of polymers in aqueous-based systems remains the preferred method of coating tablets and particles, there are disadvantages associated with both this method and also the alternative film-coating technique in which the polymer is dissolved in an organic solvent. The particular concerns with the use of organic solvents relate to their toxicity and high processing costs arising from ensuring operating safety and safe solvent recovery. Although there are fewer such issues with aqueous-based systems, the coating process uses large amounts of water and requires considerable energy to evaporate off the water during the drying stages. There will also be special problems with this method, of course, when the ingredients are susceptible to degradation in an aqueous environment or when the drug product is formulated as an amorphous solid dispersion. For these reasons, alternative methods of coating in which the use of water or organic solvents is reduced to a minimum, so-called dry-coating techniques, may be considered.

Essentially, the process of dry-powder coating follows similar steps to those of the film-coating methods outlined above, i.e. the coating material is applied to the surface; it then coalesceces and spreads over the surface to form an adhesive film. Because of the minimal amount of solvent (if any) used in applying the film-coating material, however, there is no evaporation stage in the process, as there is with the film-coating technique.

The mechanism of film formation of the powders layered on to the solid may be summarised as shown in the schematic of Fig. 1.45. The polymeric coating powder deposited on the substrate surface partially coalesces to form a film that then undergoes a levelling process in which it becomes denser and smoother as the empty spaces are removed. Finally, the film is cooled and hardened.

There are several important differences in the formulation of the coating materials for this type of coating process compared with those for film coating. To ensure uniformity of the material on the substrate surface and to improve adhesion and processing times, it is generally recommended that the particle size of the powder should be less than about 1% of the size of the substrate on which it is coated. In general, powders having a particle size below 100 μm are suitable. Also, to ensure adequate spreading of the polymeric coating material in the absence of any significant amount of solvent, it is important that the processing temperature is higher than the glass transition temperature (T_g) of the polymer so that the polymer is more 'liquid-like' and more susceptible to plastic deformation (see section 1.3). By reducing the viscosity in this way there will be adequate capillary forces to aid the spreading of this semimolten material and to ensure its adherence to the substrate surface. Hence, an important formulation requirement is the use of a polymeric coating material with a low glass transition temperature to

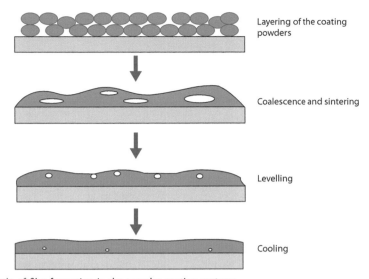

Layering of the coating powders

Coalescence and sintering

Levelling

Cooling

Figure 1.45 Schematic of film formation in dry powder coating systems.
Reproduced with permission from Felton LA, Porter SC. An update on pharmaceutical film coating for drug delivery. *Expert Opin Drug Deliv* 2013;10:421–435.

avoid the need to operate at high temperatures, which might accelerate degradation of materials. Where polymers with high glass transition temperatures ($T_g > 60°C$) are selected, plasticisers can be mixed with the polymeric materials during production to reduce the value of T_g.

Dry-coating techniques may be classified into three major types depending on the layer formation process: liquid-assisted, thermal adhesion and electrostatic.[21] Although these techniques are not widely used at present in the pharmaceutical industry, it is nevertheless interesting to review briefly the principles involved.

Liquid-assisted coating

Liquid-assisted coating techniques rely on the interfacial capillary action of liquid components of the formulation to aid adhesion of the coating layer to the core surface. The quantity of liquid included in the formulation is, however, very much less than that utilised in more conventional film-coating methods and this liquid is often intended to remain in the drug product. Similar equipment to that used for conventional strategies (particularly fluidised beds), with slight modifications, may be used for coating, although longer processing times and additional curing steps may be required. The choice of excipients will be governed by the need to ensure sufficient softening at moderate temperatures, often necessitating larger amounts of plasticiser to facilitate adequate film formation than used for liquid-based coating tech-

niques and polymers with a lower glass transition temperature. In addition, a much smaller particle size, often as low as 10 μm, is required.

Thermal adhesion

In this method of dry coating no liquid is included in the formulation and adhesion relies entirely on the thermal properties of coating powder. Removal of the liquid, however, places more exacting requirements on the formulation to ensure adequate adhesion and film formation. In particular, the amount of plasticiser becomes a critical factor in ensuring effective processing and higher levels of plasticiser than in conventional methods are usually required. Careful selection of a polymer with a suitable glass transition temperature is also important to ensure spreading and adhesion of the coating. In addition, it may be necessary to include antisticking agents such as talc to prevent the agglomeration of the powder particles during storage and during the distribution of the powders on the cores; an additional coating of talc after the curing step may be required to reduce the tackiness of the final coated tablet, particularly when the T_g of the polymer is low.

Electrostatic coating

This technique involves the deposition of charged coating powder on to the core surface and consequently it is essential that charge can be induced into the powder components so that there is an electrostatic attraction between the powder and tablet core which promotes adhesion. The process can be carried out

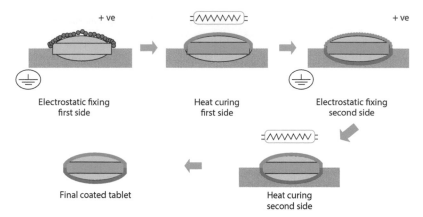

Figure 1.46 Schematic diagram of the electrostatic dry-coating process.

Reproduced with permission from Sauer D *et al.* Dry powder coating of pharmaceuticals: a review. *Int J Pharm* 2013;457:488–502. Copyright Elsevier 2013.

using specialised equipment similar to that used for the deposition of ink toner in photocopying; the essential steps in this process are shown diagrammatically in Fig. 1.46. As you can see from this figure, each side of the tablet is coated and cured separately. With this technique, the coating material can be deposited with sufficient precision to create intricate patterns on the tablet surface for brand identification purposes.

Alternatively, the electrostatic powder-coating process can be combined with the conventional liquid pan-coating technique, the polymer particles having been initially negatively charged using an electrostatic spray gun before undergoing essentially similar processes to those described above.

Key points

- Coatings may be applied to tablets to improve their appearance, to enhance chemical stability, to mask a bitter taste or unpleasant odour, to modify drug-release profiles and to protect the drug from degradation in the stomach (enteric coating).
- Tablets may be coated by film-coating (most frequently used) or dry-coating techniques.
- The *film-coating process* involves the repeated exposure of the tablets to a spray containing the polymeric coating material dissolved or suspended in a suitable solvent; the coating is then solidified by heat-ing to evaporate the solvent. The mechanism by which films are formed and the processing variables are dependent on whether the polymer is dissolved or dispersed in the spray liquid. The most commonly used processes for film coating are pan (or drum) coating and fluidised-bed coating.

- In *dry-coating techniques* the use of water or organic solvents is reduced to a minimum and the polymeric coating material is deposited on the substrate surface as a dry (or almost dry) powder rather than a spray. Dry-coating techniques may be classified into three major types depending on the layer formation process: liquid-assisted, thermal adhesion and electrostatic coating.

1.8.7 Capsule manufacture

Two types of capsules are produced as solid-dosage forms – hard and soft capsules – both usually composed of gelatin or, less commonly, hydroxypropyl-methylcellulose (hypromellose), but differing in their design and mechanical properties. Hard capsules are constructed from two cylindrical pieces sealed at one end; the shorter piece (the cap) fits over the open end of the longer piece (the body). They are generally used to deliver powders but other materials, such as pellets, granules, tablets, semisolids and non-aqueous liquids, may be filled into the hard capsules providing they do not react chemically with the gelatin or hydroxy-

Structure III Gelatin

propylmethylcellulose shells or contain free water which causes the shells to soften or distort. Soft capsules are composed of a one-piece capsule shell and are more flexible than hard capsules; they are usually filled with non-aqueous liquids in which the active ingredient is dissolved or dispersed. In this section we will look at the properties of gelatin that make it especially suitable for use in the manufacture of capsules and briefly examine how both hard and soft capsules are manufactured and filled, since this has repercussions on the ways in which capsule fillings are formulated.

Chemical and physicochemical properties of gelatin

Gelatin possesses many desirable properties, making it the material of choice for the manufacture of capsules: it is non-toxic and widely used in foodstuffs, it is capable of forming a strong flexible film, concentrated aqueous solutions of gelatin are mobile liquids above about 45°C and form gels on cooling – a property which, as we will see below, is utilised in capsule manufacture, and it is readily soluble in biological fluids at body temperature.

Gelatin (III) is a heterogeneous mixture of single or multistranded polypeptides, each containing between 50 and 1000 amino acids joined together by amide linkages to form linear polymers varying in molecular weight from 15 000 to 250 000. A typical structure is - Ala-Gly-Pro-Arg-Gly-Glu-4Hyp-Gly-Pro-.

Gelatin is prepared by the hydrolysis of collagen, which is extracted from animal skin and bones. There are two types of gelatin, depending on whether the method of extraction involves an acid or alkaline pretreatment. Type A gelatin is obtained by immersing pig skin in dilute mineral acid (pH 1–3) for approxi-

mately 24 h; the pH is then adjusted to between 3.5 and 4.0 and the gelatin is extracted by a series of hot-water washes. Type B gelatin is derived from immersion of cattle hides and bones in a calcium hydroxide (lime) slurry over a period of several months, after which time the stock is washed with cold water to remove as much of the lime as possible and then neutralised with acid before extraction with hot water, as in the acid process. In both processes the gelatin solutions are cooled to form gel sheets, which are dried and then ground to the required particle size. The two types of gelatin have differing physicochemical properties: their isoelectric points are 7–9 (Type A) and 4.7–5.3 (Type B), and their 1%w/v aqueous solutions at 25°C have pHs of 3.8–6.0 (Type A) and 5.0–7.4 (Type B). Because of the differences in isoelectric points, there is a difference in the pH dependence of solubility, but both types are poorly soluble in water at 25°C and gradually swell and soften as water is absorbed. In gastric fluid the gelatin capsules swell to release their contents rapidly. In hot water (above about 40°C), gelatin dissolves to form a mobile liquid (sol), which undergoes a reversible transition to the rigid gel state on cooling (similar in behaviour to the type II gels discussed in section 7.3.2 in Chapter 7), a property which is used in the production of gelatin capsules (see below).

The grade of gelatin is indicated by its *Bloom strength,* which is a measure of gel rigidity; it is defined as the load in grams required to push a standard plunger (diameter 12.7 mm) 4 mm into a 6.66%w/w gelatin gel that has been prepared in water and allowed to mature at 10°C. Gelatin used in the manufacture of hard capsules has a Bloom strength of 200–250 g: that suitable for soft gelatin capsules has a lower Bloom strength (150 g) because a less rigid gel is required.

Hard-capsule manufacture and filling

Manufacture

The manufacture of hard gelatin capsules makes use of the sol–gel transition occurring at about 40°C, as discussed above. A concentrated solution of gelatin (35–40%) is prepared in demineralised hot water (60–70°C) and any entrapped air is removed under vacuum. Excipients are added at this stage; these include dyes or pigments to colour the capsules for identification and aesthetic purposes, and, if necessary, wetting agents such as sodium lauryl sulfate to enhance the wetting of the shell on contact with an aqueous solution. The viscosity is now reduced to a target value by the addition of hot water. Viscosity regulates the thickness of the capsule shell during production: the higher the viscosity, the thicker is the shell. Hydroxypropyl-methylcellulose solutions do not gel (see section 7.4.2 in Chapter 7) and gelling agents such as carrageenan, together with a co-gelling agent such as potassium chloride, have to be added to their solutions when used to manufacture hard capsules.

Commercial equipment for manufacturing hard gelatin capsules consists of upper and lower sets of metal strips (bars), each containing a series of stainless-steel moulds (pins) mounted in rows: one set for the production of the cap, the other for the body of the capsule. Figure 1.47 shows diagrammatically the sequence of processes involved. The lubricated pins at room temperature are dipped into a hopper containing a fixed quantity of the gelatin solution at about 45°C, which coats each pin with a gel formed when the warm gelatin solution is cooled below the gel point on contact with the colder pins. The bar containing the pins is slowly removed from the solution and rotated to form a film of uniform thickness. The pins are then passed through a series of driers in which air at controlled humidity is blown over them to remove moisture. It is important at this stage that the water level is reduced to about 13–16% w/w, to ensure that the capsule shell is not too brittle (too low water content), or easily deformed as a result of plastic flow (too high water content). Finally, the dried films are removed from the pins, cut to size and the two halves joined together to form the complete capsules. Hydroxypropylmethylcellulose hard capsules are manufactured in a similar manner, except that the gelling step is slower, necessitating a lower machine output.

Filling of powder formulations

The hard capsules are filled by either of two main methods: a *dependent* dosing and the more widely used *independent* dosing method. In the dependent method the lower half of the capsule is placed in slots in a turntable which rotates at a range of speeds under a hopper containing the powder formulation. After

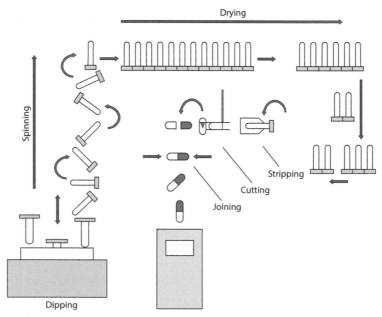

Figure 1.47 Sequence of procedures involved in the manufacture of hard gelatin capsules.

filling, the upper halves of the capsule contained in a similar turntable are brought together with the capsule bodies and the two halves sealed. In this method, the mass of powder filled into the capsule is dependent primarily by the time that the capsule body remains under the hopper, which itself is determined by the speed of rotation of the turntable. In the independent dosing method a plug of powder is formed when the open end of a dosing tube fitted with a spring-loaded piston is lowered into the powder mix. The tube containing the plug of powder is then raised from the powder bed, rotated and positioned over the lower half of the capsule, and the plug ejected into the capsule body by lowering the piston. The volume of powder filled into the capsule may be controlled by altering the position of the piston within the tube.

It is perhaps not surprising that many of the excipients used in the formulation of powder mixes for filling into hard capsules are similar to those used in the formulation of tablets, since the two dosage forms require the powder mix to have similar general properties. For example, the powder blend should have reproducible flow properties to ensure uniformity of filling and contain components of similar size distribution to ensure homogeneous mixing within the powder blend. These requirements necessitate the use of free-flowing diluents with good plug-forming properties such as lactose, starch and microcrystalline cellulose. The flow and packing properties of the powders are assessed using techniques described in section 1.8.2. Suitable flow and cohesive properties are associated with an angle of repose of approximately 25° and a Hauser ratio preferably of about 1.2, but certainly not exceeding 1.6. In addition, glidants, for example, colloidal silicon dioxide, and lubricants, particularly magnesium stearate, may be added to reduce interparticulate friction and adhesion of powder to metal surfaces. Other excipients, including disintegrants, to break up the powder mass when released in the stomach, and surfactants, to ensure powder wetting following release, may be included in the powder mix.

Filling of pellets and tablets

Pellets and granules are filled using equipment adapted from powder use and utilise a dosing system based on a chamber with an adjustable volume. Tablets are filled from hoppers into the capsule body via a gate device that controls the number of tablets allowed to pass.

Filling of liquids and semisolids

Filling of hard gelatin capsules with semisolids is usually performed using a volumetric dosing device. Where possible, semisolids are filled in the liquid state, either by heating, in the case of thermosoftening mixtures, or by stirring, in the case of thixotropic mixtures. After filling, these formulations revert to the solid state to form a plug. An important consideration when liquids are filled into capsules is the prevention of leakage; this may be achieved by applying a gelatin solution around the junction between the two halves of the capsule, which dries to form a hermetic seal, preventing liquid leakage.

The liquids in which the therapeutic agent is dissolved or dispersed must be non-aqueous and must be carefully selected to avoid any adverse effect on the stability of the capsule. Of particular concern when water-miscible liquids are used as vehicles is their effect on the moisture content of the capsule, which for optimum mechanical properties should be maintained between 13% and 16%. Suitable water-miscible liquids with low moisture uptake are higher-molecular-weight polyethylene glycols and liquid polyoxyethylene-polyoxypropylene block copolymers (see section 5.6.3). Suitable lipophilic liquids or oils are the vegetable oils such as sunflower oil and fatty-acid esters such as glyceryl monostearate.

It is important that the viscosity of liquid fill formulations is within a suitable range (between 0.1 and 25 Pa s^{-1}) for optimum filling properties: liquids with high viscosities are difficult to pump when using the volumetric dosing device, whereas liquids with very low viscosities may splash from the capsule during filling. It may be necessary when viscosities are outside these acceptable limits to include viscosity-modifying agents in the liquid formulation. Other excipients that may be required include surface-active agents for solubilisation of poorly soluble drugs or as suspending agents for suspensions, and antioxidants to stabilise the liquid formulation.

Soft gelatin (softgel) capsule manufacture and filling

It is necessary to manipulate the properties of gelatin to produce a capsule shell with a greater degree of flexibility than that of a hard capsule. Type B gelatin is most commonly used and this is modified by the addition of *plasticisers* to impart a greater pliability.

Plasticisers are selected depending on their compatibility with the capsule fill; they are usually polyhydric alcohols such as glycerol or sorbitol or their mixtures, sometimes in combination with glycerol. The amount of plasticiser incorporated affects the mechanical properties of the soft gelatin capsule and is usually within the range 20–30% of the wet mass of the mixture. At levels above this the capsules are too flexible, whereas lower concentrations produce capsules that are too brittle. The other additive influencing the flexibility of the capsule is *water*, which constitutes between 30 and 40% of the wet formulation, but reduces to an equilibrium concentration in the final capsule of 5–8% as a result of the drying process during capsule manufacture. Other excipients that may be included in the wet gel formulation include colourants, such as soluble dyes, and opacifiers, usually titanium dioxide, which are used to produce an opaque shell.

Manufacture and filling

The hot gel liquid containing the additives described above is fed into the encapsulation machine where it is cooled to the gel state and cast into two ribbons, each of which forms one-half of the capsule. So again, as with the manufacture of hard gelatin capsules, an essential stage of the process is the sol–gel transition as the hot gelatin mass is cooled below the gel point. The two ribbons are fed between two rotary dies to form pockets into which a metered dose of the liquid fill is simultaneously dispensed, as shown diagrammatically in Figure 1.48. Finally, the two halves are sealed together by the application of heat and pressure and cut automatically from the gelatin ribbon by raised rims on each die. After collection the capsules are washed in a tumble drier, spread on to trays and dried with air at 20% humidity until the water level is reduced to the required equilibrium value.

Liquid-based vehicles in which the active ingredient is dissolved or dispersed are used as the capsule fill of soft gelatin capsules. For the reasons discussed earlier, water must be avoided because of its effect on the capsule integrity. *Lipophilic liquids*, particularly vegetable oils such as soybean oil, are widely used as fill materials, although, because of their limited capacity to dissolve drugs, it may be necessary also to include cosolvents, unless the formulation is intended as a suspension, in which case a viscosity-modifying agent is included. *Water-miscible liquids* such as the poly-

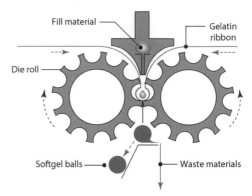

Figure 1.48 Mechanism for the manufacture of soft gelatin (softgel) capsules. Two ribbons of gelatin are fed between the rotary dies to form pockets into which a metered dose of the liquid fill is simultaneously dispensed. The two halves are then sealed together and cut from the gelatin ribbon.

ethylene glycols PEG 400 and PEG 600 are commonly used and, to a lesser extent, non-ionic surfactants, such as Tweens, and liquid polyoxyethylene-polyoxypropylene block copolymers.

Key points

- Two types of capsule are produced as solid-dosage forms – *hard capsules,* which are generally used mainly to deliver powders, pellets and granules, and *soft capsules,* which are used to deliver non-aqueous liquids in which the active ingredient is dissolved or dispersed. The shells of both types are usually composed of gelatin, although hydroxypropylmethylcellulose has also been used.
- In commercial equipment, the two halves of hard gelatin capsules are formed separately when gelatin solution, at about 45°C, is cooled below the gel point to form a film coating on a series of lubricated pins. The films are dried, removed from the pins and cut to size and the two halves are joined together to form the complete capsules.
- Soft gelatin capsules are prepared from gelatin modified by the addition of *plasticisers* (20–30%) to impart a greater pliability. Gelatin solution containing 30–40% water is cooled to the gel state

and cast into two ribbons, each of which forms one-half of the capsule. The two ribbons are fed between two rotary dies to form pockets into which a metered dose of the liquid fill (a lipophilic liquid containing dissolved or dispersed drug) is dispensed. The two halves are sealed together by the application of heat and pressure and cut automatically from the gelatin ribbon.

1.9 Solid dispersions

Over the past few years interest has been shown in *solid solutions* of drugs in attempts to change the biopharmaceutical properties of drugs that are poorly soluble or difficult to wet. The object is usually to provide a system in which the crystallinity of the drug is so altered as to change its solubility and solution rate, and to surround the drug intimately with water-soluble material. A solid solution comprises solute and solvent – a solid solute molecularly dispersed in a solid solvent. These systems are sometimes termed *mixed crystals* because the two components crystallise together in a homogeneous one-phase system. They should, however, be distinguished from cocrystals (see section 1.2.4), which are *single* crystalline forms consisting of two types of molecule. The earliest forms of solid solutions were eutectic mixtures in which the drug was dispersed as very fine particles; in later developments the poorly soluble drug was dispersed in molecular form initially in crystalline carriers and then later in amorphous carriers. We will look briefly at these types of solid solution; a review of this topic has been provided by Leuner and Dressman.[22]

1.9.1 Eutectic mixtures

In Fig. 1.49, the melting temperature of mixtures A and B is plotted against mixture composition. On addition of B to A or of A to B, melting points are reduced. At a particular composition the *eutectic point* is reached, the eutectic mixture (the composition at that point) having the lowest melting point of any mixture of A and B. Below the eutectic temperature, no liquid phase exists. The phenomenon is important because of the change in the crystallinity at this point. If we cool a solution of A and B that is richer in A than the eutectic mixture (see M in Fig. 1.49), crystals of pure A will appear. As the solution is cooled further, more and more A crystallises out and the solution becomes richer in B. When the eutectic temperature is reached, however, the remaining solution crystallises out, forming a microcrystalline mixture of pure A and pure B, differing markedly at least in superficial characteristics from either of the pure solids. This has obvious pharmaceutical possibilities. This method of obtaining microcrystalline dispersions for administration of drugs involves the formation of a eutectic

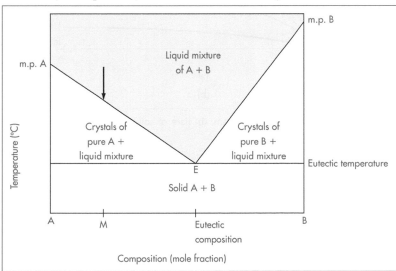

Figure 1.49 Phase diagram (temperature versus composition) showing boundaries between liquid and solid phases, and the eutectic point, E.

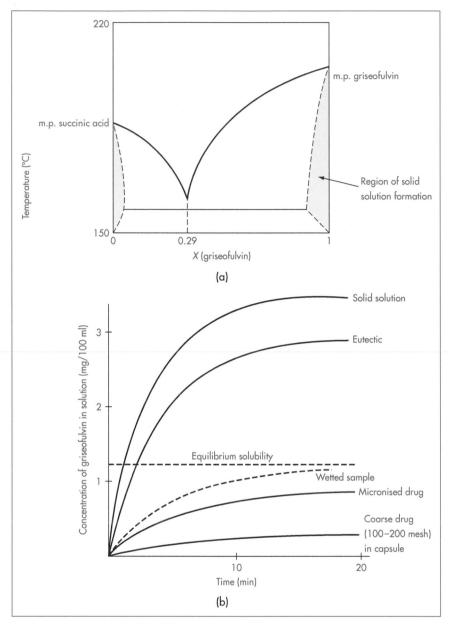

Figure 1.50 (a) Griseofulvin–succinic acid phase diagram. (b) Rate of solution of griseofulvin solid solutions, eutectic and crystalline material.

mixture composed of drug and a substance readily soluble in water. The soluble 'carrier' dissolves, leaving the drug in a fine state of solution *in vivo*, usually in a state that predisposes to rapid solution.

The simplest eutectic mixtures are usually prepared by the rapid solidification of the fused liquid mixture of components that show complete miscibility in the liquid state and negligible solid–solid solubility. In addition to the reduction in crystalline size and hence an increase in surface area, the following factors may contribute to faster dissolution rate of drugs in eutectic mixtures:

- an increase in drug solubility because of the extremely small particle size of the solid
- a possible solubilisation effect by the carrier, which may operate in the diffusion layer immediately surrounding the drug particle

- absence of aggregation and agglomeration of the particles
- improved wettability in the intimate drug–carrier mixture
- crystallisation in metastable forms.

Systems that form eutectic mixtures include chloramphenicol–urea, sulfathiazole–urea and niacinamide–ascorbic acid. The solid solution of chloramphenicol in urea was found to dissolve twice as rapidly as a physical mixture of the same composition and about four times as rapidly as the pure drug. *In vivo*, however, the system failed to display improved bioavailability. On the other hand, the eutectic mixture of sulfathiazole–urea did give higher blood levels than pure sulfonamide.

1.9.2 Solid solutions

Solid solutions are formulations in which the drug is dispersed in *molecular form* rather than as fine particles, as in the case of eutectic mixtures. The dissolution rate is now determined by that of the carrier and can be increased by up to several orders of magnitude. Figure 1.50a shows the solid solution regions for the griseofulvin–succinic acid (soluble carrier) system. In these regions one of the solid components is completely dissolved in the other solid component. Also shown is the eutectic point at 0.29 mole fraction of drug (55% w/w griseofulvin). The eutectic mixture consists here of two physically separate phases: one is almost pure griseofulvin, while the other is a saturated solid solution of griseofulvin in succinic acid. The solid solution contains about 25% griseofulvin; the eutectic mixture, which has a fixed ratio of drug to carrier, thus comprises 60% solid solution and 40% almost pure griseofulvin. As can be seen from Fig. 1.50b, which shows the solution profiles of the different forms, the solid solution dissolves 6–7 times faster than pure griseofulvin and significantly faster than the eutectic mixture.

Where more complex solubility patterns emerge, as with the griseofulvin and succinic acid phase, the phase diagram becomes correspondingly more complex. Figure 1.51 shows one example of a system in which each component dissolves in the other above and below the eutectic temperature.

The carriers of the solid solutions discussed above were in a *crystalline* state. In a development of these

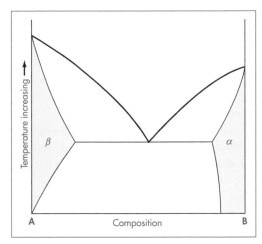

Figure 1.51 Melting point–composition plot for a system in which α and β are regions of solid-solution formation. Each component dissolves the other component to some extent above the eutectic temperature. As the temperature is lowered, the solid solution regions become narrower.

solid-solution formulations, carriers were used in an *amorphous* state, resulting in improved dissolution characteristics. In an amorphous solid solution, the drug molecules are dispersed irregularly within the amorphous solid rather than locating regularly within the crystal lattice of the carrier. Polymers such as polyvinylpyrrolidone, polyethylene glycol and various cellulose derivatives have been utilised as amorphous carriers. More recently, it has been shown that the dissolution profile can be improved if the carrier has surface-active or self-emulsifying properties, leading to the development of solid dispersions containing a surfactant carrier or a mixture of amorphous polymers and surfactants as carriers.

 Clinical point

A topical preparation for intradermal anaesthesia to reduce the pain of venepuncture is available. The cream, Emla (Eutectic Mixture of Local Anaesthetics: AstraZeneca), contains a eutectic of procaine and lidocaine.[23] The eutectic mixture (50 : 50 mixture) is an oil, which is then formulated as an oil-in-water emulsion. This allows much higher concentrations than would have been possible by using the individual drugs dissolved in an oil.

1.9.3 Eutectics and drug identification

As the eutectic temperature of a substance in mixtures with other compounds is, as a rule, different even when the other substances have the same melting point, this parameter can be used for identification purposes. Benzanilide (m.p. 163°C), phenacetin (m.p. 134.5°C) and salophen (m.p. 191°C) are often used as test substances. The eutectic temperatures of mixtures of benzanilide with various drugs are shown in Table 1.12. Substances of identical melting points can be distinguished by measurement of the eutectic temperature with another suitable compound.

Table 1.12 Eutectic temperatures of drugs with benzanilide

Compound	Melting point (°C)	Eutectic temperature (°C)
Allobarbital	173	144
Ergotamine	172–174	135
Imipramine HCl	172–174	109

Reproduced with permission from Kuhnert-Brandstatter M. *Thermomicroscopy in the Analysis of Pharmaceuticals.* New York: Pergamon Press, 1971.

Ternary eutectics are also possible. The binary eutectic points of three mixtures are as follows: for aminophenazone–phenacetin 82°C; for aminophenazone–caffeine 103.5°C; and for phenacetin–caffeine 125°C. The ternary eutectic temperature of aminophenazone–phenacetin–caffeine is 81°C. In this mixture the presence of aminophenazone and phenacetin can be detected by the mixed melting-point test, but the caffeine causes little depression of the eutectic given by the other two components.

The possibility of determining eutectic temperatures of multicomponent mixtures has practical value in another respect. During tableting, for example, heat is generated in the punch and die and in the powder compact; measurement of the eutectic temperature can give information on whether this rise in temperature is likely to cause problems of melting and fusion.

 Key points

- A solid dispersion comprises a solid solute dispersed in a solid solvent; it is designed to provide a system in which the drug is surrounded intimately with water-soluble material (carrier) and its crystallinity is so altered as to increase its solubility and solution rate.
- Mixing of the drug with a soluble carrier reduces the freezing point; the lowest temperature at which the system freezes/melts is called the eutectic point and below this point the mixture is composed of a microcrystalline dispersion of pure drug and carrier. Pharmaceutical examples of eutectic mixtures include griseofulvin–succinic acid, chloramphenicol–urea, sulfathiazole–urea and niacinamide–ascorbic acid.
- Solid solutions are formulations in which the drug is dispersed in *molecular form* rather than as fine particles, as in the case of eutectic mixtures, leading to faster dissolution rates. Further improvements in dissolution characteristics can be achieved if the carrier is in an amorphous rather than crystalline state.
- Substances having identical melting points can be distinguished by measurement of the eutectic temperature with another suitable compound.

Summary

In this chapter we have examined those aspects of the structure of crystalline and amorphous solids that influence their formulation and the properties, both physical and pharmacological, of the formulated product. We have seen that crystal lattices are constructed from repeating units called unit cells, of which there are 14 possible types (Bravais lattices) and which, for any particular compound, are all of the same size and contain the same number of molecules or ions arranged in the same way. The external appearance of the crystal, that is, its habit, is affected by the rate of crystallisation and by the presence of impurities, particularly surfactants. The habit of a crystal is of pharmaceutical importance, since it affects the compression characteristics and flow properties of the drug during tableting and also the ease with which the suspensions of insoluble drugs will pass through syringe needles. Many high-molecular-weight materials, particularly polymers, are unable to form crystals and exist as amorphous or semicrystalline solids. These materials do not have sharp melting points but change their properties at a glass transition temperature, T_g, from a glassy state below T_g to a more mobile or rubbery state as the temperature is increased.

Problems arising from the occurrence of drug polymorphs – a largely unpredictable phenomenon – have been discussed. The various polymorphs of a particular drug have different physical and chemical properties and usually exist in different habits. The transformation between polymorphic forms can cause formulation problems; phase transformations can cause changes in crystal size, which in suspensions can eventually cause caking, and in creams can cause detrimental changes in the feel of the cream. Changes in polymorphic form of vehicles, such as theobroma oil used to make suppositories, can result in unacceptable melting characteristics. Problems may also result from phase transformation when attempting to identify drugs using infrared spectroscopy. The most significant consequence of polymorphism is the possible difference in the bioavailability of the different polymorphic forms of a drug as, for example, in the case of polymorphs of chloramphenicol palmitate. The entrapment of solvent during crystallisation can result in polymorphic solvates in which the entrapped solvent becomes an integral part of the crystal structure, or pseudopolymorphic solvates, in which the solvent is not part of the crystal bonding and merely occupies voids in the crystal. Similarly, cocrystals may be formed in which a solid is hydrogen bonded to the drug. The formation of crystal solvates and cocrystals can significantly affect the aqueous solubility and also the dissolution characteristics of the drug.

The rate of absorption of many slightly soluble drugs from the gastrointestinal tract and other sites is limited by the rate of dissolution of the drug. The particle size of a drug is therefore of importance if the substance in question has a low solubility. The rate of dissolution of a solid can be increased by reduction in the particle size, providing that this does not induce changes in polymorphic form, which could alter the drug's solubility. The reduction of particle size of some drugs to below 0.1 μm can cause an increase in the intrinsic solubility. This is the basis of a method for increasing the rate of dissolution and solubility of poorly soluble drugs such as griseofulvin, by forming a eutectic mixture or solid dispersion with a highly soluble carrier compound.

Penetration of water into tablets or into granules precedes dissolution. The wettability of the powders, as measured by the contact angle (θ) of the substance with water, therefore determines the contact of solvent with the particulate mass. The contact angle is an indicator of the ability of a liquid to wet a solid surface; for complete, spontaneous wetting the contact angle should be zero. There are two types of wetting – spreading wetting, in which a liquid spreads over the surface of a solid, and immersional wetting, which is the initial wetting process that occurs when a solid is immersed in a liquid. Several pharmaceutical powders have been identified that, because of their high contact angle, present wetting problems.

We have examined the physicochemical phenomena underlying many of the unit operations involved in the manufacture of tablets and granules. We have seen how important it is that pharmaceutical powders or granules are able to flow freely into storage containers or hoppers of tablet- and capsule-filling equipment so that a uniform packing of the particles and hence a uniform tablet or capsule weight is achieved. The cohesivity of particles increases with decrease of the particle size, with consequences for the flow properties of powders; particles larger than about 250 μm are usually relatively free flowing, but very fine particles (below 10 μm) are usually extremely cohesive and have a high resistance to flow. The cohesivity of the powder may be expressed using the Hausner ratio (values of between 1.25 and 1.5 required for optimum flow properties) or the Carr's index (values of less than 25 required). Several mechanisms may be involved in the process of mixing the powdered excipients and drug(s) depending on the equipment employed: convective mixing, which is the movement of groups of particles from one region to another (as in planetary bowl mixers), shear mixing, which occurs when layers of material moving at different speeds flow over each other and mix at the layer interface (as in tumbling drum mixers) and diffusive mixing, which involves the movement of individual particles through voids created as a consequence of expansion of the powder bed (as in high-speed mixers). Segregation or demixing of powders may occur during the processing of the powder mix; this may be by trajectory segregation, in which particles with similar characteristics congregate together, and percolation segregation, in which smaller particles fall through voids created when the powder bed dilates on being disturbed by, for example, vibration or pouring. It may be prevented in tablet manufacture by granulation, the process whereby the dry-powder mix is aggregated into larger particles either by mixing with a suitable fluid (*wet granulation*) or by the application of high stresses without solvent addition (*dry granulation*).

Several bonding mechanisms operate during the various stages of wet granulation: these include adhesion and cohesion forces in the stationary films between particles; interfacial forces in mobile liquid films within the granules; and formation of solid bridges between particles. Cohesion of the particles of the powder mix in the dry granulation process is mainly due to van der Waals interactions and electrostatic forces. We have seen that in certain circumstances it may be preferable to omit the granulation stage and to compress the powder mix itself (*direct compression*). The events that occur in this process of compression include: transitional repacking of the granules after application of the initial stress; deformation under the applied stress; formation of intergranule or interparticle bonds during compaction; and stress relaxation after the release of the compaction forces on ejection of tablets. Coatings are applied to tablets and capsules for a variety of decorative, protective and functional purposes either by *film coating*, involving the repeated exposure of the tablets to a spray containing the polymeric coating material dissolved or suspended in a suitable solvent, or *dry-coating* techniques (liquid-assisted, thermal adhesion or electrostatic), in which the polymeric coating material is deposited on the substrate surface as a dry (or almost dry) powder rather than a spray.

References

1. Pilpel N. Powders – gaseous, liquid and solid. *Endeavour (NS)* 1982;6:183–188.
2. Mullin JW. *Crystallization,* 4th edn. London: Butterworth-Heinemann, 2001.
3. Michaels AS, Colville AR. The effect of surface-active agents on crystal growth rate and crystal habit. *J Phys Chem* 1960;6:413–419.
4. Vippagunta SR *et al.* Crystalline solids. *Adv Drug Deliv Rev* 2001;48:3–26.
5. Agafonov V *et al.* Polymorphism of spironolactone. *J Pharm Sci* 1991;80:181–185.
6. Nichols G, Frampton CS. Physicochemical characterization of the orthorhombic polymorph of paracetamol crystallized from solution. *J Pharm Sci* 1998;87:684–693.
7. Koda A *et al.* Characterization of chloramphenicol palmitate form C and absorption assessments of chloramphenicol palmitate polymorphs. *J Pharm Sci Technol Jpn* 2000;60:43–52.
8. Aiguiar AJ, Zelmer JE. Dissolution behaviour of polymorphs of chloramphenicol palmitate and mefanamic acid. *J Pharm Sci* 1969;58:983–987.
9. Chapman JH *et al.* Polymorphism of cephaloridine. *J Pharm Pharmacol* 1968;20:418–429.
10. Shan N *et al.* Impact of pharmaceutical cocrystals: the effect on drug pharmacokinetics. *Expert Opin Drug Metab Toxicol* 2014;10:1255–1269.
11. Volkheimer G. Persorption of particles: physiology and pharmacology. *Adv Pharmacol Chemother* 1977;14:163–187.
12. Florence AT. The oral absorption of micro- and nanoparticulates: neither exceptional nor unusual. *Pharm Res* 1997;14:259–266.
13. Atkinson RM *et al.* Effect of particle size on blood griseofulvin levels in man. *Nature* 1962;193:588–589.
14. Shaw TRD *et al.* Particle size and absorption of digoxin. *Lancet* 1973;2:209–210.
15. Nash JF *et al.* Relation between the particle size of dicoumarol and its bioavailability in dogs. I. Capsules. *Drug Dev Commun* 1975;1:443–457.
16. Fincher JH. Particle size of drugs and its relationship to absorption and activity. *J Pharm Sci* 1968;57:1825–1835.
17. Ertel KD *et al.* Determination of ibuprofen vapor pressure at temperatures of pharmaceutical interest. *J Pharm Sci* 1990;795:52.
18. Kiffmeyer TK *et al.* Vapour pressures, evaporation behaviour and airborne concentrations of hazardous drugs: implications for occupational safety. *Pharm J* 2002;268:331–337.
19. Felton LA. Mechanisms of polymeric film formation. *Int. J. Pharm* 2013;457:423–427.
20. Felton LA, Porter SC. An update on pharmaceutical film coating for drug delivery. *Expert Opin Drug Deliv* 2013;10:421–435.
21. Sauer D *et al.* Dry powder coating of pharmaceuticals: A review. *Int J Pharm* 2013;457:488–502.
22. Leuner C, Dressman J. Improving drug solubility for oral delivery using solid dispersions. *Eur J Pharm Biopharm* 2000;50:47–60.
23. Broberg BFJ, Evers HCA. *Local anaesthetic emulsion cream.* Eur Pat 0 002 425 (1981).

2

Physicochemical properties of drugs in solution

In this chapter we examine some of the important physicochemical properties of drugs in aqueous solution that are of relevance to such liquid dosage forms as injections, solutions and eye drops.

- We recount the various ways to express the strength of a solution, since it is of fundamental importance that we are able to interpret the various units used to denote solution concentration and to understand their interrelationships, not least in practice situations.
- Some basic thermodynamic concepts will be introduced, particularly that of thermodynamic activity, an important parameter in determining drug potency.
- We will see why it is important that parenteral solutions are formulated with an osmotic pressure close to that of blood serum and how this may be achieved.
- We will look at the influence of pH on the ionisation of several types of drug in solution and consider equations that allow the calculation of the pH of solutions of these drugs.
- We will examine the process whereby drugs spontaneously diffuse through solutions and between phases, an important process relevant to the dissolution of the drug and its membrane transport.

2.1 Concentration units

A wide range of units is commonly used to express solution concentration, and confusion often arises in the interconversion of one set of units to another. Wherever possible throughout this book we have used the SI system of units. Although this is the currently recommended system of units in Great Britain, other more traditional systems are still widely used. Some useful conversions between concentration units are given in Box 2.1.

2.1.1 Weight or volume concentration

Concentration is often expressed as the weight of solute in a unit volume of solution; for example, $g\,dm^{-3}$, or as % w/v, which is the number of grams of solute in 100 mL of solution. When the solute is a liquid, the concentration may also be expressed as the

Box 2.1 Conversion into SI units

- *Volume* is commonly expressed in litres (L) and millilitres (mL) rather than the SI unit of cubic metres (m^3).

  $$1\,L = 1\,dm^3 = 10^{-3}\,m^3$$
  $$1\,mL = 1\,cm^3 = 10^{-6}\,m^3$$

- *Concentration* is often given in grams per litre (g L^{-1}) rather than kilograms per cubic metre (kg m^{-3}).

  $$1\,g\,L^{-1} = 1\,g\,dm^{-3} = 1\,kg\,m^{-3}$$

  Note also that 1 mg mL^{-1} is therefore also equal to 1 kg m^{-3}.

- *Molarity* is commonly expressed as mol L^{-1} and often written using the symbol M or M; its conversion to SI units is

  $$1\,mol\,L^{-1}\ (or\ 1\,M) = 1\,mol\,dm^{-3}$$
  $$= 10^3\,mol\,m^{-3}$$

2.1.2 Molarity and molality

These two similar-sounding terms should not be confused. The *molarity* of a solution is the number of moles (gram molecular weights) of solute in 1 litre (1 dm^3) of *solution*. The *molality* is the number of moles of solute in 1 kg of *solvent*. Molality has the unit, mol kg^{-1}, which is an accepted SI unit. Molarity may be converted to SI units as shown in Box 2.1; interconversion between molarity and molality requires knowledge of the density of the solution.

Of the two units, molality is preferable for a precise expression of concentration because, unlike molarity, it does not depend on the solution temperature; also, the molality of a component in a solution remains unaltered by the addition of a second solute, whereas the molarity of the first component decreases because the total volume of solution increases following the addition of the second solute.

2.1.3 Milliequivalents

These units are commonly used clinically in expressing the concentration of an ion in solution. The term 'equivalent' or 'gram equivalent weight' is analogous to the mole or gram molecular weight. When monovalent ions are considered, these two terms are identical. A 1 molar (1 mol L^{-1}) solution of sodium bicarbonate (sodium hydrogen carbonate), $NaHCO_3$, contains 1 mol or 1 Eq of Na^+ and 1 mol or 1 Eq of HCO_3^- per litre of solution. With multivalent ions, attention must be paid to the valency of each ion; for example, 10% w/v $CaCl_2 \cdot 2H_2O$ contains 6.8 mmol or 13.6 mEq of Ca^{2+} in 10 cm^3.

The Pharmaceutical Codex[1] gives a table of milliequivalents for various ions and also a simple formula for the calculation of milliequivalents per litre (Box 2.2).

In analytical chemistry, a solution that contains 1 Eq per litre is referred to as a *normal* solution. Unfortunately the term 'normal' is also used to mean physiologically normal with reference to saline solution. In this usage, a physiologically normal saline solution contains 0.9 g NaCl in 100 cm^3 aqueous solution and not 1 equivalent (58.44 g) per litre.

volume of solute in a unit volume of solution, for example as % v/v, which is the number of mL of solute in 100 mL of solution. These are not exact methods when working at a range of temperatures, since the volume of the solution is temperature dependent and hence the weight or volume concentrations also change with temperature.

Whenever a hydrated compound is used it is important to use the correct state of hydration in the calculation of weight concentration. Thus, 10% w/v $CaCl_2$ (anhydrous) is approximately equivalent to 20% w/v $CaCl_2 \cdot 6H_2O$ and consequently the use of the vague statement '10% calcium chloride' could result in gross error.

When very dilute solutions are involved the concentration may be expressed as parts per million (or ppm), which is the number of grams in 10^6 grams of solution (which equals the number of mg per kg of solution) or, if the solute is a liquid, the number of mL in 10^6 mL (1000 litres) of solution. Since the density of very dilute aqueous solutions at room temperature approximates to 1 g mL^{-1}, a concentration of 1 ppm is approximately 1 mg of solute per litre of solution (i.e. 1 g in 10^6 mL).

Box 2.2 Calculation of milliequivalents

The number of milliequivalents in 1 g of substance is given by

$$mEq = \frac{valency \times 1000 \times no.\ of\ specified\ units\ in\ 1\ atom/molecule/ion}{atomic,\ molecular\ or\ ionic\ weight}$$

For example, $CaCl_2 \cdot 2H_2O$ (mol wt = 147.0 Da):

mEq Ca^{2+} in $1\,g\ CaCl_2 \cdot 2H_2O$

$$= (2 \times 1000 \times 1)/147.0 = 13.6\ mEq$$

and

mEq Cl^- in $1\,g\ CaCl_2 \cdot 2H_2O$

$$= (2 \times 1000 \times 2)/147.0 = 13.6\ mEq$$

that is, each gram of $CaCl_2 \cdot 2H_2O$ represents 13.6 mEq of calcium and 13.6 mEq of chloride.

2.1.4 Mole fraction

The mole fraction of a component of a solution is the number of moles of that component divided by the total number of moles present in solution. In a two-component (binary) solution, the mole fraction of solvent, x_1, is given by $x_1 = n_1/(n_1 + n_2)$, where n_1 and n_2 are, respectively, the number of moles of solvent and solute present in solution. Similarly, the mole fraction of solute, x_2, is given by $x_2 = n_2/(n_1 + n_2)$. The sum of the mole fractions of all components is, of course, unity, i.e. for a binary solution, $x_1 + x_2 = 1$.

Example 2.1 Units of concentration

Isotonic saline contains 0.9% w/v of sodium chloride (mol wt = 58.5 Da). Express the concentration of this solution as: (a) molarity; (b) molality; (c) mole fraction; and (d) milliequivalents of Na^+ per litre. Assume that the density of isotonic saline is $1\ g\ cm^{-3}$.

Answer

(a) 0.9% w/v solution of sodium chloride contains 9 g dm^{-3} = 0.154 mol dm^{-3}.

(b) 9 g of sodium chloride is dissolved in 991 g of water (assuming density = $1\ g\ cm^{-3}$).

Therefore, 1000 g of water contains 9.08 g of sodium chloride = 0.155 mol, i.e. molality = 0.155 mol kg^{-1}.

(c) Mole fraction of sodium chloride, x_1, is given by

$$x_1 = n_1/(n_1 + n_2)$$
$$= 0.154/(0.154 + 55.06)$$
$$= 2.79 \times 10^{-3}$$

(Note: 991 g of water contains 991/18 moles, i.e. $n_2 = 55.06$.)

(d) Since Na^+ is monovalent, the number of milliequivalents of Na^+ = number of millimoles.

Therefore, the solution contains 154 mEq dm^{-3} of Na^+.

2.2 Thermodynamics: a brief introduction

The importance of thermodynamics in the pharmaceutical sciences is apparent when it is realised that such processes as the partitioning of solutes between immiscible solvents, the solubility of drugs, micellisation and drug–receptor interaction can all be treated in thermodynamic terms. This brief section merely introduces some of the concepts of thermodynamics that are referred to throughout the book. Readers requiring a greater depth of treatment should consult standard texts on this subject.[2]

2.2.1 Energy

Energy is a fundamental property of a system. Some idea of its importance may be gained by considering its role in chemical reactions, where it determines what reactions may occur, how fast the reaction may proceed, and in which direction the reaction will occur. Energy takes several forms: *kinetic energy* is that which a body possesses as a result of its motion; *potential energy* is the energy a body has due to its position, whether gravitational potential energy or coulombic potential energy associated with charged particles at a given distance apart. All forms of energy are related, but in converting between the various types it is not possible to create or destroy energy. This forms the basis of the *law of conservation of energy*.

The *internal energy U* of a system is the sum of all the kinetic and potential energy contributions to the energy of all the atoms, ions and molecules in that system. In thermodynamics we are concerned with *change* in internal energy, ΔU, rather than the internal energy itself. (Notice the use of Δ to denote a finite change.) We may change the internal energy of a closed system (one that cannot exchange matter with its surroundings) in only two ways: by transferring energy as *work* (w) or as *heat* (q). An expression for the change in internal energy is

$$\Delta U = w + q \qquad (2.1)$$

If the system releases its energy to the surroundings, ΔU is negative, i.e. the total internal energy has been reduced. Where heat is absorbed (as in an endothermic process), the internal energy will increase and consequently q is positive. Conversely, in a process that releases heat (an exothermic process) the internal energy is decreased and q is negative. Similarly, when energy is supplied to the system as work, w is positive and when the system loses energy by doing work, w is negative.

It is frequently necessary to consider infinitesimally small changes in a property; we denote these by the use of d rather than Δ. Thus, for an infinitesimal change in internal energy we write equation (2.1) as

$$dU = dw + dq \qquad (2.2)$$

We can see from this equation that it does not really matter whether energy is supplied as heat or as work or as a mixture of the two: the change in internal energy is the same. Equation (2.2) thus expresses the principle of the law of conservation of energy but is much wider in its application since it involves changes in heat energy, which were not encompassed in the conservation law.

It follows from equation (2.2) that a system that is completely isolated from its surroundings, such that it cannot exchange heat or interact mechanically to do work, cannot experience any change in its internal energy. In other words, *the internal energy of an isolated system is constant* – this is the *first law of thermodynamics*.

2.2.2 Enthalpy

When a change occurs in a system at *constant pressure* as, for example, in a chemical reaction in an open vessel, the increase in internal energy is not equal to the energy supplied as heat because some energy will have been lost by the work done (against the atmosphere) during the expansion of the system. It is convenient, therefore, to consider the heat change in isolation from the accompanying changes in work. For this reason we consider a property that is equal to the heat supplied at constant pressure: this property is called the *enthalpy* (H). We can define enthalpy by

$$\Delta H = q \text{ at constant pressure} \qquad (2.3)$$

ΔH is positive when heat is supplied to a system that is free to change its volume and negative when the system releases heat (as in an exothermic reaction). Enthalpy is related to the internal energy of a system by the relationship

$$H = U + pV \qquad (2.4)$$

where p and V are the pressure and volume of the system, respectively.

Enthalpy changes accompany such processes as the dissolution of a solute, the formation of micelles, chemical reaction, adsorption on to solids, vaporisation of a solvent, hydration of a solute, neutralisation of acids and bases, and the melting or freezing of solutes.

2.2.3 Entropy

The first law, as we have seen, deals with the conservation of energy as the system changes from one state to another, but it does not specify which particular changes will occur spontaneously. The reason why some changes have a natural tendency to occur is not that the system is moving to a lower-energy state but that there are changes in the randomness of the system. This can be seen by considering a specific example: the diffusion of one gas into another occurs without any external intervention – i.e. it is spontaneous – and yet there are no differences in either the potential or kinetic energies of the system in its equilibrium state and in its initial state where the two gases are segregated. The driving force for such spontaneous processes is the tendency for an increase in the chaos of the system – the mixed system is more disordered than the original.

A convenient measure of the randomness or disorder of a system is the *entropy* (*S*). When a system becomes more chaotic, its entropy increases in line with the degree of increase in disorder caused. This concept is encapsulated in the *second law of thermodynamics*, which states that *the entropy of an isolated system increases in a spontaneous change*.

The second law, then, involves entropy change, ΔS, and this is defined as the heat absorbed in a *reversible* process, q_{rev}, divided by the temperature (in kelvins) at which the change occurred.

For a finite change,

$$\Delta S = q_{rev}/T \tag{2.5}$$

and for an infinitesimal change,

$$dS = dq_{rev}/T \tag{2.6}$$

By a 'reversible process' we mean one in which the changes are carried out infinitesimally slowly, so that the system is in equilibrium with its surroundings. In this case we infer that the temperature of the surroundings is infinitesimally higher than that of the system and consequently the heat changes are occurring at an infinitely slow rate, so that the heat transfer is smooth and uniform.

We can see the link between entropy and disorder by considering some specific examples. For instance, the entropy of a perfect gas changes with its volume V according to the relationship

$$\Delta S = nR \ln \frac{V_f}{V_i} \tag{2.7}$$

where the subscripts f and i denote the final and initial states. Note that if $V_f > V_i$ (i.e. if the gas expands into a larger volume) the logarithmic (ln) term will be positive and the equation predicts an increase of entropy. This is expected since expansion of a gas is a spontaneous process and will be accompanied by an increase in the disorder because the molecules are now moving in a greater volume.

Similarly, increasing the temperature of a system should increase the entropy because at higher tempera-

ture the molecular motion is more vigorous and hence the system is more chaotic. The equation that relates entropy change to temperature change is

$$\Delta S = C_V \ln \frac{T_f}{T_i} \tag{2.8}$$

where C_V is the molar heat capacity at constant volume. Inspection of equation (2.8) shows that ΔS will be positive when $T_f > T_i$, as predicted.

The entropy of a substance will also change when it undergoes a phase transition, since this too leads to a change in the order. For example, when a crystalline solid melts, it changes from an ordered lattice to a more chaotic liquid (Fig. 2.1) and consequently an increase in entropy is expected. The entropy change accompanying the melting of a solid is given by

$$\Delta S = \Delta H_{fus}/T \tag{2.9}$$

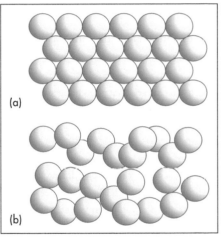

Figure 2.1 Melting of a solid involves a change from an ordered arrangement of molecules, represented by (a), to a more chaotic liquid, represented by (b). As a result, the melting process is accompanied by an increase in entropy.

where ΔH_{fus} is the enthalpy of fusion (melting) and T is the melting temperature. Similarly, we may determine the entropy change when a liquid vaporises from

$$\Delta S = \Delta H_{vap}/T \tag{2.10}$$

where ΔH_{vap} is the enthalpy of vaporisation and T now refers to the boiling point. Entropy changes accompanying other phase changes, such as change of the polymorphic form of crystals (see section 1.2.3), may be calculated in a similar manner.

At absolute zero all the thermal motions of the atoms of the lattice of a crystal will have ceased and the solid will have no disorder and hence a zero entropy. This conclusion forms the basis of the *third law of thermodynamics*, which states that *the entropy of a perfectly crystalline material is zero when T = 0.*

2.2.4 Free energy

The free energy is derived from the entropy and is, in many ways, a more useful function to use. The free energy referred to when we are discussing processes at constant pressure is the *Gibbs free energy* (G). This is defined by:

$$G = H - TS \tag{2.11}$$

The change in the free energy at constant temperature arises from changes in enthalpy and entropy and is

$$\Delta G = \Delta H - T\Delta S \tag{2.12}$$

Thus, at constant temperature and pressure,

$$\Delta G = -T\Delta S \tag{2.13}$$

from which we can see that the change in free energy is another way of expressing the change in overall entropy of a process occurring at constant temperature and pressure.

In view of this relationship, we can now consider changes in free energy that occur during a spontaneous process. From equation (2.13) we can see that ΔG will decrease during a spontaneous process at constant temperature and pressure. This decrease will occur until the system reaches an equilibrium state when ΔG becomes zero. This process can be thought of as a gradual using up of the system's ability to perform work as equilibrium is approached. Free energy can therefore be looked at in another way in that it represents the maximum amount of work, w_{max} (other than the work of expansion) that can be extracted from a system undergoing a change at constant temperature and pressure; i.e.

$$\Delta G = w_{max} \text{ at constant temperature and pressure} \tag{2.14}$$

This non-expansion work can be extracted from the system as electrical work, as in the case of a chemical reaction taking place in an electrochemical cell, or the

energy can be stored in biological molecules such as adenosine triphosphate.

When the system has attained an equilibrium state, it no longer has the ability to reverse itself. Consequently *all spontaneous processes are irreversible.* The fact that all spontaneous processes taking place at constant temperature and pressure are accompanied by a negative free-energy change provides a useful criterion of the spontaneity of any given process.

By applying these concepts to chemical equilibria we can derive (see Derivation Box 2A) the following simple relationship between free-energy change and the equilibrium constant of a reversible reaction, K:

$$\Delta G^{\ominus} = -RT \ln K \tag{2.15}$$

where the standard free energy $G^{\ominus}$ is the free energy of 1 mole of gas at a pressure of 1 bar.

A similar expression may be derived for reactions in solutions using the *activities* (see section 2.3.1) of the components rather than the partial pressures. $\Delta G^{\ominus}$ values can readily be calculated from the tabulated data and hence equation (2.15) is important because it provides a method of calculating the equilibrium constants without resort to experimentation.

A useful expression for the temperature dependence of the equilibrium constant is the *van't Hoff equation*, which may be derived as outlined in Derivation Box 2B.

A more general form of this equation is:

$$\log K = \frac{-\Delta H^{\ominus}}{2.303RT} + \text{constant} \tag{2.16}$$

Plots of $\log K$ against $1/T$ should be linear with a slope of $-\Delta H^{\ominus}/2.303R$, from which $\Delta H^{\ominus}$ may be calculated.

Equations (2.15) and (2.16) are fundamental equations that find many applications in the broad area of the pharmaceutical sciences: for example, in the determination of equilibrium constants in chemical reactions and for micelle formation; in the treatment of stability data for some solid-dosage forms (see section 3.4.3 in Chapter 3); and for investigations of drug–receptor binding.

Key points

- All forms of kinetic and potential energy can be interconverted provided that in so doing energy is neither created nor destroyed (law of conservation of energy). The internal energy change ΔU of a closed system is the sum of the changes in energy resulting from the heat q absorbed (endothermic process) or released (exothermic process) and the work w done by or on the system. When the system is completely isolated from its surrounding so that there are no changes in heat or work, then its internal energy is constant (first law of thermodynamics).

- The enthalpy H of a system is the heat supplied at constant pressure. The enthalpy change ΔH is positive when heat is supplied and negative when heat is released.

- The entropy S is related to the disorder of the system and increases when the system becomes more chaotic. Such processes are spontaneous (i.e. occur without external intervention). The entropy of an isolated system therefore increases when a reaction or change of state is spontaneous (second law of thermodynamics).

- The change in the Gibbs free energy ΔG of a system is related to changes in enthalpy and entropy by the equation, $\Delta G = \Delta H - T\Delta S$. ΔG decreases during a spontaneous change at constant temperature and pressure until the system reaches equilibrium, when ΔG becomes zero. The free energy is a measure of the work that a system can do and therefore at equilibrium the system no longer has the ability to perform any further work. Consequently, all spontaneous processes are irreversible.

2.3 Activity and chemical potential

2.3.1 Activity and standard states

The term *activity* is used in the description of the departure of the behaviour of a solution from ideality. In any real solution, interactions occur between the components which reduce the *effective concentration* of the solution. The activity is a way of describing this effective concentration. In an ideal solution or in a real solution at infinite dilution, there are no interactions between components and the activity equals the concentration. Non-ideality in real solutions at higher concentrations causes a divergence between the values of activity and concentration. The ratio of the activity to the concentration is called the *activity coefficient*, γ; that is,

$$\gamma = \text{activity/concentration} \qquad (2.17)$$

Depending on the units used to express concentration we can have a *molal* activity coefficient, γ_m, a *molar* activity coefficient, γ_c, or, if mole fractions are used, a *rational* activity coefficient, γ_x.

In order to be able to express the activity of a particular component numerically, it is necessary to define a reference state in which the activity is arbitrarily unity. The activity of a particular component is then the ratio of its value in a given solution to that in the reference state. For the solvent, the reference state is invariably taken to be the pure liquid, and, if this is at a pressure of 1 atmosphere and at a definite temperature, it is also the *standard state*. Since the mole fraction as well as the activity is unity: $\gamma_x = 1$.

Several choices are available in defining the standard state of the solute. If the solute is a liquid that is miscible with the solvent (as, for example, in a benzene–toluene mixture) then the standard state is again the pure liquid. Several different standard states have been used for solutions of solutes of limited solubility. In developing a relationship between drug activity and thermodynamic activity, the pure substance has been used as the standard state. The activity of the drug in solution was then taken to be the ratio of its concentration to its saturation solubility. The use of a pure substance as the standard state is of course of limited value since a different state is used for each compound. A more feasible approach is to use the infinitely dilute solution of the compound as the reference state. Since the activity equals the concentration in such solutions, however, it is not equal to unity as it should be for a standard state. This difficulty is overcome by defining the standard state as a hypothetical solution of unit concentration possessing, at the same time, the properties of an infinitely dilute solution. Some workers[3] have chosen to define the standard state in terms of an alkane solvent rather than water; one advantage of this solvent is the absence of specific solute–solvent interactions in the reference state that would be highly sensitive to molecular structure.

2.3.2 Activity of ionised drugs

A large proportion of the drugs that are administered in aqueous solution are salts which, on dissociation, behave as electrolytes. Simple salts such as ephedrine hydrochloride $(C_6H_5CH(OH)CH(NHCH_3)CH_3HCl)$ are 1 : 1 (or uni-univalent) electrolytes; that is, on dissociation each mole yields one cation, $C_6H_5CH(OH)CH(N^+H_2CH_3)CH_3$, and one anion, Cl^-. Other salts are more complex in their ionisation behaviour; for example, ephedrine sulfate is a 1 : 2 electrolyte, each mole giving two moles of the cation and one mole of SO_4^{2-} ions.

The activity of each ion is the product of its activity coefficient and its concentration, that is,

$$a_+ = \gamma_+ m_+ \text{ and } a_- = \gamma_- m_-$$

The anion and cation may each have a different ionic activity in solution and it is not possible to determine individual ionic activities experimentally. It is therefore necessary to use combined terms; for example, the combined activity term is the *mean ionic activity*, $a_\pm$. Similarly, we have the *mean ion activity coefficient*, $\gamma_\pm$, and the *mean ionic molality*, $m_\pm$. The relationship between the mean ionic parameters is then

$$\gamma_\pm = a_\pm / m_\pm$$

More details of these combined terms are given in Derivation Box 2C.

Values of the mean ion activity coefficient may be determined experimentally using several methods, including electromotive force measurement, solubility determinations and colligative properties. It is possible, however, to calculate $\gamma_\pm$ in very dilute solution using a theoretical method based on the Debye–Hückel theory. In this theory each ion is considered to be surrounded by an 'atmosphere' in which there is a slight excess of ions of opposite charge. The electrostatic energy due to this effect is related to the chemical potential of the ion to give a limiting expression for dilute solutions:

$$-\log \gamma_\pm = z_+ z_- A\sqrt{I} \qquad (2.18)$$

where z_+ and z_- are the valencies of the ions, A is a constant whose value is determined by the dielectric constant of the solvent and the temperature ($A = 0.509$ in water at 298 K), and I is the total ionic strength defined by

$$I = \frac{1}{2} \sum (mz^2) = \frac{1}{2}(m_1 z_1^2 + m_2 z_2^2 + \cdots) \qquad (2.19)$$

where the summation is continued over all the different species in solution. It can readily be shown from equation (2.19) that for a 1 : 1 electrolyte the ionic strength is equal to its molality; for a 1 : 2 electrolyte $I = 3m$; and for a 2 : 2 electrolyte $I = 4m$.

The Debye–Hückel expression as given by equation (2.18) is valid only in dilute solution ($I < 0.02$ mol kg^{-1}). At higher concentrations a modified expression has been proposed:

$$\log \gamma_\pm = \frac{-A z_+ z_- \sqrt{I}}{1 + a_i \beta \sqrt{I}} \qquad (2.20)$$

where a_i is the mean distance of approach of the ions or the mean effective ionic diameter, and β is a constant whose value depends on the solvent and temperature. As an approximation, the product $a_i \beta$ may be taken to be unity, thus simplifying the equation. Equation (2.20) is valid for $I < 0.1$ mol kg^{-1}.

2.3.3 Solvent activity

Although the phrase 'activity of a solution' usually refers to the activity of the *solute* in the solution, as in the preceding section, we also can refer to the activity of the *solvent*. Experimentally, solvent activity a_1 may be determined as the ratio of the vapour pressure p_1 of the solvent in a solution to that of the pure solvent $p_1^\ominus$, that is,

$$a_1 = p_1/p_1^\ominus = \gamma_1 x_1 \qquad (2.21)$$

where γ_1 is the solvent activity coefficient and x_1 is the mole fraction of solvent.

Example 2.2 Calculation of mean ionic activity coefficient

Calculate the mean ionic activity coefficient of: (a) 0.002 mol kg^{-1} aqueous solution of ephedrine sulfate; (b) an aqueous solution containing 0.002 mol kg^{-1} ephedrine sulfate and 0.01 mol kg^{-1} sodium chloride. Both solutions are at 25°C.

Answer

(a) Ephedrine sulfate is a 1:2 electrolyte and hence the ionic strength is given by equation (2.19) as

$$I = \frac{1}{2}[(0.002 \times 2 \times 1^2) + (0.002 \times 2^2)] = 0.006 \text{ mol kg}^{-1}$$

From the Debye–Hückel equation (equation 2.18),

$$-\log \gamma_{\pm} = 0.509 \times 1 \times 2 \times \sqrt{0.006}$$
$$\log \gamma_{\pm} = -0.0789$$
$$\gamma_{\pm} = 0.834$$

(b) Ionic strength of 0.01 mol kg^{-1} NaCl = ½(0.01 × 1^2) + (0.01 × 1^2) = 0.01 mol kg^{-1}

$$-\log \gamma_{\pm} = 0.509 \times 2 \times \sqrt{0.016}$$
$$\log \gamma_{\pm} = -0.1288$$
$$\gamma_{\pm} = 0.743$$

The relationship between the activities of the components of the solution is expressed by the Gibbs–Duhem equation:

$$x_1 \, d(\ln a_1) + x_2 \, d(\ln a_2) = 0 \qquad (2.22)$$

which provides a way of determining the activity of the solute from measurements of vapour pressure. An example of the role of water activity in inhibiting bacterial growth in wounds is given below.

Water activity and inhibition of bacterial growth

When thinking about the role of water activity in determining bacterial growth it is useful, but not strictly correct, to picture water activity as a measure of the amount of 'available' water in a system; this is not the total amount but the quantity that is free to act as a solvent. Some of the water may be unavailable because it is bound, either chemically or physically, to solutes present in the system; this water has different properties to free water and is biologically unavailable for microbial growth. Consequently, when the aqueous solution in the environment of a microorganism is concentrated by the addition of solutes such as

sucrose, the consequences for microbial growth result mainly from a change in the amount of free water which is reflected in a change in the water activity a_w. Every microorganism has a limiting a_w below which it will not grow. The minimum a_w levels for growth of human bacterial pathogens such as streptococci, *Klebsiella, Escherichia coli, Corynebacterium, Clostridium perfringens* and other clostridia, and *Pseudomonas* is 0.91.[4] *Staphylococcus aureus* can proliferate at an a_w as low as 0.86. Figure 2.2 shows the influence of a_w, adjusted by the addition of sucrose, on the growth rate of this microorganism at 35°C and pH 7.0. The control medium, with a water activity value of $a_w = 0.993$, supported the rapid growth of the test organism. Reduction of a_w of the medium by addition of sucrose progressively increased generation times and lag periods and lowered the peak cell counts. Complete growth inhibition was achieved at an a_w of 0.858 (195 g sucrose per 100 g water) with cell numbers declining slowly throughout the incubation period.

An *in vitro* study has been reported[5] of the efficacy of thick sugar pastes, and also of those prepared using xylose as an alternative to sucrose, in inhibiting the growth of bacteria commonly present in infected

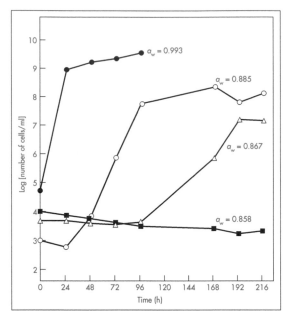

Figure 2.2 Staphylococcal growth at 35°C in medium alone (a_w = 0.993) and in media with a_w values lowered by additional sucrose.

Reproduced with permission from Chirife J et al. Scientific basic for use of granulated sugar in treatment of infected wounds. Lancet 1982;319:560–561.

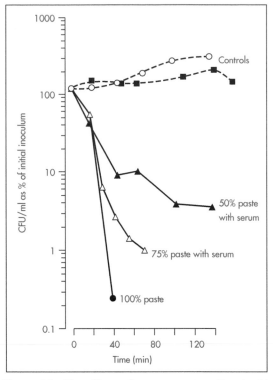

Figure 2.3 The effects of sucrose pastes diluted with serum on the colony-forming ability in Colony Forming Units (CFU) of Proteus mirabilis.

Reproduced with permission from Ambrose U et al. In vitro studies of water activity and bacterial growth inhibition of sucrose-polyethylene glycol 400-hydrogen peroxide and xylose-polyethylene glycol 400-hydrogen peroxide pastes used to treat infected wounds. Antimicrob Agents Chemother 1991;35:1799–1803.

wounds. Polyethylene glycol was added to the pastes as a lubricant and hydrogen peroxide was included in the formulation as a preservative. To simulate the dilution that the pastes invariably experience as a result of fluid being drawn into the wound, serum was added to the formulations in varying amounts. Figure 2.3 illustrates the effects of these sucrose pastes on the colony-forming ability of *Proteus mirabilis* and shows the reduction in efficiency of the pastes as a result of dilution and the consequent increase of their water activity from a value of 0.50 at 90% to 0.86 at 50% v/v paste in serum. It is clear that *P. mirabilis* was susceptible to the antibacterial activity of the pastes, even when they were diluted by

50%. It was reported that, although a_w may not be maintained at less than 0.86 (the critical level for inhibition of growth of *S. aureus*) for more than 3 h after packing of the wound, nevertheless clinical experience had shown that twice-daily dressing was adequate to remove infected slough from dirty wounds within a few days.

Clinical point

These results explain why the old remedy of treating infected wounds with sugar, honey or molasses is successful. When the wound is filled with sugar, the sugar dissolves in the tissue water, creating an environment of low a_w, which inhibits bacterial growth. However, the difference in water activity between the tissue and the concentrated sugar solution causes migration of water out of the tissue, hence diluting the sugar and raising a_w. Further sugar must then be added to the wound to maintain growth inhibition. Sugar may be applied as a paste with a consistency appropriate to the wound characteristics; thick sugar paste is suitable for cavities with wide openings, whereas a thinner paste with the consistency of thin honey is more suitable for instillation into cavities with small openings.

Water activity and assessment of pharmaceutical products

As we have discussed above, there is a link between water activity and microbial growth. However, because water activity can be thought of as a measure of the free (i.e. unbound) water in the system, it also indicates the ability of water to act as a solvent and to migrate within the system; this has several other implications relating to, for example, chemical degradation, dissolution of solids and moisture-induced phase changes such as those which occur in amorphous systems. Consequently, the measurement of the total water content by, for example, Karl Fischer analysis does not provide information on the 'availability' of the water; determination of the water activity would enable better correlations to biological and chemical reaction rates within the formulation. Despite this, there is a currently a general reluctance to utilise water activity measurements in the assessment of pharmaceutical products. Recent guidance provided by the regulatory bodies' International Conference on Harmonisation may provide an impetus to begin effectively using water activity in pharmaceutical quality programs.[6]

2.3.4 Chemical potential

Properties such as volume, enthalpy, free energy and entropy that depend on the quantity of substance are called *extensive* properties. In contrast, properties such as temperature, density and refractive index that are independent of the amount of material are referred to as *intensive* properties. The quantity denoting the rate of increase in the magnitude of an extensive property with increase in the number of moles of a substance added to the system at constant temperature and pressure is termed a *partial molar quantity*. Such quantities are distinguished by a bar above the symbol for the particular property. For example:

$$\left(\frac{\partial V}{\partial n_2}\right)_{T,P,n_1} = \overline{V}_2 \tag{2.23}$$

Note the use of the symbol ∂ to denote a partial change, which, in this case, occurs under conditions of constant temperature, pressure and number of moles of solvent (denoted by the subscripts outside the brackets).

In practical terms the partial molar volume, $\overline{V}$, represents the change in the total volume of a large amount of solution when one additional mole of solute is added – it is the effective volume of 1 mole of solute in solution.

Of particular interest is the partial molar free energy, $\overline{G}$, which is also referred to as the *chemical potential*, μ, and is defined for component 2 in a binary system by

$$\left(\frac{\partial G}{\partial n_2}\right)_{T,P,n_1} = \overline{G}_2 = \mu_2 \tag{2.24}$$

Partial molar quantities are of importance in the consideration of open systems, that is, those involving transference of matter as well as energy. For an open system involving two components,

$$dG = \left(\frac{\partial G}{\partial T}\right)_{P,n_1,n_2} dT + \left(\frac{\partial G}{\partial P}\right)_{T,n_1,n_2} dP$$
$$+ \left(\frac{\partial G}{\partial n_1}\right)_{T,P,n_2} dn_1 + \left(\frac{\partial G}{\partial n_2}\right)_{T,P,n_1} dn_2 \tag{2.25}$$

At constant temperature and pressure equation (2.25) reduces to

$$dG = \mu_1 \, dn_1 + \mu_2 \, dn_2 \tag{2.26}$$

Thus,

$$G = \int dG = \mu_1 n_1 + \mu_2 n_2 \tag{2.27}$$

The chemical potential therefore represents the contribution per mole of each component to the total free energy. It is the effective free energy per mole of each component in the mixture and is always less than the free energy of the pure substance.

It can be readily shown (see Derivation Box 2D) that the chemical potential of a component in a two-phase system (for example, oil and water) at equilibrium at a fixed temperature and pressure is identical in both phases, i.e.

$$\mu_a = \mu_b \tag{2.28}$$

where a and b are two immiscible phases.

Because of the need for equality of chemical potential at equilibrium, a substance in a system that is not at equilibrium will have a tendency to diffuse spontaneously from a phase in which it has a high chemical potential to another in which it has a low chemical potential. In this respect, the chemical *potential* resembles electrical *potential* and hence its name is an apt description of its nature.

Chemical potential of a component in solution

Where the component of the solution is a *non-electrolyte*, its chemical potential in dilute solution at a molality m can be calculated from

$$\mu_2 = \mu^\ominus + RT \ln m \qquad (2.29)$$

where

$$\mu^\ominus = \mu_2^\ominus + RT \ln M_1 - RT \ln 1000$$

and M_1 is the molecular weight of the solvent.

At higher concentrations, the solution generally exhibits significant deviations from ideality and the concentration must be replaced by activity

$$\mu_2 = \mu_2^\ominus + RT \ln a_2 \qquad (2.30)$$

In the case of *strong electrolytes*, the chemical potential is the sum of the chemical potential of the ions. For the simple case of a 1 : 1 electrolyte, the chemical potential is given by

$$\mu_2 = \mu_2^\ominus + 2RT \ln m\gamma_\pm$$

The derivations of these equations are given in Derivation Box 2E.

Key points

- The activity a of an *ideal* solution is equal to the solution concentration. The activity is reduced when there are interactions between the components of the solution (a *non-ideal* or real solution). The degree of non-ideality is expressed by the activity coefficient γ which is the ratio of the activity to the concentration. In an electrolyte solution each ion has an activity and the mean ion activity coefficient of the solution is the ratio of the mean ion activity to the mean ion molality.

- The chemical potential of a component of a mixture is its effective free energy per mole when in the mixture, which, because of interactions in the mixture, is less than its molar free energy in its pure state. The chemical potential of a component in a two-phase system (for example, oil and water) is identical in both phases of the system when it is at equilibrium at a fixed temperature and pressure. A component in a two-phase system that is not at equilibrium will have a tendency to diffuse spontaneously from a phase in which it has a high chemical potential to another in which it has a low chemical potential. The difference in chemical potential is the driving force for diffusion between the two phases.

2.4 Osmotic properties of drug solutions

A non-volatile solute added to a solvent affects not only the magnitude of the vapour pressure above the solvent but also the freezing point and the boiling point to an extent that is proportional to the relative number of solute molecules present, rather than to the weight concentration of the solute. Properties that are dependent on the number of molecules in solution in this way are referred to as *colligative* properties, and the most important of such properties from a pharmaceutical viewpoint is the osmotic pressure.

2.4.1 Osmotic pressure

Whenever a solution is separated from a solvent by a membrane that is permeable only to solvent molecules (referred to as a *semipermeable membrane*), there is a passage of solvent across the membrane into the solution. This is the phenomenon of *osmosis*. If the solution is totally confined by a semipermeable membrane and immersed in the solvent, a pressure differential develops across the membrane, which is referred to as the *osmotic pressure*. Solvent passes through the membrane because of the inequality of the chemical potentials on either side of the membrane. Since the chemical potential of a solvent molecule in solution is less than that in pure solvent, solvent will spontaneously enter the solution until this inequality is removed. The equation that relates the osmotic pressure of the solution, Π, to the solution concentration is the *van't Hoff equation*:

$$\Pi V = n_2 RT \qquad (2.31)$$

On application of the van't Hoff equation to the drug molecules in solution, consideration must be made of any ionisation of the molecules, since osmotic pressure, being a colligative property, will be dependent on the total number of particles in solution (including the free counterions). To allow for what was at the time considered to be anomalous behaviour of electrolyte solutions, van't Hoff introduced a correction factor, i. The value of this factor approaches a number equal to that of the number of ions, v, into which each molecule dissociates as the solution is progressively diluted. The ratio i/v is termed the *practical osmotic coefficient*, ϕ.

For non-ideal solutions, the activity and osmotic pressure are related by the expression

$$\ln a_1 = \frac{-vmM_1}{1000}\phi \tag{2.32}$$

where M_1 is the molecular weight of the solvent and m is the molality of the solution. The relationship between the osmotic pressure and the osmotic coefficient is thus

$$\Pi = \left(\frac{RT}{\overline{V}_1}\right)\frac{vmM_1}{1000}\phi \tag{2.33}$$

where $\overline{V}_1$ is the partial molal volume of the solvent.

2.4.2 Osmolality and osmolarity

The experimentally derived osmotic pressure is frequently expressed as the *osmolality* ξ_m, which is the mass of solute that when dissolved in 1 kg of water will exert an osmotic pressure, Π', equal to that exerted by a mole of an ideal un-ionised substance dissolved in 1 kg of water. The unit of osmolality is the osmole (abbreviated as osmol), which is the amount of substance that dissociates in solution to form one mole of osmotically active particles, thus 1 mole of glucose (not ionised) forms 1 osmole of solute, whereas 1 mole of NaCl forms 2 osmoles (1 mole of Na^+ and 1 mole of Cl^-). In practical terms, this means that a 1 molal solution of NaCl will have (approximately) twice the osmolality (osmotic pressure) as a 1 molal solution of glucose.

According to the definition $\xi_m = \Pi/\Pi'$, the value of Π' may be obtained from equation (2.33) by noting that, for an ideal un-ionised substance $v = \phi = 1$, and since m is also unity, equation (2.33) becomes

$$\Pi' = \left(\frac{RT}{\overline{V}_1}\right)\frac{M_1}{1000}$$

Thus

$$\xi_m = vm\phi \tag{2.34}$$

Example 2.3 Calculation of osmolality

A 0.90% w/w solution of sodium chloride (mol wt = 58.5 Da) has an osmotic coefficient of 0.928. Calculate the osmolality of the solution.

Answer
Osmolality is given by equation (2.34) as

$$\xi_m = vm\phi$$

so

$$\xi_m = 2 \times (9.0/58.5) \times 0.928$$
$$= 286 \text{ mosmol kg}^{-1}$$

Pharmaceutical labelling regulations sometimes require a statement of the osmolarity; for example, the USP 27 requires that sodium chloride injection should be labelled in this way. *Osmolarity* is defined as the mass of solute which, when dissolved in 1 litre of solution, will exert an osmotic pressure equal to that exerted by a mole of an ideal un-ionised substance dissolved in 1 litre of solution. The relationship between osmolality and osmolarity has been discussed by Streng *et al.*[7]

Table 2.1 lists the osmolalities of commonly used intravenous (IV) fluids.

2.4.3 Clinical relevance of osmotic effects

Tonicity

Osmotic effects are particularly important from a physiological viewpoint since biological membranes, notably the red blood cell membrane, behave in a manner similar to that of semipermeable membranes. Consequently, when red blood cells are immersed in a solution of greater osmotic pressure than that of their contents, they shrink as water passes out of the cells in an attempt to reduce the chemical potential gradient across the cell membrane. Conversely, on placing the cells in an aqueous environment of lower osmotic

Table 2.1 Tonicities (osmolalities) of intravenous fluids

Solution	Tonicity (mosmol kg^{-1})
Vamin 9	700
Vamin 9 Glucose	1350
Vamin 14	1145
Vamin 14 Electrolyte-free	810
Vamin 18 Electrolyte-free	1130
Vaminolact	510
Vitrimix KV	1130
Intralipid 10% Novum	300
Intralipid 20%	350
Intralipid 30%	310
Intrafusin 22	1400
Hyperamine 30	1450
Gelofusine	279[a]
Lipofundin MCT/LCT 10%	345[a]
Lipofundin MCT/LCT 20%	380[a]
Nutriflex 32	1140[a]
Nutriflex 48	1400[a]
Nutriflex 70	2100[a]
Sodium Bicarbonate Intravenous Infusion BP	
8.4% w/v	2000[a]
4.2% w/v	1000[a]

[a] Osmolarity (mosmol dm^{-3}).

pressure, the cells swell as water enters and eventually lysis may occur. It is an important consideration, therefore, to ensure that the *effective* osmotic pressure of a solution for injection is approximately the same as that of blood serum. This effective osmotic pressure, which is termed the *tonicity*, is not always identical to the osmolality because it is concerned only with those solutes in solution that can exert an effect on the passage of water through the biological membrane. Solutions that have the same tonicity as blood serum are said to be *isotonic* with blood. Solutions with a higher tonicity are *hypertonic* and those with a lower tonicity are termed *hypotonic* solutions. Similarly, in order to avoid discomfort on administration of solu-

tions to the delicate membranes of the body, such as the eyes, these solutions are made isotonic with the relevant tissues.

The osmotic pressures of many of the products in Table 2.1 are in excess of that of plasma (291 mosmol dm^{-3}). It is generally recommended that any fluid with an osmotic pressure above 550 mosmol dm^{-3} should not be infused rapidly as this would increase the incidence of venous damage. The rapid infusion of marginally hypertonic solutions (in the range 300–500 mosmol dm^{-3}) would appear to be clinically practicable; the higher the osmotic pressure of the solution within this range, the slower should be its rate of infusion to avoid damage. Patients with centrally inserted lines are not normally affected by limits on tonicity as infusion is normally slow and dilution is rapid.

 Clinical point

Certain oral medications commonly used in the intensive care of premature infants have very high osmolalities. The high tonicity of enteral feedings has been implicated as a cause of necrotising enterocolitis (NEC). A higher frequency of gastrointestinal illness including NEC has been reported[8] among premature infants fed undiluted calcium lactate than among those fed no supplemental calcium or calcium lactate diluted with water or formula. White and Harkavy[9] have discussed a similar case of the development of NEC following medication with calcium glubionate elixir.

White and Harkavy[9] have measured osmolalities of several medications by freezing-point depression and compared these with the osmolalities of analogous IV preparations (Table 2.2). Except in the case of digoxin, the osmolalities of the IV preparations were very much lower than those of the corresponding oral preparations despite the fact that the IV preparations contained at least as much drug per millilitre as did the oral forms. This striking difference may be attributed to the additives such as ethyl alcohol, sorbitol and propylene glycol, which make a large contribution to the osmolalities of the oral preparations. The vehicle

Table 2.2 Measured and calculated osmolalities of drugs

Drug (route)	Concentration of drug	Mean measured osmolality (mosmol kg^{-1})	Calculated available milliosmoles in 1 kg of drug preparation[a]
Theophylline elixir (oral)	80 mg/15 cm^3	>3000	4980
Aminophylline (IV)	25 mg cm^{-3}	116	200
Calcium glubionate (oral)	115 mg/5 cm^3	>3000	2270
Calcium gluceptate (IV)	90 mg/5 cm^3	507	950
Digoxin elixir	25 mg dm^{-3}	>3000	4420
Digoxin (IV)	100 mg dm^{-3}	>3000	9620
Dexametasone elixir (oral)	0.5 mg/5 cm^3	>3000	3980
Dexametasone sodium phosphate (IV)	4 mg cm^{-3}	284	312

[a]This would be the osmolality of the drug if the activity coefficient were equal to 1 in the full-strength preparation. The osmolalities of serial dilutions of the drug were plotted against the concentrations of the solution, and a least-squares regression line was drawn. The value for the osmolality of the full-strength solution was then estimated from the line. This is the 'calculated available milliosmoles'.
Reproduced with permission from White KC, Harkavy KL (1982). Hypertonic formula resulting from added oral medications. *Am J Dis Child*; 136:931–933.

for the IV digoxin consists of 40% propylene glycol and 10% ethyl alcohol with calculated osmolalities of 5260 and 2174 mosmol kg^{-1} respectively, thus explaining the unusually high osmolality of this IV preparation. These authors have recommended that extreme caution should be exercised in paediatric and neonatal therapy in the administration of these oral preparations and perhaps any medication in a syrup or elixir form when the infant is at risk from NEC.

Clinical point

The osmolarity of preparations for oral administration to premature infants should be less than 400–500 mosmol dm^{-3} to limit stress imposed on the gastrointestinal system, which could lead to *pneumatosis intestinalis*.[10] Many drugs administered to preterm infants, however, have osmolarities greatly exceeding this limit, for example, paracetamol (acetaminophen) solutions have osmolarities of 10 000–16 000 mosmol dm^{-3}.

Where no suitable alternative drugs are available, it may be possible to reduce osmolarity by administering the drugs by mixing with an infant formula. In such cases the final osmolarity of the mixture (OM) is calculated from

$$OM = \frac{(OD \times VD) + (OF \times VF)}{VD + VF} \quad (2.35)$$

where OD and OF are the osmolarities of drug and infant formula, respectively, and VD and VF are the volumes of drug solution and infant formula, respectively. Example 2.4 (taken from reference 10) illustrates the use of this equation.

Example 2.4 Reduction of osmolarity by mixing with an infant formula

A 0.25 mL solution of Fer-In-Sol drops has an approximate osmolarity of 5010 mosmol dm^{-3}; calculate the final osmolarity of the preparation obtained when this dose is added to 15 mL of Premature Enfamil Formula (osmolarity 305 mosmol dm^{-3}).

Answer
Substitution in equation (2.35) gives

$$OM = \frac{(5010 \times 0.00025) + (305 \times 0.015)}{0.00025 + 0.015}$$

$$= 382 \text{ mosmol dm}^{-3}$$

Note that the volumes are converted to litres (dm^{-3}) before substitution.

In some cases the osmolality of the elixir is so high that even mixing with infant formula does not reduce the osmolality to a tolerable level. For example, when a clinically appropriate dose of dexamethasone elixir was mixed in volumes of formula appropriate for a single feeding for a 1500 g infant, the osmolalities of the mixes increased by at least 300% compared to formula alone (Table 2.3).

Table 2.3 Osmolalities of drug–infant formula mixtures

Drug (dose)	Volume of drug (cm^3) + volume of formula (cm^3)	Mean measured osmolality (mosmol kg^{-1})
Infant formula	–	292
Theophylline elixir, 1 mg kg^{-1}	0.3 + 15	392
	0.3 + 30	339
Calcium glubionate syrup, 0.5 mmol kg^{-1}	0.5 + 15	378
	0.5 + 30	330
Digoxin elixir, 5 µg kg^{-1}	0.15 + 15	347
	0.15 + 30	322
Dexamethasone elixir, 0.25 mg kg^{-1}	3.8 + 15	1149
	3.8 + 30	791

Reproduced with permission from White KC, Harkavy KL (1982). Hypertonic formula resulting from added oral medications. *Am J Dis Child*; 136:931–933.

Volatile anaesthetics

The aqueous solubilities of several volatile anaesthetics can be related to the osmolarity of the solution.[11] The inverse relationship between solubility (expressed as the liquid/gas partition coefficient) of those anaesthetics and the osmolarity is shown in Table 2.4.

These findings have practical applications for the clinician. Although changes in serum osmolarity within the physiological range (209–305 mosmol dm^{-3}) have only a small effect on the liquid/gas partition coefficient, changes in the serum osmolarity and the concentration of serum constituents at the extremes of the physiological range may significantly decrease the liquid/gas partition coefficient. For example, the blood/gas partition coefficient of isoflurane decreases significantly after an infusion of mannitol. This decrease may be attributed to both a transient increase in the osmolarity of the blood and a more prolonged decrease in the concentration of serum constituents caused by the influx of water due to the osmotic gradient.

Rehydration solutions

An interesting application of the osmotic effect has been in the design of rehydration solutions. During the day the body moves many litres of fluid from the blood into the intestine and back again. The inflow of water into the intestine, which aids the breakdown of food, is an osmotic effect arising from the secretion of Cl$^-$ ions by the crypt cells of the intestinal lining (see section 8.2.2) into the intestine. Nutrients from the food are taken up by the villus cells in the lining of the small intestine. The villus cells also absorb Na$^+$ ions, which they pump out into the extracellular spaces, from where they return to the circulation. As a consequence of this flow of Na$^+$, water and other ions follow by osmotic flow and hence are also transferred to the

Table 2.4 Liquid/gas partition coefficients of anaesthetics in four aqueous solutions at 37°C

Solution	Osmolarity (mosmol dm^{-3})	Partition coefficient			
		Isoflurane	Enflurane	Halothane	Methoxyflurane
Distilled H$_2$O	0	0.626 ± 0.05	0.754 ± 0.06	0.859 ± 0.02	4.33 ± 0.5
Normal saline	308	0.590 ± 0.01	0.713 ± 0.01	0.825 ± 0.02	4.22 ± 0.30
Isotonic heparin (1000 U cm^{-3})	308	0.593 ± 0.01	0.715 ± 0.01	–	4.08 ± 0.22
Mannitol (20%)	1098	0.476 ± 0.023	0.575 ± 0.024	0.747 ± 0.03	3.38 ± 0.14

Reproduced with permission from Lerman J *et al*. Osmolarity determines the solubility of anesthetics in aqueous solutions at 37°C. *Anesthesiology* 1983;59:554–558.

blood. This normal functioning is disrupted by diarrhoea-causing microorganisms, which either increase the Cl^--secreting activity of the crypt cells or impair the absorption of Na^+ by the villus cells, or both. Consequently, the fluid that is normally returned to the blood across the intestinal wall is lost in watery stool. If untreated, diarrhoea can eventually lead to a severe decline in the volume of the blood, the circulation may become dangerously slow, and death may result.

Oral rehydration therapy

Treatment of dehydration by oral rehydration therapy (ORT) is based on the discovery that the diarrhoea-causing organisms do not usually interfere with the

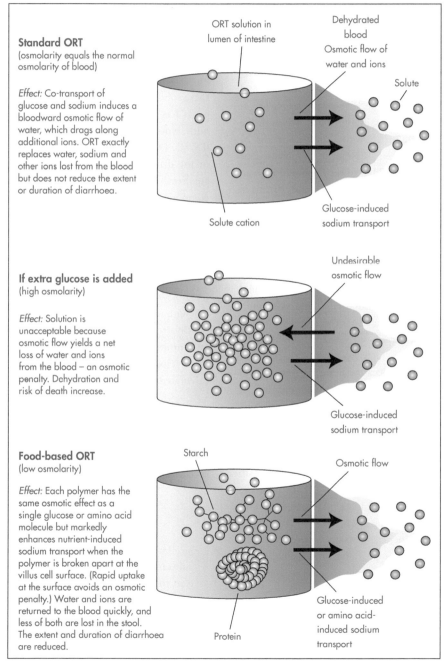

Standard ORT
(osmolarity equals the normal osmolarity of blood)

Effect: Co-transport of glucose and sodium induces a bloodward osmotic flow of water, which drags along additional ions. ORT exactly replaces water, sodium and other ions lost from the blood but does not reduce the extent or duration of diarrhoea.

If extra glucose is added
(high osmolarity)

Effect: Solution is unacceptable because osmotic flow yields a net loss of water and ions from the blood – an osmotic penalty. Dehydration and risk of death increase.

Food-based ORT
(low osmolarity)

Effect: Each polymer has the same osmotic effect as a single glucose or amino acid molecule but markedly enhances nutrient-induced sodium transport when the polymer is broken apart at the villus cell surface. (Rapid uptake at the surface avoids an osmotic penalty.) Water and ions are returned to the blood quickly, and less of both are lost in the stool. The extent and duration of diarrhoea are reduced.

ORT solution in lumen of intestine

Dehydrated blood
Osmotic flow of water and ions
Solute
Solute cation
Glucose-induced sodium transport

Undesirable osmotic flow
Glucose-induced sodium transport

Starch
Osmotic flow
Protein
Glucose-induced or amino acid-induced sodium transport

Figure 2.4 How osmosis affects the performance of solutions used in oral rehydration therapy (ORT).

carrier systems that bring sodium and glucose simultaneously into the villus cells from the intestinal cavity. This 'co-transport' system only operates when both sodium and glucose are present. The principle behind ORT is that if glucose is mixed into an electrolyte solution it activates the co-transport system, causing electrolyte and then water to pass through the intestinal wall and to enter the blood, so minimising the dehydration.

ORT requires administration to the patient of small volumes of fluid throughout the day (to prevent vomiting); it does not reduce the duration or severity of the diarrhoea, it simply replaces lost fluid and electrolytes. Let us examine, using the principles of the osmotic effect, two possible methods by which the process of fluid uptake from the intestine might be speeded up. It might seem reasonable to suggest that more glucose should be added to the formulation in an attempt to enhance the co-transport system. If this is done, however, the osmolarity of the glucose will become greater than that of normal blood, and water would now flow from the blood to the intestine and so exacerbate the problem. An alternative is to substitute starches for simple glucose in the ORT. When these polymer molecules are broken down in the intestinal lumen, they release many hundreds of glucose molecules, which are immediately taken up by the co-transport system and removed from the lumen. The effect is therefore as if a high concentration of glucose were administered, but because osmotic pressure is a *colligative* property (dependent on the *number* of molecules rather than the mass of substance), there is no associated problem of a high osmolarity when starches are used. The process is summarised in Fig. 2.4. A similar effect is achieved by the addition of proteins, since there is also a co-transport mechanism whereby amino acids (released on breakdown of the proteins in the intestine) and Na^+ ions are simultaneously taken up by the villus cells.

This process of increasing water uptake from the intestine has an added appeal since the source of the starch and protein can be cereals, beans and rice, which are likely to be available in the parts of the world where problems arising from diarrhoea are most prevalent. Food-based ORT offers additional advantages: it can be made at home from low-cost ingredients and can be cooked, which kills the pathogens in the water.

2.4.4 Preparation of isotonic solutions

Since osmotic pressure is not a readily measurable quantity, it is usual to make use of the relationship between the colligative properties and to calculate the osmotic pressure from a more easily measured property such as the freezing-point depression. In so doing, however, it is important to realise that the red blood cell membrane is not a perfect semipermeable membrane and allows through small molecules such as urea and ammonium chloride. Therefore, although the quantity of each substance required for an isotonic solution may be calculated from freezing-point depression values, these solutions may cause cell lysis when administered.

It has been shown that a solution that is isotonic with blood has a freezing-point depression, ΔT_f, of 0.52°C. One has therefore to adjust the freezing point of the drug solution to this value to give an isotonic solution. Freezing-point depressions for a series of compounds are given in reference texts[1,12] and it is a simple matter to calculate the concentration required for isotonicity from these values. For example, a 1% NaCl solution has a freezing-point depression of 0.576°C. The percentage concentration of NaCl required to make isotonic saline solution is therefore $(0.52/0.576) \times 1.0 = 0.90\%$ w/v.

With a solution of a drug, it is of course not possible to alter the drug concentration in this manner, and an adjusting substance must be added to achieve isotonicity. The quantity of adjusting substance can be calculated as shown in Box 2.3.

Box 2.3 Preparation of isotonic solutions

If the drug concentration is x g per 100 cm^3 solution, then

ΔT_f for drug solution
$= x \times (\Delta T_f$ of 1% drug solution)
$= a$

Similarly, if w is the weight in grams of adjusting substance to be added to 100 cm^3 of drug solution to achieve isotonicity, then

ΔT_f for adjusting solution
$= w \times (\Delta T_f$ of 1% adjusting substance)
$= w \times b$

For an isotonic solution, $a + (w \times b) = 0.52$. Therefore,

$$w = \frac{0.52 - a}{b} \qquad (2.36)$$

Example 2.5 Isotonic solutions

Calculate the amount of sodium chloride that should be added to 50 cm^3 of a 0.5% w/v solution of lidocaine hydrochloride to make a solution isotonic with blood serum.

Answer

From reference lists, the values of b for sodium chloride and lidocaine hydrochloride are 0.576°C and 0.130°C, respectively.

From equation (2.36) we have

$$a = 0.5 \times 0.13 = 0.065$$

Hence,

$$w = (0.52 - 0.065)/0.576 = 0.790\,g$$

Therefore, the weight of sodium chloride to be added to 50 cm^3 of solution is 0.395 g.

Key points

- Parenteral solutions should be of approximately the same tonicity as blood serum. The amount of adjusting substance which must be added to a formulation to achieve isotonicity can be calculated from

$$w = \frac{0.52 - a}{b}$$

where w is the weight in grams of adjusting substance to be added to 100 mL of drug solution to achieve isotonicity, a is the number of grams of drug in 100 mL of solution multiplied by the freezing-point depression ΔT_f of a 1% drug solution, and b is ΔT_f of 1% adjusting substance.

2.5 Ionisation of drugs in solution

Many drugs are either weak organic acids (for example, acetylsalicylic acid (aspirin)), or weak organic bases (for example, procaine), or their salts (for example, ephedrine hydrochloride). The degree to which these drugs are ionised in solution is highly dependent on the pH. The exceptions to this general statement are the non-electrolytes, such as the steroids, and the quaternary ammonium compounds, which are completely ionised at all pH values and in this respect behave as strong electrolytes.

2.5.1 Clinical relevance of drug ionisation

The extent of ionisation of a drug has an important effect on its absorption, distribution and elimination and there are many examples of the alteration of pH to change these properties. The pH of urine may be adjusted (for example, by administration of ammonium chloride or sodium bicarbonate) in cases of overdosing with amphetamines, barbiturates, narcotics and salicylates, to ensure that these drugs are completely ionised and hence readily excreted. Conversely, the pH of the urine may be altered to prevent ionisation of a drug in cases where reabsorption is required for therapeutic reasons. Sulfonamide crystalluria may also be avoided by making the urine alkaline. An understanding of the relationship between pH and drug ionisation is of use in the prediction of the causes of precipitation in admixtures, in the calculation of the solubility of drugs, and in the attainment of optimum bioavailability by maintaining a certain ratio of ionised to un-ionised drug. Table 2.5 shows the nominal pH values of some body fluids and sites, which are useful in the prediction of the percentage ionisation of drugs *in vivo*.

2.5.2 Dissociation of weakly acidic and basic drugs and their salts

According to the Lowry–Brønsted theory of acids and bases, an acid is a substance that will donate a proton and a base is a substance that will accept a proton. Thus the dissociation of acetylsalicylic acid, a weak acid, could be represented as in Scheme 2.1. In this equilibrium, acetylsalicylic acid acts as an acid because it donates a proton, and the acetylsalicylate ion acts as

Table 2.5 Nominal pH values of some body fluids and sites

Site	Nominal pH
Aqueous humour	7.21
Blood, arterial	7.4
Blood, venous	7.39
Blood, maternal umbilical	7.25
Cerebrospinal fluid	7.35
Duodenum	5.5
Faeces[a]	7.15
Ileum, distal	8.0
Intestine, microsurface	5.3
Lacrimal fluid (tears)	7.4
Milk, breast	7.0
Muscle, skeletal[b]	6.0
Nasal secretions	6.0
Prostatic fluid	6.45
Saliva	6.40
Semen	7.2
Stomach	1.5
Sweat	5.4
Urine, female	5.8
Urine, male	5.7
Vaginal secretions, premenopause	4.5
Vaginal secretions, postmenopause	7.0

Reproduced from Newton DW, Kluza RB. *Drug Intell Clin Pharm* 1978;12:547.
[a] Value for normal soft, formed stools; hard stools tend to be more alkaline, whereas watery, unformed stools are acidic.
[b] Studies conducted intracellularly in the rat.

a base because it accepts a proton to yield an acid. An acid and base represented by such an equilibrium is said to be a *conjugate acid–base pair*.

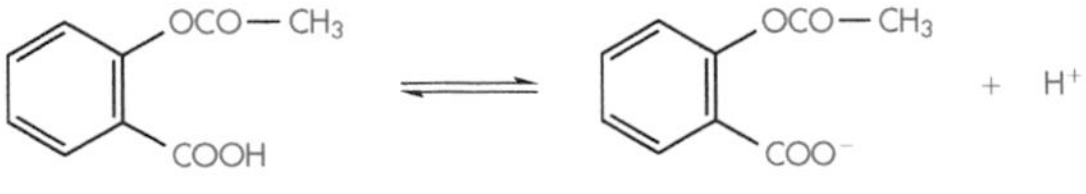

Scheme 2.1

Scheme 2.1 is not a realistic expression, however, since protons are too reactive to exist independently and are rapidly taken up by the solvent. The proton-accepting entity, by the Lowry–Brønsted definition, is a base, and the product formed when the proton has been accepted by the solvent is an acid. Thus a second acid–base equilibrium occurs when the solvent accepts the proton, and this may be represented by

$$H_2O + H^+ \rightleftharpoons H_3O^+$$

The overall equation on summing these equations is shown in Scheme 2.2, or, in general,

$$HA + H_2O \rightleftharpoons A^- + H_3O^+$$

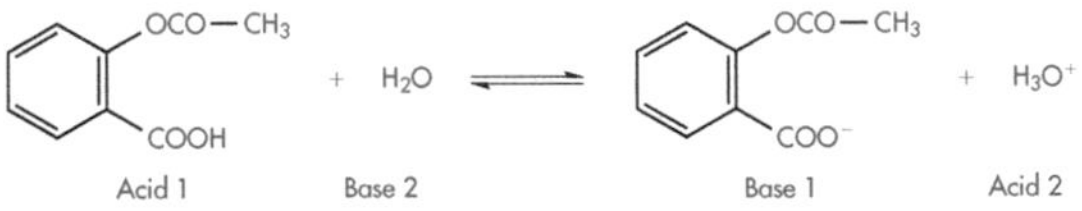

Scheme 2.2

By a similar reasoning, the dissociation of benzocaine, a weak base, may be represented by the equilibrium

$$\underset{\text{base 1}}{NH_2C_6H_5\ COOC_2H_5} + \underset{\text{acid 2}}{H_2O}$$
$$\rightleftharpoons \underset{\text{acid 1}}{NH_3^+\ C_6H_5\ COOC_2H_5} + \underset{\text{base 2}}{OH^-}$$

or, in general,

$$B + H_2O \rightleftharpoons BH^+ + OH^-$$

Comparison of the two general equations shows that H_2O can act as either an acid or a base. Such solvents are called *amphiprotic* solvents.

Salts of weak acids or bases are essentially completely ionised in solution. For example, ephedrine hydrochloride (salt of the weak base ephedrine, and the strong acid HCl) exists in aqueous solution in the form of the conjugate acid of the weak base, $C_6H_5CH(OH)$ $CH(CH_3)N^+H_2CH_3$, together with its Cl^- counterions. In a similar manner, when sodium salicylate (salt of the weak acid salicylic acid, and the strong base NaOH) is dissolved in water, it ionises almost entirely into the conjugate base of salicylic acid, $HOC_6H_5COO^-$, and Na^+ ions.

The conjugate acids and bases formed in this way are, of course, subject to acid–base equilibria described by the general equations above.

2.5.3 The effect of pH on the ionisation of weakly acidic or basic drugs and their salts

If the ionisation of a weak acid is represented as described above, we may express an equilibrium constant as follows:

$$K_a = \frac{a_{H_3O^+} \times a_{A^-}}{a_{HA}} \qquad (2.37)$$

Assuming the activity coefficients approach unity in dilute solution, the activities may be replaced by concentrations:

$$K_a = \frac{[H_3O^+][A^-]}{[HA]} \qquad (2.38)$$

K_a is variously referred to as the *ionisation constant*, *dissociation constant* or *acidity constant* for the weak acid. The negative logarithm of K_a is referred to as pK_a, just as the negative logarithm of the hydrogen ion concentration is called the pH. Thus

$$pK_a = -\log K_a \qquad (2.39)$$

Similarly, the *dissociation constant* or *basicity constant* for a weak base is

$$K_b = \frac{a_{OH^-} \times a_{BH^+}}{a_B} \approx \frac{[OH^+][BH^+]}{[B]} \qquad (2.40)$$

and

$$pK_b = -\log K_b \qquad (2.41)$$

The pK_a and pK_b values provide a convenient means of comparing the strengths of weak acids and bases. The lower the pK_a, the stronger the acid; the lower the pK_b, the stronger is the base. The pK_a values of a series of drugs are given in Table 2.6. pK_a and pK_b values of conjugate acid–base pairs are linked by the expression

$$pK_a + pK_b = pK_w \qquad (2.42)$$

where pK_w is the negative logarithm of the dissociation constant for water, K_w. K_w is derived from consideration of the equilibrium

$$H_2O + H_2O \rightleftharpoons H_3O^+ + OH^-$$

Table 2.6 pK_a values of some medicinal compounds[a]

Compound	Acid	Base	Compound	Acid	Base
Acebutolol		9.4	Amiodorone		6.6 (5.6)[b]
Acetazolamide		7.2, 9.0	Amoxicillin	2.4	7.4, 9.6
Acetylsalicylic acid	3.5		Amoxapine		7.6
Aciclovir		2.3, 9.3	Ampicillin	2.7	7.2
Adrenaline	9.9	8.5	Apomorphine	8.9	7.0
Adriamycin		8.2	Atenolol		9.6
Allopurinol	10.2		Ascorbic acid	4.2, 11.6	
Alphaprodine		8.7	Astemizole		8.4
Alprazolam		2.4	Atropine		9.9
Alprenolol		9.6	Azapropazone		6.6
Amikacin		8.1	Azathioprine	8.2	
p-Aminobenzoic acid	4.9	2.4	Azelastine		9.5
Aminophylline		5.0	Benazepril	3.1	5.3
p-Aminosalicylic acid	3.2		Benzylpenicillin	2.8	
Amitriptyline		9.4	Benzocaine		2.8

Table 2.6 *(continued)*

Compound	pK_a Acid	pK_a Base	Compound	pK_a Acid	pK_a Base
Bupivacaine		8.1	Dibucaine		8.3
Bupropion		7.9	Diclofenac	4.0	
Captopril	3.5		Diethylpropion		8.7
Carteolol		9.7	Diltiazem		8.0
Cefadroxil	7.6	2.7	Diphenhydramine		9.1
Cefalexin	7.1	2.3	Dithranol		9.4
Cefaclor	7.2	2.7	Doxepin		8.0
Celiprolol		9.7	Doxorubicin		8.2,10.2
Cetirizine	2.9	2.2, 8.0	Doxycycline	7.7	3.4, 9.3
Chlorambucil	4.5 (4.9)[b]	2.5	Enalapril		5.5
Chloramphenicol		5.5	Enoxacin	6.3	8.6
Chlorcyclizine		8.2	Epirubicin		8.1
Chlordiazepoxide		4.8	Ergometrine		6.8
Chloroquine		8.1, 9.9	Ergotamine		6.4
Chlorothiazide	6.5	9.5	Erythromycin		8.8
Chlorphenamine		9.0	Famotidine		6.8
Chlorpromazine		9.3	Fenoprofen	4.5	
Chlorpropamide		4.9	Flucloxacillin	2.7	
Chlorprothixene		8.8	Flufenamic acid	3.9	
Cilazapril		6.4	Flumequine	6.5	
Cimetidine		6.8	Fluopromazine		9.2
Cinchocaine		8.3	Fluorouracil	8.0, 13.0	
Clarithromycin		8.3	Fluphenazine		3.9, 8.1
Clindamycin		7.5	Flurazepam	8.2	1.9
Cocaine		8.5	Flurbiprofen	4.3	
Codeine		8.2	Furosemide	3.9	
Cyclopentolate		7.9	Glibenclamide	5.3	
Daunomycin		8.2	Guanethidine		11.9
Desipramine		10.2	Guanoxan		12.3
Dextromethorphan		8.3	Halofantrine		9.7
Diamorphine		7.6	Haloperidol		8.3
Diazepam		3.4	Hexobarbital	8.3	

Table 2.6 (continued)

Compound	pK_a		Compound	pK_a	
	Acid	Base		Acid	Base
Hydralazine		0.5, 7.1	Novobiocin	4.3, 9.1	
Ibuprofen	4.4		Ofloxacin	6.1	8.3
Imipramine		9.5	Oxolinic acid	6.6	
Indometacin	4.5		Oxprenolol		9.5
Ketoprofen	4.0		Oxybutynin		6.9
Labetalol	7.4	9.4	Oxycodone		8.9
Levamisole		8.0	Oxytetracycline	7.3	3.3, 9.1
Levodopa	2.3, 9.7, 13.4		Paroxetine		9.9
Lidocaine		7.94 (26°C), 7.55 (36°C)	Penbutolol		9.3
Lincomycin		7.5	Pentazocine		8.8
Loxoprofen	4.2		Pethidine		8.7
Maprotiline		10.2	Phenazocine		8.5
Meclofenamic acid	4.0		Phenytoin	8.3	
Metoprolol		9.7	Physostigmine		2.0, 8.1
Methadone		8.3	Pilocarpine		1.6, 7.1
Methotrexate	3.8, 4.8	5.6	Pindolol		8.8
Metronidazole		2.5	Piperazine		5.6, 9.8
Minocycline	7.8	2.8, 5.0, 9.5	Piroxicam	2.3	
Minoxidil		4.6	Polymyxin B		8.9
Morphine	8.0 (phenol)	9.6 (amine)	Prazosin		6.5
Nadolol		9.7	Procaine		8.8
Nafcillin	2.7		Prochlorperazine		3.7, 8.1
Nalidixic acid	6.4		Promazine		9.4
Nalorphine		7.8	Promethazine		9.1
Naloxone		7.9	Propofol	11.0	
Naltrexone	9.5	8.1	Propranolol		9.5
Naproxen	4.3		Quinapril		2.8, 5.4
Nitrofurantoin		7.2	Quinidine		4.2, 8.3
Nitrazepam	10.8	3.2 (3.4)[b]	Quinine		4.2, 8.8
Norfloxacin	6.2	8.6	Ranitidine		2.7, 8.2
Nortriptyline		9.7	Sotalol	8.3	9.8

Table 2.6 *(continued)*

Compound	pK$_a$		Compound	pK$_a$	
	Acid	Base		Acid	Base
Sulfadiazine	6.5	2.0	Thiopental	7.5	
Sulfaguanidine	12.1	2.8	Ticlopidine		7.6
Sulfamerazine	7.1	2.3	Timolol		9.2 (8.8)[b]
Sulfathiazole	7.1	2.4	Tolrestat	3.0	
Tamoxifen		8.9	Tolbutamide	5.3	
Temazepam		1.6	Triflupromazine		9.2
Tenoxicam	1.1	5.3	Trimethoprin		7.3
Terazosin		7.1	Triprolidine		9.3
Terfenadine		9.5 (8.6)[b]	Valproate	5.0	
Tetracaine		8.4	Verapamil		8.8
Tetracycline	7.7	3.3, 9.5	Warfarin	5.1	
Theophylline	8.6	3.5	Zidovudine		9.7

[a]For a more complete list, which critically examines cited values in the literature to 2000, see Prankerd RJ. Critical compilation of pK$_a$ values for pharmaceutical substances. In: Britain HG (ed.) *Profiles of Drug Substances, Excipients and Related Methodology*, vol. 33. London: Academic Press, 2007.
[b]Values in parentheses represent alternative values from the literature.

where one molecule of water is behaving as the weak acid or base and the other is behaving as the solvent. Then

$$K = \frac{a_{H_3O^+} \times a_{OH^-}}{a_{H_2O}^2} \approx \frac{[H_3O^+][OH^-]}{[H_2O]^2} \quad (2.43)$$

The concentration of molecular water is considered to be virtually constant for dilute aqueous solutions. Therefore,

$$K_w = [H_3O^+][OH^-] \quad (2.44)$$

where the dissociation constant for water (the *ionic product*) now incorporates the term for molecular water and has the values given in Table 2.7.

When the pH of an aqueous solution of the weakly acidic or basic drug approaches the pK$_a$ or pK$_b$, there is a very pronounced change in the ionisation of that drug. Expressions that enable predictions of the pH dependence of the degree of ionisation to be made are given in the following sections.

Weak acids

Taking logarithms of the expression for the dissociation constant (equation 2.38) gives

$$pH = pK_a + \log \frac{[A^-]}{[HA]} \quad (2.45)$$

Table 2.7 Ionic product for water

Temperature (°C)	$K_w \times 10^{14}$	pK$_w$
0	0.1139	14.94
10	0.2920	14.53
20	0.6809	14.17
25	1.008	14.00
30	1.469	13.83
40	2.919	13.54
50	5.474	13.26
60	9.614	13.02
70	15.1	12.82
80	23.4	12.63

which can be rearranged to give

$$\text{percentage ionisation} = \frac{100}{1 + \text{antilog} \ (pK_a - pH)}$$
(2.46)

Weak bases

Taking logarithms of the expression for the dissociation constant (equation 2.40) gives

$$pH = pK_w - pK_b - \log \frac{[BH^+]}{[B]}$$
(2.47)

which can be rearranged to give

$$\text{percentage ionisation} = \frac{100}{1 + \text{antilog} \ (pH - pK_w + pK_b)}$$
(2.48)

These equations may be derived as shown in Derivation Box 2F. The influence of pH on the percentage ionisation may be determined for drugs of known pK_a using Table 2.8.

 Example 2.6 Calculation of percentage ionisation

Calculate the percentage of cocaine existing as the free base in a solution of cocaine hydrochloride at pH 4.5, and at pH 8.0. The pK_b of cocaine is 5.6.

Answer
From equation (2.48):
 At pH 4.5:

Percentage ionisation

$$= \frac{100}{1 + \text{antilog} \ (4.5 - 14.0 + 5.6)}$$
$$= 100/1.000126$$
$$= 99.99\%$$

Thus the percentage existing as cocaine base = 0.01%.

At pH 8.0:

Percentage ionisation

$$= \frac{100}{1 + \text{antilog} \ (8.0 - 14.0 + 5.6)}$$
$$= 100/1.398$$
$$= 71.53\%$$

Thus the percentage existing as cocaine base = 28.47%

If we carry out calculations such as those of Example 2.6 over the whole pH range for both acidic and basic drugs, we arrive at the graphs shown in Fig. 2.5. Notice from this figure that:

- A basic drug is virtually completely ionised at pH values up to 2 units below its pK_a, and virtually completely un-ionised at pH values greater than 2 units above its pK_a.
- An acidic drug is virtually completely un-ionised at pH values up to 2 units below its pK_a and virtually completely ionised at pH values greater than 2 units above its pK_a.
- Both acidic and basic drugs are exactly 50% ionised at their pK_a values.

2.5.4 Ionisation of amphoteric drugs

Ampholytes (amphoteric electrolytes) can function as either weak acids or weak bases in aqueous solution and have pK_a values corresponding to the ionisation of each group. They may be conveniently divided into two categories – ordinary ampholytes and zwitterionic ampholytes – depending on the relative acidity of the two ionisable groups.[13,14]

Ordinary ampholytes

In this category of ampholytes, the pK_a of the acidic group, pK_a^{acidic}, is higher than that of the basic group, pK_a^{basic}, and consequently the first group that loses its proton as the pH is increased is the basic group. Table 2.6 includes several examples of this type of ampholyte. We will consider, as a simple example, the ionisation of *m*-aminophenol (I), which has $pK_a^{\text{acidic}} = 9.8$ and $pK_a^{\text{basic}} = 4.4$.

Table 2.8 Percentage ionisation of anionic and cationic compounds as a function of pH

At pH above pK_a			At pH below pK_a		
pH – pK_a	If anionic	If cationic	pK_a – pH	If anionic	If cationic
6.0	99.999 90	0.000 099 9	0.1	44.27	55.73
5.0	99.999 00	0.000 999 9	0.2	38.68	61.32
4.0	99.990 0	0.009 999 0	0.3	33.39	66.61
–	–	–	0.4	28.47	71.53
–	–	–	0.5	24.03	75.97
3.5	99.968	0.031 6	–	–	–
3.4	99.960	0.039 8	–	–	–
3.3	99.950	0.050 1	0.6	20.07	79.93
3.2	99.937	0.063 0	0.7	16.63	83.37
3.1	99.921	0.079 4	0.8	13.70	86.30
–	–	–	0.9	11.19	88.81
–	–	–	1.0	9.09	90.91
3.0	99.90	0.099 9	–	–	–
2.9	99.87	0.125 7	–	–	–
2.8	99.84	0.158 2	1.1	7.36	92.64
2.7	99.80	0.199 1	1.2	5.93	94.07
2.6	99.75	0.250 5	1.3	4.77	95.23
–	–	–	1.4	3.83	96.17
–	–	–	1.5	3.07	96.93
2.5	99.68	0.315 2	–	–	–
2.4	99.60	0.396 6	–	–	–
2.3	99.50	0.498 7	1.6	2.450	97.55
2.2	99.37	0.627 0	1.7	1.956	98.04
2.1	99.21	0.787 9	1.8	1.560	98.44
–	–	–	1.9	1.243	98.76
–	–	–	2.0	0.990	99.01
2.0	99.01	0.990	–	–	–
1.9	98.76	1.243	–	–	–
1.8	98.44	1.560	2.1	0.787 9	99.21
1.7	98.04	1.956	2.2	0.6270	99.37
1.6	97.55	2.450	2.3	0.498 7	99.50
–	–	–	2.4	0.396 6	99.60
–	–	–	2.5	0.315 2	99.68

Table 2.8 *(continued)*					
At pH above pK_a			**At pH below pK_a**		
pH – pK_a	**If anionic**	**If cationic**	**pK_a – pH**	**If anionic**	**If cationic**
1.5	96.93	3.07	–	–	–
1.4	96.17	3.83	–	–	–
1.3	95.23	4.77	2.6	0.250 5	99.75
1.2	94.07	5.93	2.7	0.199 1	99.80
1.1	92.64	7.36	2.8	0.158 2	99.84
			2.9	0.125 7	99.87
1.0	90.91	9.09	3.0	0.099 9	99.90
0.9	88.81	11.19	–	–	–
0.8	86.30	13.70	3.1	0.079 4	99.921
0.7	83.37	16.63	3.2	0.063 0	99.937
0.6	79.93	20.07	3.3	0.050 1	99.950
–	–	–	3.4	0.039 8	99.960
0.5	75.97	24.03	3.5	0.031 6	99.968
0.4	71.53	28.47	–	–	–
0.3	66.61	33.39	4.0	0.009 999 0	99.990 0
0.2	61.32	38.68	5.0	0.000 999 9	99.999 00
0.1	55.73	44.27	6.0	0.000 099 9	99.999 90
0	50.00	50.00	–	–	–

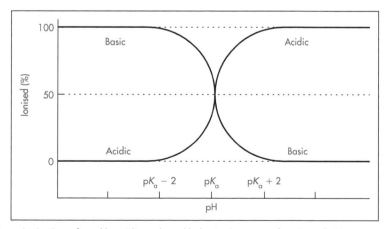

Figure 2.5 Percentage ionisation of weakly acidic and weakly basic drugs as a function of pH.

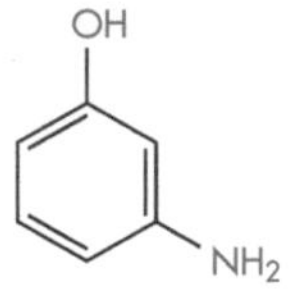

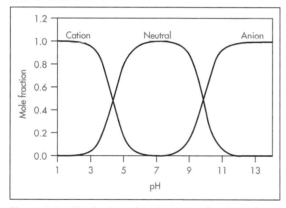

Structure I *m*-Aminophenol

The steps of the ionisation on increasing pH are shown in the following equilibria:

$$NH_3{}^+C_6H_4OH \rightleftharpoons NH_2C_6H_4OH \rightleftharpoons NH_2C_6H_5O^-$$

This compound can exist as a cation, as an un-ionised form, or as an anion depending on the pH of the solution, but because the difference between $pK_a{}^{acidic}$ and $pK_a{}^{basic}$ is > 2, there will be no simultaneous ionisation of the two groups and the distribution of the species will be as shown in Fig. 2.6. The ionisation pattern will become more complex, however, with drugs in which the difference in pK_a of the two groups is much smaller because of overlapping of the two equilibria.

Figure 2.6 Distribution of ionic species for the ordinary ampholyte *m*-aminophenol.

Zwitterionic ampholytes

This group of ampholytes is characterised by the relation $pK_a{}^{acidic} < pK_a{}^{basic}$. The most common examples of zwitterionic ampholytes are the amino acids, peptides and proteins. There are essentially two types of zwitterionic electrolyte depending on the difference ΔpK_a between the $pK_a{}^{acidic}$ and $pK_a{}^{basic}$ values.

Large ΔpKₐ

The simplest type to consider is that of compounds having two widely separated pK_a values, for example, glycine. The pK_a values of the carboxylate and amino groups on glycine are 2.34 and 9.6, respectively, and the changes in ionisation as the pH is increased are described by the following equilibria:

$$HOOCCH_2 \cdot NH_3^+ \rightleftharpoons {}^-OOCCH_2NH_3^+ \rightleftharpoons$$
$${}^-OOCCH_2NH_2$$

Over the pH range 3–9, glycine exists in solution predominantly in the form $^-OOCCH_2\,NH_3{}^+$. Such a structure, having both positive and negative charges on the same molecule, is referred to as a zwitterion and can react as an acid,

$$^-OOCCH_2NH_3^+ + H_2O \rightleftharpoons {}^-OOCCH_2NH_2 + H_3O^+$$

or as a base,

$$^-OOCCH_2NH_3^+ + H_2O \rightleftharpoons$$
$$HOOCCH_2NH_3^+ + OH^-$$

This compound can exist as a cation, a zwitterion and an anion depending on the pH of the solution. The two pK_a values of glycine are > 2 pH units apart and hence the distribution of the ionic species will be similar to that shown in Fig. 2.6.

At a particular pH, known as the *isoelectric pH* or *isoelectric point*, pH_i, the effective net charge on the molecule is zero. pH_i can be calculated from

$$pH_i = \frac{pK_a{}^{acidic} + pK_a{}^{basic}}{2} \tag{2.49}$$

Small ΔpKₐ

In cases where the two pK_a values are ≪ 2 pH units apart there is overlap of the ionisation of the acidic and basic groups, with the result that the zwitterionic electrolyte can exist in four different electrical states – the cation, the un-ionised form, the zwitterion and the anion (Scheme 2.3).

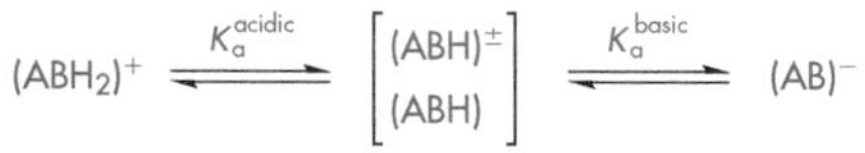

$$(ABH_2)^+ \underset{}{\overset{K_a{}^{acidic}}{\rightleftharpoons}} \begin{bmatrix} (ABH)^\pm \\ (ABH) \end{bmatrix} \underset{}{\overset{K_a{}^{basic}}{\rightleftharpoons}} (AB)^-$$

Scheme 2.3

In Scheme 2.3, $(ABH)^\pm$ is the zwitterion and, although possessing both positive and negative charges, is essentially neutral. The un-ionised form, (ABH), is of course also neutral and can be regarded as a tautomer of the zwitterion. Although only two dissociation constants K_a^{acidic} and K_a^{basic} (*macrodissociation constants*) can be determined experimentally, each of these is composed of individual *microdissociation constants* because of simultaneous ionisation of the two groups (see section 2.5.6). These microdissociation constants represent equilibria between the cation and zwitterion; the anion and the zwitterion; the cation and the un-ionised form; and the anion and the un-ionised form. At pH_i, the un-ionised form and the zwitterion always coexist, but the ratio of the concentrations of each will vary depending on the relative magnitude of the microdissociation constants. The distribution of the ionic species for labetalol which has $pK_a^{acidic} = 7.4$ and $pK_a^{basic} = 9.4$ is shown in Fig. 2.7.

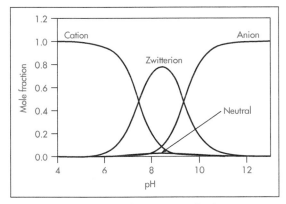

Figure 2.7 Distribution of ionic species for the zwitterionic ampholyte labetalol.

Reprinted with permission from Pagliara A *et al.* Lipophilicity profiles of ampholytes. *Chem. Rev.* 1997;97:3385. Copyright 1997 American Chemical Society.

Examples of zwitterionic drugs with both large and small ΔpKa values are given in Box 2.4; others can be noted in Table 2.6.

2.5.5 Ionisation of polyprotic drugs

In the examples we have considered so far, the acidic drugs have donated a single proton. There are several acids, for example citric, phosphoric and tartaric acids, that are capable of donating more than one proton; these compounds are referred to as *polyprotic* or *polybasic* acids. Similarly, a polyprotic base is one capable of accepting two or more protons. Many examples of both types of polyprotic drugs can be found in Table 2.6, including the polybasic acids

amoxicillin and fluorouracil, and the polyacidic bases pilocarpine, doxorubicin and aciclovir. Each stage of the dissociation may be represented by an equilibrium expression and hence each stage has a distinct pK_a or pK_b value. The dissociation of phosphoric acid, for example, occurs in three stages; thus:

$$H_3PO_4 + H_2O \rightleftharpoons H_2PO_4^- + H_3O^+ \quad K_1 = 7.5 \times 10^{-3}$$

$$H_2PO_4^- + H_2O \rightleftharpoons H_2PO_4^{2-} + H_3O^+ \quad K_2 = 6.2 \times 10^{-8}$$

$$HPO_4^{2-} + H_2O \rightleftharpoons PO_4^{3-} + H_3O^+ \quad K_3 = 2.1 \times 10^{-13}$$

2.5.6 Microdissociation constants

The experimentally determined dissociation constants for the various stages of dissociation of polyprotic and zwitterionic drugs are referred to as macroscopic values. However, it is not always easy to assign macroscopic dissociation constants to the ionisation of specific groups of the molecule, particularly when the pK_a values are close together, as discussed in section 2.5.5. The diprotic drug morphine has macroscopic pK_a values of 8.3 and 9.5, arising from ionisation of amino and phenolic groups. Experience suggests that the first pK_a value is probably associated with the ionisation of the amino group and the second with that of the phenolic group; but it is not possible to assign the values of these groups unequivocally, and for a more complete picture of the dissociation it is necessary to take into account all possible ways in which the molecule may be ionised and all the possible species present in solution. We may represent the most highly protonated form of morphine, ^+HMOH, as $+O$, where the '+' refers to the protonated amino group and the O refers to the uncharged phenolic group. Dissociation of the amino proton only produces an uncharged form MOH, represented by OO, while dissociation of the phenolic proton gives a zwitterion $^+HMO^-$ represented by '+−'. The completely dissociated form MO^- is represented as O−. The entire dissociation scheme is given in Scheme 2.4.

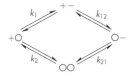

Scheme 2.4

Box 2.4 Chemical structures and pK_a values of some zwitterionic drugs

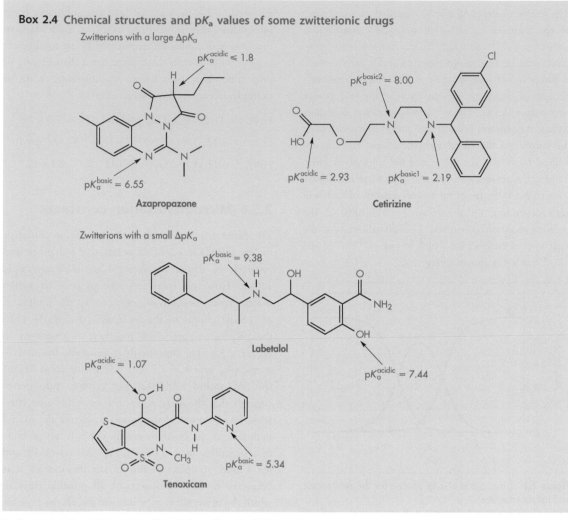

Pagliara A et al. Lipophilicity profiles of ampholytes. *Chem Rev* 1997;97:3385–3400.

The constants K_1, K_2, K_{12} and K_{21} are termed micro-dissociation constants and are defined by

$$k_1 = \frac{[+-][H_3O^+]}{[+O]} \qquad k_2 = \frac{[OO][H_3O^+]}{[+O]}$$

$$k_{12} = \frac{[O-][H_3O^+]}{[+-]} \qquad k_{21} = \frac{[O-][H_3O^+]}{[OO]}$$

The micro- and macrodissociation constants are related by the following expressions:

$$K_1 = k_1 + k_2 \tag{2.50}$$

$$\frac{1}{K_2} = \frac{1}{k_{12}} + \frac{1}{k_{21}} \tag{2.51}$$

$$K_1 K_2 = k_1 k_{12} = k_2 k_{21} \tag{2.52}$$

Various methods have been proposed whereby the microdissociation constants for the morphine system may be evaluated.[15] Other drugs for which microdissociation constants have been derived include the tetracyclines,[16] doxorubicin,[17] cephalosporin,[18] dopamine[19] and the group of drugs shown in Box 2.4.

2.5.7 pK_a values of proteins

The pK_a values of ionisable groups in proteins and other macromolecules can be significantly different from those of the corresponding groups when they are isolated in solution. The shifts in pK_a values between native and denatured states or between bound and free forms of a complex can cause changes in binding constants or stability of the protein due to pH effects. For example, the acid denaturation of proteins may be a consequence of anomalous shifts of the pK_a values of a small number of amino acids in the native protein.[20] Several possible causes of such shifts have been proposed. They may arise from interactions between ionisable groups on the protein molecule; for example, an acidic group will have its pK_a lowered by interactions with basic groups. Other suggested cases of shifts of pK_a include hydrogen-bonding interactions with non-ionisable groups and the degree of exposure to the bulk solvent; for example, an acidic group will have its pK_a increased if it is fully or partially removed from solvent, but the effect may be reversed by strong hydrogen-bonding interactions with other groups.

The calculation of pK_a values of protein molecules thus requires a detailed consideration of the environment of each ionisable group, and is consequently highly complex. An additional complication is that a protein with N ionisable residues has 2^N possible ionisation states; the extent of the problem is apparent when it is realised that a moderately sized protein may contain as many as 50 ionisable groups.

2.5.8 Calculation of the pH of drug solutions

We have considered above the effect on the ionisation of a drug of buffering the solution at given pH values. When these weakly acidic or basic drugs are dissolved in water they will, of course, develop a pH value in their own right. In this section we examine how the pH of drug solutions of known concentration can be simply calculated from a knowledge of the pK_a of the drug. We will consider the way in which one of these expressions may be derived from the expression for the ionisation in solution; the derivation of the other expressions follows a similar route and you may wish to derive these for yourselves.

Weakly acidic drugs

The pH of a solution of a weakly ionised acidic drug is given by

$$pH = \frac{1}{2}pK_a - \frac{1}{2}\log c \qquad (2.53)$$

The derivation of this expression is given in Derivation Box 2G.

Example 2.7 Calculation of the pH of a weak acid

Calculate the pH of a 50 mg cm^{-3} solution of ascorbic acid (mol wt = 176.1 Da; $pK_a = 4.17$).

Answer
For a weakly acidic drug,

$$pH = \frac{1}{2}pK_a - \frac{1}{2}\log c$$

$$c = 50\,\text{mg cm}^{-3} = 50\,\text{g dm}^{-3}$$

$$= 0.2839\,\text{mol dm}^{-3}$$

$$\therefore pH = 2.09 + 0.273 = 2.36$$

Weakly basic drugs

We can show by a similar derivation to that of Derivation Box 2G that the pH of aqueous solutions of weakly basic drugs will be given by

$$pH = \frac{1}{2}pK_w + \frac{1}{2}pK_a + \frac{1}{2}\log c \qquad (2.54)$$

Example 2.8 Calculation of the pH of a weakly basic drug

Calculate the pH of a saturated solution of codeine monohydrate (mol wt = 317.4 Da) given that its pK_a is 8.2 and its solubility at room temperature is 1 g in 120 cm^3 water.

Answer
Codeine is a weakly basic drug and hence its pH will be given by

$$pH = \frac{1}{2}pK_w + \frac{1}{2}pK_a + \frac{1}{2}\log c$$

where $c = 1$ g in 120 cm^3 = 8.33 g dm^{-3} = 0.02633 mol dm^{-3}.

$$\therefore pH = 7.0 + 4.1 - 0.790 = 10.31$$

Drug salts

Because of the limited solubility of many weak acids and weak bases in water, drugs of these types are commonly used as their salts; for example, sodium salicylate is the salt of a weak acid (salicylic acid) and a strong base (sodium hydroxide). The pH of a solution of this type of salt is given by

$$pH = \frac{1}{2}pK_w + \frac{1}{2}pK_a + \frac{1}{2}\log c \qquad (2.55)$$

Alternatively, a salt may be formed between a weak base and a strong acid; for example, ephedrine hydrochloride is the salt of ephedrine and hydrochloric acid. Solutions of such drugs have a pH given by

$$pH = \frac{1}{2}pK_a - \frac{1}{2}\log c \qquad (2.56)$$

Finally, a salt may be produced by the combination of a weak base and a weak acid, as in the case of codeine phosphate. Solutions of such drugs have a pH given by

$$pH = \frac{1}{2}pK_w + \frac{1}{2}pK_a - \frac{1}{2}pK_b \qquad (2.57)$$

Note that this equation does not include a concentration term and hence the pH is independent of concentration for such drugs.

2.5.9 Buffer solutions

A mixture of a weak acid and its salt (that is, a conjugate base) or of a weak base and its conjugate acid has the ability to reduce the large changes in pH that would otherwise result from the addition of small amounts of acid or alkali to the solution. The reason for the buffering action of a weak acid HA and its

---

Example 2.9 Calculation of the pH of drug salts

Calculate the pH of the following solutions:
- (a) 5% oxycodone hydrochloride ($pK_a = 8.9$, mol wt = 405.9 Da).
- (b) 600 mg of benzylpenicillin sodium ($pK_a = 2.76$, mol wt = 356.4 Da) in 2 cm^3 of water for injection.
- (c) 100 mg cm^{-3} chlorphenamine maleate (mol wt = 390.8 Da) in water for injection (pK_b chlorphenamine = 5.0, pK_a maleic acid = 1.9).

Answer

(a) Oxycodone hydrochloride is the salt of a weak base and a strong acid, hence

$$pH = \frac{1}{2}pK_a - \frac{1}{2}\log c$$

where $c = 50$ g dm^{-3} = 0.1232 mol dm^{-3}.

$$\therefore pH = 4.45 + 0.45 = 4.90$$

(b) Benzylpenicillin sodium is the salt of a weak acid and a strong base, hence

$$pH = \frac{1}{2}pK_w + \frac{1}{2}pK_a + \frac{1}{2}\log c$$

where $c = 600$ mg in 2 cm^3 = 0.842 mol dm^{-3}.

$$\therefore pH = 7.00 + 1.38 - 0.037 + 8.34$$

(c) Chlorphenamine maleate is the salt of a weak acid and a weak base, hence

$$pH = \frac{1}{2}pK_w + \frac{1}{2}pK_a - \frac{1}{2}pK_b$$

$$\therefore pH = 7.00 + 0.95 - 2.5 = 5.45$$

Key points

- While some drugs such as tadalafil have no ionisable groups, many drugs are either weak organic acids (for example, acetylsalicylic acid (aspirin)), or weak organic bases (for example, procaine), or their salts (for example, ephedrine hydrochloride); the degree to which these drugs are ionised in solution is highly dependent on the pH. The exceptions to this general statement are the non-electrolytes, such as the steroids, and the quaternary ammonium compounds, which are completely ionised at all pH values and in this respect behave as strong electrolytes.

- The negative logarithm of the dissociation constant K_a of a weakly acidic drug is the pK_a and that of a weakly basic drug is the pK_b; the sum of pK_a and pK_b values of conjugate acid–base pairs is equal to the negative logarithm of the dissociation constant for water, pK_w (see Table 2.7 for values).

- *Acidic drugs* are completely un-ionised at pH values up to 2 units below their pK_a and completely ionised at pH values greater than 2 units above their pK_a. Conversely, *basic drugs* are completely ionised at pH values up to 2 units below their pK_a and completely un-ionised when the pH is more than 2 units above their pK_a. Both types of drug are exactly 50% ionised at their pK_a values.

- *Salts of weak acids or bases* are essentially completely ionised in solution; for example, when sodium salicylate (salt of the weak acid, salicylic acid, and the strong base NaOH) is dissolved in water, it ionises almost entirely into the conjugate base of salicylic acid, $HOC_6H_5COO^-$, and Na^+ ions. The conjugate acids or bases formed in this way are subject to the usual acid–base equilibria.

- *Amphoteric drugs* can function as either weak acids or weak bases in aqueous solution depending on the pH and have pK_a values corresponding to the ionisation of each group. Depending on the relative acidity of the two ionisable groups, they may be ordinary ampholytes (when the pK_a of the acidic group, pK_a^{acidic}, is higher than that of the basic group, pK_a^{basic}) or zwitterionic ampholytes (when $pK_a^{acidic} < pK_a^{basic}$). Ordinary ampholytes exist in solution as a cation, an un-ionised form and an anion. Zwitterionic ampholytes exist in solution as a cation, a zwitterion (having both positive and negative charges) and an anion depending on the pH of the solution.

- Several acids, for example citric, phosphoric and tartaric acid, are capable of donating more than one proton and these compounds are referred to as *polyprotic* or *polybasic* acids. Similarly, polyprotic bases are capable of accepting two or more protons. Each stage of the dissociation of the drug may be represented by an equilibrium expression and hence each stage has a distinct pK_a or pK_b value. In cases where the dissociation constants of each dissociation stage are less than about 2 pH units apart, it is necessary to take into account all possible ways in which the molecule may be ionised and all the possible species present in solution. In this case the constants are called *microdissociation constants*.

- The pH of aqueous solutions of each of these types of drug and their salts can be calculated from their pK_a and the concentration c of the drug:
  - *Weakly acidic drugs:* $pH = \frac{1}{2} pK_a - \frac{1}{2} \log c$
  - *Weakly basic drugs:* $pH = \frac{1}{2} pK_w + \frac{1}{2} pK_a + \frac{1}{2} \log c$
  - *Drug salts:*
    - Salts of a weak acid and a strong base: $pH = \frac{1}{2} pK_w + \frac{1}{2} pK_a + \frac{1}{2} \log c$
    - Salts of a weak base and a strong acid: $pH = \frac{1}{2} pK_a - \frac{1}{2} \log c$
    - Salts of a weak acid and a weak base: $pH = \frac{1}{2} K_w + \frac{1}{2} pK_a - \frac{1}{2} pK_b$ (Note that there is no concentration term in this equation, meaning that the pH does not vary with concentration.)

ionisable salt (for example, NaA) is that the A^- ions from the salt combine with the added H^+ ions, removing them from solution as an undissociated weak acid:

$$A^- + H_3O^+ \rightleftharpoons H_2O + HA$$

Added OH^- ions are removed by combination with the weak acid to form undissociated water molecules:

$$HA + OH^- \rightleftharpoons H_2O + A^-$$

The buffering action of a mixture of a weak base and its salt arises from a removal of H^+ ions by the base B to form the salt and removal of OH^- ions by the salt to form undissociated water:

$$B + H_2O^+ \rightleftharpoons H_2O + BH^+$$
$$BH^+ + OH^- \rightleftharpoons H_2O + B$$

The concentration of buffer components required to maintain a solution at the required pH may be calculated using equation (2.45). Since the acid is weak and therefore only very slightly ionised, the term [HA] in this equation may be equated with the total acid concentration. Similarly, the free A^- ions in solution may be considered to originate entirely from the salt and the term $[A^-]$ may be replaced by the salt concentration.

Equation (2.45) now becomes

$$pH = pK_a + \log\frac{[salt]}{[acid]} \tag{2.58}$$

By a similar reasoning, equation (2.47) may be modified to facilitate the calculation of the pH of a solution of a weak base and its salt, giving

$$pH = pK_w - pK_b + \log\frac{[base]}{[salt]} \tag{2.59}$$

Equations (2.58) and (2.59) are often referred to as the *Henderson–Hasselbalch equations*.

Equations (2.58) and (2.59) are also useful in calculating the change in pH that results from the addition of a specific amount of acid or alkali to a given buffer solution, as seen from the calculation in Example 2.11.

 Example 2.10 Buffer solutions

Calculate the amount of sodium acetate to be added to 100 cm^3 of a 0.1 mol dm^{-3} acetic acid solution to prepare a buffer of pH 5.20.

Answer
The pK_a of acetic acid is 4.76. Substitution in equation (2.58) gives

$$5.20 = 4.76 + \log\frac{[salt]}{[acid]}$$

The molar ratio of [salt]/[acid] is 2.754. Since 100 cm^3 of 0.1 mol dm^{-3} acetic acid contains 0.01 mol, we would require 0.02754 mol of sodium acetate (2.258 g), ignoring dilution effects.

 Example 2.11 Calculation of the pH change in buffer solutions

Calculate the change in pH following the addition of 10 cm^3 of 0.1 mol dm^{-3} NaOH to the buffer solution described in Example 2.10.

Answer
The added 10 cm^3 of 0.1 mol dm^{-3} NaOH (equivalent to 0.001 mol) combines with 0.001 mol of acetic acid to produce 0.001 mol of sodium acetate. Reapplying equation (2.58) using the revised salt and acid concentrations gives

$$pH = 4.76 + \log\frac{(0.02754 + 0.001)}{(0.01 - 0.001)}$$
$$= 5.26$$

The pH of the buffer has been increased by only 0.06 units following the addition of the alkali.

Buffer capacity

The effectiveness of a buffer in reducing changes in pH is expressed as the buffer capacity, β. The buffer capacity is defined by the ratio

$$\beta = \frac{dc}{d(pH)} \tag{2.60}$$

where dc is the number of moles of alkali (or acid) needed to change the pH of 1 litre of solution by an amount $d(pH)$. If the addition of 1 mol of alkali to 1 litre of buffer solution produces a pH change of 1 unit, the buffer capacity is unity.

The capacity of a buffer of total initial concentration c_0 can be readily calculated from the pK_a value of the component weak acid using equation (2.61), the derivation of which is given in Derivation Box 2H.

$$\beta = \frac{2.303 c_0 \, K_a \, [H_3O^+]}{([H_3O^+] + K_a)^2} \tag{2.61}$$

Example 2.12 Calculation of buffer capacity

Calculate the buffer capacity of the acetic acid–acetate buffer of Example 2.10 at pH 4.0.

Answer

The total amount of buffer components in 100 cm³ of solution = 0.01 + 0.02754 = 0.03754 mol. Therefore,

$$c_0 = 0.3754 \, \text{mol dm}^{-3}$$

The pK_a of acetic acid = 4.76. Therefore,

$$K_a = 1.75 \times 10^{-5}$$

The pH of the solution = 4.0. Therefore,

$$[H_3O^+] = 10^{-4} \, \text{mol dm}^{-3}$$

Substituting in equation (2.61):

$$\beta = \frac{2.303 \times 0.3754 \times 1.75 \times 10^{-5} \times 10^{-4}}{(10^{-4} + 1.75 \times 10^{-5})^2}$$

$$= 0.1096$$

The buffer capacity of the acetic acid–acetate buffer is 0.1096 mol dm⁻³ per pH unit.

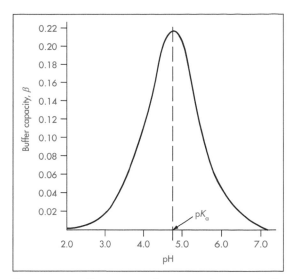

Figure 2.8 Buffer capacity of acetic acid–acetate buffer (initial concentration = 0.3754 mol dm⁻³) as a function of pH.

Figure 2.8 shows the variation of buffer capacity with pH for the acetic acid–acetate buffer used in the numerical examples above ($c_0 = 0.3754 \, \text{mol dm}^{-3}$), as calculated from equation (2.61). It should be noted that β is at a maximum when pH = pK_a (that is, at pH 4.76). When selecting a weak acid for the preparation of a buffer solution, therefore, the chosen acid should have a pK_a as close as possible to the pH required. Substituting pH = pK_a into equation (2.61) gives the useful result that the maximum buffer capacity, β_{max}, is

$$\beta_{max} = 0.576 c_0 \tag{2.62}$$

where c_0 is the total buffer concentration.

Buffer solutions are widely used in pharmacy to adjust the pH of aqueous solutions to that required for maximum stability or that needed for optimum physiological effect. Solutions for application to delicate tissues, particularly the eye, should also be formulated at a pH not too far removed from that of the appropriate tissue fluid, as otherwise irritation may be caused on administration. The pH of tears lies between 7 and 8, with an average value of 7.4. Fortunately, the buffer capacity of tears is high, and provided that the solutions to be administered have a low buffer capacity, a reasonably wide range of pH may be tolerated, although there is a difference in the irritability of the various ionic species that are commonly used as buffer components. As explained below, the pH of blood is maintained at about 7.4 by primary buffer components in the plasma (carbonic acid–carbonate and the acid–sodium salts of phosphoric acid) and secondary buffer components in the erythrocytes. Values of 0.025 and 0.039 mol dm^{-3} per pH unit have been quoted for the buffer capacity of whole blood. Parenteral solutions are not normally buffered, or alternatively are buffered at a very low capacity, since the buffers of the blood are usually capable of bringing them within a tolerable pH range.

 Clinical point

The normal pH of arterial blood is 7.4, while that of venous blood and of interstitial fluids is about 7.35, because of extra quantities of carbon dioxide that form carbonic acid in these fluids. A person is considered to have *acidosis* whenever the pH of blood plasma falls below 7.35; in this state the central nervous system becomes depressed, causing symptoms such as confusion, disorientation and coma. If the pH rises above 7.45 the person is said to have *alkalosis*, a condition characterised by overstimulation of the skeletal muscles causing muscle spasms, convulsion or respiratory paralysis. The importance of control of the pH of arterial blood is apparent when it is realised that the lower pH limit at which a person can survive for more than a few hours is about 7.0 and the upper limit approximately 7.7; the situation quickly becomes fatal if pH falls below 6.8 or rises above 8.0.

Physiological regulation of acid–base balance

Several control mechanisms are available to prevent acidosis and alkalosis. All the body fluids are supplied with acid–base buffer systems that immediately combine with any acid or alkali and thereby prevent excessive changes in hydrogen ion concentration. These *chemical* buffer systems are discussed in more detail below. In addition, if the hydrogen ion concentration does change measurably, two *physiological* buffer mechanisms – the respiratory and urinary systems – come into operation. These systems are appreciably slower to react to changes in pH than

the chemical buffers, which can respond within a fraction of a second. The basis of the buffering action of the *respiratory* system is an immediate alteration of the rate of pulmonary ventilation and consequently the rate of removal of carbon dioxide from the body fluids – a process that takes 2–3 minutes to restore the pH to normal. The *urinary* buffer system operates differently from the other buffering systems in that the hydrogen ions are actually expelled from the body in the urine, thereby readjusting their concentration in body fluids to normal. Although the kidneys are more effective in restoring pH than the other buffering mechanisms, the process is considerably slower, taking several hours to readjust the hydrogen ion concentration.

The three major *chemical* buffers are the bicarbonate, phosphate and protein systems. Each of these performs major buffering functions under different conditions.

The *bicarbonate* buffer system consists of a solution of the weak acid carbonic acid (pK_a 6.1) and its salt sodium bicarbonate.

$$H_2CO_3 \rightleftharpoons HCO_3^- + H^+$$

An acidic substance added to the blood would be neutralised by the bicarbonate ions and the carbon dioxide produced excreted by the lungs.

$$HCO_3^- + H^+ \rightleftharpoons H_2CO_3 \rightleftharpoons H_2O + CO_2$$

A base added to the blood would be neutralised by the reaction

$$H_2CO_3 + OH^- \rightleftharpoons HCO_3^- + H_2O$$

This might seem, at first sight, to be a rather ineffective system for two reasons. Firstly, the buffer is operating at a pH (7.4) well away from its maximum buffering capacity which, as we have already discussed, is at the pK_a (6.1). Secondly, the concentrations of the bicarbonate buffer are relatively low. The buffer system is, however, extremely efficient because it is self-regulating; carbonic acid is replenished by carbon dioxide from respiration, and bicarbonate ions by the kidneys.

The *phosphate* buffer system operates in the internal fluid of all cells and consists of dihydrogen phosphate ions ($H_2PO_4^-$) as hydrogen-ion donor (acid) and hydrogen phosphate ions (HPO_4^{2-}) as hydrogen-ion acceptor (base). These two ions are in equilibrium with each other, as indicated by the chemical equation

$$H_2PO_4^- \rightleftharpoons H^+ + HPO_4^{2-}$$

If additional hydrogen ions enter the cellular fluid, they are consumed in the reaction with HPO_4^{2-}, and the equilibrium shifts to the left. If additional hydroxide ions enter the cellular fluid, they react with $H_2PO_4^-$, producing HPO_4^{2-}, and shifting the equilibrium to the right. The pK_a of this equilibrium, 7.2, is closer to the physiological pH than that of the bicarbonate buffer, but its concentration in the extracellular fluids is only one-sixth of this buffer.

The *protein* buffer system accounts for about 75% of all chemical buffering ability of the body fluids. The buffering ability of proteins is due to the dissociation of the acidic –COOH groups of the amino acid residues to –COO⁻ and H⁺, and the dissociation of the basic –NH₃OH groups of the amino acids into NH_3 and OH⁻. Furthermore, the pK_a values of the amino acids are not far from 7.4, making the protein buffering systems by far the most powerful of the body.

Universal buffers

We have seen from Fig. 2.8 that the buffer capacity is at a maximum at a pH equal to the pK_a of the weak acid used in the formulation of the buffer system and decreases appreciably as the pH extends more than 1 unit either side of this value. If, instead of a single weak monobasic acid, a suitable mixture of polybasic and monobasic acids is used, it is possible to produce a buffer that is effective over a wide pH range. Such solutions are referred to as *universal buffers*. A typical example is a mixture of citric acid ($pK_{a1} = 3.06$, $pK_{a2} = 4.78$, $pK_{a3} = 5.40$), Na_2HPO_4 (pK_a of conjugate acid, $H_2PO_4^- = 7.2$), diethylbarbituric acid ($pK_{a1} = 7.43$) and boric acid ($pK_{a1} = 9.24$). Because of the wide range of pK_a values involved, each associated with a maximum buffer capacity, this buffer is effective over a correspondingly wide pH range (pH 2.4 – 12).

2.6 Diffusion of drugs in solution

Diffusion is the process by which a concentration difference is reduced by a spontaneous flow of matter. Consider the simplest case of a solution containing a

Key points

- Buffers are usually mixtures of a weak acid and its salt (conjugate base), or a weak base and its conjugate acid.
- The concentration of buffer components required to maintain a solution at the required pH may be calculated from the *Henderson–Hasselbalch equations*:
  - Weak acid and its salt:

  $$pH = pK_a + \log \frac{[\text{salt}]}{[\text{acid}]}$$

  - Weak base and its salt:

  $$pH = pK_w - pK_b + \log \frac{[\text{base}]}{[\text{salt}]}$$

- The effectiveness of a buffer in reducing changes in pH is greatest at a pH equal to the pK_a of the weak acid component of the buffer; the maximum buffer capacity, β_{max}, is $0.576c_0$ where c_0 is the total initial buffer concentration.
- Mixtures of polybasic and monobasic acids with a wide range of pK_a values act as universal buffers that are effective over a wide pH range.

single solute. The solute will spontaneously diffuse from a region of high concentration to one of low concentration. Strictly speaking, the driving force for diffusion is the gradient of chemical potential, but it is more usual to think of the diffusion of solutes in terms of the gradient of their concentration. Imagine the solution to be divided into volume elements. Although no individual solute particle in a particular volume element shows a preference for motion in any particular direction, a definite fraction of the molecules in this element may be considered to be moving in, say, the x direction. In an adjacent volume element, the same fraction may be moving in the reverse direction. If the concentration in the first volume element is greater than that in the second, the overall effect is that more particles are leaving the first element for the second and hence there is a net flow of solute in the x direction, the direction of decreasing concentration.

The expression that relates the flow of material to the concentration gradient (dc/dx) is referred to as *Fick's first law*:

$$J = -D(dc/dx) \qquad (2.63)$$

where J is the flux of a component across a plane of unit area and D is the diffusion coefficient (or diffusivity). The negative sign indicates that the flux is in the direction of decreasing concentration. J is in units of $mol\ m^{-2}\ s^{-1}$, c is in $mol\ m^{-3}$ and x is in metres; therefore, the units of D are $m^2\ s^{-1}$.

The relationship between the radius, a, of the diffusing molecule and its diffusion coefficient (assuming spherical particles or molecules) is given by the *Stokes–Einstein equation* as

$$D = \frac{RT}{6\pi\eta a N_A} \qquad (2.64)$$

Table 2.9 shows diffusion coefficients of some *p*-hydroxybenzoate (paraben) preservatives and typical proteins in aqueous solution. Although the trend for a decrease of D with increase of molecular size (as predicted by equation 2.64) is clearly seen from the data of this table, it is clear that other factors such as branching of the *p*-hydroxybenzoate molecules (as with the isoalkyl derivatives) also affect the diffusion coefficients. The diffusion coefficients of more complex molecules such as proteins will also be affected by the shape of the molecule, more asymmetric molecules having a greater resistance to flow.

The diffusional properties of a drug have relevance in pharmaceutical systems in consideration of processes such as the dissolution of the drug and transport through artificial (e.g. polymer) or biological membranes. Diffusion in tissues such as the skin or in tumours is a process that relies on the same criteria as discussed above, even though the diffusion takes place in complex media. Diffusion is discussed in several other chapters e.g. Chapter 13 which discusses therapeutic peptides and proteins and Chapter 14 on nanotechnology.

Summary

This chapter has dealt with several physicochemical properties of drugs of relevance to their formulation in aqueous solution and their biological activity. Of

Table 2.9 Effect of molecular weight on diffusion coefficient (25°C) in aqueous media

Compound	Molecular weight	D $(10^{-10}\ m^2\ s^{-1})$
p-Hydroxybenzoates[a]		
Methyl hydroxybenzoate	152.2	8.44
Ethyl hydroxybenzoate	166.2	7.48
n-Propyl hydroxybenzoate	180.2	6.81
Isopropyl hydroxybenzoate	180.2	6.94
n-Butyl hydroxybenzoate	194.2	6.31
Isobutyl hydroxybenzoate	194.2	6.40
n-Amyl hydroxybenzoate	208.2	5.70
Proteins[b]		
Cytochrome c (horse)	12 400	1.28
Lysozyme (chicken)	14 400	0.95
Trypsin (bovine)	24 000	1.10
Albumin (bovine)	66 000	0.46

[a] From Seki T *et al.* Measurement of diffusion coefficients of parabens by the chromatographic broadening method. *J Pharm Sci Technol Jpn* 2000;60:114–117.
[b] From Baden N, Terazima M. A novel method for measurement of diffusion coefficients of proteins and DNA in solution. *Chem Phys Lett* 2004;393:539–545; see also Chapter 13 for further values of therapeutic peptides and proteins.

primary importance is their ionisation in solution since this influences such important physicochemical properties as their osmolarity, solubility and activity, and their *in vivo* absorption, distribution and elimination. We have seen how the extent of ionisation of the large number of drugs that are weak acids or bases or salts of acids or bases is dependent on pH and can be predicted from the pK_a value. Acidic drugs are completely un-ionised at pH values up to 2 units below their pK_a and completely ionised at pH values greater than 2 units above their pK_a. Conversely, basic drugs are completely ionised at pH values up to 2 units below their pK_a and completely un-ionised when the pH is more than 2 units above their pK_a. Both types of drug are exactly 50% ionised at their pK_a values.

The pH of liquid formulations may be confined to within narrow limits through the use of buffers consisting of mixtures of weak acids or bases and their salts and we have seen how to formulate buffer systems effective at a chosen pH or, in the case of universal buffers, over a wide range of pH values. In a clinical setting, drug ionisation may be altered by adjustment of, for example, the pH of urine with the aim of increasing the excretion of toxic substances.

Osmotic effects are important from a physiological viewpoint since the red blood cell membrane acts as a semipermeable membrane, with implications for the integrity of red blood cells when immersed in solutions of osmotic pressures which differ from that of their contents. A simple equation (the Henderson–Hasselbalch equation) for the calculation of the amount of adjusting substance required to ensure the isotonicity of a drug solution has been proposed. Additives, such as ethyl alcohol, sorbitol and propylene glycol make a large contribution to the osmolarities of oral formulations, which must be recognised when these are administered to infants at risk from necrotising enterocolitis. Applications of the osmotic effect in the design of rehydration solutions and in oral rehydration therapy have been discussed.

The driving force for the spontaneous diffusion of drugs in solution is the difference in concentration, or more precisely, the chemical potential gradient between different regions of the system. For example, a drug will transfer between two immiscible phases until its chemical potential is the same in both phases, when a state of equilibrium will be reached. The diffusional properties of a drug are relevant to processes such as the dissolution of the drug and its membrane transport.

References

1. *The Pharmaceutical Codex*, 12th edn. London: Pharmaceutical Press, 1994.
2. Atkins PW, de Paula J. *Atkins' Physical Chemistry,* 8th edn. Oxford: Oxford University Press, 2006.
3. Rytting JH *et al.* Suggested thermodynamic standard state for comparing drug molecules in structure–activity studies. *J Pharm Sci* 1972;61:816–818.
4. Christian JHB. Specific solute effects on microbial water relations. In: Rockland LB, Stewart GF (eds) *Water Activity: Influences on Food Quality.* New York: Academic Press, 1981: 825.
5. Ambrose U *et al. In vitro* studies of water activity and bacterial growth inhibition of sucrose-polyethylene glycol 400-hydrogen peroxide and xylose-polyethylene glycol 400-hydrogen peroxide pastes used to treat infected wounds. *Antimicrob Agents Chemother* 1991;35:1799–1803.
6. Hussong D. Water activity and pharmaceutical manufacturing; a regulatory microbiology perspective. In Cundell A, Fontana A (eds) *Water Activity Applications in the Pharmaceutical Industry.* River Grove, IL: Davis Healthcare International Publishing, 2009: 253–257.
7. Streng WH *et al.* Relationship between osmolality and osmolarity. *J Pharm Sci* 1978;67:384–386.
8. Willis DM *et al.* Unsuspected hyperosmolality of oral solutions contributing to necrotizing enterocolitis in very-low-birth-weight infants. *Pediatrics* 1977;60:535–538.
9. White KC, Harkavy KL. Hypertonic formula resulting from added oral medications. *Am J Dis Child* 1982;136:931–933.
10. Luedtke SA. Pediatric and neonatal therapy. In: Helms RA, Quan DJ (eds) *Textbook of Therapeutics: Drug and Disease Management,* 8th edn. Philadelphia: Lippincott, Williams and Wilkins, 2006: 325–340.
11. Lerman J *et al.* Osmolarity determines the solubility of anesthetics in aqueous solutions at 37°C. *Anesthesiology* 1983;59:554–558.
12. *The Merck Index,* 15th edn. London: Royal Society of Chemistry Publishing, 2013.
13. Pagliara A *et al.* Lipophilicity profiles of ampholytes. *Chem Rev* 1997;97:3385–3400.
14. Bouchard G *et al.* Theoretical and experimental exploration of the lipophilicity of zwitterionic drugs in 1,2-dichloroethane/water system. *Pharm Res* 2002;19:1150–1159.
15. Niebergall PJ *et al.* Spectral determination of microdissociation constants. *J Pharm Sci* 1972;61:232–234.
16. Leeson LJ *et al.* Structural assignment of the second and third acidity constants of tetracycline antibiotics. *Tetrahedron Lett* 1963;18:1155–1160.
17. Sturgeon RJ, Schulman SG. Electronic absorption spectra and protolytic equilibriums of doxorubicin: direct spectrophotometric determination of microconstants. *J Pharm Sci* 1977;66:958–961.
18. Streng WH *et al.* Ionization constants of cephalosporin zwitterionic compounds. *J Pharm Sci* 1976;65:1034–1038; 1977;66:1357.
19. Ishimitsu T *et al.* Microscopic acid dissociation constants of 3,4-dihydroxyphenethylamine (dopamine). *Chem Pharm Bull* 1978;26:74–78.
20. Honig B, Nicholls A. Classical electrostatics in biology and chemistry. *Science* 1995;268:1144–1149.

3

Drug stability

In this chapter we will:

- identify those classes of drugs that are particularly susceptible to chemical breakdown and examine some of the precautions that can be taken to minimise the loss of activity
- look at how reactions can be classified into various 'orders', and how we can calculate the rate constant for a reaction under a given set of environmental conditions
- consider the various factors that accelerate the decomposition of drugs in both liquid and solid states and see how far it is possible to manipulate these to achieve optimum stability
- examine methods for accelerating the drug breakdown using elevated temperatures. We will see how it is possible to estimate the stability of the drug for the required storage conditions from these measurements and so determine a time interval over which the drug retains sufficient potency for it to be used. Although such experiments cannot replace the rigorous stability-testing procedures on the product in the form in which it is finally to be marketed, they do lead to considerable saving of time at the product development stage when it is necessary to identify rapidly a formulation in which the stability is at an acceptable level.

The stability of proteins will be considered separately in Chapter 13.

3.1 The chemical decomposition of drugs

Many drugs are susceptible to some form of chemical decomposition when formulated in either liquid or even solid-dosage forms. Such degradation can lead to

rejection of a drug product for one or more of the following reasons.

- Chemical degradation of the active drug can lead to a substantial lowering of the quantity of the therapeutic agent in the dosage form. Many drugs, including for example digoxin and theophylline, have narrow therapeutic indices, and they need to be carefully titrated in individual patients so that serum levels are neither so high that they are potentially toxic, nor so low that they are ineffective. For these drugs, it is important that the dosage form reproducibly delivers the same amount of drug.

- Although chemical degradation of the active drug may not be extensive, a toxic product may be formed in the decomposition process. There are several examples in which the products of degradation are significantly more toxic than the original therapeutic agent. For example, the conversions of tetracycline to epianhydrotetracycline, of arsphenamine to oxophenarsine and of *p*-aminosalicylic acid to *m*-aminophenol in dosage forms give rise to potentially toxic agents that, when ingested, can cause undesirable effects.

- A substantial lowering in the therapeutic efficacy of the dosage form may occur as a consequence of physical or chemical changes in the excipients present in the dosage form, irrespective of any changes in the active drug.

- There may be noticeable changes in the physical appearance of the dosage form, for example, discoloration following the photochemical decomposition of the drug; mottling of tablets; creaming of emulsions and caking of suspensions. Although such changes may not affect therapeutic efficacy, they may lead to a loss of confidence by the patient in the product.

In this section we examine various ways in which drugs in both liquid and solid formulations can lose their activity, so that we can be aware of those chemical groups that when present in drug molecules can cause stability problems. We will later see how to prevent or minimise the chemical breakdown for each type of decomposition process. Although each decomposition scheme is considered separately, it should be noted that with some drug molecules more than one type of decomposition may be occurring at the same time; this, of course, complicates the analysis of the system.

3.1.1 Hydrolysis

Drugs susceptible to hydrolytic degradation

How can we tell whether a drug is likely to be susceptible to this type of degradation? If the drug is a derivative of carboxylic acid or contains functional groups based on this moiety, for example an ester, amide, lactone, lactam, and imide or carbamate (see Scheme 3.1), then we are dealing with a drug that is liable to undergo hydrolytic degradation. We will consider some examples.

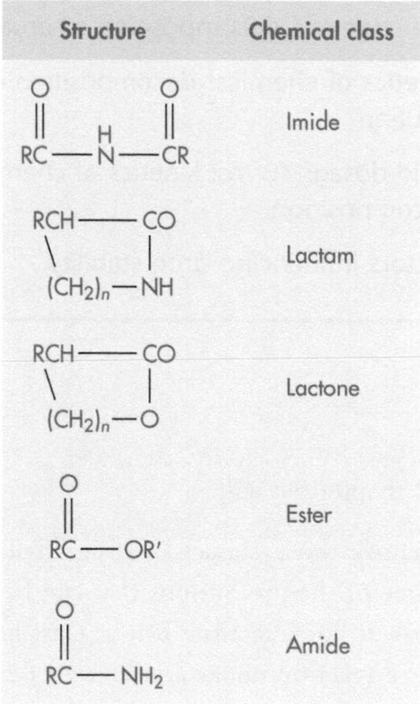

Structure	Chemical class
$\overset{O}{\underset{\|}{R C}} - \overset{H}{\underset{\|}{N}} - \overset{O}{\underset{\|}{C R}}$	Imide
RCH——CO \ | (CH$_2$)$_n$—NH	Lactam
RCH——CO \ | (CH$_2$)$_n$—O	Lactone
$\overset{O}{\underset{\|}{R C}} - OR'$	Ester
$\overset{O}{\underset{\|}{R C}} - NH_2$	Amide

Scheme 3.1 Examples of chemical groups susceptible to hydrolysis.

Drugs that contain ester linkages include acetylsalicylic acid, physostigmine, methyldopa, tetracaine and procaine. Ester hydrolysis is usually a bimolecular reaction involving acyl-oxygen cleavage. For example, the hydrolysis of procaine is shown in Scheme 3.2.

The hydrolysis of amides involves the cleavage of the amide linkage as, for example, in the breakdown of the local anaesthetic cinchocaine (Scheme 3.3). This type of link is also found in drugs such as chloramphenicol, ergometrine and benzylpenicillin sodium.

As examples of lactam ring hydrolysis we can consider the decomposition of nitrazepam and chlordiazepoxide, which is discussed in more detail

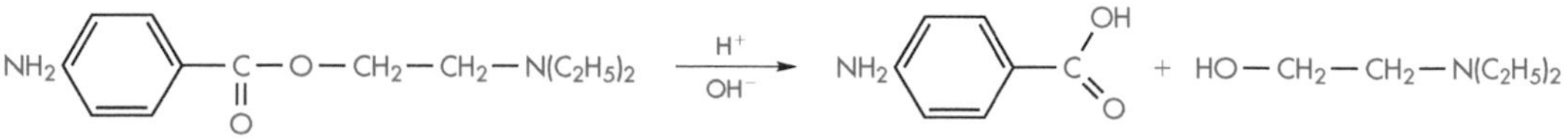

$$NH_2-\underset{}{\bigcirc}-\underset{\underset{O}{\|}}{C}-O-CH_2-CH_2-N(C_2H_5)_2 \xrightarrow[\mathrm{OH^-}]{\mathrm{H^+}} NH_2-\underset{}{\bigcirc}-\underset{\underset{O}{\diagdown}}{\overset{\overset{OH}{\diagup}}{C}} + HO-CH_2-CH_2-N(C_2H_5)_2$$

Scheme 3.2 Hydrolysis of the ester group of procaine.

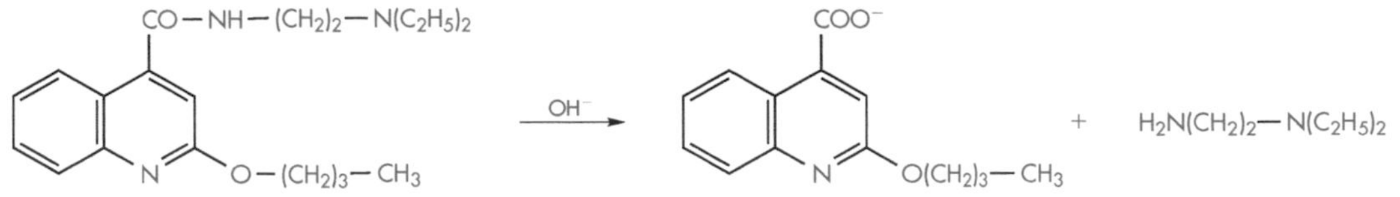

Scheme 3.3 Hydrolysis of the amide linkage of cinchocaine.

later (section 3.2.7). Other drugs, apart from the benzodiazepines, which are susceptible to lactam-ring hydrolysis include the penicillins and cephalosporins. The lactones pilocarpine and spironolactone are susceptible to hydrolysis, as are the imides glutethimide and ethosuximide.

A review by LePree and Connors[1] gives a detailed account of the mechanisms involved in the hydrolytic degradation of drugs.

Controlling drug hydrolysis in solution

Optimisation of formulation

Hydrolysis is frequently catalysed by hydrogen ions (specific acid catalysis) or hydroxyl ions (specific base catalysis) and also by other acidic or basic species that are commonly encountered as components of buffers. This latter type of catalysis is referred to as general acid–base catalysis. Both types of catalysis will be dealt with in greater depth in section 3.4.1. Several methods are available to stabilise a solution of a drug that is susceptible to acid–base-catalysed hydrolysis. The usual method is to determine the pH of maximum stability from kinetic experiments at a range of pH values and to formulate the product at this pH (section 3.4.1). Alteration of the dielectric constant by the addition of non-aqueous solvents such as alcohol, glycerin or propylene glycol may in many cases reduce hydrolysis (section 3.4.1).

Since only that portion of the drug which is in solution will be hydrolysed, it is possible to suppress degradation by making the drug less soluble. The stability of penicillin in procaine penicillin suspensions was significantly increased by reducing its solubility by using additives such as citrates, dextrose, sorbitol and gluconate. Adding a compound that forms a complex with the drug can increase stability. The addition of caffeine to aqueous solutions of benzocaine, procaine and tetracaine was shown to decrease the base-catalysed hydrolysis of these local anaesthetics in this way. In many cases, solubilisation of a drug by surfactants protects against hydrolysis, as discussed in section 3.4.1.

Modification of chemical structure of drug

The control of drug stability by modifying chemical structure using appropriate substituents has been suggested for drugs for which such a modification does not reduce therapeutic efficiency. The *Hammett linear free-energy relationship* for the effect of substituents on the rates of aromatic side-chain reactions, such as the hydrolysis of esters, is given by

$$\log k = \log k_0 + \sigma\rho \qquad (3.1)$$

where k and k_0 are the rate constants for the reaction of the substituted and unsubstituted compounds, respectively, σ is the Hammett substituent constant (which is determined by the nature of the substituents and is independent of the reaction) and ρ is the reaction constant, which is dependent on the reaction, the conditions of reaction and the nature of the side-chains undergoing reaction. Thus, a plot of $\log k$ against the Hammett constant (values are readily available in the literature[2]) is linear if this relationship is obeyed, with a slope of ρ. This concept has been used, for example, in the production of the best substituents for allylbarbituric acids to obtain optimum stability.[3]

3.1.2 Oxidation[4]

After hydrolysis, oxidation is the next most common pathway for drug breakdown. However, whereas the hydrolytic degradation of drugs has been thoroughly studied, their oxidative degradation has received comparatively little attention. Indeed, in cases where simultaneous hydrolytic and oxidative degradation can occur, the oxidative process has usually been eliminated by storage under anaerobic conditions without an investigation of the oxidative mechanism.

Oxidation processes

Oxidation involves the removal of an electropositive atom, radical or electron, or the addition of an electronegative atom or radical. Oxidative degradation can occur by *autoxidation*, in which a reaction is uncatalysed and proceeds quite slowly under the influence of molecular oxygen, or may involve *chain processes* consisting of three concurrent reactions – initiation, propagation and termination. Initiation can be via free radicals formed from organic compounds by the action of light, heat or transition metals such as copper and iron that are present in trace amounts in almost every buffer. The propagation stage of the reaction involves the combination of molecular oxygen with the free radical $R^{\bullet}$ to form a peroxy radical $ROO^{\bullet}$, which then removes H from a molecule of the organic compound to form a hydroperoxide, ROOH, and in so doing creates a new free radical (Scheme 3.4).

Initiation: $X^{\bullet} + RH \longrightarrow R^{\bullet} + XH$

Propagation: $R^{\bullet} + O_2 \longrightarrow ROO^{\bullet}$

$ROO^{\bullet} + RH \longrightarrow ROOH + R^{\bullet}$

Termination: $ROO^{\bullet} + ROO^{\bullet} \longrightarrow$ stable product

$ROO^{\bullet} + R^{\bullet} \longrightarrow$ stable product

$R^{\bullet} + R^{\bullet} \longrightarrow$ stable product

Scheme 3.4 Simplified oxidation scheme involving a chain process.

The reaction proceeds until the free radicals are destroyed by inhibitors or by side-reactions that eventually break the chain. The rancid odour that is a characteristic of oxidised fats and oils is due to aldehydes, ketones and short-chain fatty acids, which are the breakdown products of the hydroperoxides. Peroxides (ROOR′) and hydroperoxides (ROOH) are photolabile, breaking down to hydroxyl ($HO^{\bullet}$) and/or alkoxyl ($RO^{\bullet}$) radicals, which are themselves highly oxidising species. The presence of residual peroxides in polyoxyethylene glycols is a cause for concern when these excipients are used in formulation, as for example in the case of fenprostalene.[5]

Drugs susceptible to oxidation

We will consider some examples of drugs and excipients that are subject to oxidative degradation owing to the possession of functional groups that are particularly sensitive to oxidation.

Steroids and sterols represent an important class of drugs that are subject to oxidative degradation through the possession of carbon–carbon double bonds (alkene moieties) to which peroxyl radicals can readily add. Similarly, *polyunsaturated fatty acids*, commonly used in drug formulations, are particularly susceptible to oxidation and care must be exercised to minimise degradation in formulations containing high concentrations of, for example, vegetable oils.[6] For drugs such as the cholesterol-lowering agent *simvastatin* (**I**) that contain conjugated double bonds, addition of peroxyl radicals may lead to the formation of polymeric peroxides (simvastatin polymerises up to a pentamer[7]), cleavage of which produces epoxides which may further degrade into aldehydes or ketones.

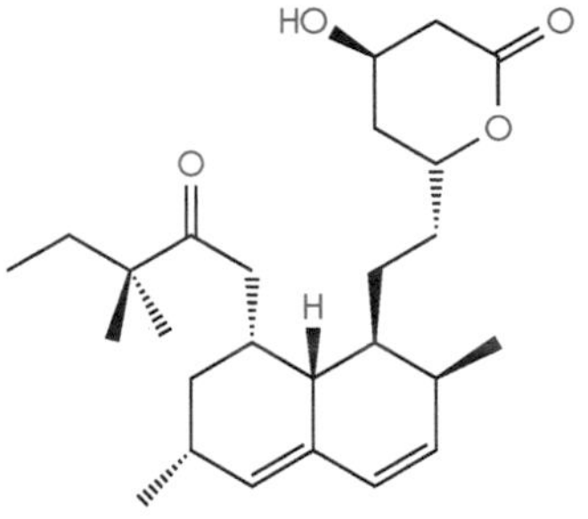

Structure I Simvastatin

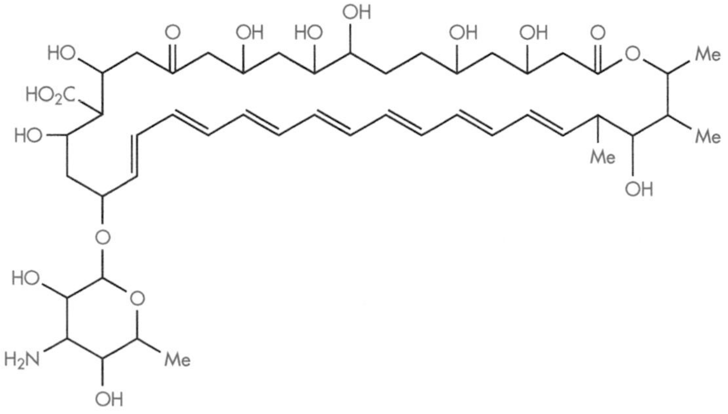

Structure II Amphotericin B

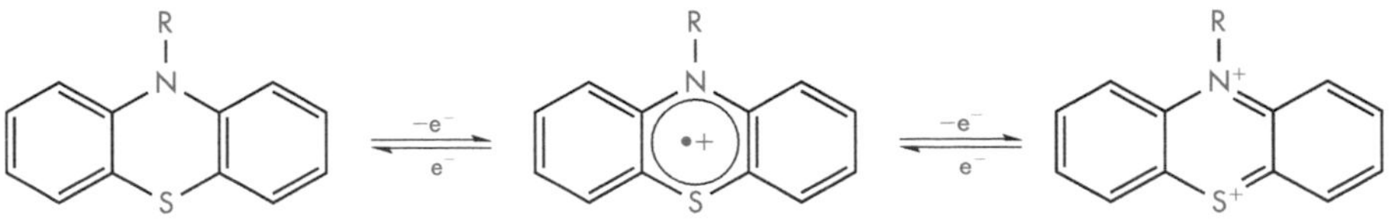

Scheme 3.5 Oxidation of phenothiazines.

Polyene antibiotics, such as amphotericin B (**II**), which contains seven conjugated double bonds (heptaene moiety), are subject to attack by peroxyl radicals, leading to aggregation and loss of activity.[8]

The oxidation of *phenothiazines* to the sulfoxide involves two single-electron transfer reactions involving a radical cation intermediate, as shown in Scheme 3.5. The sulfoxide is subsequently formed by reaction of the cation with water.

The ether group in drugs such as *econazole nitrate* (**III**) and *miconazole nitrate* (**IV**) is susceptible to oxidation. The process involves removal of hydrogen from the C–H bonds in the α-position to the oxygen to produce a radical, which further degrades to α-hydroperoxides and eventually to aldehydes, ketones, alcohols and carboxylic acids.

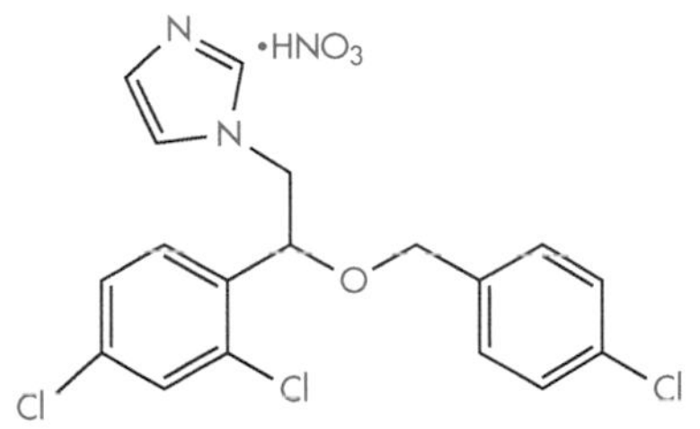

Structure III Econazole nitrate

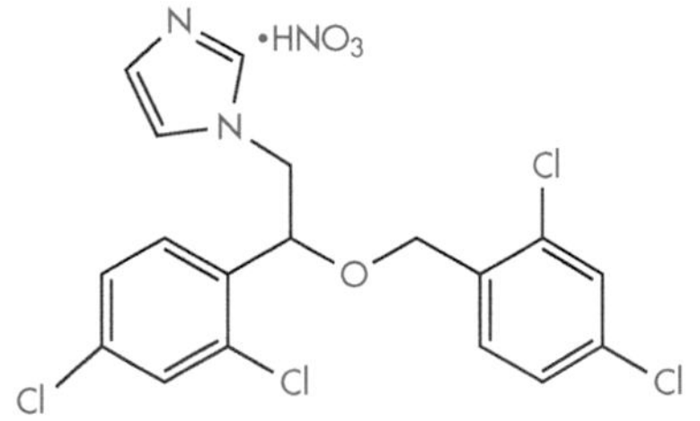

Structure IV Miconazole nitrate

Stabilisation against oxidation

Various precautions should be taken during manufacture and storage to minimise oxidation. The oxygen in pharmaceutical containers should be replaced with nitrogen or carbon dioxide; contact of the drug with heavy-metal ions such as iron, cobalt or nickel that catalyse oxidation should be avoided; and storage should be at reduced temperatures.

Antioxidants

It is very difficult to remove all of the oxygen from a container and even traces of oxygen are sufficient to initiate the oxidation chain. The propagation of the chain reaction may be prevented or delayed by adding low concentrations of compounds that act as inhibitors. Such compounds are called *antioxidants* and interrupt the propagation by interaction with the free radical. The antioxidant free radical so formed is not sufficiently reactive to maintain the chain reaction and is eventually annihilated. The structures of some commonly used antioxidants are given in Scheme 3.6. Reducing agents such as sodium metabisulfite may also be added to formulations to prevent oxidation. These compounds are more readily oxidised than the drug and so protect it from oxidation by consuming the oxygen. They are particularly effective in closed systems in which the oxygen cannot be replaced once it has been consumed. Chelating agents, such as ethylenediaminetetraacetic acid derivatives, may also protect the drug from autoxidation. These act by forming complexes with the heavy-metal ions that are often required to initiate oxidation reactions. Oxidation is catalysed by unprotonated amines such as aminophylline, and hence admixture of susceptible drugs with such compounds should be avoided.

3.1.3 Isomerisation

Isomerisation is the process of conversion of a drug into its optical or geometric isomers. Since the various isomers of a drug are frequently of different activities, such a conversion may be regarded as a form of degradation, often resulting in a serious loss of therapeutic activity. For example, the appreciable loss of activity of solutions of adrenaline at low pH has been attributed to *racemisation* – the conversion of the therapeutically active form, in this case the levorotatory form, into its less-active isomer.

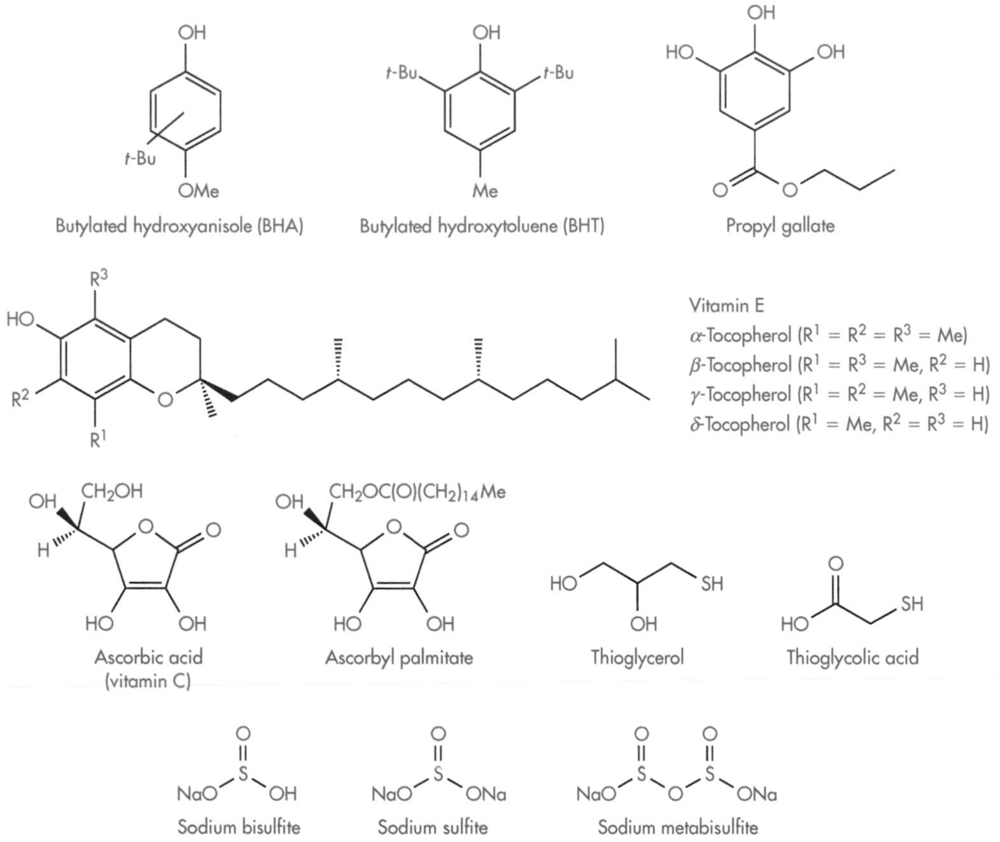

Scheme 3.6 Structures of some common antioxidants.

In acidic conditions the tetracyclines undergo *epimerisation* – a change of configuration at only one chiral centre. In this case, the change of configuration occurs at carbon atom 4 to form an equilibrium mixture of tetracycline and the epimer, 4-epi-tetracycline (Scheme 3.7). The 4-epi-tetracycline is toxic and its content in medicines is restricted to not more than 3%. The epimerisation follows the kinetics of a first-order reversible reaction (see equation 3.16). The degradation rate is pH-dependent (maximum epimerisation occurring at pH 3.2) and is also catalysed by phosphate and citrate ions.

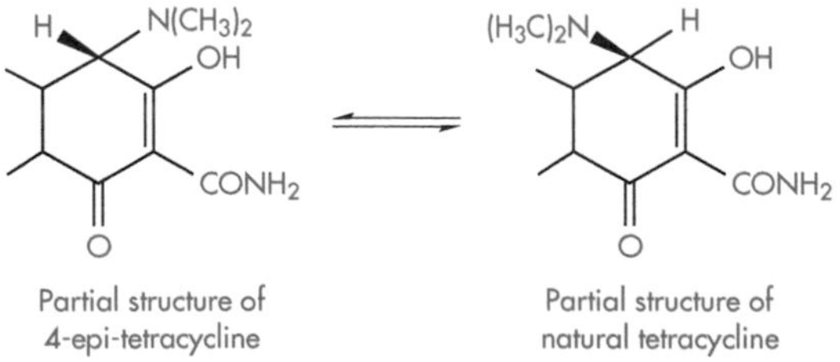

Scheme 3.7 Epimerisation of tetracyclines.

Although limits are set by pharmacopoeias on the level of the toxic 4-epi-anhydrotetracycline in tetracycline products, there may still be a problem when generic products are synthesised. As discussed in Chapter 16, even if the limit on these toxic impurities is very low (say, 0.005%), there may be three products (or the same product in different batches) with levels of such an impurity at 0.0048%, 0.004% and 0.002%.

Docetaxel is approved by the US Food and Drug Administration for treatment of locally advanced or metastatic breast cancer, head and neck cancer, gastric cancer, hormone-refractory prostate cancer and non-small-cell lung cancer. One of the principal paths of degradation of docetaxel is the epimerisation of the hydroxyl group at position 7, which results in the formation of 7-epidocetaxol (Scheme 3.8). The products of degradation have reduced activity or are completely inactive; these products demonstrate pharmacological and toxicological profiles which may be completely different from docetaxel.[9]

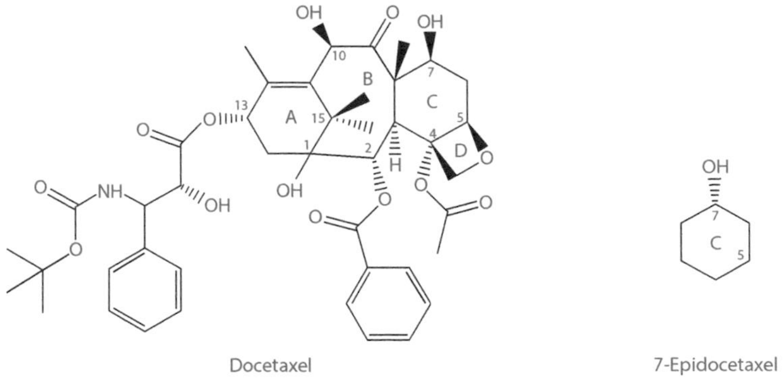

Scheme 3.8   Epimerisation of the hydroxyl group at position 7 of docetaxel to form 7-epidocetaxel.

Cephalosporin esters are widely used as intermediates in cephalosporin synthesis and as prodrugs for oral administration of parenteral cephalosporins. These esters undergo reversible base-catalysed isomerisation according to the mechanism shown in Scheme 3.9. A proton in the 2-position is abstracted by a base (B) and the resulting carbanion can be reprotonated in the 4-postion, giving a Δ^2-ester. On hydrolysis, Δ^2-cephalosporin esters yield Δ^2-cephalosporins, which are biologically inactive.

Cis-trans isomerisation may be a cause of loss of potency of a drug if the two geometric isomers have different therapeutic activities. Vitamin A (all-*trans*-retinol) is enzymatically oxidised to the aldehyde and then isomerised to yield 11-*cis*-retinal (Scheme 3.10), which has a decreased activity compared with the all-*trans* molecule.

3.1.4 Photochemical decomposition[10]

Many pharmaceutical compounds, including the phenothiazine tranquillisers, hydrocortisone, prednisolone, riboflavin, ascorbic acid and folic acid, degrade when exposed to light. As a result there will be a loss of potency of the drug, often accompanied by changes in the appearance of the product, such as discoloration or formation of a precipitate. Photodecomposition might occur not only during storage but also during usage of the product. For example, sunlight is able to penetrate the skin to a sufficient depth to cause photodegradation of drugs circulating in the surface capillaries or in the eyes of patients receiving the drug. Phototoxic dermatitis may occur when the allergen or irritant is activated by sunlight, as discussed in Chapter 12.

Primary photochemical reaction occurs when the wavelength of the incident light is within the wavelength range of absorption of the drug (usually within the ultraviolet range, unless the drug is coloured), so that the drug molecule itself absorbs radiation and degrades. Photodegradation may also occur with drugs that do not directly absorb the incident radiation, as a consequence of absorption of radiation by excipients in the formulation (*photosensitisers*) that transfer the absorbed energy to the drug, causing it to degrade. In assessing the photostability of a product it is therefore necessary to consider the final formulation rather than simply the drug itself. The rate of the photodegradation is dependent on the rate at which light is absorbed by the system and also the efficiency of the photochemical process. In formulations that contain low drug concentrations, the primary photochemical reaction follows first-order kinetics; the kinetics are more complicated at higher concentrations and in the solid

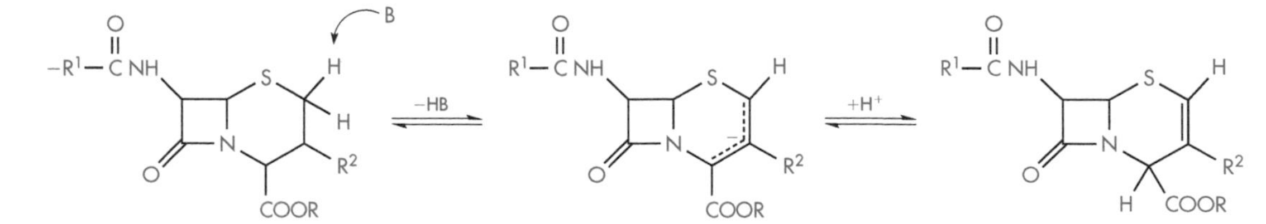

Scheme 3.9   Proposed mechanism for the base-catalysed isomerisation of cephalosporin esters.

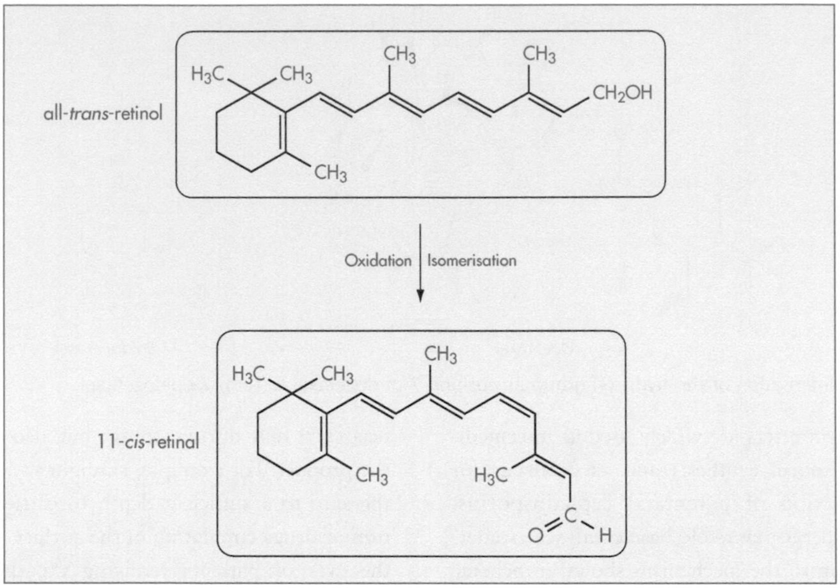

Scheme 3.10 Isomerisation of vitamin A.

state because most of the light is then absorbed near the surface of the product.

Although it is difficult to predict which drugs are likely to be prone to photodegradation, there are certain chemical functions that are expected to introduce photoreactivity, including carbonyl, nitroaromatic and N-oxide functions, aryl halides, alkenes, polyenes and sulfides.[11] The mechanisms of photodegradation are of such complexity as to have been fully elucidated in only a few cases. We will consider two examples – chlorpromazine and ketoprofen.

The phenothiazine *chlorpromazine* is rapidly decomposed under the action of ultraviolet light, the decomposition being accompanied by discoloration of the solutions (Scheme 3.11).

Chlorpromazine behaves differently towards ultraviolet irradiation under anaerobic conditions. A polymerisation process has been proposed[12] that involves the liberation of HCl in its initial stages. The polymer (**V**) was isolated and upon intracutaneous injection produced a bluish-purple discoloration typical of that observed in some patients receiving prolonged chlorpromazine medication. It was suggested that the skin

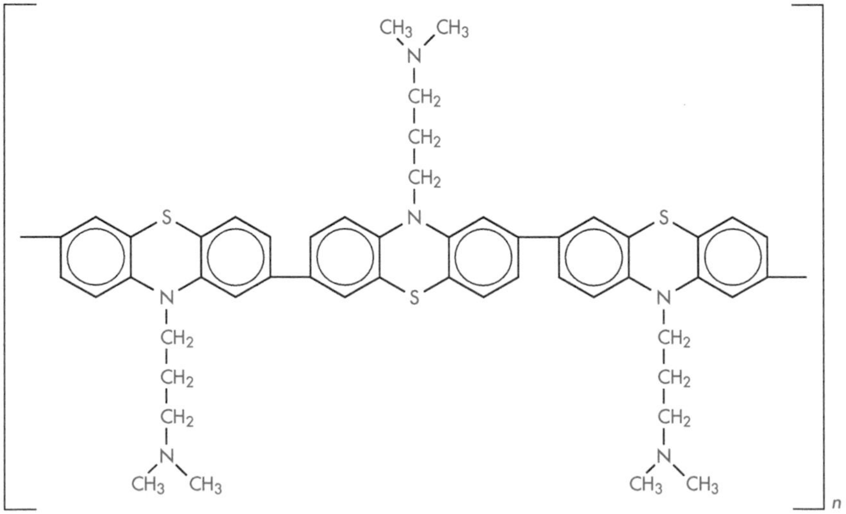

Structure V Polymer produced by the ultraviolet irradiation of chlorpromazine under anaerobic conditions.

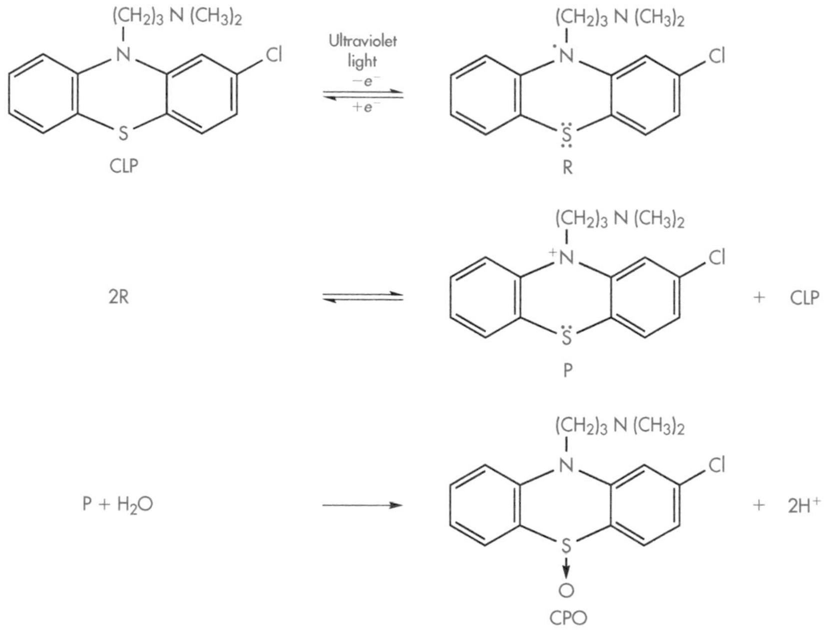

Scheme 3.11 Mechanism proposed for the effect of ultraviolet light on chlorpromazine (CLP). The first step of the photodegradation is the loss of an electron to yield the semiquinone free radical R. Further stages in the degradation yield the phenazathonium ion P, which is thought to react with water to yield chlorpromazine sulfoxide (CPO). The chlorpromazine sulfoxide is itself photolabile and further decomposition occurs. Other products of the photooxidation include chlorpromazine N-oxide and hydroxychlorpromazine.

Reproduced from Merkle FH, Discher CA. Electrochemical oxidation of chlorpromazine hydrochloride. *J Pharm Sci* 1964;53:620. Copyright Wiley-VCH Verlag GmbH & Co. KGaA. Reproduced with permission.

irritation that accompanies the discoloration may be a result of the HCl liberation during photodecomposition.

The photodegradation of *ketoprofen* can involve decarboxylation to form an intermediate that then undergoes reduction, or dimerisation of the ketoprofen itself, as illustrated in Scheme 3.12.

Stabilisation against photochemical decomposition

Pharmaceutical products can be adequately protected from photo-induced decomposition by the use of coloured-glass containers and storage in the dark. Amber glass excludes light of wavelength <470 nm and so affords considerable protection of compounds sensitive to ultraviolet light. Coating tablets with a

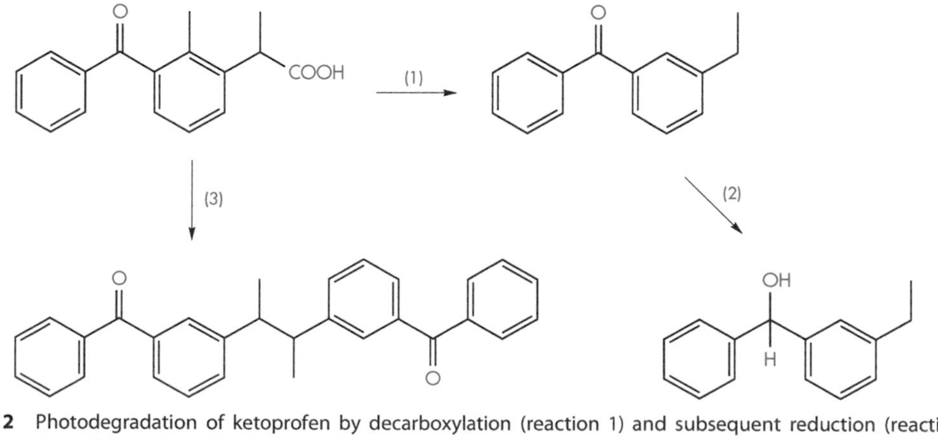

Scheme 3.12 Photodegradation of ketoprofen by decarboxylation (reaction 1) and subsequent reduction (reaction 2), and also by dimerisation of the ketoprofen (reaction 3).

Reproduced from Tønnesen HH. *Int J Pharm* 2001;225:1.

polymer film containing ultraviolet absorbers has been suggested as an additional method for protection from light. In this respect, a film coating of vinyl acetate containing oxybenzone as an ultraviolet absorber has been shown[13] to be effective in minimising the discoloration and photolytic degradation of sulfasomidine tablets.

3.1.5 Polymerisation

Polymerisation is the process by which two or more identical drug molecules combine together to form a complex molecule. It has been demonstrated that a polymerisation process occurs during the storage of concentrated aqueous solutions of aminopenicillins, such as ampicillin sodium. The reactive β-lactam bond of the ampicillin molecule is opened by reaction with the side-chain of a second ampicillin molecule and a dimer is formed (Scheme 3.13). The process can continue to form higher polymers. Such polymeric substances have been shown to be highly antigenic in animals and they are considered to play a part in eliciting penicilloyl-specific allergic reactions to ampicillin in humans. The dimerising tendency of the aminopenicillins increases with the increase in the basicity of the side-chain group, the order in terms of increasing rates being:

cyclacillin ≪ ampicillin < epicillin < amoxicillin.

Impurities in amoxicillin samples can include the dimer, trimer and other oligomers which, as discussed in Chapter 12, are possibly prime culprits in penicillin allergies as they are formed with peptide bonds and resemble peptides.

The hydrate of formaldehyde, $HOCH_2OH$, may under certain conditions polymerise in aqueous solution to form paraformaldehyde, $HOCH_2(OCH_2)_nO-CH_2OH$, which appears as a white deposit in the solution. The polymerisation may be prevented by adding to the solution 10–15% of methanol.

3.2 Kinetics of chemical decomposition in solution

Before we can predict the shelf-life of a dosage form it is essential to determine the kinetics of the breakdown of the drug under carefully controlled conditions. Unfortunately, drug decomposition often does not follow simple reaction schemes and in this section we will look not only at the traditional ways of classifying reactions but also at some of the complications that can arise with pharmaceutical preparations, which confuse this simple classification.

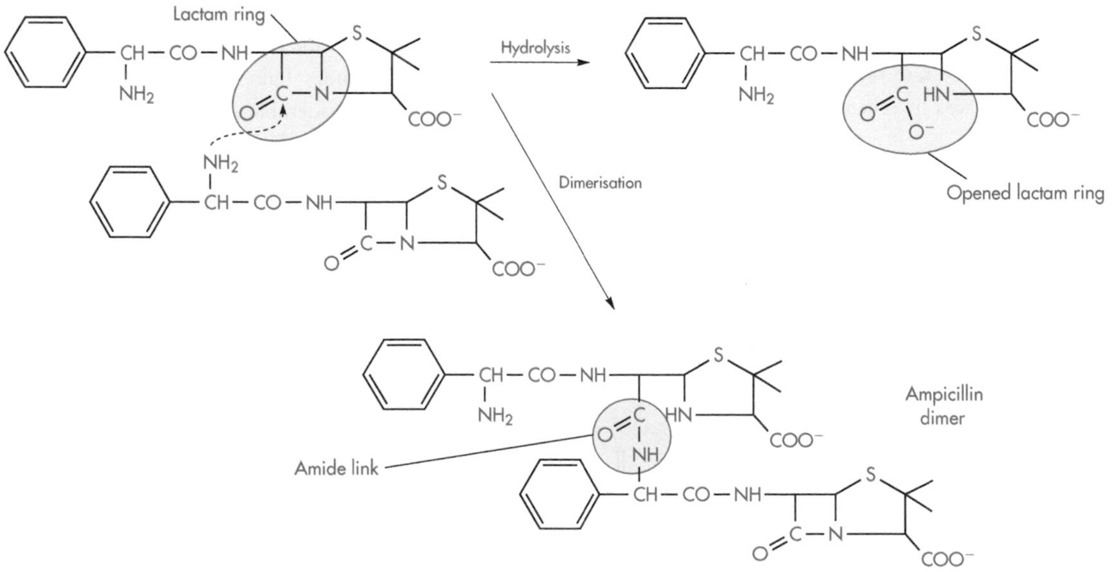

Scheme 3.13 Dimerisation and hydrolysis of ampicillin.

Reproduced with permission from Bundgaard H. Polymerization of penicillins: kinetics and mechanism of di- and polymerization of ampicillin in aqueous solution. *Acta Pharm Suec* 1976;13:9.

Key points

- The most common cause of degradation of drugs in aqueous systems is hydrolysis and the most susceptible drugs are those containing ester, amide, lactone, lactam, imide or carbamate groups. Hydrolytic breakdown is catalysed by hydrogen and/or hydroxyl ions and consequently the extent of hydrolysis may be reduced by formulating the product at the pH of maximum stability. The inclusion into the formulation of non-aqueous solvents may, in some cases, reduce hydrolysis by alteration of the dielectric constant. It may also be possible to achieve stability by modification of the chemical structure of the drug.
- Oxidative degradation is the second most common cause of drug breakdown and can occur by autoxidation, in which the reaction is uncatalysed and proceeds quite slowly under the influence of molecular oxygen, or may involve chain processes consisting of three concurrent reactions: initiation, propagation and termination. Oxidative degradation is a problem with drugs possessing carbon–carbon double bonds, such as the steroids, polyunsaturated fatty acids and polyene antibiotics. Such drugs can be stabilised by replacing the oxygen in the system with inert gases such as nitrogen; by avoiding contact with metals such as iron, cobalt and nickel; and by adding antioxidants or reducing agents to the solution. Some oxidative reactions are pH-dependent, in which case the product can be stabilised by buffering the system.
- Loss of activity of solutions of some drugs such as the tetracyclines can occur because of epimerisation of the drug molecule, while others such as vitamin A lose activity because of geometrical isomerisation.
- Photochemical decomposition can be a problem with drugs such as the phenothiazine tranquillisers and can cause discoloration of the solution and loss of activity. Formulations containing light-sensitive drugs have to be stored in amber glass containers, which remove the ultraviolet components of light.

3.2.1 Classifying reactions: the order of reaction

Reactions are classified according to the number of reacting species whose concentration determines the rate at which the reaction occurs, i.e. the *order of reaction*. We will concentrate mainly on *zero-order* reactions, in which the breakdown rate is independent of the concentration of any of the reactants; *first-order* reaction, in which the reaction rate is determined by one concentration term; and *second-order* reactions, in which the rate is determined by the concentrations of two reacting species.

Experimentally we can monitor the rate of breakdown of the drug either by its decrease in concentration with time or alternatively by the rate of appearance of one of the breakdown products. If we represent the initial concentration of drug A as a mol dm^{-3} and if we find experimentally that x mol dm^{-3} of the drug has reacted in time t, then the amount of drug remaining at a time t is $(a - x)$ mol dm^{-3} and the rate of reaction is

$$\frac{-d[A]}{dt} = \frac{-d(a - x)}{dt} = dx/dt \qquad (3.2)$$

Notice that the term a is a constant and therefore disappears during differentiation. We will use dx/dt to describe the reaction rate in this section.

If we assume that a typical reaction between a drug molecule A and a reactant B occurs when two molecules are in collision, then we might expect that the number of collisions, and hence the reaction rate, would be proportional to the concentration of the two reacting molecules, i.e.

Rate $\propto$ [A][B]

or

$$\frac{dx}{dt} = k[A][B] \qquad (3.3)$$

where the proportionality constant, k, is called the *rate constant*. The order of reaction is the sum of the exponents of the concentration terms in the rate equation and so this is an example of a *second-order* reaction. As we will see (section 3.4.1), many hydrolysis reactions are catalysed by H^+, OH^- or buffer components and so we can write equation (3.3) as, for example,

$$\frac{dx}{dt} = k_2[A][H^+] \tag{3.4}$$

k_2 is a second-order rate constant and has units of (concentration)$^{-1}$(time)$^{-1}$, for example (mol dm^{-3})$^{-1}$ min^{-1}. When the solution is buffered at constant pH, $[H^+]$ is now constant and we can write equation (3.4) as

$$\frac{dx}{dt} = k_1[A] = k_1(a - x) \tag{3.5}$$

where $k_1 = k_2[H^+]$. Since the rate of reaction now effectively depends on one concentration term it is a *first-order* reaction or, more correctly in this case, a *pseudo first-order* reaction (see section 3.2.3). The majority of decomposition reactions involving drugs fall into this category, either because the species reacting with the drug is maintained constant by buffering or because, as in the case of uncatalysed hydrolysis reactions, the water is in such large excess that any change in its concentration is negligible.

If as well as maintaining a constant amount of water in a reaction, we also maintain a fixed drug concentration, then equation (3.3) becomes

$$\frac{dx}{dt} = k_0 \tag{3.6}$$

where $k_0 = k_1[A] = k_2[A][B]$.

This type of reaction, which is called a *zero-order* reaction, can often occur in suspensions of poorly soluble drugs. In these systems the suspended drug slowly dissolves as the drug decomposes and so a constant drug concentration in solution is maintained.

We will now examine the ways in which we can determine the rate constants for these three types of reaction.

3.2.2 Zero-order reactions

In this type of reaction the decomposition proceeds at a constant rate and is independent of the concentrations of any of the reactants. The rate equation is given by equation (3.6) as

$$\frac{dx}{dt} = k_0$$

Integration of this equation (see Derivation Box 3A) gives

$$x = k_0 t \tag{3.7}$$

A plot of the amount remaining (as ordinate) against time (as abscissa) is linear with a slope of k_0 (concentration × time^{-1}).

Many decomposition reactions in the solid phase (section 3.3), or in suspensions, apparently follow zero-order kinetics. Figure 3.1 shows the hydrolysis of a suspension of acetylsalicylic acid.

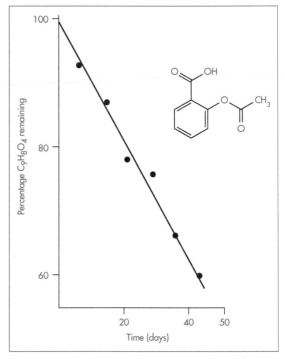

Figure 3.1 Hydrolysis of a suspension of acetylsalicylic acid at 34°C.

Reproduced from James KC. The hydrolysis of acetylsalicylic acid from aqueous suspension. *J Pharm Pharmacol* 1958;10:363. Copyright Wiley-VCH Verlag GmbH & Co. KGaA. Reproduced with permission.

3.2.3 First-order reactions

The rate of first-order reactions is determined by one concentration term and may be written using equation (3.5) as

$$\frac{dx}{dt} = k_1(a - x)$$

Integration of this equation (see Derivation Box 3A) gives

$$t = \frac{2.303}{k_1} \log a - \frac{2.303}{k_1} \log (a - x) \qquad (3.8)$$

According to equation (3.8), a plot of the logarithm of the amount of drug remaining (as ordinate) as a function of time (as abscissa) is linear if the decomposition follows first-order kinetics. The first-order rate constant may be obtained from the gradient of the plot (gradient = $-k_1/2.303$). k_1 has the dimensions of time^{-1}.

The time taken for half of the reactant to decompose is referred to as the *half-life* of the reaction, $t_{0.5}$. The half-life of a first-order reaction may be calculated from equation (3.9) (Derivation Box 3A)

$$t_{0.5} = \frac{0.693}{k_1} \qquad (3.9)$$

The half-life is therefore independent of the initial concentration of reactants. Example 3.1 shows the method of determination of rate constant and half-life for a drug which hydrolyses by first-order kinetics.

Even in the case of a reaction involving more than one reacting species, the rate may still follow first-order kinetics. The most common example of this occurs when one of the reactants is in such a large excess that any change in its concentration is negligible compared with changes in the concentration of the other reactants. This type of reaction is termed a *pseudo first-order reaction*. Such reactions are often met in stability studies of drugs that hydrolyse in solution, the water being in such excess that changes in its concentration are negligible and hence the rate of reaction is dependent solely on the drug concentration.

e.g. **Example 3.1 Calculation of first-order rate constant and half-life**

The following data were obtained for the hydrolysis of homatropine in 0.226 mol dm^{-3} HCl at 90°C:

Percentage homatropine remaining	93.4	85.2	75.9	63.1	52.5	41.8
Time (h)	1.38	3.0	6.0	8.6	12	17

Show that the hydrolysis follows first-order kinetics and calculate: (a) the rate constant; and (b) the half-life.

Answer

(a) The reaction will be first-order if a plot of the logarithm of the amount of homatropine remaining against time is linear.

Log percentage remaining	1.97	1.93	1.88	1.80	1.72	1.62
Time (h)	1.38	3.0	6.0	8.6	12	17

Figure 3.2 shows a linear plot with a gradient = $-(1.96 - 1.55)/(20 - 2) = -2.278 \times 10^{-2}$ h^{-1}.

Gradient = $-k_1/2.303$

Therefore,

$k_1 = 5.25 \times 10^{-2}$ h^{-1}

(b) From equation (3.9),

$t_{0.5} = 0.693/k_1 = 13.2$ h

The half-life of the reaction is 13.2 h.

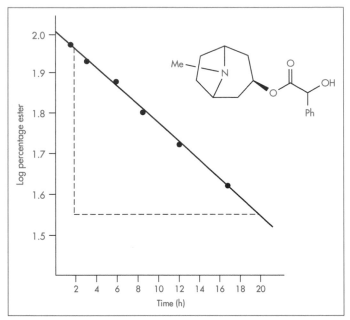

Figure 3.2 First-order plot for hydrolysis of homatropine in hydrochloric acid (0.226 mol dm^{-3}) at 90°C.
Data from Krasowska MH *et al.* Stability of homatropine in aqueous solution. *Dansk Tidsskr Farm* 1968;42:170, with permission.

3.2.4 Second-order reactions

The rate of a second-order reaction is determined by the concentrations of two reacting species. The general rate equation is given by equation (3.3) as

$$\frac{dx}{dt} = k_2[A][B]$$

In most second-order reactions the reactants have different initial concentrations, in which case the rate equation is given by

$$\frac{dx}{dt} = k_2(a - x)(b - x) \tag{3.10}$$

Integration of this equation, as shown in Derivation Box 3A, yields

$$t = \frac{2.303}{k_2(a - b)} \log \frac{b}{a} + \frac{2.303}{k_2(a - b)} \log \frac{(a - x)}{(b - x)} \tag{3.11}$$

from which it is seen that k_2 can then be obtained from the gradient, $2.303/k_2(a - b)$, of a plot of t (as ordinate) against $\log[(a - x)/(b - x)]$ (as abscissa).

An examination of equation (3.11) shows that the second-order rate constant is dependent on the units used to express concentration; the units of k_2 are concentration^{-1} time^{-1}.

For second-order reactions in which both concentration terms refer to the same reactant or in which the initial concentrations of the two reactants are the same we may write

$$\frac{-d[A]}{dt} = k_2[A]^2 \text{ and } \frac{dx}{dt} = k_2(a - x)^2$$

Integration as shown in Derivation Box 3A yields

$$t = \frac{1}{k_2}\left[\frac{1}{a - x} - \frac{1}{a}\right] = \frac{x}{k_2 a(a - x)} \tag{3.12}$$

from which it is seen that a plot of t (ordinate) against $x/[a(a - x)]$ (abscissa) yields a linear plot of gradient $1/k_2$.

The half-life of a reaction that follows equation (3.12) is given by

$$t_{0.5} = 1/(k_2 a) \tag{3.13}$$

Unlike $t_{0.5}$ for first-order reactions, the half-life of the second-order reaction is dependent on the initial concentration of reactants. It is not possible to derive a simple expression for the half-life of a second-order reaction with unequal initial concentrations.

3.2.5 Third-order reactions

Third-order reactions are only rarely encountered in drug stability studies involving, as they do, the simultaneous collision of three reactant molecules. The overall rate of ampicillin breakdown by simultaneous hydrolysis and polymerisation may be represented by an equation of the form

$$\frac{-d[A]}{dt} = k_a[A] + k_b[A]^2 + k_c[A]^3 \qquad (3.14)$$

where k_a, k_b and k_c are the pH-dependent apparent rate constant for hydrolysis, uncatalysed polymerisation and the general acid–base-catalysed polymerisation of ampicillin, respectively.[14] As seen from equation (3.14), the decomposition rate shows both second-order and third-order dependency on the total ampicillin concentration [A].

3.2.6 Determination of the order of reaction

The most obvious method of determining the order of a reaction is to determine the amount of drug decomposed after various intervals and to substitute the data into the integrated equations for zero-, first- and second-order reactions. The equation giving the most consistent value of k for a series of time intervals is that corresponding most closely to the order of the reaction. Alternatively, the data may be displayed graphically according to the linear equations for the various orders of reactions until a straight-line plot is obtained. Thus, for example, if the data yield a linear graph when plotted as t against $\log(a - x)$, the reaction is then taken to be first-order.

Fitting data to the standard rate equations may, however, produce misleading results if a fractional order of reaction applies. An alternative method of determining the order of reaction, which avoids this problem, is based on equation (3.15):

$$\log t_{0.5} = \log\left[\frac{2^{n-1} - 1}{k(n - 1)}\right] + (1 - n)\log C_0 \qquad (3.15)$$

The half-life of the reaction is determined for a series of initial drug concentrations, C_0, and the order, n, is calculated from the slope of plots of $\log t_{0.5}$ as a function of $\log C_0$. The method of determination of order or reaction using equation (3.15) is shown by Example 3.2.

3.2.7 Complex reactions

There are many examples of drugs in which decomposition occurs simultaneously by two or more pathways, or involves a sequence of decomposition steps or a reversible reaction. Indeed, the degradation pathways of some drugs include examples of each of these types of complex reactions. Modification of the rate equations is necessary whenever such reactions are encountered.

Reversible reactions

Treatment of the kinetics of a reversible reaction involves two rate constants: one, k_f, to describe the rate of the forward reaction, and the other, k_r, to describe the rate of the reverse reaction. For the simplest example in which both of these reactions are first-order, that is

$$A \; \frac{k_f}{k_r} \; B$$

the rate of decomposition of reactant is given by equation (3.16) (Derivation Box 3B):

$$\frac{-d[A]}{dt} = k_f[A] - k_r[B] \qquad (3.16)$$

If the initial concentration, $[A]_0$, the concentration at time t, $[A]$ and the equilibrium concentration of reactant A, $[A]_{eq}$, are known, then, as explained in Derivation Box 3B, plots of t (as ordinate) against $\log [([A]_0 - [A]_{eq})/([A] - [A]_{eq})]$ should be linear with a gradient of $2.303/(k_f + k_r)$, from which values of the sum of the equilibrium constants k_f and k_r may be determined. Individual values of k_f and k_r can then be evaluated by combining this sum with the equilibrium constant K, which is the ratio of the concentration of products formed by each reaction at equilibrium,

$$K = \frac{[B]_{eq}}{[A]_{eq}} = \frac{1 - [A]_{eq}}{[A]_{eq}} = \frac{k_f}{k_r} \qquad (3.17)$$

The epimerisation of tetracycline (see section 3.1.3) follows first-order reversible decomposition kinetics; Example 3.3 shows how to calculate rate constants for the epimerisation of this drug.

Example 3.2 Determination of the order of reaction

The kinetics of decomposition of a drug in aqueous solution were studied using a series of solutions of different initial drug concentrations, C_0. For each solution the time taken for half the drug to decompose (that is, $t_{0.5}$) was determined with the following results:

C_0 (mol dm^{-3})	4.625	1.698	0.724	0.288
$t_{0.5}$ (min)	87.17	240.1	563.0	1414.4

Determine the order of reaction and calculate the rate constant.

Answer

Application of equation (3.15) requires values for $\log C_0$ and $\log t_{0.5}$; thus

$\log C_0$	0.665	0.230	−0.140	−0.540
$\log t_{0.5}$	1.94	2.38	2.75	3.15

A plot of $\log t_{0.5}$ against $\log C_0$ is linear (Fig. 3.3) with gradient $(1 - n) = -1.01$. Hence $n = 2.01$, i.e. the reaction is second-order.

The intercept of the graph (that is, the value of $\log t_{0.5}$ at $\log C_0 = 0$) is 2.60. Thus, from equation (3.15),

$$\log[(2 - 1)/k] = 2.60$$

and

$$k = 2.51 \times 10^{-3}(\text{mol dm}^{-3})^{-1}\,\text{min}^{-1}$$

Example 3.3 Determination of rate constants for a reversible first-order reaction

The reversible epimerisation of tetracycline to 4-epi-tetracycline in 0.10 M phosphate buffer at pH 4 and 23°C was shown to follow first-order kinetics (Remmers *et al. J Pharm Sci* 1963;52:752). The gradient of a plot of t against $\log[([A]_0 - [A]_{eq})/([A] - [A]_{eq})]$ was 41.15 h and the equilibrium ratio R was 0.614. Calculate the value of the rate constants k_f and k_r.

Answer

$K = k_f/k_r = 0.614$, therefore $k_f = 0.614\,k_r$

Gradient $= 2.303/(k_f + k_r)$

$= 2.303/(0.614\,k_r + k_r) = 41.15$ h

Therefore

$k_r = 0.035$ h^{-1} and $k_f = 0.056 - 0.035$

$= 0.021$ h^{-1}

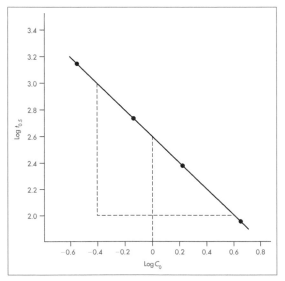

Figure 3.3 Plot of log of half-life ($t_{0.5}$) against log of initial drug concentration (C_0) (see Example 3.2).

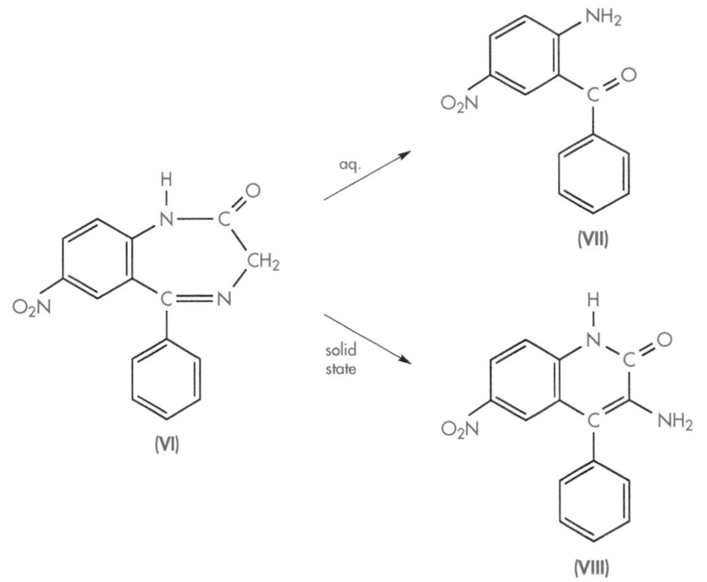

Scheme 3.14 Simplified decomposition scheme for nitrazepam (**VI**) in the solid state and aqueous solution. The main decomposition product is 2-amino-5-nitrobenzophenone (**VII**) in aqueous solution and 3-amino-6-nitro-4-phenyl-2(1*H*)-quinolone (**VIII**) in the solid state.

Reproduced with permission from Meyer W *et al.* Analysis and stability of various pharmaceutically interesting benzodiazepines. 1. Diazepam and nitrazepam, course of hydrolysis and determination of a circle contraction to isomeric quinolone derivatives. *Pharmazie* 1972;27:32.

Parallel reactions

The decomposition of many drugs involves two or more pathways, the preferred route of reaction being dependent on reaction condition. Nitrazepam (**VI**) decomposes in two pseudo first-order parallel reactions, giving different breakdown products in solution and in the solid state, as illustrated in Scheme 3.14. Decomposition of nitrazepam tablets in the presence of moisture will occur by both routes, the ratio of the two products being dependent on the amount of water present.

In other cases decomposition may occur simultaneously by two different processes, as in the simultaneous hydrolysis and epimerisation of pilocarpine (Example 3.4).

The overall rate equation for a parallel reaction is the sum of the constants for each pathway. For example, for a decomposition of a drug X involving two pathways, each of which is first-order,

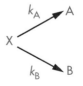

the rate equation is given by

$$\frac{-\mathrm{d}[X]}{\mathrm{d}t} = (k_A + k_B)[X] = k_{exp}[X] \tag{3.18}$$

where k_A and k_B are the rate constants for the formation of A and B, respectively, and k_{exp} is the experimentally determined rate constant. Values of the rate constants k_A and k_B may be evaluated separately from plots of [A] or [B] against $(1 - e^{-k_{exp}t})$ which have gradients of $k_A[X]_0/k_{exp}$ and $k_B[X]_0/k_{exp}$, respectively, as explained in Derivation Box 3B, or from the ratio R of the concentration of products formed by each reaction at equilibrium using

$$k_A = k_{exp} \frac{R}{(R+1)} \tag{3.19}$$

and

$$k_B = \frac{k_{exp}}{(R+1)} \tag{3.20}$$

Consecutive reactions

The simplest example of a consecutive reaction is that described by a sequence

$$A \xrightarrow{k_A} B \xrightarrow{k_B} C$$

Example 3.4 Calculation of rate constants of parallel reactions

Pilocarpine has been shown to undergo simultaneous hydrolysis and epimerisation in aqueous solution. The experimentally determined rate constant, k_{exp}, at 25°C is 6.96×10^2 $(mol\ dm^{-3})^{-1}\ h^{-1}$. Analysis has shown that at equilibrium the percentage of the epimerised form of pilocarpine (isopilocarpine) at 25°C is 20.6%. Calculate the rate constants for hydrolysis, k_H, and epimerisation, k_E.

Answer

The ratio R of pilocarpine to isopilocarpine is

$$R = 79.38/20.62 = 3.85$$

From equation (3.19),

$$k_H = (6.96 \times 10^2)(3.85/4.85)$$

i.e.

$$k_H = 5.48 \times 10^2\ (mol\ dm^{-3})^{-1}\ h^{-1}$$

From equation (3.20),

$$k_E = (6.96 \times 10^2)/4.85$$

i.e.

$$k_E = 1.44 \times 10^2\ (mol\ dm^{-3})^{-1}\ h^{-1}$$

The rate constants for hydrolysis and epimerisation are 5.48×10^2 and 1.44×10^2 $(mol\ dm^{-3})^{-1}\ h^{-1}$, respectively.

where each step is a non-reversible first-order reaction. The hydrolysis of chlordiazepoxide follows a first-order decomposition scheme similar to that described in this equation (Scheme 3.15).

The rate constants k_A and k_B and also the concentration of the breakdown product C may be estimated using equations given in Derivation Box 3B (equations 3B.16, 3B.18 and 3B.20).

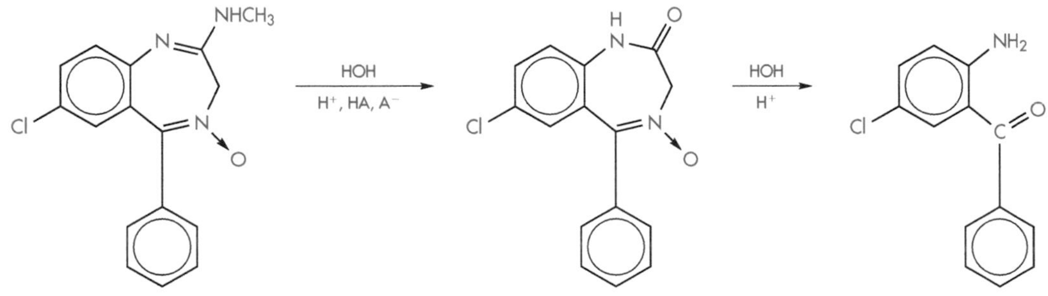

Scheme 3.15 Decomposition scheme for chlordiazepoxide. The neutral or cationic chlordiazepoxide (**IX** or **IXH⁺**) is transformed to the lactam (**X**) and, finally, in acidic solutions, to the yellow benzophenone (**XI**).

Reproduced from Maudling HV et al. Practical kinetics III: benzodiazepine hydrolysis. J Pharm Sci 1975;64:278. Copyright Wiley-VCH Verlag GmbH & Co. KGaA. Reproduced with permission.

Key points

- Reactions may be classified according to the order of reaction, which is the number of reacting species whose concentrations determine the rate at which the reaction occurs.
- The most important orders of reaction are zero-order (breakdown rate is independent of the concentration of any of the reactants), first-order (reaction rate is determined by one concentration term) and second-order (rate is determined by the concentrations of two reacting species). In solutions containing two reactants, the reaction rate may still follow first-order kinetics if one of the reactants (usually water) is in such large excess that changes in its concentration are negligible; such reactions are called pseudo first-order reactions. The breakdown of drugs in the majority of preparations in which the drug is dissolved in aqueous solution follows first-order or pseudo first-order kinetics.
- The rate constant of a reaction is determined graphically by substitution of experimental data in the linear equations for the appropriate order of reaction:
- Zero-order: $x = k_0 t$
- First-order: $t = \dfrac{2.303}{k_1} \log a - \dfrac{2.303}{k_1} \log(a - x)$
- Second-order: $t = \dfrac{2.303}{k_2(a - b)} \log\dfrac{b}{a} + \dfrac{2.303}{k_2(a - b)} \log\dfrac{(a - x)}{(b - x)}$
- The order of reaction is usually determined by plotting data according to the equations for each of the main types of reaction, linearity of the plot being indicative of the applicability of that order of reaction. This method is not suitable if decomposition follows fractional-order kinetics and in such cases an alternative method in which the half-life is plotted as a function of initial drug concentration may be used.
- The half-life of a reaction is the time taken for half of the reactant to decompose; the half-life of a first-order reaction is given by $t_{0.5} = 0.693/k_1$.
- The decomposition of many drugs can occur simultaneously by two or more pathways (parallel reactions), or may involve a sequence of decomposition steps (consecutive reactions) or may be a reversible reaction.

3.3 Solid-dosage forms: kinetics of chemical decomposition

In spite of the importance of solid-dosage forms, there have been relatively few attempts to evaluate the detailed kinetics of decomposition. Most of the earlier work was carried out with the sole objective of predicting stability, and data were treated using the rate equations derived for reaction in solution. More recently, the mechanisms that were developed to describe the kinetics of decomposition of pure solids have been applied to pharmaceutical systems and some rationalisation of decomposition behaviour has been possible. A comprehensive account of this topic has been presented by Carstensen,[15,16] on which the following summary is based.

It is convenient to divide single-component systems into two categories – those solids that decompose to a solid product and a gas, and those that decompose to give a liquid and a gas.

3.3.1 Solids that decompose to give a solid and a gas

An example of this category is p-aminosalicylic acid, which decomposes to a solid (p-aminophenol) and a gas (carbon dioxide):

$$NH_2C_6H_3(OH)COOH \rightarrow NH_2C_6H_4OH + CO_2$$

The decomposition curves that result from such a reaction show either (a) an initial rapid decomposition followed by a more gradual decomposition rate, or (b) an initial lag period, giving a sigmoidal appearance.

The shape produced by (a) can usually be accounted for by *topochemical* (or contracting geometry) reactions and that produced in (b) by *nucleation* theories.

The model used in the treatment of topochemical decomposition is that of a cylinder or sphere (Fig. 3.4), in which it is assumed that the radius, r, of the intact chemical substance decreases linearly with time, t, i.e., $r = r_0 - kt$, where r_0 is the initial radius. For the contracting cylinder model, the mole fraction x decomposed at time t is given by

$$(1 - x)^{1/2} = 1 - (k/r_0)t \qquad (3.21)$$

For the contracting sphere model,

$$(1 - x)^{1/3} = 1 - (k/r_0)t \qquad (3.22)$$

There are a few pharmaceutical examples of compounds that decompose by topochemical reaction. Thus, the decomposition of aspirin at elevated temperatures has been shown to conform to equation (3.21) (Fig. 3.5).

A similarity between equations (3.21) and (3.22) and the first-order rate equations was pointed out by Carstensen,[15] who suggested that this similarity might account for the fact that many decompositions in solid-dosage forms appear to follow first-order kinetics.

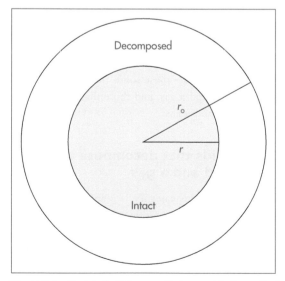

Figure 3.4 Model of sphere or cylinder used in theoretical treatment of topochemical reactions.

Reproduced from Carstensen JT. Stability of solids and solid dosage forms. *J Pharm Sci* 1974;63:1. Copyright Wiley-VCH Verlag GmbH & Co. KGaA. Reproduced with permission.

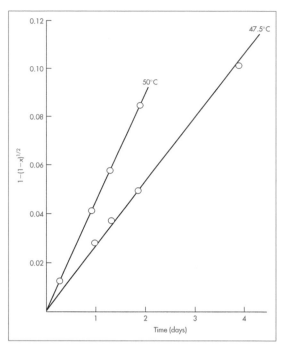

Figure 3.5 Decomposition of aspirin at elevated temperatures in tablets containing sodium bicarbonate, plotted according to equation (3.21).

Reproduced from Nelson E *et al.* Topochemical decomposition patterns of aspirin. *J Pharm Sci* 1974;63:755. Copyright Wiley-VCH Verlag GmbH & Co. KGaA. Reproduced with permission.

The sigmoidal decomposition curves can be interpreted using the Prout and Tompkins model. This model assumes that the decomposition is governed by the formation and growth of active nuclei that occur on the surface as well as inside the crystals. The formation of product molecules sets up further strains in the crystal since the surface array of product molecules has a different unit cell from the original substance. The strains are relieved by the formation of cracks. Reaction takes place at the mouth of these cracks owing to lattice imperfections and spreads down into the crevices. Decomposition on these surfaces produces further cracking and so the chain reaction spreads.

The equation proposed to describe decomposition by this process is of the form

$$\ln\left[\frac{x}{(1 - x)}\right] = \frac{k}{r_0}t + C \qquad (3.23)$$

where C is a lag-time term.

The decomposition curves of *p*-aminosalicylic acid are sigmoidal (Fig. 3.6) and linear plots are produced when the data are plotted according to equation (3.23).

Stability measurements made inadvertently in the lag periods of this type of decomposition would suggest zero-order kinetics.

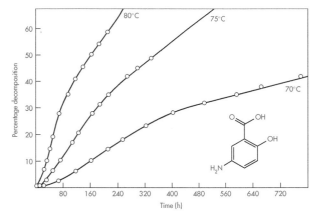

Figure 3.6 Degradation of powdered *p*-aminosalicylic acid in a dry atmosphere at elevated temperatures.

Reproduced from Kornblum SS, Sciarrone BJ. Decarboxylation of *p*-aminosalicylic acid in the solid state. *J Pharm Sci* 1964;53:935. Copyright Wiley-VCH Verlag GmbH & Co. KGaA. Reproduced with permission.

3.3.2 Solids that decompose to give a liquid and a gas

An example of a solid in this category is *p*-aminobenzoic acid, which decomposes into aniline and carbon dioxide. Decomposition causes a layer of liquid to form around the solid, which dissolves the solid. The decomposition curves show an initial lag period (Fig. 3.7) that corresponds to the establishment of the liquid

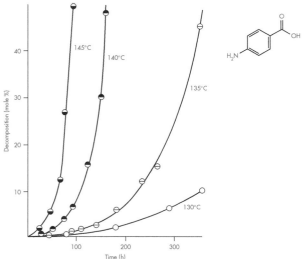

Figure 3.7 Decomposition curves of *p*-aminobenzoic acid at temperatures in the range 130–145°C showing the initial lag phase in *p*-aminobenzoic acid decomposition.

Reproduced from Carstensen JT, Musa MN. *J Pharm Sci* 1972;61:1113.

layer. Beyond this region, the plot represents first-order decomposition of the solid in solution in its liquid decomposition products. There are thus two rate constants, that for the initial decomposition of the solid itself, and that for the decomposition of the solid in solution.

3.4 Factors influencing drug stability

Before we can suggest ways in which we might prevent the decomposition of drugs, we should first consider the various factors that accelerate the decomposition processes. For convenience we will consider liquid and solid-dosage forms separately, although, as we will see, there are similarities in the influence of several factors on drug breakdown in both.

3.4.1 Liquid-dosage forms

pH

pH is perhaps the most important parameter that affects the hydrolysis rate of drugs in liquid formulations; it is certainly the one that has been most widely examined.

Studying the influence of pH on degradation rate is not as simple as might at first be imagined. If the hydrolysis rate of the drug in a series of solutions buffered to the required pH is measured and the hydrolytic rate constant is then plotted as a function of pH, a pH–rate profile will be produced, but this will almost certainly be influenced by the buffers used to prepare the solutions. It is probable that a different pH–rate profile would be obtained using a different buffer. To understand why this should be, we have to consider not only the catalytic effect of hydrogen and hydroxyl ions, which is called *specific acid–base catalysis*, but also the possible accelerating effect of the components of the buffer system, which we refer to as *general acid–base catalysis*. These two types of acid–base catalysis can be combined together in a general expression as follows:

$$k_{obs} = k_0 + k_{H^+}[H^+] + k_{OH^-}[OH^-] \\ + k_{HX}[HX] + k_{X^-}[X^-] \tag{3.24}$$

In this equation, k_{obs} is the experimentally determined hydrolytic rate constant, k_0 is the uncatalysed or solvent catalysed rate constant, k_{H^+} and k_{OH^-} are the specific acid and base catalysis rate constants respectively, k_{HX} and k_{X^-} are the general acid and base catalysis rate constants, respectively, and [HX] and [X$^-$] denote the concentrations of protonated and unprotonated forms of the buffer.

For a complete evaluation of the stability of the drug we need to evaluate the catalytic coefficients for specific acid and base catalysis and also to determine the catalytic coefficients of possible buffers that we might wish to use in the formulation.

First we will examine how to achieve a buffer-independent pH–rate profile, since this will show us at which pH the stability is greatest. By way of illustration we can consider a specific example of a stability study that has been reported for the antihypertensive vasodilator ciclosidomine. Experiments carried out at constant temperature and constant ionic strength using a series of different buffers over the pH range 3–6 produced the graphs shown in Fig. 3.8. These plots show that an increase of buffer concentration, particularly at pH 3, had a marked effect on the hydrolysis rate. The effect of the phosphate buffer on this system became less pronounced with increase of pH and was found to have a negligible effect above pH 7.5.

To remove the influence of the buffer, the reaction rate should be measured at a series of buffer concentrations at each pH and the data extrapolated back to zero concentration, as shown in Fig. 3.8. If these extrapolated rate constants are plotted as a function of pH, the required buffer-independent pH–rate profile will be obtained. Figure 3.9 illustrates the simple type of pH–rate profile that is obtained with codeine sulfate.

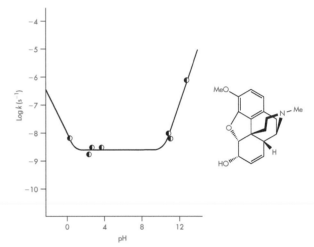

Figure 3.9 Log rate–pH profile for the degradation of codeine sulfate in buffer-free solutions at 60°C.

Reproduced from Powell MF. Enhanced stability of codeine sulfate: effect of pH, buffer, and temperature on the degradation of codeine in aqueous solution. *J Pharm Sci* 1986;75:901. Copyright Wiley-VCH Verlag GmbH & Co. KGaA. Reproduced with permission.

As we can see from Fig. 3.9, this drug is very stable in unbuffered solution over a wide pH range but degrades relatively rapidly in the presence of strong acids or bases. Since the influence of buffer components has been removed, this plot allows us to calculate the rate constants for specific acid and base catalysis. Removing the terms for the effect of buffer from equation (3.24) we have

$$k_{obs} = k_0 + k_{H^+}[H^+] + k_{OH^-}[OH^-] \qquad (3.25)$$

and consequently a plot of measured rate constant k_{obs} against the hydrogen ion concentration [H$^+$] at low pH will have a gradient equal to the rate constant for acid catalysis. Similarly, of course, if we plot k_{obs} against [OH$^-$] at high pH, the gradient will be the rate constant for base-catalysed hydrolysis. Example 3.5 illustrates the calculation of these catalytic coefficients.

The degradation of codeine is particularly susceptible to the effects of buffers. Its hydrolysis rate in 0.05 mol dm^{-3} phosphate buffer at pH 7 is almost 20 times

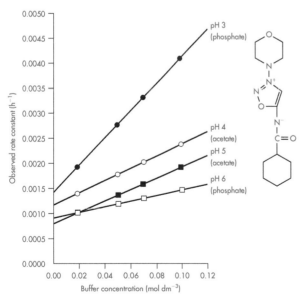

Figure 3.8 Effect of buffer concentration on the hydrolytic rate constant for ciclosidomine at 60°C as a function of pH.

Reproduced from Carney CF. Solution stability of ciclosidomine. *J Pharm Sci* 1987;76:393. Copyright Wiley-VCH Verlag GmbH & Co. KGaA. Reproduced with permission.

Example 3.5 Calculation of rate constants for base-catalysed hydrolysis

The following data were obtained for the hydrolytic rate constant, k_{obs}, of codeine sulfate in aqueous buffer-free solution at 80°C:

$10^7 k_{obs}$ (s^{-1})	5.50	4.40	2.30	1.25	0.70
pH	11.63	11.53	11.23	10.93	10.63

Determine graphically (a) the catalytic coefficient for base catalysis, k_{OH^-}, and also (b) the coefficient for solvent catalysis, k_0.

Answer

At high pH,

$$k_{obs} = k_0 + k_{OH^-}[OH^-]$$

where $[OH^-]$ is calculated from

$$p[OH^-] = -\log[OH^-] = 12.63 - pH$$

(Note: $pK_w = 12.63$ at 80°C.)

A plot of k_{obs} against $[OH^-]$ has a gradient of k_{OH^-} and an intercept of k_0.

From a graph of the above data,

$$k_0 = 2.0 \times 10^{-8}\,\text{s}^{-1}$$

$$k_{OH^-} = 5.2 \times 10^{-6}\,(\text{mol dm}^{-3})^{-1}\,\text{s}^{-1}$$

faster than in unbuffered solution at this pH, so this is a good drug to use as an example of the determination of the influence of buffer components on the breakdown rate.

In phosphate buffers of neutral pH, the major buffer species are $H_2PO_4^-$ and HPO_4^{2-}, either of which may act as a catalyst for codeine degradation. To find out which of these is the stronger catalyst, we can treat the experimental data in the following way. In neutral pH solutions we can write the following expression for the observed rate constant,

$$k_{obs} = k_0 + k_{H_2PO_4^-}[H_2PO_4^-] + k_{HPO_4^{2-}}[HPO_4^{2-}] \tag{3.26}$$

or

$$k_{obs} = k_0 + k'B_T \tag{3.27}$$

where $k_{H_2PO_4^-}$ and $k_{HPO_4^{2-}}$ are the rate constants for catalysis by $H_2PO_4^-$ and HPO_4^{2-} ions, respectively, and B_T is the total concentration of phosphate buffer. Notice that the terms for specific acid and base catalysis have little effect at this pH and we need not consider them in this treatment.

From equation (3.27), a plot of k_{obs} against B_T will have an intercept k_0 and a gradient k'. To find values for the catalytic coefficients, we rearrange the equation into the following linear form:

$$k' = \frac{(k_{obs} - k_0)}{B_T}$$
$$= \frac{k_{H_2PO_4^-}[H_2PO_4^-]}{B_T} + k_{HPO_4^{2-}}\left(\frac{B_T - [H_2PO_4^-]}{B_T}\right) \tag{3.28}$$

We can now see that a second plot of the apparent rate constant k' against the fraction of the acid buffer component present, i.e. $[H_2PO_4^-/B_T]$, will have an intercept at $[H_2PO_4^-/B_T] = 0$ equal to $k_{HPO_4^{2-}}$. Furthermore, the k' value at $[H_2PO_4^-/B_T] = 1$ is the other catalytic coefficient, $k_{H_2PO_4^-}$.

The relationship between the ability of a buffer component to catalyse hydrolysis, denoted by the catalytic coefficient, k, and its dissociation constant, K, may be expressed by the Brønsted catalysis law as

$$k_A = aK_A^\alpha \quad \text{for a weak acid} \tag{3.29}$$

and

$$k_B = bK_B^\beta \quad \text{for a weak base} \tag{3.30}$$

where a, b, α and β are constants characteristic of the solvent and temperature. α and β are positive and vary between 0 and 1.

In our treatment of the degradation of codeine sulfate we have not yet considered any effect that changes in its ionisation might have on its stability. Codeine has a pK_a of 8.2 at 25°C and so its ionisation state will change over the pH range 6–10. With this particular drug, the stability was not affected by any such changes. This is not the case with many drugs, however, and complex pH–rate profiles are often produced because of the differing susceptibility of the unionised and ionised forms of the drug molecule to hydrolysis.

By way of illustration we will look at the case of the hydrolysis of mecillinam (**XII**), which is an

Example 3.6 Calculation of the catalytic coefficients for buffer species

The following data were obtained for the hydrolytic rate constant k of codeine sulfate at 100°C in phosphate buffers of varying total concentration B_T at pH values of 6 and 8:

B_T (mol dm^{-3})	0.03	0.06	0.09	0.12
$10^7 k$ (s^{-1}) at pH 6	6.1	11.2	16.3	21.4
$10^7 k$ (s^{-1}) at pH 8	12.9	25.0	37.0	49.0

If the fraction of $[H_2PO_4^-]$ present in buffer solutions at pH 6 is 0.74 and at pH 8 is 0.23, determine graphically the catalytic coefficients for the buffer species (a) $H_2PO_4^-$ and (b) HPO_4^{2-}.

Answer

From equation (3.27), a plot of k_{obs} against B_T has an intercept k_0 and a gradient k'.

Therefore, plot k_{obs} against B_T from the given data at each pH and measure the gradient of the graph.

From the graph:

$$k' \text{ at pH } 6 = 1.7 \times 10^{-5} \, (\text{mol dm}^{-3})^{-1} \, \text{s}^{-1}$$

$$k' \text{ at pH } 8 = 4.0 \times 10^{-5} \, (\text{mol dm}^{-3})^{-1} \, \text{s}^{-1}$$

From equation (3.28), a plot of k' against the fraction of acidic buffer component, $[H_2PO_4^-]/B_T$, has an intercept of $k_{HPO_4^{2-}}$.

Also when $[H_2PO_4^-]/B_T = 1$,

$$k' = k_{H_2PO_4^-}$$

From the graph:

$$k_{HPO_4^{2-}} = 5.1 \times 10^{-5} \, (\text{mol dm}^{-3})^{-1} \, \text{s}^{-1}$$

$$k_{H_2PO_4^-} = 0.5 \times 10^{-5} \, (\text{mol dm}^{-3})^{-1} \, \text{s}^{-1}$$

varying extents and so each contributes to the overall profile shown in Fig. 3.10.

The various reactions thought to occur are

$$MH_2^+ + H^+ \xrightarrow{k_H} \text{products} \quad 1$$

$$MH^\pm + H^+ \xrightarrow{k_H'} \text{products} \quad 2$$

$$MH^\pm + H_2O \xrightarrow{k_0} \text{products} \quad 3$$

$$MH^\pm + OH^- \xrightarrow{k_{OH}'} \text{products} \quad 4$$

$$M^- + OH^- \xrightarrow{k_{OH}} \text{products} \quad 5 \quad (3.31)$$

The part of the pH–rate profile at very low pH (below pH 1.5) is given entirely by reaction (1). This is because the mecillinam exists as the cation MH_2^+, the hydrolysis of which will be acid-catalysed over this pH

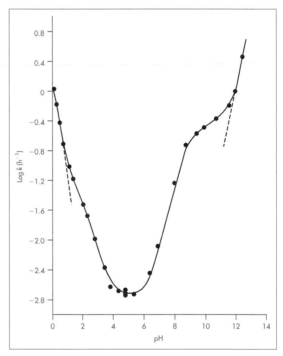

Figure 3.10 Log k–pH profile for the degradation of mecillinam in aqueous solution at 35°C (ionic strength = 0.5), where k is the apparent first-order rate constant for degradation in buffer-free solutions or in buffers showing no effect on rate of degradation.
Reproduced from Larsen C, Bundgaard H. *Arch Pharm Chem* 1977;5:66.

antimicrobially active amidopenicillamic acid. This amphoteric drug can exist as a cation, which we can write as MH_2^+, a zwitterion $MH^\pm$ or an anion M^-. Figure 3.10 shows the pH–rate profile at zero buffer concentration. The reason this plot is so much more complex than that of codeine sulfate is that each of the species present in solution can undergo specific to

Structure XII Mecillinam

range. The shoulder in the pH–rate profile at around pH 2 coincides approximately with the first pK_a value of mecillinam and indicates an increased acid catalysis of the zwitterion relative to the cationic species. The decrease of hydrolysis rate constant with increasing pH up to pH 4 can be explained by assuming that both reactions (1) and (2) are occurring. We can see from Fig. 3.10 that the hydrolysis rate is almost constant between pH 4 and 6, and this suggests that the hydrolysis is water-catalysed (reaction 3) over this pH region. The hydrolysis rate now starts to increase with increasing pH, which indicates that base catalysis is now the dominating factor. Between pH 6.5 and the pK_a for ionisation of the amidino side-chains ($pK_{a2} = 8.79$), it is reaction (4) that describes the hydrolysis rate. The plot changes slope at around pH 8 because it is affected by the changes that are occurring in the state of ionisation of the amidino side-chain. Above pH 12, the mecillinam exists in solution as the anion and this final part of the graph is described entirely by the base catalysis of this species (reaction 5).

Even though we may not always be able to explain the pH–rate profile as completely as we can for mecillinam, we can still, of course, choose the pH at which to buffer the drug solution for maximum stability. In the case of mecillinam this would be between pH 4 and 6.

We should also note that the *oxidative degradation* of some drugs in solution may be pH-dependent; for example, the oxidation of prednisolone is base-catalysed. Similarly, the oxidation of morphine occurs more rapidly in alkaline or neutral solution than in acid solution. The reason for this may be the effect of pH on the oxidation–reduction potential, E_0, of the drug.

The *photodegradation* of several drugs is also pH-dependent. For example, the photochemical decomposition of the benzodiazepine derivative midazolam (**XIII**) increases with pH,[17] and ciprofloxacin (**XIV**) is most sensitive to photodegradation at slightly basic pH at which the drug is in zwitterionic form, the stability increasing when the pH is lowered to 3–4[18] (Fig. 3.11).

During use, parenteral solutions may be exposed to light due to the low drug concentration and a large surface to volume ratio. Protection of infusion sets by a coloured or non-transparent outer package (e.g. foil) should always be considered, especially in the case of long-term infusion regimes.

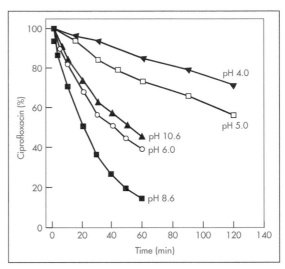

Figure 3.11 The effect of pH on the photodegradation of ciprofloxacin. Radiation source: mercury lamp at wavelength 313 nm.

Reproduced from Torniainen K *et al. Int J Pharm* 1996;132:53.

Structure XIII Midazolam

Structure XIV Ciprofloxacin

Temperature

Increase in temperature usually causes a very pronounced increase in the hydrolysis rate of drugs in solution, a fact which is used to good effect in the experimental studies of drug stability described above. Such studies are usually carried out at high temperatures, say 60°C or 80°C, because the hydrolysis rate is greater at these temperatures and can therefore be measured more easily. Of course, if a formulation has to be heat sterilised then its stability will, in any case, have to be measured at elevated temperatures. Figure 3.12 shows the pH–rate profiles for the degradation of codeine sulfate at several temperatures and also the calculated values at 25°C. We will now see how these calculated values can be obtained.

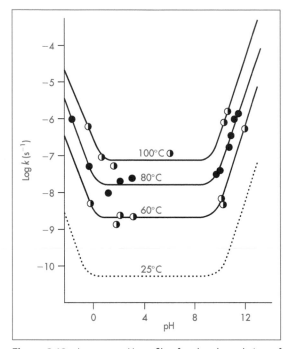

Figure 3.12 Log rate–pH profiles for the degradation of codeine sulfate in buffer-free solutions at several temperatures. The dashed line is the log rate–pH profile calculated from the Arrhenius equation.

Reproduced from Powell MF. Enhanced stability of codeine sulfate: effect of pH, buffer, and temperature on the degradation of codeine in aqueous solution. *J Pharm Sci* 1986;75:901. Copyright Wiley-VCH Verlag GmbH & Co. KGaA. Reproduced with permission.

The equation that describes the effect of temperature on decomposition, and which shows us how to calculate the rate of breakdown at room temperature from measurements at much higher temperatures, is the *Arrhenius equation*.

$$\log k = \log A - \frac{E_a}{2.303RT} \qquad (3.32)$$

In this equation, E_a is the activation energy, which is the energy barrier that has to be overcome if reaction is to occur when two reactant molecules collide. A is the frequency factor and this is assumed to be independent of temperature for a given reaction. R is the gas constant (8.314 J mol^{-1} K^{-1}) and T is the temperature in kelvins. We can see from equation (3.32) that a plot

of the log rate constant, k, against the reciprocal of the temperature should be linear with a gradient of $-E_a/2.303R$. Therefore, assuming that there is not a change in the form of the reaction as the temperature is changed, we can extrapolate plots of log k against $1/T$ to any required temperature and so determine the rate of breakdown at that temperature. We can also, of course, calculate the activation energy from the gradient of this plot. Figure 3.13 shows Arrhenius plots for the breakdown of the drug ciclosidomine at several pH values.

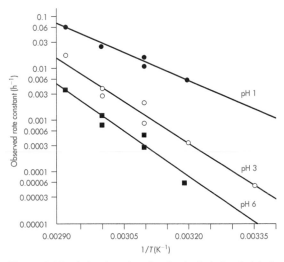

Figure 3.13 Arrhenius plots for the hydrolysis of ciclosidomine in buffer solutions at several pH values.

Reproduced from Carney CF. Solution stability of ciclosidomine. *J Pharm Sci* 1987;76:393. Copyright Wiley-VCH Verlag GmbH & Co. KGaA. Reproduced with permission.

When it is clear from stability determinations that a drug is particularly unstable at room temperature, then of course it will need to be labelled with instructions to store in a cool place. This is the case, for example, with injections of penicillin, insulin, oxytocin and vasopressin.

Ionic strength

We often need to add electrolytes to drug solutions, for example to control their tonicity. Consequently we must pay particular attention to any effect they may have on stability. In fact, the stability experiments that we considered earlier in this section should all be carried out at constant electrolyte concentration to avoid any confusion arising from possible differences in electrolyte effects between different systems.

Example 3.7 Calculation using the Arrhenius equation

The following values were determined for the specific acid-catalytic constants k_{H+} for an anti-inflammatory drug:

Temperature (°C)	95	90	85	75	65
$10^3 k_{H+}$ (mol dm^{-3})$^{-1}$ s^{-1}		8.15	4.85	2.76	1.02	0.29

Determine graphically: (a) the rate constant for acid-catalysis at 25°C; (b) the activation energy.

Answer

According to the Arrhenius equation, a plot of $\log k$ against $1/T$ has a gradient of $-E_a/2.303R$. From the graph:

(a) At $1/T = 3.356 \times 10^{-3}$ K^{-1}, $\log k = -5.85$.

Therefore, k at 25°C $= 1.41 \times 10^{-6}$ (mol dm^{-3})$^{-1}$ s^{-1}.

(b) Gradient $= -5.91 \times 10^3$ K.

Therefore $E_a = 113$ kJ mol^{-1}.

The equation that describes the influence of electrolyte on the rate constant is the *Brønsted–Bjerrum equation*,

$$\log k = \log k_0 + 2A z_A z_B \mu^{1/2} \quad (3.33)$$

In this equation, z_A and z_B are the charge numbers of the two interacting ions and A is a constant for a given solvent and temperature ($A = 0.509$ in water at 298K). μ is the ionic strength of the solution, which we can calculate from

$$\mu = \frac{1}{2} \sum (mz^2)$$
$$= \frac{1}{2}(m_A z_A^2 + m_B z_B^2 + \cdots) \quad (3.34)$$

For example, if we have a monovalent drug ion of concentration 0.01 mol kg^{-1} in the presence of 0.001 mol kg^{-1} of Ca^{2+} ions then the ionic strength of the solution will be

$$\mu = \frac{1}{2}[(0.01 \times 1^2) + (0.001 \times 2^2)]$$
$$= 0.007 \text{ mol kg}^{-1}$$

If the drug ion and the electrolyte ion are both monovalent, then the ionic strength will be equal to the total molality of the solution.

We can see from equation (3.33) that if we determine the rate constant of a reaction in the presence of a series of different concentrations of the same electrolyte and plot $\log k$ against $\mu^{1/2}$, then the plot should be linear with an intercept of $\log k_0$ and a gradient of $2A z_A z_B$. This is frequently found to be the case even in solutions of high ionic strength, although equation (3.33) is strictly valid only for ionic strengths of less than 0.01 mol kg^{-1}. At higher ionic strengths (up to about 0.1 mol kg^{-1}) it is preferable to use the following modified form of the Brønsted–Bjerrum equation in which we plot $\log k$ against $\mu^{1/2}/(1 + \mu^{1/2})$.

$$\log k = \log k_0 + 2A z_A z_B \left[\frac{\mu^{1/2}}{(1 + \mu^{1/2})} \right] \quad (3.35)$$

Figure 3.14 shows the degradation of phentolamine hydrochloride at two different pH values plotted according to equation (3.35). The gradients of these plots should be proportional to the product of the charge carried by the reactive species. Whether or not the gradient is positive or negative depends on the reaction involved. Reactions between ions of similar charge, for example, the acid-catalysed hydrolysis of a cationic drug ion, will produce plots of positive slope (i.e. the reaction rate will be increased by electrolyte addition), whereas the base-catalysed hydrolysis of positively charged drug species will produce negative gradients. Investigations of the influence of ionic strength on reaction rate may therefore be used to provide confirmation of the type of reaction that is occurring. For example, the gradients of the two plots of Fig. 3.14 are 0.260 and −1.759 at pH 3.1 and 7.2, respectively. Since the value of $2A$ at 90°C is 1.174, we can calculate values of the product $z_A z_B$ of 0.221 and −1.498 at pH 3.1 and 7.2, respectively. These values are not integers as they should be if the reactions involved were simple acid- and base-catalysed reactions. This has been explained by suggesting complex reactions between the buffer species and the phentolamine at each pH.

Solvent effects

Since we are considering the hydrolysis of drugs it might seem that an obvious way to reduce the breakdown would be to replace some or all of the water in

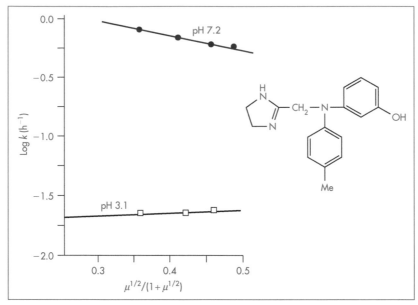

Figure 3.14 The effect of ionic strength, μ, on the hydrolytic rate constant, k, for phentolamine hydrochloride in buffer solutions of pH 3.1 and 7.2 at 90°C.

e.g. Example 3.8 Calculation using the Brønsted–Bjerrum equation

The following values of the rate constant, k, were obtained at 60°C for the hydrolysis of penicillin in phosphate buffer at pH 8.8 in a series of solutions of varying ionic strength, μ:

| k (h^{-1}) | 0.078 | 0.068 | 0.056 | 0.049 |
| μ (mol kg^{-1}) | 0.49 | 0.38 | 0.27 | 0.20 |

Plot the data in accordance with the modified Brønsted–Bjerrum equation (equation 3.35) and determine the gradient of the plot. Comment on whether this value would be expected for the acid catalysis of the protonated penicillin ion. (Note: assume a value of unity for A at this temperature.)

Answer

The gradient of the plot of $\log k$ against $\mu^{1/2}/(1 + \mu^{1/2})$ is +2.0. As expected for a reaction between ions of like charge (acid and protonated penicillin ion), the gradient is positive.

the system with a solvent such as alcohol or propylene glycol. As we will see in this section, however, this is effective only in certain systems and in others it can, in fact, increase the rate of breakdown. The equation that allows us to predict the effect of the solvent on the hydrolysis rate is

$$\log k = \log k_{\varepsilon = \infty} - \frac{K z_A z_B}{\varepsilon} \tag{3.36}$$

In this equation, K is a constant for a given system at a given temperature. We can see that a plot of $\log k$ as a function of the reciprocal of the dielectric constant, ε, of the solvent should be linear with a gradient of $-K z_A z_B$ and an intercept equal to the logarithm of the rate constant in a theoretical solvent of infinite dielectric constant. If the charges on the drug ion and the interacting species are the same, then we can see that the gradient of the line will be negative. In this case, if we replace the water with a solvent of lower dielectric constant then we will achieve the desired effect of reducing the reaction rate. If the drug ion and the interacting ion are of opposite signs, however, then the slope will be positive and the choice of a non-polar solvent will only result in an increase of decomposition.

Oxygen

Since molecular oxygen is involved in many oxidation schemes, we could use oxygen as a challenge to find out whether a particular drug is likely to be affected by oxidative breakdown. We would do this by storing solutions of the drug in ampoules purged with oxygen and then comparing their rate of breakdown with similar solutions stored under nitrogen. Formulations that are shown to be susceptible to oxidation can be stabilised by replacing the oxygen in the storage containers with nitrogen or carbon dioxide, by avoiding contact with heavy-metal ions and by adding antioxidants (see section 3.1.2).

Light

Photolabile drugs are usually stored in containers that exclude ultraviolet light, since exposure to light in this wavelength range is the most usual cause of photodegradation (see section 3.1.4). Amber glass is particularly effective in this respect because it excludes light of wavelength of less than about 470 nm. As an added precaution, it is always advisable to store photolabile drugs in the dark.

Surfactants

As might be expected, the presence of surfactants in micellar form has a modifying effect on the rate of hydrolysis of drugs. The magnitude of the effect depends on the difference in the rate constant when the drug is in aqueous solution and when it is solubilised within the micelle, and also on the extent of solubilisation. Thus

$$k_{obs} = k_m f_m + k_w f_w \tag{3.37}$$

where k_{obs}, k_m and k_w are the observed, micellar and aqueous rate constants, respectively, and f_m and f_w are the fractions of drug associated with the micelles and aqueous phase, respectively. The value of k_m is dependent on the location of the drug within the micelle. A solubilisate may be incorporated into the micelle in a variety of locations. Non-polar compounds are thought to be solubilised within the lipophilic core and, as such, are likely to be more effectively removed from the attacking species than those compounds that are located close to the micellar surface. Where the drug is located near to the micellar surface, and therefore still susceptible to attack, the ionic nature of the surfactant is an important influence on decomposition

rate. For base-catalysed hydrolysis, solubilisation into anionic micelles affords an effective stabilisation due to repulsion of OH^- by the micelles. Conversely, solubilisation into cationic micelles might be expected to cause an enhanced base-catalysed hydrolysis.

Many drugs associate to form micelles in aqueous solution (see section 5.3 in Chapter 5) and several studies have been reported of the effect of this self-association on stability. In micellar solutions of benzylpenicillin (500 000 units cm^{-3}) the apparent rate of the hydrogen ion-catalysed degradation was increased twofold, but that of water and hydroxide ion-catalysed hydrolysis was decreased two- to threefold.[19] Consequently, the pH profile was shifted to higher pH values and the pH of minimum degradation was found to be 7.0, compared with 6.5 for monomeric solution (8000 units cm^{-3}). When compared at the respective pH–rate profile minima, micellar benzylpenicillin was reported to be 2.5 times more stable as the monomeric solutions under conditions of constant pH and ionic strength.

3.4.2 Semisolid-dosage forms

The chemical stability of active ingredients incorporated into ointments or creams is frequently dependent on the nature of the ointment or cream base used in the formulation. Hydrocortisone in a series of commercially available bases exhibits maximum decomposition in polyethylene glycol base.[20,21] The reported shelf-life was only 6 months in this base, which makes manufacture on a commercial basis an unreasonable proposition, considering the length of time involved in distribution of the drug from wholesaler to patient.

Not only should possible stability problems be borne in mind in the choice of ointment base at the formulation stage, but also similar care should be exercised if the ointment is diluted at a later stage. Such dilution is, unfortunately, common practice in cases where the practitioner wishes to reduce the potency of highly active topical preparations, particularly steroids. The pharmaceutical and biopharmaceutical dangers of this procedure have been stressed.[22] Of particular interest here are the problems of drug stability, which can occur through the use of unsuitable diluents. An example has been cited of the dilution of betamethasone valerate cream with a cream base having a neutral to alkaline pH. Under such conditions, conversion of the 17-ester to the less-active betamethasone 21-ester can occur. Similarly, diluents containing oxidising agents could cause chemical degradation of fluocinolone acetate to less-active compounds.

Incorporation of drugs into gel structures frequently leads to a change in their stability, such as increased degradation of benzylpenicillin sodium in hydrogels of various natural and semisynthetic polymers.[23] At pH 6 in Carbopol hydrogels, the percentage of undecomposed pilocarpine at equilibrium is a simple function of the apparent viscosity of the medium.[24] The rate constant for degradation was not, however, significantly affected by changes in viscosity. Little influence of viscosity on the rate of oxidation of ascorbic acid in gels of polysorbate 80 has been noted.[25]

3.4.3 Solid-dosage forms

Moisture

Water-soluble drugs present in a solid-dosage form will dissolve in any moisture that has adsorbed on the solid surface. The drug will now be in an aqueous environment and its decomposition could be influenced by many of the factors we have already discussed when dealing with liquid-dosage forms. For example, decom-

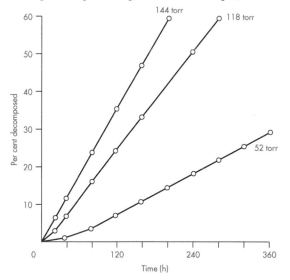

Figure 3.15 The effect of water vapour pressure on the decomposition of aminosalicylic acid.

Reproduced from Kornblum SS, Sciarrone BJ. Decarboxylation of *p*-aminosalicylic acid in the solid state. *J Pharm Sci* 1964;53:935. Copyright Wiley-VCH Verlag GmbH & Co. KGaA. Reproduced with permission.

position could now occur by hydrolytic cleavage of ester or amide linkages in the drug molecule and hence will be affected by the pH of the adsorbed moisture film. It is not surprising, therefore, that moisture is considered to be one of the most important factors that must be controlled in order to minimise decomposition.

We can get an idea of the extent to which moisture adsorption affects stability from the results shown in Fig. 3.15. We can see from this figure that an increase in the water vapour pressure (and therefore an increase in the amount of moisture associated with the drug) greatly increases the percentage decomposition at any given time. The problem is even more pronounced with drugs that are hygroscopic or that decompose to give hygroscopic products. In such cases it is worth trying to prepare a less hygroscopic salt of the drug.

In all cases it is important to minimise access of moisture during manufacture and storage. The correct selection of packaging is obviously important, although this is not as straightforward as you might at first think. For example, tablets containing a water-labile drug were found to be more stable in a water-permeable blister package at 50°C than in a sealed glass bottle and yet the situation was reversed at room temperature and 70% relative humidity.[26] The reason for this behaviour was attributed to the loss of considerable amounts of water through the film at 50°C, so improving stability, and the reverse diffusion at room temperature, so decreasing stability.

Excipients

One of the main ways in which the excipients of the solid-dosage form can affect the degradation of drugs is by increasing the moisture content of the preparation. Excipients such as starch and povidone have particularly high water contents (povidone contains about 28% equilibrium moisture at 75% relative humidity). However, whether this high moisture level has an effect on stability depends on how strongly it is bound and whether the moisture can come into contact with the drug. Magnesium trisilicate causes increased hydrolysis of aspirin in tablet form because, it is thought, of its high water content.

Many examples of the effects of tablet excipients on drug decompositions are reported in the pharmaceutical literature. Chemical interaction between components in solid-dosage forms may lead to increased

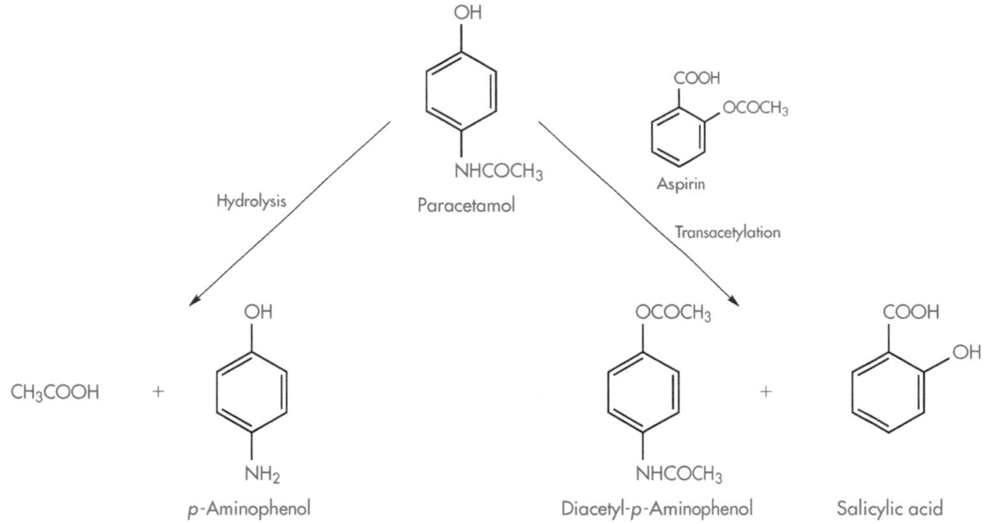

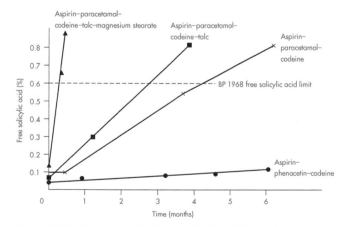

Scheme 3.16 Reactions showing the postulated transacetylation between aspirin and paracetamol and the direct hydrolysis of paracetamol.

Reproduced from Boggianno BG *et al. Aust J Pharm* 1970;51:S14.

decomposition. Replacement of the phenacetin in compound codeine and APC tablets by paracetamol in NHS formulations in Australia in the 1960s (because of the undesirable side-effects of phenacetin) led to an unexpected decreased stability of the tablets. The cause was later attributed to a transacetylation reaction between aspirin and paracetamol and also a possible direct hydrolysis of the paracetamol (Scheme 3.16).

Figure 3.16 shows the increased generation of free salicylic acid at 37°C in the tablets containing paracetamol. It is interesting to note from this figure the effect on stability of tablet excipients. Addition of 1% talc caused only a minimal increase in the decompos-

ition, while 0.5% magnesium stearate increased the breakdown rate dramatically.

Other studies on the influence of tablet excipients on drug decomposition have identified problems with stearate salts and it has been suggested that these salts should be avoided as tablet lubricants if the active component is subject to hydroxide ion-catalysed degradation. The degradative effect of the alkali stearates is inhibited in the presence of malic, hexamic or maleic acid owing, it is thought, to competition for the lubricant cation between the drug and the additive acid.

The base used in the formulation of suppositories can often affect the rate of decomposition of the active ingredients. Aspirin decomposes in several polyoxyethylene glycols that are often incorporated into suppository bases.[27] Degradation was shown to be due in part to transesterification, giving the decomposition products salicylic acid and acetylated polyethylene glycol. The rate of decomposition, which followed pseudo first-order kinetics, was considerably greater than when a fatty base such as cocoa butter was used.[28] Analysis of commercial batches of 100 mg indometacin–polyethylene glycol suppositories[29] showed that approximately 2%, 3.5% and 4.5% of the original amount of indometacin was esterified with polyoxyethylene glycol 300 (**XV**) after storage times of 1, 2 and 3 years, respectively.

Figure 3.16 Development of free salicylic acid in aspirin–paracetamol–codeine and aspirin–phenacetin–codeine tablets at 37°C.

Reproduced from Boggianno BG *et al. Aust J Pharm* 1970;51:S14.

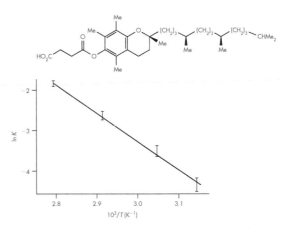

Structure XV Polyethylene glycol esters of indometacin identified in stored suppositories (n = number of ethylene oxide units).

Excipients present in tablet formulations can have an impact on the photostability of the product, the effect arising in many cases from impurities present in the excipients.[10] For example, free radical reactions involving phenolic impurities in tablet-binding agents such as povidone, disintegrants such as crospovidone, and viscosity-modifying agents such as alginates can lead to photodegradation. Similarly, coloured products may be formed by the reaction of aldehydes formed during spray drying or autoclaving of lactose with primary amine groups in the product.

Temperature

Investigation of the effect of temperature change on the stability of solid-dosage forms can be complicated for many possible reasons. The drug or one of the excipients may, for example, melt or change its polymorphic form as temperature is increased, or it may contain loosely bound water that is lost at higher temperatures. We should also remember that the relative humidity will change with temperature and so we must take care to keep this at a constant value.

Despite these possible complications, many authors have found that the effect of temperature on decomposition rate can be described by an Arrhenius-type equation; i.e. plots of log k against $1/T$ are linear. This then enables the stability to be predicted at room temperature from measurements made at elevated temperatures. Although we can calculate an apparent activation energy, E_a, from the gradient of the plots, we must remember that this does not have the same meaning as the activation energy for reactions in solution. The E_a value in the solid state is affected, for example, by changes not only in the solubility of

the drug in the moisture layer but also in the intrinsic rate of reaction. We cannot, however, use the Arrhenius equation in cases where decomposition shows an approach to equilibrium. Examples of such systems include vitamin A in gelatin beadlets and vitamin E in lactose based tablets. In these cases we can often use the van't Hoff equation to describe the effect of temperature on breakdown. We determine the equilibrium concentrations of products and reactants at a series of temperatures and then plot the logarithm of the equilibrium constant, K, against the reciprocal of the temperature (Fig. 3.17) according to the equation

$$\ln K = \frac{-\Delta H}{RT} + \text{constant} \tag{3.38}$$

Figure 3.17 Van't Hoff plot for vitamin E succinate decomposition in lactose base tablets.

Reproduced from Carstensen JT et al. Equilibrium phenomena in solid dosage forms. *J Pharm Sci* 1968;57:23. Copyright Wiley-VCH Verlag GmbH & Co. KGaA. Reproduced with permission.

Light and oxygen

We have examined above the stability problems that arise with drugs that are susceptible to photodecomposition or oxidation. We will not reconsider them here but merely re-emphasise that we should take all the necessary precautions to exclude light or oxygen when storing these drugs. In this respect we should remember that water contains dissolved oxygen and so the presence of moisture on the surface of solid preparations may increase the oxidation of susceptible drugs; such drugs must, therefore, be stored under dry conditions.

Key points

- The rate of hydrolysis of drugs in liquid-dosage forms is strongly influenced by the pH of the solution and can be catalysed not only by H^+ and OH^- ions (specific acid–base catalysis) but also by the components of the buffer used (general acid–base catalysis). To remove the influence of the buffer, the reaction rate is measured at a series of buffer concentrations at each pH and the data extrapolated back to zero concentration. These extrapolated rate constants are then plotted as a function of pH to give a buffer-independent pH–rate profile from which the pH of maximum stability of the solution can be determined and the rate constants for specific acid–base catalysis calculated.

- Temperature increase usually causes a pronounced increase of hydrolytic degradation. The hydrolytic rate constant at room temperature is determined by extrapolation of data at elevated temperatures using the Arrhenius equation,

$$\log k = \log A - \frac{E_a}{2.303RT}$$

- The effect of addition of electrolyte on the hydrolysis rate is determined from the Brønsted–Bjerrum equation, $\log k = \log k_0 + 2Az_A z_B \mu^{1/2}$. The reaction will be increased by electrolyte addition when it involves the interaction of the drug ion with an ion of the same charge and decreased when reaction is between ions of opposite charge.

- The effect of solvent on hydrolysis rate is determined by the equation $\log k = \log k_{\varepsilon=\infty} - Kz_A z_B/\varepsilon$; a change of solvent to one of lower dielectric constant will only stabilise reaction between ions of the same charge.

- Formulations that are shown to be susceptible to oxidation can be stabilised by replacing the oxygen in the storage containers with nitrogen or carbon dioxide, by avoiding contact with heavy-metal ions and by adding antioxidants. Photolabile drugs should be stored in containers that exclude ultraviolet light.

- The bases used for the preparation of ointments and creams should be chosen carefully to avoid possible drug stability problems. Care should also be taken with the choice of bases if it is necessary to dilute these semisolid-dosage forms.

- In solid-dosage forms containing drugs that are susceptible to hydrolysis, decomposition of the drug can occur if moisture is allowed to adsorb on the surface of the dosage form. Careful selection of packaging is important to reduce this possibility. The stability of drugs that dissolve in this surface layer will be affected by many of the factors that influence their decomposition in liquid-dosage forms. Excipients of the solid-dosage form can affect the drug breakdown by increasing the moisture content of the dosage form.

- Temperature increase causes an increase in the rate of breakdown of drugs in solid-dosage forms, which can often be described by the Arrhenius equation, although the effect of temperature change is usually far more complicated than for simple liquid formulations. This equation cannot be used for systems that show an approach to equilibrium. The van't Hoff equation, $\ln K = -\Delta H/RT + \text{constant}$, is often useful to describe the effect of temperature on the decomposition of these systems.

3.5 Stability testing and prediction of shelf-life

It is clearly most important to be able to ensure that a particular formulation when packaged in a specific container will remain within its physical, chemical, microbiological, therapeutic and toxicological specifications on storage for a specified period. In order to make such an assurance, we obviously need to conduct a rigorous stability-testing programme on the product in the form that is finally to be marketed. Since the testing period can be as long as 2 years, it has become essential to devise a more rapid technique that can be used during product development to speed up the identification of the most suitable formulation. In this section we shall examine ways of predicting the chemical stability of a formulation during preformulation studies using accelerated storage tests. We will not be considering the toxicological or microbiological studies or the determination of physical stability, all of which are essential elements in the overall stability testing of the formulation, but which are outside the scope of this chapter. Although most of this section will be concerned with the prediction of the effect of temperature on drug decomposition, other environmental factors will also be briefly considered.

3.5.1 Effect of temperature on stability

We have already considered the basic method of accelerating the chemical decomposition by raising the temperature of the preparations. We shall briefly reconsider essential steps in the process. The order of reaction can be determined by plotting stability data at several elevated temperatures according to the equations relating decomposition to time for each of the orders of reaction, until linear plots are obtained. We can now calculate values of rate constant at each temperature from the gradient of these plots, and plot the logarithm of k against reciprocal temperature according to the Arrhenius equation

$$\log k = \log A - \frac{E_a}{2.303RT} \tag{3.39}$$

The required value of k can be interpolated from this plot at room temperature, and the activation energy E_a calculated from the gradient, which is $-E_a/2.303R$. Values of E_a are usually within the range $50-96$ kJ mol^{-1}.

A convenient, approximate method that is useful for estimation of decomposition rates at room temperature makes use of the ratio of rate constants at room temperature (T_1) and a higher temperature (T_2). If we subtract the Arrhenius equations at temperatures T_1 and T_2, assuming that the log A term is the same at each temperature, we obtain

$$\log \left[\frac{k_2}{k_1} \right] = -\frac{E_a}{2.303R} \left[\frac{1}{T_2} - \frac{1}{T_1} \right] \tag{3.40}$$

 Example 3.9 Application of the Arrhenius equation

The first-order rate constant for the hydrolysis of sulfacetamide at 120°C is 9×10^{-6} s^{-1} and the activation energy is 94 kJ mol^{-1}. Calculate the rate constant at 25°C.

Answer

Using equation (3.41) with an E_a value of 94 kJ mol^{-1} we have

$$\log \left[\frac{k_{120}}{k_{25}} \right] = \frac{94 \times 10^3 \times (393 - 298)}{2.303 \times 8.314 \times (393 \times 298)}$$
$$= 3.98$$

Removing the logarithms, $k_{120}/k_{25} = 9.55 \times 10^3$.

Therefore, $k_{25} = 9 \times 10^{-6}/9.55 \times 10^3 = 9.4 \times 10^{-10}$ s^{-1}.

or

$$\log \left[\frac{k_2}{k_1} \right] = \frac{E_a(T_2 - T_1)}{2.303RT_2T_1} \tag{3.41}$$

We must, of course, have a value of E_a in order to be able to use these equations for the calculation of the room temperature rate constant k_1. If we only require a rough estimation of k_1 then we can assume a mid-range value of E_a, say 75 kJ mol^{-1}, for these calculations.

An alternative method of data treatment is to plot the logarithm of the half-life, $t_{0.5}$, as a function of reciprocal temperature. From equation (3.9), $t_{0.5} = 0.693/k$. Therefore,

$$\log k = \log 0.693 - \log t_{0.5} \tag{3.42}$$

and substituting into equation (3.32) gives

$$\log t_{0.5} = \log 0.693$$
$$- \log A + (E_a/2.303RT) \tag{3.43}$$

Once the rate constant is known at the required storage temperature it is a simple matter to calculate a shelf-life for the product based on an acceptable degree of decomposition. The equations we can use for 10% loss of activity are obtained by substituting

> ### e.g. Example 3.10 Calculation of expiry date
>
> The initial concentration of active principle in an aqueous preparation was 5.0×10^{-3} g cm^{-3}. After 20 months the concentration was shown by analysis to be 4.2×10^{-3} g cm^{-3}. The drug is known to be ineffective after it has decomposed to 70% of its original concentration. Assuming that decomposition follows first-order kinetics, calculate the nominal expiry date of the drug preparation.
>
> **Answer**
>
> Substituting into the first-order equation (equation 3.8)
>
> $$k = (2.303/20)$$
> $$\times \log[(5 \times 10^{-3})/(4.2 \times 10^{-3})]$$
> $$k = 8.719 \times 10^{-3} \text{ month}^{-1}$$
>
> 70% of the initial concentration = 3.5×10^{-3} g cm^{-3}.
>
> $$t = (2.303/8.719 \times 10^{-3})$$
> $$\times \log[(5 \times 10^{-3})/(3.5 \times 10^{-3})]$$
> $$t = 40.9 \text{ months}$$
>
> The nominal expiry date is thus 40.9 months after initial preparation (although in practice the shelf-life would probably be calculated for a decomposition to 95% of its value).

$x = 0.1a$ in the zero- and first-order equations (equations 3.7 and 3.8), giving

$$t_{0.9} = 0.1 \frac{[\text{D}]_0}{k_0} \qquad \text{(zero order)} \qquad (3.44)$$

and

$$t_{0.9} = \frac{0.105}{k_1} \qquad \text{(first order)} \qquad (3.45)$$

where $[\text{D}_0]$ is the initial concentration of drug. Although $t_{0.9}$ is usually used as an estimate of shelf-life, other percentage decompositions may be required, for example when the decomposition products produce discoloration or have undesirable side-effects. The required equations for these may be derived by substituting in the relevant rate equations.

Although accelerated storage testing based on the use of the Arrhenius equation has resulted in a very significant saving of time, it still involves the time-consuming step of the initial determination of the order of reaction for the decomposition. While most investigators have emphasised the need for a knowledge of the exact kinetic pathway of degradation, some have bypassed this initial step by assuming a particular decomposition model. At less than 10% degradation and within the limits of experimental error involved in stability studies, it is not possible to distinguish between zero-, first- or simple second-order kinetics using curve-fitting techniques; consequently the assumption of first-order kinetics for any decomposition reaction should involve minimum error. In fact, it was shown that there was a linear relationship between the logarithm of $t_{0.9}$ (the time taken for the concentration of the reactant to decompose to 90% of its original value) and the reciprocal temperature, which was independent of the order of reaction for the decomposition of a series of drugs.[30] On the basis of these findings it was suggested that the use of such linear plots to determine $t_{0.9}$ at the required temperature would provide a rapid, and yet sufficiently accurate, means of studying decomposition rate during the development stage.

Even with the modifications suggested above, the method of stability testing based on the Arrhenius equation is still time-consuming, involving as it does the separate determination of rate constants at a series of elevated temperatures. Experimental techniques have been developed[31,32] that enable the decomposition rate

Example 3.11 Accelerated storage testing using temperature–time programme

In a study of the first-order decomposition of riboflavine in 0.05 mol dm^{-3} NaOH using accelerated storage techniques, the temperature was programmed to rise from 12.5 to 55°C using a programme constant, b, of 2.171×10^{-4} K^{-1}. The initial concentration, c_0, of riboflavine was 10^{-4} mol dm^{-3}, and the concentration remaining at time t, c_t, was as follows:

t (h)	0.585	0.996	1.512	2.163	2.982	4.013	5.312	6.946
$10^5 c_t$ (mol dm^{-3})	9.881	9.763	9.532	9.109	8.371	6.902	4.931	2.435

Calculate the activation energy and the rate constant at 20°C.

Answer

For first-order reactions the data are plotted as log f(c) against log(1 + t) where f(c) = 2.303 log (c_0/c_t)

t	log(1 + t)	log[2.303 log(c_0/c_t)]
0.585	0.2	−1.94
0.996	0.3	−1.62
1.512	0.4	−1.32
2.163	0.5	−1.03
2.982	0.6	−0.75
4.013	0.7	−0.43
5.321	0.8	−0.15
6.946	0.9	+0.15

A plot of log[2.303 log(c_0/c_t)] against log(1 + t) is linear (Fig. 3.18) with a gradient of 2.95. Since

$$\text{Gradient} = 1 + \frac{E_a b}{R}$$

Therefore,

$$E_a = (1.95 \times 8.314)/(2.171 \times 10^{-4})$$
$$= 74.68 \text{ kJ mol}^{-1}$$

Intercept at log(1 + t) = 0 is −2.55. As seen from equation (3C.6) (Derivation Box 3C), an approximate equation for the intercept is

$$\text{Intercept} = \log k_0 - \log \left[1 + \frac{E_a b}{R}\right]$$

Therefore,

$$\log k_0 = -2.55 + \log 2.95 = -2.08$$

and

$$k_0 = 0.0083 \text{ h}^{-1}$$

That is, the rate constant at temperature T_0 (12.5°C) is 0.0083 h^{-1}.

The rate constant at 20°C may then be calculated from the Arrhenius equation in the form of equation (3.40):

$$\log k_t = -2.08 + [74\,680/(2.303 \times 8.314)][(1/285.5) - (1/293)]$$
$$= -2.08 + 0.3497 = -1.730$$

and

$$k_t = 1.86 \times 10^{-2} \text{ h}^{-1}$$

The rate constant at 20°C is thus 0.0186 h^{-1}.

to be determined from a single experiment. Such methods involve raising the temperature of the product in accordance with a predetermined temperature–time programme and are consequently referred to as non-isothermal stability studies. Any suitable temperature–time programme may be used; Derivation Box 3C illustrates the method proposed by Rogers[31] in which the rise of temperature was programmed so that the reciprocal of the temperature varied logarithmically with time. In this method data are plotted as log $f(c)$ against $\log(1 + t)$, where $f(c) = 2.303 \log (c_0/c_t)$ and c_0 and c_t are the concentrations at zero time and at time t, respectively. The gradient of this plot is $(1 + E_a b/R)$, where b is any suitable proportionality constant, enabling E_a to be determined. The rate constant k_0 at an initial time T_0 may then be calculated from the intercept when $\log(1 + t) = 0$, which is equal to $\log k_0 - \log(1 + E_a b/R)$. The rate constant at any other temperature may be calculated from k_0 and E_a.

The advantages of the method shown in Derivation Box 3C over the conventional method of stability testing are that: (a) the data required to calculate the stability are obtained in a single 1-day experiment rather than from a series of experiments that might last for several weeks; (b) no preliminary experiments are required to determine the optimum temperatures for the accelerated storage test; and (c) the linearity of the plot of log $f(c)$ against $\log(1 + t)$ confirms that the correct order of reaction has been assumed.

Several improvements on the original non-isothermal stability-testing methods have been suggested. Rather than subjecting the drug formulation to a predetermined fixed time–temperature profile, the temperature may be changed during the course of the experiment at a rate consistent with the analytical results from the experiment.[32] The resultant time–temperature data are fitted to a polynomial expression of sufficient degree to describe the changes. This relationship and the experimental data are then combined and used to compute a series of degradation pathways corresponding to a series of values of activation energy. The curves are matched with the experimental analytical data to obtain the correct activation energy for the reaction. Using this activation energy and the analytical data, the reaction rate and stability may be calculated. Computational procedures whereby the activation energy and frequency factor of the Arrhenius equation may be determined from simple non-isothermal experiments with a fixed temperature–time profile have been described.[33,34]

An improvement in the design of stability tests has been suggested that avoids the difficulties inherent in the non-linear curve-fitting procedures outlined above.[35] The experimental procedure involves changing the temperature of the samples being studied until degradation is rapid enough to proceed at a convenient rate for isothermal studies to be carried out. The analytical information obtained during the non-isothermal and isothermal portions of the experiment is used in calculating the activation energy and determining the order of reaction and the reaction rate and predicting stability at any required temperature.

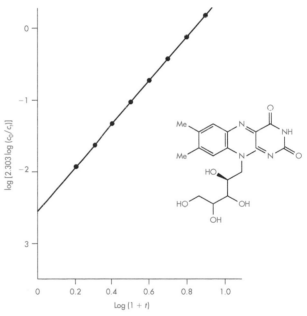

Figure 3.18 Example 3.11: Accelerated storage plot for the decomposition of riboflavin in 0.05 mol dm^{-3} NaOH using data from reference 31.

Although accelerated storage testing has proved invaluable in the development of stable formulations, it is important that we consider some of the limitations of this technique. We must take care that the order of reaction is not different at the higher temperatures from that which occurs at room temperature. There are several cases where this might be so. For example, with complex decomposition processes involving parallel or consecutive reactions, there may be a change in the relative contributions of the component reactions as the temperature is increased.

Suspensions

One complication that arises when we are carrying out stability testing of suspensions is the changes in the solubility of the suspended drug with increase in temperature. With suspensions, the concentration of the drug in solution usually remains constant because, as the decomposition reaction proceeds, more of the drug dissolves to keep the solution saturated. As we have seen, this situation usually leads to zero-order release kinetics. If the actual decomposition of dissolved drug is first-order, then we can express the decrease of concentration, c, with time, t, as

$$-\frac{\mathrm{d}c}{\mathrm{d}t} = k_0 \qquad (3.46)$$

where $k_0 = k_1 S$ and S is the solubility of the drug.

The problem that arises with these systems is that an increase of temperature causes not only the usual increase in rate constant, but also an increase in solubility. Application of the Arrhenius equation to the data involves the measurement of the changes in solubility of the drug over the temperature range involved. An alternative method that does not necessitate the determination of solubility uses the relationship between solubility and temperature:

$$\log S = -\frac{\Delta H_f}{2.303RT} + \text{constant} \qquad (3.47)$$

Since $k_0 = k_1 S$,

$$\log k_0 = \log k_1 + \log S$$

If we substitute for $\log k_1$, using the Arrhenius equation, we obtain

$$\log k_0 = \frac{(-E_a + \Delta H_f)}{2.303RT} + \text{constant} \qquad (3.48)$$

where ΔH_f is the molar heat of fusion. You can now see that we can plot $\log k_0$ against $1/T$ and extrapolate to give a room temperature value of k_0. It is important we remember that this treatment assumes that drug degradation in solution follows first-order kinetics and that the kinetics are not limited by the dissolution rate.

Solid state

The main problems arising in stability testing of solid-dosage forms are[26]: (a) that the analytical results tend to have more scatter because tablets and capsules are distinct dosage units rather than the true aliquots encountered with stability studies on drugs in solution, and (b) that these dosage forms are heterogeneous systems often involving a gas phase (air and water vapour), a liquid phase (adsorbed moisture) and the solid phase itself. The compositions of all of these phases can vary during an experiment.

The first of these problems can be overcome by ensuring uniformity of the dosage form before commencing the stability studies. The problems arising from the heterogeneity are more difficult to overcome. The main complicating factor is associated with the presence of moisture. As we have seen in section 3.4.3, moisture can have a significant effect on the kinetics of decomposition and this may produce many experimental problems during stability testing. For example, with gelatin capsules the water in the capsule shell must equilibrate with that in the formulation and surrounding air and this may require an appreciable time. The prediction of stability is difficult in solid-dosage forms in which there is chemical interaction between components, or chemical equilibrium phenomena. In fact, the data for stability studies involving the latter are often plotted using a van't Hoff plot rather than an Arrhenius plot.

To reduce some of these problems, particularly those associated with moisture, during stability testing, the following have been suggested[26]: (a) the use of tightly sealed containers, except where the effect of packaging is to be investigated; (b) that the amount of water present in the dosage form should be determined, preferable at each storage temperature, and (c) that a separate, sealed ampoule should be taken for each assay point and water determination, thus avoiding disturbance of water equilibrium on opening the container.

As has been discussed above, we can often use the Arrhenius equation to predict stability in the solid state, even though the kinetics of breakdown are different from those in solution. The exception to this is when equilibrium reactions occur, in which case we can often use the van't Hoff equation (equation 3.38) to predict room-temperature stability.

3.5.2 Other environmental factors affecting stability

Light

Photostability testing of drug substances usually involves the initial stress testing of the drug to determine its overall photostability and the identification of any degradation products. In this process the sample is irradiated at all absorbing wavelengths using a broad-spectrum light source. Those drugs or formulations that are shown to be photosensitive are then subjected to more formal photostability testing in which they are challenged with light of wavelength comparable to that to which the formulations are exposed in practical situations. During their shelf-life it is most likely that the products will be exposed to fluorescent light, direct daylight and daylight filtered through window glass, and the stability-testing procedures are designed to cover these possibilities. A specific protocol for testing the photostability of new drugs and products is described in the International Conference on Harmonisation (ICH) Guideline.[36]

Oxygen

The stability of an oxidisable drug in a liquid-dosage form is generally a function of the efficiency of any antioxidant included in the formulation. Exaggeration of the effect of oxygen on stability may be achieved by an increase in the partial pressure of oxygen in the system. It is not often easy, however, to make decisions on what would be the normal access of oxygen during storage and a meaningful extrapolation of the acquired data may be difficult.

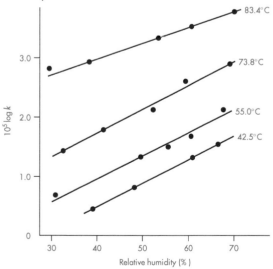

Figure 3.19 Logarithm of the nitrazepam decomposition constant, k, as a function of relative humidity at various temperatures.

Reproduced from Genton D, Kesselring UW. Effect of temperature and relative humidity on nitrazepam stability in solid state. *J Pharm Sci* 1977;66:676. Copyright Wiley-VCH Verlag GmbH & Co. KGaA. Reproduced with permission.

Moisture content

The stability of solid-dosage forms is usually very susceptible to the moisture content of the atmosphere in the container in which they are stored (see section 3.4.3) A linear relationship between log k and the water vapour pressure for vitamin A palmitate beadlets in sugar-coated tablets has been found.[37] Similarly, a linear relationship has been established between the

Key points

- It is most important to be able to ensure that a particular formulation when packaged in a specific container will remain within its physical, chemical, microbiological, therapeutic and toxicological specifications on storage for a specified time period. In order to make such an assurance we need to conduct a rigorous stability-testing programme on the product in the form that is finally to be marketed.

- To calculate the shelf-life it is necessary to know the rate constant at the storage temperature. However, the rate of breakdown of most pharmaceutical products is so slow that it would take many months to determine this at room temperature and it has become essential to devise a more rapid technique that can be used during product development to speed up the identification of the most suitable formulation.

- The method that is used for accelerated storage testing is based on the Arrhenius equation, $\log k = \log A - (E_a/2.303RT)$.

- The shelf-life for first-order reactions assuming 10% loss of activity, i.e. $t_{0.9}$, is calculated from the rate constant at the storage temperature k_1 using $t_{0.9} = 0.105/k_1$.

- Non-isothermal stability-testing methods may be used to reduce further the time taken to conduct stability studies; in these methods the temperature is usually increased in accordance with a predetermined temperature–time programme.

logarithm of the rate constant for the decomposition of nitrazepam in the solid state and the relative humidity (Fig. 3.19). The need for consideration of the effect of moisture on stability has been stressed by Carstensen,[15] who stated that stability programmes should always include samples that have been artificially stressed by addition of moisture. One purpose of a stability programme should be to define the stability of the dosage form as a function of moisture content.

3.5.3 Protocol for stability testing

A stability-testing requirement for a Registration Application agreed within the three areas of the EC, Japan and the USA exemplifies the core stability data package required for new drug substances and associated drug products.[38] Under this agreement, information on stability generated in any one of these three areas that meets the appropriate requirements of this guideline is mutually acceptable in both of the other two areas. The following summarises some of the main points of the guideline as it affects the stability testing of both drug substances and drug products; the original document should of course be consulted if a more detailed account is required.

Drug substances

Stability information from accelerated and long-term testing is required to be provided on at least three batches manufactured to a minimum of pilot plant scale by the same synthetic route and using a method of manufacture and procedure that simulates the final process to be used on a manufacturing scale. In this context, 'pilot plant scale' is taken to mean a minimum scale of one-tenth that of the full production process. The containers to be used in the long-term evaluation should be the same as, or simulate, the actual packaging used for storage and distribution. The overall quality of the batches of drug substance subjected to stability testing should be representative of both the quality of the material used in preclinical and clinical studies and the quality of material to be made on a manufacturing scale.

The testing should be designed to cover those features susceptible to change during storage and likely to influence quality, safety and/or efficacy, including, as necessary, the physical, chemical and microbiological characteristics. The length of the studies and the storage conditions should be sufficient to cover storage, shipment and subsequent use. The specifications for the long-term testing are a temperature of $25 \pm 2°C$ and $60\% \pm 5\%$ relative humidity for a period of 12 months. For accelerated testing the temperature is specified as $40 \pm 2°C$ and $75\% \pm 5\%$ relative humidity for a period of 6 months. Other storage conditions are allowable if justified; in particular, temperature-sensitive drugs should be stored at a lower temperature, which then becomes the designated long-term testing temperature. The 6-month accelerated testing should then be carried out at a temperature at least 15°C above this designated temperature together with the relative humidity appropriate to that temperature. Where 'significant change' occurs during the 6 months' accelerated storage testing, additional testing at an intermediate temperature (such as $30 \pm 2°C/60\% \pm 5\%$ relative humidity) should be conducted for drug substances to be used in the manufacture of dosage forms tested for long-term stability at 25°C/60% relative humidity. 'Significant change' at 40°C/75% relative humidity or 30°C/60% relative humidity is defined as failure to meet the specification.

The long-term testing is required to be continued for a sufficient period of time beyond 12 months to cover all appropriate retest periods. The frequency of testing should be sufficient to establish the stability characteristics of the drug substance; under the long-term conditions this will normally be every 3 months over the first year, every 6 months over the second year, and then annually.

Drug product

The design of the stability programme for the finished product is based on the knowledge of the behaviour and properties of the drug substance and the experience gained from clinical formulation studies and from stability studies on the drug substance. Stability information from long-term and accelerated testing is required to be presented on three batches of the same formulation and dosage form in the containers and closure proposed for marketing. Two of the three batches should be at least pilot-scale; the third batch may be smaller, for example 25 000–50 000 tablets or capsules for solid-dosage forms. Data on laboratory-scale batches are not acceptable as primary stability information. It is stipulated that the manufacturing process to be used should meaningfully simulate that which would be applied to large-scale batches for marketing and should provide product of the same quality intended for marketing, and meeting the same quality specification as to be applied for release of material. Where possible, batches of the finished product should be manufactured using identifiably different batches of drug substance.

As with the stability testing of drug substance, the testing of the product should cover those features susceptible to change during storage and likely to influence quality, safety and/or efficacy. The range of testing should cover not only chemical and biological stability but also loss of preservative, physical properties and characteristics, organoleptic properties and, where required, microbiological attributes.

The conditions and time periods for long-term and accelerated storage testing are the same as those outlined above for drug substances but with special considerations arising from the nature of the drug product. If it is necessary to store the product at a lower temperature because of its heat sensitivity, then consideration should be given to any physical or chemical change in the product that might occur at this temperature; for example, suspensions or emulsions may sediment or cream, while oils and semisolid preparations may show an increased viscosity. Storage under conditions of high relative humidity applies particularly to solid-dosage forms. For products such as solutions and suspensions contained in packs designed to provide a permanent barrier to water loss, specific storage under conditions of high relative humidity is not necessary, but the same range of temperatures should be applied. It is recognised that low relative humidity (10–20%) can adversely affect products packed in semipermeable containers such as solutions in plastic bags and nose drops in small plastic containers, and consideration should be given to appropriate testing under such conditions.

In the case of drug products, 'significant change' at the accelerated condition is defined as:

- a 5% potency loss from the initial assay value of a batch
- any specified degradant exceeding its specification limit
- the product exceeding its pH limits
- dissolution exceeding the specification limits for 12 capsules or tablets

- failure to meet specifications for appearance and physical properties, e.g. colour, phase separation, resuspendability, delivery per actuation, caking and hardness.

If significant change occurs at 40°C/75% relative humidity then it is necessary to submit a minimum of 6 months' data from an ongoing 1-year study at 30°C/60% relative humidity using the same criteria for 'significant change'.

Summary

In this chapter we have examined the various ways in which drugs can chemically break down in both liquid and solid-dosage forms and discussed possible means of preventing or minimising this loss of activity. The most common cause of degradation of drugs in aqueous solution is the hydrolysis of groups such as esters, amides, lactones, lactams, imides or carbamates. The stability of solutions of drugs containing these groups can be improved by formulation at the pH of maximum stability. Care must be taken, however, in the choice of buffer used because hydrolysis is catalysed not only by hydrogen or hydroxyl ions (specific acid–base hydrolysis) but also by the components of buffer solutions (general acid–base catalysis). Drugs possessing carbon–carbon double bonds, such as the steroids, polyunsaturated fatty acids and polyene antibiotics, are susceptible to oxidative degradation; liquid formulations of these drugs may be stabilised by replacing the oxygen in the system with inert gases such as nitrogen; by avoiding contact with metals such as iron, cobalt and nickel; and by adding antioxidants or reducing agents to the solution. Some oxidative reactions are pH-dependent, in which case the product can be stabilised by buffering the system. Other less common types of drug decomposition include photochemical breakdown (necessitating storage in amber containers), epimerisation and polymerisation.

We have seen how reactions may follow zero-, first- and second-order kinetics and examined how to determine the rate constant, and in some cases the half-life, of the decomposition process. With this information we are able to make a prediction of the shelf-life of the product, which is usually the time taken for the drug to be reduced to 95% of its original potency. Although the breakdown of most drugs in solution follows first-order or pseudo first-order kinetics, the decomposition process may be complicated by more complex breakdown schemes involving parallel, reversible or consecutive reactions.

Assessment of the optimum pH for formulation of liquid-dosage forms is greatly speeded up by measuring the hydrolysis rate at a series of elevated temperatures and extrapolating to room temperature using the Arrhenius equation. A protocol for stability testing that has been agreed in the EC, Japan and the USA has been described.

The kinetics of drug decomposition in solid-dosage forms is less well understood. Decomposition of drugs susceptible to hydrolysis can occur if moisture is allowed to adsorb on to the surface of the dosage form and the packaging should be selected to minimise this effect. Excipients of the solid-dosage form can affect drug breakdown by increasing the moisture content of the dosage form. Film coating of tablets can markedly reduce moisture ingress, as discussed in Chapter 1.

Some final points on the stability of drugs

Given that the explicit aim of an understanding of the stability of drug molecules is to ensure the quality of medicines and to avoid the presence of toxic and other degradants, is it worth remembering the wide relevance of stability at various stages of drug development and use.

- It is important at the drug discovery stage to ensure that drugs injected into animals or tissues in culture are indeed stable in the medium used in pharmacology laboratories, where the media used may have suboptimal pH for drug solubility or stability. This is to ensure that the drug being studied is indeed the one intended.

- It is, of course, vital that different routes of synthesis of new (and established) molecules are evaluated in terms of which route produces the purest molecules with minimal impurities caused by side-reactions or residual solvents and catalysts.

- Many protein-based therapeutics have complex pathways of production, discussed briefly in Chapters 13 and 16; these molecules can be fragile

and suffer not only chemical instability but also physical (such as conformational) instabilities.

- There are many possibilities for drugs to interact with formulation components, as we have discussed; there are examples of drugs such as doxorubicin interacting with components of microspheres and nanoparticles, or reacting with chemicals such as glutaraldehyde used in the preparation of, for example, albumin microspheres. Sadly, in these days where counterfeiting is becoming a greater problem not only in the developing world but also in Europe, the analysis of drug content and quality can often distinguish those drugs which are genuine and those which are counterfeit. Often it is the impurity profile which provides the fingerprint to aid detection.

Historical examples of instability, interactions and adverse effects are very much worthy of study as they can aid us in predicting the likelihood of these events with novel drug molecules. This requires us, as we point out in the Introduction to this book, to have a feeling for the chemistry of drugs and thus the ability to extrapolate sensibly from known scenarios to new and uncertain cases.

References

1. LePree JM, Connors KA. Hydrolysis of drugs. In: Swarbrick J (ed.) *Encyclopedia of Pharmaceutical Technology*, 3rd edn. New York: Informa Healthcare; 2006: 2040–2047.
2. Wells PR. Linear free energy relationships. *Chem Rev* 1963;63:171–219.
3. Cartensen JT *et al*. Use of Hammett graphs in stability programs. *J Pharm Sci* 1964;53:1547–1548.
4. Hovorka SW, Schöneich C. Oxidative degradation of pharmaceuticals: theory, mechanisms and inhibition. *J Pharm Sci* 2001;90:253–269.
5. Johnson DM, Taylor WF. Degradation of fenprostalene in polyethylene glycol 400 solution. *J Pharm Sci* 1984;73:1414–1417.
6. Halbaut L *et al*. Oxidative stability of semi-solid excipient mixtures with corn oil and its implication in the degradation of vitamin A. *Int J Pharm* 1997;147:31–40.
7. Smith GB *et al*. Autooxidation of simvastatin. *Tetrahedron* 1993;49:4447–4462.
8. Lamy-Freund MT *et al*. Effect of aggregation on the kinetics of autoxidation of the polyene antibiotic amphotericin B. *J Pharm Sci* 1993;82:162–166.
9. Manjappa AS *et al*. Is an alternative drug delivery system needed for docetaxel? The role of controlling epimeriza-

tion in formulations and beyond. *Pharm Res* 2013;30:2675–2693.

10. Tønnesen HH. Formulation and stability testing of photolabile drugs. *Int J Pharm* 2001;225:1–14.

11. Greenhill JV, McLelland MA. Photodecomposition of drugs. *Prog Med Chem* 1990;27:51–121.

12. Huang CL, Sands FL. Effect of ultraviolet irradiation on chlorpromazine. II. Anaerobic condition. *J Pharm Sci* 1967;56:259–264.

13. Matsuda Y *et al.* Stabilization of sulfisomidine tablets by use of film coating containing UV absorber: protection of coloration and photolytic degradation from exaggerated light. *J Pharm Sci* 1978;67:196–201.

14. Bundgaard H. Polymerization of penicillins: kinetics and mechanism of di- and polymerization of ampicillin in aqueous solution. *Acta Pharm Suec* 1976;13:9–26.

15. Carstensen JT. Stability of solids and solid dosage forms. *J Pharm Sci* 1974;63:1–14.

16. Carstensen JT. *Drug Stability. Principles and Practices,* 2nd edn. New York: Marcel Dekker; 1995.

17. Andersin R, Tammilehto S. Photochemical decomposition of midazolam. IV. Study of pH-dependent stability by high-performance liquid chromatography. *Int J Pharm* 1995;123:229–235.

18. Torniainen K *et al.* The effect of pH, buffer type and drug concentration on the photodegradation of ciprofloxacin. *Int J Pharm* 1996;132:53–61.

19. Ong JTH, Kostenbauder HB. Effect of self-association on rate of penicillin G degradation in concentrated aqueous solutions. *J Pharm Sci* 1975;64:1378–1380.

20. Allen AE, Das Gupta V. Stability of hydrocortisone in polyethylene glycol ointment base. *J Pharm Sci* 1974;63:107–109.

21. Das Gupta V. Effect of vehicles and other active ingredients on stability of hydrocortisone. *J Pharm Sci* 1978;67:299–302.

22. Busse MJ. Dangers of dilution of topical steroids. *Pharm J* 1978;220:25.

23. Ullmann E *et al.* The stability of sodium penicillin G in the presence of ionic surfactants, organic gel formers, and preservatives. *Pharm Acta Helv* 1963;38:577–586.

24. Testa B, Etter JC. Hydrolysis of pilocarpine in Carbopol hydrogels. *Can J Pharm Sci* 1975;10:16–20.

25. Poust RI, Colaizzi JC. Copper-catalyzed oxidation of ascorbic acid in gels and aqueous solutions of polysorbate 80. *J Pharm Sci* 1968;57:2119–2125.

26. Tingstad J, Dudzinski J. Preformulation studies. II. Stability of drug substances in solid pharmaceutical systems. *J Pharm Sci* 1973;62:1856–1860.

27. Jun HW *et al.* Decomposition of aspirin in polyethylene glycols. *J Pharm Sci* 1972; 61:1160–1162.

28. Whitworth CW *et al.* Stability of aspirin in liquid and semisolid bases. II. Effect of fatty additives on stability in a polyethylene glycol base. *J Pharm Sci* 1973; 62:1372–1374.

29. Ekman R *et al.* Formation of indomethacin esters in polyethylene glycol suppositories. *Acta Pharm Suec* 1982;19:241–246.

30. Amirjahed AK. Simplified method to study stability of pharmaceutical preparations. *J Pharm Sci* 1977;66:785–789.

31. Rogers AR. An accelerated storage test with programmed temperature rise. *J Pharm Pharmacol* 1963;15:101T.

32. Maudling HV, Zoglio MA. Flexible nonisothermal stability studies. *J Pharm Sci* 1970;59:333–337.

33. Madsen BW *et al.* Integral approach to nonisothermal estimation of activation energies. *J Pharm Sci* 1974;63:777–781.

34. Kay AI, Simon TH. Use of an analog computer to simulate and interpret data obtained from linear nonisothermal stability studies. *J Pharm Sci* 1971;60:205–208.

35. Zoglio MA *et al.* Nonisothermal kinetic studies III: rapid nonisothermal–isothermal method for stability prediction. *J Pharm Sci* 1975;64:1381–1383.

36. ICH Harmonised Tripartite Guideline. Q1B: photostability testing of new drug substances and products. *Federal Register* 1997;62:27115.

37. Lachman L. Physical and chemical stability testing of tablet dosage forms. *J Pharm Sci* 1965;54:1519–1526.

38. Note for Guidance on Stability Testing: *Stability Testing of New Drug Substances and Products (ICH).* CPMP/ICH/2736/99. London: Medicines Control Agency; 1999 (adopted 2003).

4

The solubility of drugs

There are many reasons why it is vital to understand the way in which drugs dissolve in solution and the factors that maintain solubility or cause drugs to come out of solution, that is, to precipitate. For example, many drugs are formulated as solutions or are added in powder or solution form to the liquids, such as infusion fluids, in which they must remain in solution for a given period. In whatever way drugs are presented to the body, they must usually be in a molecularly dispersed form (that is, in solution) before they can be absorbed across biological membranes.* The solution process will precede absorption unless the drug is administered as a solution, but even solutions may precipitate in the stomach contents or in blood, and the precipitated drug will then have to redissolve before being absorbed. Similarly, a knowledge of factors influencing solubility is important if we are to address the problems in relation to the formulation and bioavailability of drugs of low aqueous solubility (e.g. Taxol).

In this chapter we will:

- consider the factors controlling the solubility of drugs in solution, in particular the nature of the drug molecule and the crystalline form in which it exists, its hydrophobicity, its shape, its surface area, its state of ionisation, the influence of pH of the medium and the importance of the pK_a of the drug
- see how to predict the solubility of a drug from a knowledge of its chemical structure, recognising hydrophilic and hydrophobic groups and their influence on solubility
- discuss how additives such as salts, cosolvents, water-miscible solvents, hydrotropes and cyclodextrins may be used to increase the water solubility of the drug and to what extent their effects may be predicted from theory, bearing in mind the complexity of many formulations

---

* In section 8.2.1 we discuss the special circumstances under which nanoparticulate materials can be taken up by specialised cells in the gut and, by way of the lymphatic circulation, reach the liver and blood and other organs. It may be that very insoluble colloidal drug suspensions are absorbed to an extent by this route also.

- examine how the choice of a particular salt of a drug for use in formulations can have a marked effect on the solubility of that drug
- look at experimental methods of measurement of solubility which are essential in drug development
- see how the partitioning of a drug or solute between two immiscible phases may be quantified in the partition coefficient of the compound and how this may be correlated with the biological activity.

4.1 Definitions

A *solution* can be defined as a system in which molecules of a solute (such as a drug or protein) are dissolved in a solvent vehicle. When a solution contains a solute at the limit of its solubility at any given temperature and pressure, it is said to be *saturated*. If the solubility limit is exceeded, solid particles of solute may be present and the solution phase will be in equilibrium with the solid, although under certain circumstances *supersaturated* solutions may be prepared, where the drug exists in solution above its normal solubility limit.

The maximum *equilibrium solubility* of a drug in a given medium is of practical pharmaceutical interest because it dictates the *rate of solution (dissolution)* of the drug (the rate at which the drug dissolves from the solid state). The higher the solubility, the more rapid is the rate of solution when no chemical reaction is involved.

4.1.1 Expressions of solubility

The solubility of a solute in a solvent can be expressed quantitatively in several ways (see Chapter 2, section 2.1). The British Pharmacopoeia and other chemical and pharmaceutical compendia frequently use less specific forms of noting solubility, such as parts per parts of solvent (for example, parts per million, ppm) and also the expressions 'insoluble', 'very highly soluble' and 'soluble'. These are imprecise and often not very helpful. For quantitative work, specific concentration terms must be used.

Most substances have at least some degree of solubility in water and, while they may appear to be 'insoluble' by a qualitative test, their solubility can be measured and quoted precisely. In aqueous media at pH 10, chlorpromazine base has a solubility of $8 \times 10^{-6}\ \text{mol dm}^{-3}$, that is, it is very slightly soluble, but it might be considered to be 'insoluble' if judged visually by the lack of disappearance of solid placed in a test tube of water.

4.2 Factors influencing solubility

Progress has been made in ways of predicting the solubility of solutes in aqueous media, both from estimates of their molecular surface area and from the nature of the key chemical groups in the parent structure.

4.2.1 Structural features and aqueous solubility

Size and shape

The importance of the surface area, which is a function of size and shape, becomes clear if we think of the processes involved in the dissolution of a crystal (Fig. 4.1). The process can be considered simplistically in three stages:

1. A solute (drug) molecule is 'removed' from its crystal.
2. A cavity for the molecule is created in the solvent.
3. The solute molecule is inserted into this cavity.

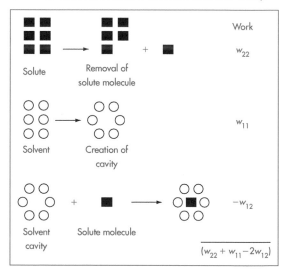

Figure 4.1 Diagrammatic representation of the three processes involved in the dissolution of a crystalline solute: the expression for the work involved is $w_{22} + w_{11} - 2w_{12}$ (solute–solvent interaction in the last stage is $-2w_{12}$ as bonds are made with one solute and two solvent molecules).

Table 4.1 Experimental aqueous solubilities, boiling points, surface areas and predicted aqueous solubilities

Compound	Solubility (mol kg^{-1})	Surface area (nm^2)	Boiling point (°C)	Predicted solubilities (mol kg^{-1})
1-Butanol	1.006	2.721	117.7	0.821
1-Pentanol	2.5×10^{-1}	3.039	137.8	2.09×10^{-1}
1-Hexanol	6.1×10^{-2}	3.357	157	5.32×10^{-2}
1-Heptanol	1.55×10^{-2}	3.675	176.3	1.36×10^{-2}
Cyclohexanol	3.83×10^{-1}	2.905	161	4.3×10^{-1}
1-Nonanol	1×10^{-3}	4.312	213.1	0.88×10^{-3}

The first stage of the process involves the breaking of bonds within the crystal lattice, for example, overcoming the attractive electrostatic forces in a drug crystal consisting of cations and anions. The work required to achieve this may be written as w_{22}; the subscript 2 is used for the solute and hence w_{22} implies solute–solute interaction. Work is also required in the creation of a cavity in the solvent to accommodate the displaced solute molecule; this may be written as w_{11} since now the process involves a solvent–solvent interaction (solvent is denoted by subscript 1). Placing the solute molecule in the solvent cavity requires a number of solute–solvent contacts; the larger the solute molecule, the more contacts are created. If the surface area of the solute molecule is A, the solute–solvent interface increases by $\sigma_{12}A$, where σ_{12} is the interfacial tension between the solvent and the solute. σ is a parameter not readily obtained for solid interfaces on the molecular scale, but reasonable estimates can be made from knowledge of the interfacial tensions of molecules at normal interfaces.[1–5]

The number of solvent molecules that can pack around the solute molecule is considered in calculations of the thermodynamic properties of the solution. The molecular surface area of the solute is therefore the key parameter and good correlations can be obtained between aqueous solubility and this parameter.[4,5] Chain branching of hydrophobic groups also influences aqueous solubility, as shown by the solubilities of a series of straight and branched-chain alcohols in Table 4.1.

Of course, most drugs are not simple non-polar hydrocarbons and we have to consider polar molecules and weak organic electrolytes. The term w_{12} in Fig. 4.1, a measure of solute–solvent interactions, has to be further divided to take into account the interactions involving the non-polar part and the polar portion of the solute. The molecular surface area of each portion can be considered separately: the greater the area of the hydrophilic portion relative to the hydrophobic portion, the greater is the aqueous solubility. For a hydrophobic molecule of area A, the free-energy change in placing the solute in the solvent cavity is $-\sigma_{12}A$. Indeed, it can be shown that the reversible work of solution is $(w_{11} + w_{22} - 2w_{12})A$.

Implicit in this derivation is the assumption that the solution formed is dilute, so that solute–solute interactions are unimportant. The success of the molecular area approach is evidenced by the fact that equations can be written to relate solubility to surface area. For example, equation (4.1) has been shown to hold for a range of 55 compounds (some of which are listed in Table 4.1):

$$\ln S = -4.3A + 11.78 \qquad (4.1)$$

where S is the molal (not molar) solubility, and A is the total surface area in nm^2.

The compounds in Table 4.1 are liquids, so the process of dissolution is simpler than that outlined in Fig. 4.1.

Melting point and boiling point

Interactions between non-polar groups and water were discussed above, where the importance of both size and shape was indicated. What other predictors of solubility might there be? The boiling point of liquids and the melting point of solids are useful in that both reflect the strengths of interactions between the molecules in the pure liquid or the solid state. Boiling point correlates with total surface area, and in a large enough

Table 4.2 Solubilities of pentanol isomers in water

Compound	Solubility (molality, m)	Surface area (nm^2)	Boiling point (°C)	Structure
1-Pentanol	2.6×10^{-1}	3.039	137.8	
3-Methyl-1-butanol	3.11×10^{-1}	2.914	131.2	
2-Methyl-1-butanol	3.47×10^{-1}	2.894	128.7	
2-Pentanol	5.3×10^{-1}	2.959	119.0	
3-Pentanol	6.15×10^{-1}	2.935	115.3	
3-Methyl-2-butanol	6.67×10^{-1}	2.843	111.5	
2-Methyl-2-butanol	1.403	2.825	102.0	

Reproduced from Amidon GL *et al*. Solubility of nonelectrolytes in polar solvents. II. Solubility of aliphatic alcohols in water. *J Pharm Sci* 1974;63:1858–1866. Copyright Wiley-VCH Verlag GmbH & Co. KGaA. Reproduced with permission.

range of compounds we can detect the trend of decreasing aqueous solubility with increasing boiling point (see data in Table 4.2).

As boiling points of liquids and melting points of solids are indicators of molecular cohesion, these can be useful indicators of trends in a series of similar compounds. There are other empirical correlations that are useful. Melting points, even of compounds that form non-ideal solutions, can be used as a guide to the order of solubility in a closely related series of compounds, as can be seen in the properties of sulfonamide derivatives listed in Table 4.3. Such correlations depend on the relatively greater importance of w_{22} in the solution process in these compounds.

The relationship between the molar solubility of a drug in water, S_w, at a temperature T (in kelvins), and the melting point T_m, for a non-ideal solution may be written as

$$\log S_w = -\frac{\Delta S_{fus}(T_m - T)}{2.303} + \log \gamma_w + \log \overline{V} \quad (4.2)$$

Table 4.3 Correlation between melting points of sulfonamide derivatives and aqueous solubility

Compound	Melting point (°C)	Solubility
Sulfadiazine	253	1 g in 13 dm^3 (0.077 g dm^{-3})
Sulfamerazine	236	1 g in 5 dm^3 (0.20 g dm^{-3})
Sulfapyridine	192	1 g in 3.5 dm^3 (0.29 g dm^{-3})
Sulfathiazole	174	1 g in 1.7 dm^3 (0.59 g dm^{-3})

where ΔS_{fus} is the entropy of fusion (melting), γ is the activity coefficient and $\overline{V}$ is the molar volume of the solvent. Equation (4.2) shows an increase of solubility as the melting point decreases.

Substituents

The influence of substituents on the solubility of molecules in water can be due to their effect on the properties of the solid or liquid (for example, on its molecular cohesion) or to the effect of the substituent on its interaction with water molecules. It is not easy to predict what effect a particular substituent will have on crystal properties, but as a guide to the solvent interactions, substituents can be classified as either hydrophobic or hydrophilic, depending on their polarity (Table 4.4). The position of the substituent on the molecule can influence its effect, however. This can be seen in the aqueous solubilities of o-, m- and p-dihydroxybenzenes; as expected, all are much greater than that of benzene, but they are not the same, being 4, 9 and 0.6 mol dm^{-3}, respectively. The relatively low solubility of the *para* compound is due to its greater stability. The melting points of the derivatives indicate that is so, as they are 105°C, 111°C and 170°C, respectively. In the case of the *ortho* derivative, the possibility of intramolecular hydrogen bonding in aqueous solution, decreasing the ability of the OH group to interact with water, may explain why its solubility is lower than that of its *meta* analogue.

One can best illustrate the use of the information in Table 4.4 by considering the solubility of a series of substituted acetanilides, data for which are provided in Table 4.5. The strong hydrophilic characteristics of polar groups capable of hydrogen bonding with water molecules are evident. The presence of hydroxyl groups can therefore markedly change the solubility characteristics of a compound; phenol, for example, is 100 times more soluble in water than is benzene. In the case of phenol, where there is considerable hydrogen-bonding capability, the solute–solvent interaction (w_{12}) outweighs other factors (such as w_{22} or w_{11}) in the solution process. But, as we have discovered, the position of any substituent on the parent molecule will affect its contribution to solubility.

Steroid solubility

The steroids as a group tend to be poorly soluble in water. Their complex structure makes prediction of solubility somewhat difficult, but one can generally rationalise, *post hoc*, the solubility values of related steroids. Table 4.6 gives solubility data for 14 steroids. As examples, the substitution of an ethinyl group has conferred increased solubility on the estradiol molecule, as would be expected. Estradiol benzoate with its 3-OH substituent is much less soluble than the parent estradiol because of the loss of the hydroxyl and

Table 4.4 Substituent group classification

Substituent	Classification
—CH$_3$	Hydrophobic
—CH$_2$—	Hydrophobic
—Cl, —Br, —F	Hydrophobic
—N(CH$_3$)$_2$	Hydrophobic
—SCH$_3$	Hydrophobic
—OCH$_2$CH$_3$	Hydrophobic
—OCH$_3$	Slightly hydrophilic
—NO$_2$	Slightly hydrophilic
—CHO	Hydrophilic
—COOH	Slightly hydrophilic
—COO$^-$	Very hydrophilic
—NH$_2$	Hydrophilic
—NH$_3^+$	Very hydrophilic
—OH	Very hydrophilic

Table 4.5 The effect of substituents on solubility of acetanilide derivatives in water

Derivative	X	Solubility (mg dm^{-3})
NHCOCH$_3$ (structure) X	H	6.38
	Methyl	1.05
	Ethoxyl	0.93
	Hydroxyl	13.9
	Nitro	15.98
	Aceto	9.87

its substitution with a hydrophobic group. The same relationships are seen in testosterone and testosterone propionate. As both estradiol benzoate and testosterone propionate are oil soluble, they are used as solutions in castor oil and sesame oil for intramuscular and subcutaneous injection (see Chapter 9).

Methyltestosterone might be expected to be less soluble in water than is testosterone, but in fact it is not; this demonstrates again the importance of crystal properties in determining solubility. The methyl compound is more soluble because of the smaller heat of

Table 4.6 Steroid structure and solubility in water

Structure	Compound	Solubility ($\mu g\,cm^{-3}$)
(I)	Estradiol (I)	5
(II)	Ethinylestradiol (II)	10
(III)	Estradiol benzoate (III)	0.4
(IV)	Testosterone (IV) Testosterone propionate	24 0.4
(V)	Methyltestosterone (V)	32
(VI)	Prednisolone (VI)	215

(continued overleaf)

Table 4.6 *(continued)*

Structure	Compound	Solubility (μg cm^{-3})
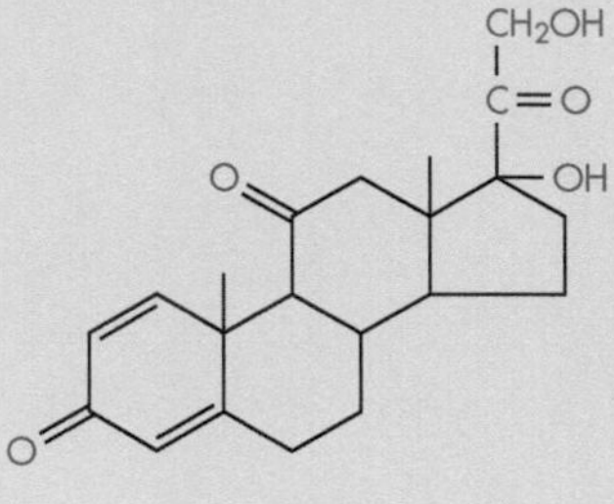 (VII)	Prednisone (**VII**) Prednisone acetate	115 23
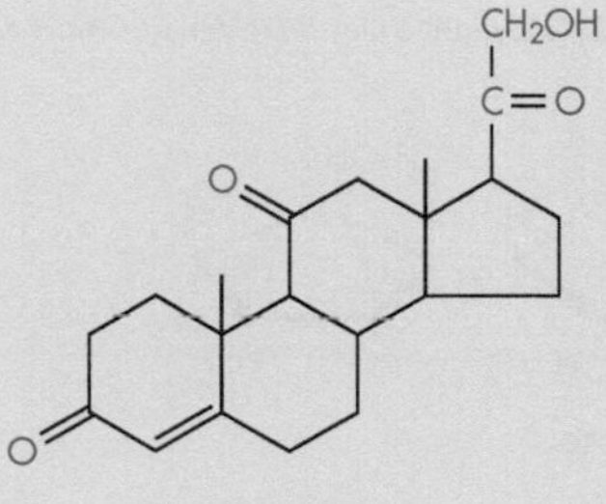 (VIII)	Cortisone (**VIII**)	230
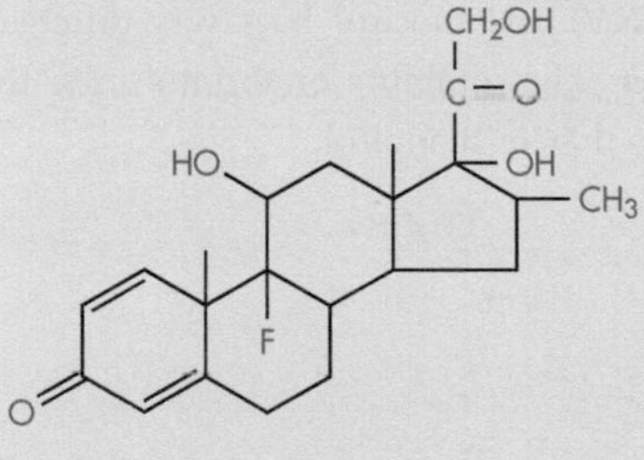 (IX)	Dexamethasone (**IX**)	84
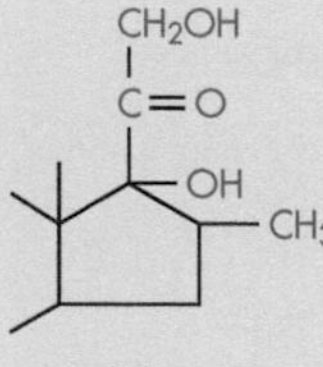 (X)	Betamethasone (**X**)	58
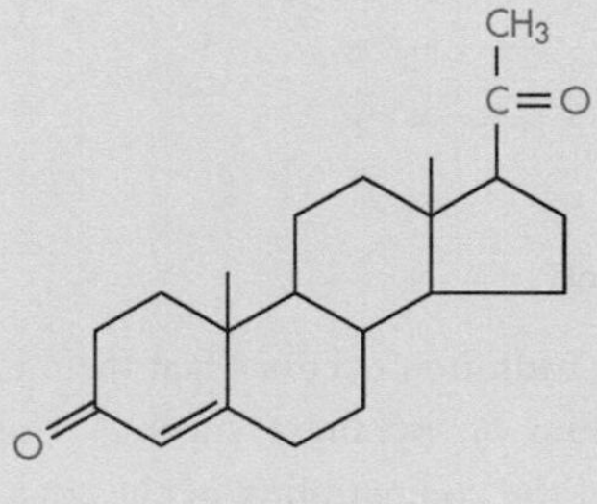 (XI)	Progesterone (**XI**)	9

(continued overleaf)

Table 4.6 *(continued)*		
Structure	Compound	Solubility ($\mu g\ cm^{-3}$)
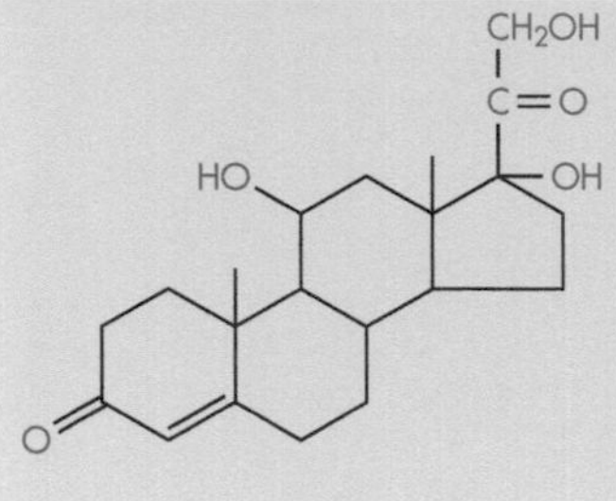 (XII)	Hydrocortisone (**XII**)	285

Reproduced from Kabasakalian P *et al.* Solubility of some steroids in water. *J Pharm Sci* 1966;55:642. Copyright Wiley-VCH Verlag GmbH & Co. KGaA. Reproduced with permission.

fusion of this derivative, hence the solid state more readily 'disintegrates' in the solvent.

Dexamethasone and betamethasone are isomeric fluorinated derivatives of methylprednisolone, but their solubilities are not identical, which might be a crystal property or a solution property. A simpler example of differences in isomeric solubility is that of the o-, m- and p-dihydroxybenzenes referred to above. A steric argument may be applied to the case of dexamethasone, water molecules being less able to move close to the 17-OH group than in the case of betamethasone.

4.2.2 Hydration and solvation

The way in which solute molecules interact with the water molecules of the solvent is crucial to determining their affinity for the solvent. Ionic groups and electrolytes interact avidly with the polar water molecules, but non-electrolytes also do not leave the structure of water unchanged, nor even do non-polar groups and molecules such as the hydrocarbons.

Hydration of non-electrolytes

Solvation is the general term used to describe the process of binding of solvent to solute molecules. If the solvent is water, the process is hydration. In a solution of sucrose (**XIII**), six water molecules are bound to each sucrose molecule with such avidity that the water and sucrose move as a unit in solution, and the extent of hydration can therefore be measured by hydrodynamic techniques.

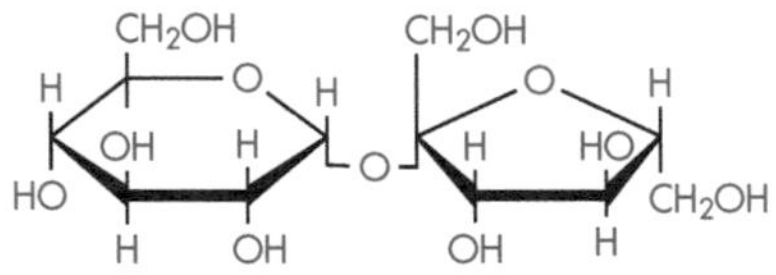

Structure XIII Sucrose

Chemically very similar molecules such as mannitol (**XIV**), sorbitol (**XV**) and inositol have very different affinities for water. The solubility of sorbitol in water is about 3.5 times that of mannitol.

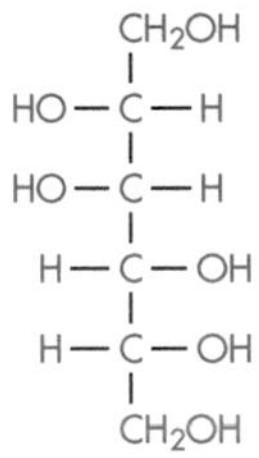

Structure XIV Mannitol

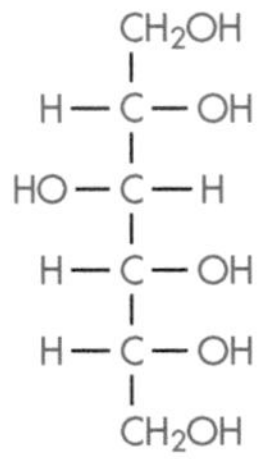

Structure XV Sorbitol

Most favourable hydration occurs when there is an equatorial –OH group on pyranose sugars.[6] This is thought to be due to the compatibility of the equatorial –OH with the organised structure of water in bulk. Axial hydroxyl groups cannot bond on to the water 'lattice' without causing it to distort considerably. This may be one explanation of the difference, although differences in the lattice energies of the crystals may also contribute.

Hydration of ionic species: water structure breakers and structure makers

The study of ionic solvation is complicated but is relevant in pharmaceutics because of the effect ions have on the solubility of other species. The forces between cations and water molecules are so strong that the cations may retain a layer of water molecules in their crystals. The effect of ions on water structure is complex and variable. All ions in water possess a layer of tightly bound water – the water molecules being directionally oriented. Four water molecules are in the bound layer of most monovalent, monatomic ions. The firmly held layer can be regarded as being in a 'frozen' condition around a positive ion. The water molecules could be oriented with all the hydrogen atoms of the water molecules pointing outwards (Fig. 4.2). Because of this and because their orientation depends on the

ion size, they cannot all participate in the normal tetrahedral arrangements of bulk water (see section 5.3.1 in Chapter 5). For this to be feasible, two of the water molecules must be oriented with the hydrogens of the water molecules pointing in towards the ion. Inevitably, then, with cations and many small anions there tends to be a layer of water around the bound layer which is *less ordered* than bulk water (Fig. 4.2). Such ions, which include all the alkali and halide ions except Li^+ and F^-, are called *structure breakers*. The size of the ion is important, as the surface area of the ion determines the constraints on the polarised water molecules. Many polyvalent ions, for example Al^{3+}, increase the structured nature of water beyond the immediate hydration layer, and are therefore *structure makers*.

Hydration numbers

Hydration numbers (the number of water molecules in the primary hydration layer) can be determined by

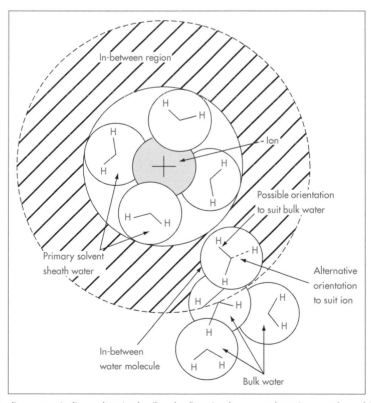

Figure 4.2 Schematic diagram to indicate that, in the (hatched) region between the primary solvated ion and bulk water, the orientation of the 'in-between' water molecules must be a compromise between that which suits the ion (oxygen-facing ion) and that which suits the bulk water (hydrogen-facing ion).

Reproduced with permission from Bockris JO'M, Reddy AKN. *Modern Electrochemistry*, vol. 1. London: MacDonald, 1970.

various physical techniques (for example, compressibility) and the values obtained tend to differ depending on the method used. The overall total action of the ion on water may be replaced conceptually by a strong binding between the ion and some effective number (solvation number) of solvent molecules; this effective number may well be almost zero in the case of large ions such as iodide, caesium and tetraalkylammonium ions. The solvation numbers decrease with increase of ionic radius because the ionic force field diminishes with increasing radius, and consequently water molecules are less inclined to be abstracted from their position in bulk water.

Hydrophobic hydration

Water is associated in a dynamic manner with non-polar groups, but only in rare cases (where crystalline clathrates can be formed) is this water able to be isolated along with the hydrophobic groups. The phrase 'hydrophobic hydration' is used to describe this layer of water. The motion of water molecules is slowed down in the vicinity of non-polar groups. Hydrophobic groups induce structure formation in water, hence the negative entropy ($-\Delta S$) of their dissolution in water and the positive entropy ($+\Delta S$) gained on their removal. In the discussion of hydrophobic bonding (see section 5.3.1 in Chapter 5) and non-polar interactions, this special relationship between water and hydrocarbon chains is elaborated.

The solubility of inorganic materials in water

While a minority of therapeutic agents are inorganic electrolytes, it is nevertheless pertinent to consider the manner of their interaction with water. Electrolytes are, of necessity, components of replacement fluids, injections and eye drops and many other formulations. An increasing number of metal-containing compounds are used in diagnosis and therapy, some of which have interesting solution behaviour.

First consider the simpler salts. What determines the solubility of a salt such as sodium chloride and its solubility in relation to, say, silver chloride? The solubility of NaCl is in excess of $5 \, mol \, dm^{-3}$ while the solubility of AgCl is 500 000 times less. The heats of solution ($\Delta H_{solution}$) are $62.8 \, kJ \, mol^{-1}$ for silver chloride and $4.2 \, kJ \, mol^{-1}$ for sodium chloride, suggesting a substantial difference either in the crystal properties or in the interaction of the ions with water. In fact the very great strength of the silver chloride crystal is due to the high polarisability of the silver ion. The heat of solution of an ionic solute can be written as

$$\Delta H_{solution} = \Delta H_{sublimation} - \Delta H_{hydration} \tag{4.3}$$

Conceptually, the solid salt (sodium chloride, for instance) is converted to the gaseous (g) state, $Na^+(g) + Cl^-(g)$, and each unit is then hydrated to form the species $Na^+(aq)$ and $Cl^-(aq)$. If the heat of hydration is sufficient to provide the energy needed to overcome the lattice forces, the salt will be freely soluble at a given temperature and the ions will readily dislodge from the crystal lattice. If the partial molal enthalpy of solution of the substance is positive, the solubility will increase with increasing temperature; if it is negative the solubility will decrease, in agreement with Le Chatelier's principle.

4.2.3 The effect of simple additives on solubility

Solubility products

For poorly soluble materials such as silver chloride and barium sulfate the concept of the solubility product can be used. The following equilibrium exists in solution between crystalline silver chloride $AgCl_c$ and ions in solution:

$$AgCl_c \rightleftharpoons Ag^+ + Cl^- \tag{4.4}$$

An equilibrium constant K can be defined as

$$K = \frac{[Ag^+][Cl^-]}{[AgCl_c]} \tag{4.5}$$

Strictly, K should be written in terms of thermodynamic activities and not concentrations, but activities can be replaced by concentrations (denoted by square brackets) because of the low solubilities involved (see section 2.3.1 in Chapter 2). At saturation the concentration of the crystalline silver chloride $[AgCl_c]$ is essentially constant and the solubility product, K_{sp}, may therefore be written

$$K_{sp} = [Ag^+][Cl^-] \tag{4.6}$$

The sparingly soluble compound silver chloride is an example of a 1:1 salt, i.e. each molecule ionises to give one ion of Ag^+ and one of Cl^-. When a compound has more than one ion of each type, for example, the poorly soluble salt calcium hydroxide $Ca(OH)_2$, then the solubility product is defined as the product of each ion raised to the appropriate power. Calcium hydroxide ionises to give one ion of Ca^{2+} and two OH^- ions and the solubility product becomes

$$K_{sp} = [Ca^{2+}][OH^-]^2$$

Some values of solubility products are quoted in Table 4.7.

Table 4.7 Solubility products of some inorganic salts	
Compound	K_{sp} (mol^2 dm^{-6})
AgCl	1.25×10^{-10}
Al(OH)$_3$	7.7×10^{-13}
BaSO$_4$	1.0×10^{-10}

Common ion effect

The solubility product is useful for evaluating the influence of other species on the solubility of salts of low aqueous solubility. One of the most important influences on the solubility of poorly soluble salts occurs on addition of another compound that has an identical ion to one of those of the salt. For example, if sodium chloride is added to a saturated solution of silver chloride, the concentration of Cl^- ions in solution will be increased, as therefore will the product $[Ag^+][Cl^-]$. Consequently, to maintain K_{sp} constant the concentration of Ag^+ in solution will decrease, i.e. solid AgCl will be precipitated. This effect, whereby the solubility of a sparingly soluble salt is decreased by the addition of another compound having an ion in common, is referred to as the *common ion effect*. Several examples of the influence of the common ion effect on drug solubilities *in vivo* are discussed in section 4.7.2.

Salting in and salting out

In general, additives may either increase or decrease the solubility of a solute in a given solvent. The effect that they have will depend on several factors:

- the effect the additive has on the structure of water
- the interaction of the additive with the solute

- the interaction of the additive with the solvent.

The effect of a solute additive on the solubility of another solute may be quantified by the Setschenow equation:

$$\log \frac{S}{S_a} = kc_a \tag{4.7}$$

where S_a is the solubility in the presence of an additive, S is the solubility in its absence, c_a is the concentration of additive and k is the salting coefficient. The sign of k is positive when the activity coefficient is increased; it is negative if the activity coefficient is decreased by the additive. The Setschenow equation frequently holds up to additive concentrations of $1 \, mol \, dm^{-3}$, a measure of the sensitivity of the activity coefficient of the solute towards the salt.

Salts that increase solubility are said to *salt in* the solute and those that decrease solubility *salt out* the solute. Salting out may result from the removal of water molecules that can act as solvent because of competing hydration of the added ion. The opposite effect, salting in, can occur when salts with large anions or cations that are themselves very soluble in water are added to the solutions of non-electrolytes. Sodium benzoate and sodium *p*-toluenesulfonate are good examples of such agents and are referred to as *hydrotropic salts*; the increase in the solubility of other solutes is known as *hydrotropy*. Values of k (in $(mol \, dm^{-3})^{-1}$) for three salts added to benzoic acid in aqueous solution are 0.17 for NaCl; 0.14 for KCl; and -0.22 for sodium benzoate. That is, NaCl and KCl decrease the solubility of benzoic acid, and sodium benzoate increases it.

4.2.4 The effect of pH on the solubility of ionisable drugs

pH is one of the primary influences on the solubility of most drugs that contain ionisable groups. As the great majority of drugs are organic electrolytes, there are four parameters that determine their solubility:

1. their degree of ionisation
2. their molecular size
3. interactions of substituent groups with solvent
4. their crystal properties.

In this section consideration is given to the solubility of weak electrolytes and the influence of pH on aqueous solubility, important in both formulation and dissolution of drugs *in vivo*, and ultimately and importantly their biological activity.

Acidic drugs

Acidic drugs, such as the non-steroidal anti-inflammatory agents, are less soluble in acidic solutions than in alkaline solutions because the predominant undissociated species cannot interact with water molecules to the same extent as the ionised form, which is readily hydrated. Equation (4.8), which is a form of the Henderson–Hasselbalch equation relating drug solubility to the pH of the solution and to the pK_a of the drug, is derived in Derivation Box 4A.

$$pH - pK_a = \log\left(\frac{S - S_0}{S_0}\right) \quad (4.8)$$

where S is the total saturation solubility of the drug and S_0 is the solubility of the undissociated species. Examples of the use of equation (4.8) to calculate the effect of pH on the solubility of acidic drugs are given below.

Basic drugs

Basic drugs such as ranitidine are more soluble in acidic solutions, where the ionised form of the drug is predominant. If S_0 is the solubility of an undissociated

Example 4.2 Calculation of the effect of pH on the solubility of an acidic drug

What is the solubility of benzylpenicillin G at a pH sufficiently low to allow only the non-dissociated form of the drug to be present?

The pK_a of benzylpenicillin G is 2.76 and the solubility of the drug at pH 8.0 is 0.174 mol dm^{-3}. (From Notari RE. *Biopharmaceutics and Pharmacokinetics*, 2nd edn. New York: Marcel Dekker, 1978.)

Answer

If only the undissociated form is present at low pH then we need to find S_0. This can be obtained from the information given using equation (4.8):

$$pH - pK_a = \log\left(\frac{S - S_0}{S_0}\right)$$

Therefore,

$$8.0 - 2.76 = \log\left(\frac{0.174 - S_0}{S_0}\right)$$

i.e.

$$5.24 = \log\left(\frac{0.174 - S_0}{S_0}\right)$$

Therefore, $S_0 = 1 \times 10^{-6}$ mol dm^{-3}.

Example 4.1 Calculation of the effect of pH on the solubility of an acidic drug

What is the pH below which sulfadiazine ($pK_a = 6.48$) will begin to precipitate in an infusion fluid, when the initial molar concentration of sulfadiazine sodium is 4×10^{-2} mol dm^{-3} and the solubility of sulfadiazine is 3.07×10^{-4} mol dm^{-3}?

Answer

The pH below which the drug will precipitate is calculated using equation (4.8):

$$pH = 6.48 + \log\frac{(4.00 \times 10^{-2}) - (3.07 \times 10^{-4})}{3.07 \times 10^{-4}}$$

$$= 8.60$$

base, RNH_2, the Henderson–Hasselbalch expression for the solubility (S) as a function of pH (see Derivation Box 4B) is

$$pH - pK_a = \log\left(\frac{S_0}{S - S_0}\right) \quad (4.9)$$

Solubility–pH profiles of a basic drug (chlorpromazine) and an acidic drug (indometacin) and values for the more complex profile of the amphoteric drug oxytetracycline are plotted in Fig. 4.3.

In general, this approach is valid in dilute ideal solutions for which the solubility of the ionised species is much greater than that of the uncharged species. Despite its widespread use to predict the pH dependence of drug solubility, a study of the accuracy of equation (4.9) in predicting the solubility of a series of cationic drugs as a function of pH in divalent buffer

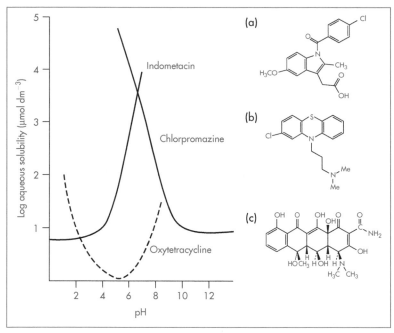

Figure 4.3 Solubility of (a) indometacin, (b) chlorpromazine and (c) oxytetracycline as a function of pH, plotted as logarithm of the solubility.

systems mimicking the intestinal fluid highlighted some limitations of this equation and the authors cautioned against its uncritical use.[7]

Example 4.3 Calculation of the effect of pH on the aqueous solubility of a basic drug

A drug is found to have the following saturation solubilities at room temperature:

pH	S (μmol dm^{-3})
7.4	205.0
9.0	10.0
10.0	5.5
12.0	5.0

What type of compound is it likely to be and what is its pK_a?

Answer

As the solubility decreases with increasing pH, the compound is a base. At pH 12 the solubility quoted is likely to be the solubility of the unprotonated species, that is, S_0. Using the figures given, we can apply a re-arranged form of equation (4.9) at each of the other pH values:

$$pK_a = pH + \log\left(\frac{S - S_0}{S_0}\right)$$
$$= 7.4 + \log\frac{200}{5}$$
$$= 7.4 + \log 40 = 7.4 + 1.602 = 9.0$$
$$pK_a = 9.0 + \log\frac{10 - 5}{5} = 9.0 + \log 1 = 9.0$$
$$pK_a = 10.0 + \log\frac{5.5 - 5}{5} = 10.0 + \log 0.1 = 9.0$$

The drug has a pK_a value of 9.0 and is thus likely to be an amine.

Amphoteric drugs

Several drugs and amino acids, peptides and proteins are amphoteric, displaying both basic and acidic characteristics. Frequently encountered drugs in this category are the sulfonamides and the tetracyclines. If, for simplicity, we were to use a generalised structure for an amphoteric compound

$$R - X - COOH$$
$$| $$
$$NH_2$$

and if the solution equilibrium between the species were written down, we would obtain the following equations relating solubility to pH (see Derivation Box 4C).

$$pH - pK_a = \log\left(\frac{S_0}{S - S_0}\right) \qquad (4.10)$$

at pH values below the isoelectric point, and

$$pH - pK_a = \log\left(\frac{S - S_0}{S_0}\right) \qquad (4.11)$$

at pH values above the isoelectric point.

Table 4.8 gives solubility data for oxytetracycline (**XVI**) as a function of pH. Oxytetracycline has three pK_a values: $pK_{a1} = 3.27$, $pK_{a2} = 7.32$ and $pK_{a3} = 9.11$, corresponding to the regions 1, 2 and 3 in the structure shown.

Structure XVI Oxytetracycline

The equations for the solubilities of acidic, basic and zwitterionic drugs (equations 4.8, 4.9, 4.10 and 4.11) can all be used to calculate the pH at which a drug will precipitate from solution of a given concentration (or the concentration at which a drug will reach its maximum solubility at a given pH). This is especially important in determining the maximum allowable levels of a drug in infusion fluids or formulations. Some idea of the range of pH values encountered in common infusion fluids can be seen from the data of Tse et al.[8] Typical examples include: Ringer's solution (pH 7.0), 1 L of Ringer's solution containing 2 cm^3 vitamins (pH 5.5), normal saline (pH 5.4), 5% dextrose in water (pH 4.4), 1 L of 5% dextrose containing 100 mg of thiamine hydrochloride (pH 3.9).

The variation in pH between preparations and within batches of the same infusion fluid (the monograph for Dextrose Infusion BP allows a pH ranging

Table 4.8 Oxytetracycline: pH dependence of solubility at 20°C	
pH	**Solubility (g dm^{-3})**
1.2	31.4
2	4.6
3	1.4
4	0.85
5	0.5
6	0.7
7	1.1
8	28.0
9	38.6

Data from the *United States Dispensatory*, 25th edn.

from 3.5 to 5.5) means that the fluids vary considerably in their solvent capacity for weak electrolytes.

Not only is it important to consider the pH of the formulation when deciding on the concentration of drug that can be incorporated, it is equally important to bear in mind possible changes in pH that might occur following administration of the formulation as these might be responsible for drug precipitation from formulations in which the drug concentration is close to the solubility limit. Several examples of the precipitation of drugs *in vivo* resulting from alteration of pH are considered in Chapter 11 and we will consider here only one example, that of precipitation from eye drop formulations containing amphoteric fluoroquinolone drugs.

Rule of thumb

From the above equations it is seen that, as a rough guide, the solubility of drugs with un-ionised species of low solubility varies by a factor of 10 for each pH unit change. A compilation of the pKa values of drugs is given in Chapter 2 (Table 2.6).

Clinical point

Eye drops containing norfloxacin (Chibroxin), ciprofloxacin (Ciloxan) and ofloxacin (Ocuflox) are used for the treatment of external ocular infection and corneal ulcer. Although these products are all formulated as sterile, isotonic, aqueous solutions, preserved with benzalkonium chloride, and all contain 0.3% of the respective fluoroquinolone drug, there have been observations of crystallised corneal deposits only following the clinical use of Ciloxan. The reason for the precipitation of this drug is seen from a consideration of differences in the pH of the formulations (Chibroxin 5.2, Ciloxan 4.5 and Ocuflox 6.4) and also the solubilities of the three fluoroquinolones. As we have seen above, solubility of this class of drug generally exhibits a minimum near physiological pH corresponding to the zwitterionic form of the drug; ciprofloxacin is the least soluble of the commercially available fluoroquinolones, with particularly low solubility near the pH of tears. Figure 4.4 shows the solubility–pH plots for the three drugs up to pH 7.5 (the solubility would, of course, increase at higher pH values as the compounds are amphoteric) and provides an explanation for the precipitation of ciprofloxacin. The pH of the tear film immediately following instillation of the eye drops is determined by the pH of the formulation but returns to the physiological value (pH 6.8) within 15 minutes due to tear turnover and drainage.

Superimposed on the solubility profile of each drug in Fig. 4.4 are the total drug concentration and the concentration of drug dissolved in the tear fluid. The decrease of total drug concentration with time is a result of tear turnover and drainage. Following dosing of ofloxacin and norfloxacin (Fig. 4.4a, b), the soluble drug concentration is identical to the total drug concentration at all time points and the tear solution remains clear and particulate-free. Following ciprofloxacin dosing (Fig. 4.4c), however, the soluble drug concentration falls significantly below the total drug concentration at approximately 8 minutes after drug addition (tear pH 6.1). At this pH the drug concentration exceeds the solubility limit, a supersaturated solution is formed and precipitation of ciprofloxacin occurs, producing a milky-white tear solution. At approximately 12 minutes post dose (tear pH 6.6), the soluble ciprofloxacin concentration is reduced to almost half (54%) of the total drug concentration due to continued precipitation.

Example 4.4 Calculation of the solubility of an amphoteric drug

Tryptophan has two pK_a values, 2.4 and 9.4, and an isoelectric point of 5.9. Calculate the solubility of tryptophan at pH 2 and at pH 10, given that the solubility of the compound in neutral solutions, S_0, is $2 \times 10^{-2}\,mol\,dm^{-3}$.

Answer

At pH 2.0: This pH is below the isoelectric point so we must use equation (4.10):

$$pH - pK_a = \log\left(\frac{S_0}{S - S_0}\right)$$

$$2 - 2.4 = \log\left(\frac{2 \times 10^{-2}}{S - (2 \times 10^{-2})}\right)$$

Rearranging,

$$\log\left(\frac{S - (2 \times 10^{-2})}{2 \times 10^{-2}}\right) = 0.4$$

That is,

$$\frac{S - (2 \times 10^{-2})}{2 \times 10^{-2}} = 2.5118$$

Therefore, $S = (5.02 \times 10^{-2}) + (2 \times 10^{-2}) = 7.02 \times 10^{-2}\,mol\,dm^{-3}$.

At pH 10 (using equation 4.11):

$$10 - 9.4 = \log\left(\frac{S - (2 \times 10^{-2})}{2 \times 10^{-2}}\right)$$

That is,

$$\left(\frac{S - (2 \times 10^{-2})}{2 \times 10^{-2}}\right) = 3.981$$

Therefore, $S = (7.96 \times 10^{-2}) + (2 \times 10^{-2}) = 9.96 \times 10^{-2}\,mol\,dm^{-3}$.

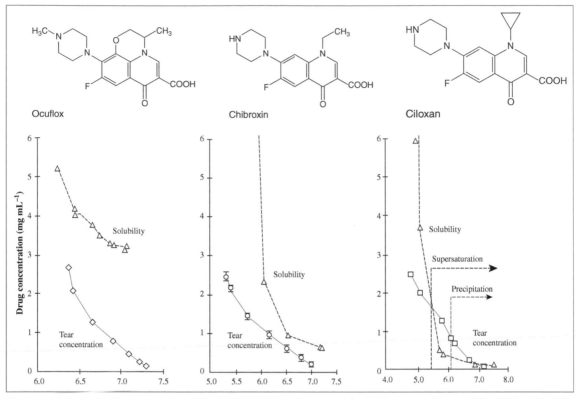

Figure 4.4 Relationship between drug concentration in a tear turnover model (solid lines) and drug solubility (dashed lines) for (a) ofloxacin (Ocuflox); (b) norfloxacin (Chibroxin); and (c) ciprofloxacin (Ciloxan).

Reproduced with permission from Firestone BA *et al.* Solubility characteristics of three fluoroquinolone ophthalmic solutions in an *in vitro* tear model. *Int J Pharm* 1998;164:119. Copyright Elsevier 1998.

Example 4.5 Calculation of the effect of pH on solubility

Calculate the pH at which the following drugs will precipitate from solution given the information supplied.

Drug	pK_a	Solubility of un-ionised species	Concentration of solution
(a) Thioridazine HCl (mol wt 407 Da)	9.5	1.5×10^{-6} mol dm^{-3}	0.407% w/v
(b) Oxytetracycline HCl	3.3, 7.3 and 9.1	0.5 g dm^{-3}	1.4 mg cm^{-3}

The isoelectric point of oxytetracycline HCl is at approx. pH = 5.

Answer

(a) We use equation (4.9) to calculate the pH above which thioridazine will precipitate:

$$pH = pK_a + \log\left(\frac{S_0}{S - S_0}\right)$$

The concentration of solution is the saturation solubility at the point of precipitation. 0.407% w/v = 1×10^{-2} mol dm^{-3} = S. $S_0 = 1.5 \times 10^{-6}$ mol dm^{-3}.

$$pH = 9.5 + \log\left(\frac{1.5 \times 10^{-6}}{(1 \times 10^{-2}) - (1.5 \times 10^{-6})}\right)$$

$$= 9.5 + \log\left(\frac{1.5 \times 10^{-6}}{1.0 \times 10^{-2}}\right)$$

$$= 9.5 - 3.284$$

$$= 5.68$$

(b) The concentration of solution is 1.4 mg cm^{-3}, which is 1.4 g dm^{-3}. $S_0 = 0.5$ g dm^{-3}.

At pH values below the isoelectric point, the pH at which S is the maximum solubility is given by eq (4.10)

$$pH = pK_a + \log\left(\frac{S_0}{S - S_0}\right)$$
$$= 3.3 + \log(0.556)$$
$$= 3.3 - 0.255$$
$$= 3.05$$

At pH values above the isoelectric point, the pH at which S is the maximum value is given by eq (4.11)

$$pH = 7.3 + \log(1.8)$$
$$= 7.3 + 0.255$$
$$= 7.56$$

Thus at pH values between 3.05 and 7.56 the solution containing $1.4\,mg\,cm^{-3}$ will precipitate.

4.3 Measurement of solubility

In the traditional method of determining drug solubility, often referred to as the 'shake flask' method, the drug is added to a standard buffer solution until saturation occurs, indicated by undissolved excess drug. The pH is remeasured and, if necessary, readjusted with dilute acid or alkali. The flasks are then shaken for a minimum of 24 h and the amount of dissolved drug is determined by a suitable assay of the supernatant solution after filtration. This method is, however, manually intensive and time-consuming, and several alternative procedures have been proposed.

A simple turbidimetric method for the determination of the solubility of acids and bases in buffers of different pH can be used.[9] Solutions of the hydrochloride (or other salt) of a basic drug, or the soluble salt of an acidic compound, are prepared in water over a range of concentrations. Portions of each solution are added to buffers of known pH and the turbidity of the solutions is determined in the visible region. Typical results are shown in Fig. 4.5. Below the solubility limit there is no turbidity. As the solubility limit is progressively exceeded, the turbidity rises. The solubility can be determined by extrapolation, as shown in Fig. 4.5. Table 4.9 shows results obtained by this method for some phenothiazines and tricyclic antidepressant compounds. Determination of the solubility of weak electrolytes at several pH values provides one method of

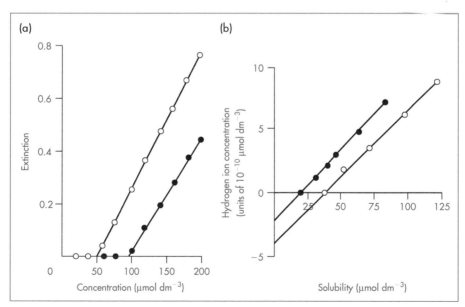

Figure 4.5 (a) Plot of extinction against concentration of amitriptyline hydrochloride at pH 9.78 (○) and pH 9.20. (b) (●) Relationship between hydrogen ion concentration and solubility of pecazine (●) and amitriptyline (○).

Reproduced from Green AL. Ionisation constants and water solubilities of some aminoalkyl phenothiazine tranquillizers and related compounds. *J Pharm Pharmacol* 1967;19:10–16. Copyright Wiley-VCH Verlag GmbH & Co. KGaA. Reproduced with permission.

Table 4.9 Water solubilities and pK_a values of aminoalkylphenothiazines and related compounds

Structure	Approved name	pK_a, solubility method	pK_a, Chatten–Harris[a]	Solubility (μ mol dm^{-3})	Calculated relative solubility at pH 7.4
R=H;R'=CH$_2$CH(Me)·NMe$_2$	Promethazine	9.1	9.1	55	4.5
R=H;R'=[CH$_2$]$_3$·NMe$_2$	Promazine	9.4	–	50	8.0
R=Cl; R'=[CH$_2$]$_3$·NMe$_2$	Chlorpromazine	9.3	9.2	8	1.0
R=CF$_3$; R'=[CH$_2$]$_3$·NMe$_2$	Triflupromazine	9.2	9.4	5	0.4
R = H; R'= CH$_2$	Pecazine	9.7	–	18	5.0
R = SMe; R'= [CH$_2$]$_2$	Thioridazine	9.5	9.2	1.5	0.3

Reproduced from Green AL. Ionisation constants and water solubilities of some aminoalkyl phenothiazine tranquillizers and related compounds. *J Pharm Pharmacol* 1967;19:10–16. Copyright Wiley-VCH Verlag GmbH & Co. KGaA. Reproduced with permission.
[a]Data from Chatten LG, Harris LE. *Anal Chem* 1962;34:1495.

obtaining the dissociation constant of the drug substance. For basic drugs,

$$pH = pK_a + \log\left(\frac{S_0}{S - S_0}\right)$$

S_0, the solubility of the undissociated species (base), is determined at high pH, and S is determined at several different lower pH values. A plot of $\log[S_0/(S - S_0)]$ versus pH will have the pK_a as the intercept on the pH axis.

Alternatively, S may be plotted against $[H^+]$, as in Fig. 4.5b. The dissociation of a basic drug in water may be written as (see Derivation Box 4B)

$$\frac{K_b}{[OH^-]} = \frac{[H^+]}{K_a} = \frac{S - S_0}{S_0} \tag{4.12}$$

which can be rearranged to

$$[H^+] = \left(\frac{K_a S}{S_0}\right) - K_a \tag{4.13}$$

Plotting data as in Fig. 4.5b yields S_0 when the line crosses the x-axis as $[H^+] = 0$ (and $S = S_0$). The intercept on the y-axis gives $-K_a$ and the slope of the line is K_a/S_0.

4.4 The solubility parameter

Regular solution theory characterises non-polar solvents in terms of solubility parameter, δ_1, which is defined as

$$\delta_1 = \left(\frac{\Delta U}{V}\right)^{1/2} = \left(\frac{\Delta H - RT}{V}\right)^{1/2} \tag{4.14}$$

where ΔU is the molar energy and ΔH is the molar heat of vaporisation of the solvent. ΔH is determined by calorimetry at temperatures below the boiling point at constant volume. V is the molar volume of the solvent. The solubility parameter is thus a measure of the intermolecular forces within the solvent and gives us information on the ability of the liquid to act as a solvent. Table 4.10 gives the solubility parameters of some common solvents calculated using equation (4.14).

$\Delta U/V$ is the liquid's *cohesive energy density*, a measure of the attraction of a molecule from its own liquid, which is the energy required to remove it from the liquid and is equal to the energy of vaporisation per unit volume. Because cavities have to be formed in a solvent, by separating other solvent molecules, to accommodate solute molecules (as discussed earlier)

Table 4.10 Solubility parameters of common solvents	
Solvent	**δ_1 (cal$^{1/2}$ cm$^{-3/2}$)^a**
Methanol	14.50
Ethanol	12.74
1-Propanol	11.94
2-Propanol	11.56
1-Butanol	11.40
1-Octanol	10.24
Ethyl acetate	8.58
Isoamyl acetate	8.07
Hexane	7.30
Hexadecane	8
Carbon disulfide	10
Membrane (erythrocytes)	10.3 ± 0.40
Cyclohexane	8.2
Benzene	9.2

^{a}The solubility parameter is commonly expressed in hildebrand units:
1 hildebrand unit = 1 (cal cm^{-3})$^{1/2}$.
1 cal = 4.18 J.

the solubility parameter δ_1 enables predictions of solubility to be made in a semiquantitative manner, especially in relation to the solubility parameter of the solute, δ_2.

By itself the solubility parameter can explain the behaviour of only a relatively small group of solvents – those with little or no polarity and those unable to participate in hydrogen-bonding interactions. The difference between the solubility parameters expressed as $(\delta_1 - \delta_2)$ will give an indication of solubility relationships.

For solid solutes a hypothetical value of δ_2 can be calculated from $(U/V)^{1/2}$, where U is in this case the lattice energy of the crystal. In a study of the solubility of ion pairs in organic solvents it has been found that the logarithm of the solubility (log S) correlates well with $(\delta_1 - \delta_2)^2$.

4.4.1 Solubility parameters and biological processes

The solubility of small molecules in biological membranes is of importance from pharmacological, physio-logical and toxicological viewpoints. Biological membranes are not simple solvents – the bilayer has an interior core of hydrocarbon chains about 2.5–3.5 nm thick – and therefore one would not expect simple solution theory to hold. Regular solution theory has been applied to biomembranes to obtain a value of δ_1 for a membrane.[10] From experimental solubility data for anaesthetic gases in erythrocyte ghosts, mean empirical solubility parameters of 10.3 ± 0.40 for the whole membrane and 8.7 ± 1.03 for membrane lipid were calculated. The values compare with solubility parameters of 7.3 for hexane and 8.0 for hexadecane. The value for the whole membrane (10.3) is very close to the solubility parameter of 1-octanol (10.2), a solvent that is used widely in partition coefficient work to simulate biological lipid phases.

Solubility parameters of drugs (δ_2) have also been correlated with membrane absorption rates in model systems. A reasonable relationship was obtained between δ_2 and a logarithmic absorption term, thus providing one predictive index of absorption. Scott[11] has said of solubility parameters and equations employing them that 'the theory offers a useful initial approach to a very wide area of solutions. Like a small-scale map for a very broad long-distance view of a sub-continent they are unlikely to prove highly accurate when a small area is examined carefully, but they are equally unlikely to prove completely absurd.'

4.5 Solubility in mixed solvents: use of cosolvents

The device of using mixed solvents (cosolvents) is resorted to when drug solubility in one solvent is limited or perhaps when the stability characteristics of soluble salts forbid the use of single solvents. Cosolvent use is widespread during the screening of new molecular entities as potential drug candidates where large numbers of molecules need to be brought into solution to be tested for biological activity. For such testing in tissue culture or in experimental animals it is important that the drug does not precipitate in the system under study, as this will affect the apparent activity. Common water-miscible solvents used in pharmaceutical formulations include glycerol, propylene glycol, ethyl alcohol and polyoxyethylene glycols, particularly polyoxyethylene glycol 400 (PEG

400). Ethanol is frequently combined with propylene glycol in cosolvent mixtures, for example phenobarbital is solubilised in a cosolvent mixture of 68–75% propylene glycol and 10% ethanol; pentobarbital sodium, phenytoin sodium and digoxin are all solubilised in solutions with 40% propylene glycol and 10% ethanol. Cosolvent formulations often contain several organic cosolvents; for example, the sparingly water-soluble antineoplastic agent etoposide is solubilised in a cosolvent mixture of PEG 400, glycerin and water; digoxin is solubilised in a cosolvent mixture of propylene glycol, PEG 400 and ethanol; parenteral solutions of diazepam contain propylene glycol, ethanol and benzyl alcohol. As can be imagined, the addition of another component complicates any system and explanations of the often complex solubility patterns are not easy. Toxicity considerations are, of course, a constraint on the choice of solvent for products for administration by any route.

The range of solubilty of phenobarbital in common mixed solvents is seen from the data of Krause et al.[12] Phenobarbital dissolves up to 0.12% w/v in water at 25°C. Glycerol, even in high concentrations, does not significantly increase the solubility of the drug (the solubility increases to only 1% w/v in 100% glycerol). Ethanol is a much more efficient cosolvent than glycerol as it is less polar. Phenobarbital solubility reaches a maximum of 13.4% w/v at 90% ethanol in ethanol–water mixtures, and 16% w/v at 80% ethanol in ethanol–glycerol mixtures. Adding an organic cosolvent to water makes the solvating environment less polar, resulting in a more favourable mixing (solvation) of a hydrophobic solute in the liquid phase. One key aspect of drug solubilisation with the aid of cosolvents is to create a solvent mixture that closely matches the polarity of the hydrophobic solute. In general, the more hydrophobic the solute, the greater the solubilising effect produced by an organic cosolvent that is less polar than water.

A proposed model for prediction of the solubility, S_m, of organic compounds in mixed solvents composed of water and an organic cosolvent, the log-linear cosolvency model, assumes that the solubility in the water–cosolvent mixture, S_m, increases logarithmically with a linear increase in the fraction of organic solvent according to

$$\log S_m = f_c \log S_c + f_w \log S_w \tag{4.15}$$

where f_c and f_w are the volume-fraction concentrations of the organic cosolvent and water, respectively, and S_c and S_w, are the solubilities in pure cosolvent and water, respectively. The model is based on the assumption that the free energy of solution of the mixture corresponds to the (volume-fraction) weighted average of the free energy of solution in the pure solvent components.

Rearranging equation (4.15) and noting that $f_w = 1 - f_c$ gives

$$\log S_m = f_c \sigma + \log S_w \tag{4.16}$$

where $\sigma = \log (S_c/S_w)$ or, more correctly, $\log (\gamma_w/\gamma_c)$ where γ_w and γ_c are the activity coefficients of the solute in water and pure organic solvent, respectively. The model therefore predicts a linear relationship between the logarithm of the solubility in the mixed solvent and the volume fraction of the cosolvent in the mixed solvent. The gradient of the plot is σ and the intercept is the logarithm of the solubility of the drug in water.

The σ term is often referred to as the cosolvency power, since it provides a measure of the inherent ability of the particular cosolvent to solubilise the solute in relation to its solubility in water. The σ parameter has the properties of a hypothetical partition coefficient. For example, for a given organic solvent, the σ parameter of different solutes is linearly related to their octanol–water partition coefficient, such that σ estimates can be made from the σ values of other solutes in the same cosolvent.

The model assumes that the solute–water and solute–cosolvent interactions are present in the water–cosolvent mixture in direct proportion to the respective concentration of each of the solvents in the solvent blend. The model also assumes that no additional interactions exist in the solvent mixture apart from these. The polarity match predicted by the log-linear model has been shown to apply when polar cosolvents such as aliphatic alcohols (methanol, ethanol, propanol) are used but is less predictable with less polar cosolvents such as tetraglycol, Labrasol and 1-methyl-2-pyrrolidone, because of cosolvent–water interactions.[13]

The situation becomes more complex when additives are included in the formulation as these will influence solute–solvent interfacial energies or dissociation of electrolytes through changes in dielectric constant. A reduction in ionisation through a decrease in dielectric constant will favour decreased solubility, but this effect may be counterbalanced by the greater affinity of the undissociated species in the presence of the cosolvent.

Problems which may arise from precipitation of poorly water-soluble drugs during the administration of mixed-solvent systems are discussed in the following clinical point and in more detail in Chapter 11 (section 11.2).

Room-temperature ionic liquids

An interesting class of solvents with potential application for the solubilisation of poorly water-soluble drugs are the room-temperature ionic liquids (RTILs).[14] These are organic salts comprising a relatively large asymmetric organic cation (e.g. alkyl pyridinium and dialkyl imidazolium ions) combined with an inorganic or organic anion (e.g. halide, hexafluorophosphate and tetrafluoroborate) which, as the name implies, are liquid at ambient temperature. Their versatility as solvents arises from the wide range of possible combinations of the constituent anions and cations providing a correspondingly wide variation of acidity, basicity, hydrophilicity/hydrophobicity and water miscibility. Typical examples are given in Structure **XVII** which shows RTILs based on 1-alkyl-3-methylimidazolium cations combined with PF_6^-, Cl^-, BF_4^- and Br^- anions. The ability of some of these RTILs to act as solvents for the poorly water-soluble drugs albendazole and danazol is shown in Table 4.11 from which it is seen that the longer the alkyl chain of the cation (i.e. the greater the hydrophobicity), the greater is the solubility enhancement.

Structure XVII Room-temperature ionic liquids based on 1-alkyl-3-methylimidazolium cations

The miscibility of RTILs with water can be improved by inclusion of a second RTIL enabling their application as cosolvents in aqueous systems. For example, the solubility of albendazole in mixtures of water/ C_4H_9imidazolium PF_6^-/ C_6H_{13}imidazolium Cl^- at a 1/1/1 molar ratio was 7.95 mmol/L compared to a water solubility of 0.002 mmol/L.

Clinical point

A potential problem associated with the administration of mixed-solvent formulations of poorly water-soluble drugs is drug precipitation when these preparations are added to an aqueous solution such as blood plasma. For example, precipitation of the relatively water-insoluble diazepam has been reported when formulations of this drug in a mixed-solvent solution containing propylene glycol (40%) and alcohol (10%) are administered by injection using an intravenous (IV) infusion set, rather than directly into the vein of the patient,

	Albendazole	Danazol
[bmim] BF$_4^-$	1.49 ± 0.02	18.9 ± 0.6
[hmim] BF$_4^-$	2.97 ± 0.04	ND
[omim] BF$_4^-$	7.2 ± 0.3	>59
[bmim] PF$_6^-$	29 ± 9	11.9 ± 0.2
[hmim] PF$_6^-$	53 ± 4	ND
[omim] PF$_6^-$	>75	35 ± 5
Water	0.00200 ± 0.00008	0.00030 ± 0.00006

Table 4.11 Solubility (mmol/L, mean ± SD, $n = 3$) of two model drugs in room-temperature ionic liquids based on the 1-alkyl-3-methylimidazolium cations (**XVII**) with alkyl chain lengths: R = C_4H_9 [bmim]; C_6H_{13} [hmim]; C_8H_{17} [omim]. ND = not determined.

Reproduced from Mizuuchi H *et al*. Room temperature ionic liquids and their mixtures: potential pharmaceutical solvents. *Eur J Pharm Sci* 2008;33:326–331.

as instructed by the supplier. Precipitation occurs because of changes in the proportions of the solvents on dilution with plasma in the infusion set; we discuss this problem in more detail in Chapter 11 (section 11.2).

Precipitation of a poorly water-soluble drug during IV injection may also be a consequence of a rapid infusion rate or abnormally slow venous flow rate, both of which result in unfavourable changes in solvent composition. The critical parameters that determine whether a drug will precipitate during IV injection are its solubility in plasma, the drug dose and the plasma flow rate in the vein. The maximum infusion rate ($mg\,min^{-1}$) is the product of the plasma solubility ($mg\,cm^{-3}$) and the venous flow rate (normally between 40 and $60\,cm^3\,min^{-1}$). Example 4.6 shows the calculation of minimum injection times for a poorly water-soluble drug and illustrates the influence of the rate of venous flow on the time required to prevent precipitation of drug in the plasma. Note that in this calculation it is assumed that the injected solution mixes instantaneously with the plasma; in practice longer injection times should be used to ensure safety.

Example 4.6 Calculation of minimum injection times for poorly water-soluble drugs

What is the minimum time required for the IV injection of a 20 mg dose of a poorly water-soluble drug (solubility in plasma $= 0.60\,mg\,cm^{-3}$) to ensure that precipitation does not occur? Assume a venous flow rate of (a) $60\,cm^3\,min^{-1}$ and (b) $40\,cm^3\,min^{-1}$.

Answer

(a) Maximum infusion rate $=$ plasma solubility $\times$ venous flow rate:

$$= 0.60 \times 60 = 36.0\,mg\,min^{-1}$$

Therefore, a 20 mg dose should be injected over a period of at least 33 seconds to avoid drug precipitation.

(b) Maximum infusion rate $= 0.60 \times 40 = 24.0\,mg\,min^{-1}$.

Therefore, at least 50 seconds should be allowed for injection at this venous flow rate.

4.6 Cyclodextrins as solubilising agents

Solubilisation by surface-active agents is discussed in Chapter 5. Alternatives to micellar solubilisation (or solubilisation in vesicles) include the use of the cyclodextrin (CD) family. When the first edition of this book was published in 1981 (and a diagram of a CD–drug complex was used to adorn the cover), the use of CDs was in its infancy. Attention was then focused around α-, β- and γ-CDs, but a veritable industry has grown up with an array of derivatives that can lend useful new properties to the complexes they form. For example, 10% of the CD derivative Encapsin HPB (hydroxypropyl-β-cyclodextrin) can enhance the aqueous solubility of betamethasone 118 times, of diazepam 21 times and of ibuprofen 55 times. The solubilising capacities of a range of CDs and their derivatives have been reviewed.[15] An idea of the extent to which natural CDs and their derivatives are currently included in marked pharmaceutical products is seen from Table 4.12, which details just some of the estimated 35 different commercial formulations. This topic has been comprehensively reviewed by Kurkov and Loftsson.[16]

CDs are enzymatically modified starches. Their glucopyranose units form a ring: α-CD a ring of 6 units; β-CD a ring of 7 units; and γ-CD a ring of 8 units (Table 4.13; Fig. 4.6). The 'ring' is cylindrical, the outer surface being hydrophilic and the internal surface of the cavity being non-polar. Appropriately sized lipophilic molecules can be accommodated wholly or partially in the complex, in which the host–guest ratio is usually 1:1 (Fig. 4.7), although other stoichiometries are possible, one, two or three CD molecules complexing with one or more drug molecules. The dissolution–dissociation–crystallisation process that can occur on dissolution is illustrated in Fig. 4.8.

Not all CDs are free of adverse effects; di-O-methyl β-CD, for example, has a strong affinity for cholesterol and is haemolytic. It is also one of the best solubilisers technically.

Table 4.12 Marketed pharmaceutical products which include natural cyclodextrins (αCD, and βCD) and the cyclodextrin derivatives 2-hydroxypropyl-β-cyclodextrin (HPβCD), sulfobutylether β-cyclodextrin sodium salt (SBEβCD) and 2-hydroxypropyl-γ-cyclodextrin (HP γCD)

Drug/cyclodextrin	Therapeutic usage	Formulation	Trade name
αCD			
Alprostadill	Treatment of erectile dysfunction	Intracavernous solution	CaverJect Dual
βCO			
Cetirzine	Antibacterial agent	Chewing tablets	Cetrizin
Dexamethasone	Anti-Inflammatory steroid	Ointment, tablets	Glymesason
Nicotine	Nicotine replacement product	Sublingual tablets	Nicorette
Nimesulide	Non-steroidal anti-inflammatory drug	Tablets	Nimedex
Piroxicam	Non-steroidal anti-inflammatory drug	Tablets, suppository	Brexin
HPβCD			
Indomethacin	Non-steroidal anti-inflammatory drug	Eye drop solution	Indocid
Itraconazole	Antifungal agent	Oral and IV solutions	Sporanox
Mitomycin	Anticancer agent	IV infusion	MitoExtra
SBEβCD			
Aripiprazole	Antipsychotic drug	IM solution	Abllify
Maropitant	Anti-emetic drug (motion sickness in dogs)	Parenteral solution	Cerenia
Voriconazole	Antifungal agent	IV solution	Vfend
Ziprasidone mesylate	Antipsychotic drug	IM solution	Geodon
HPγCD			
Diclofenac sodium salt	Non-steroidal anti-Inflammatory drug	Eye drop solution	Voltaren Ophtha
Tc-99 Teoboroxime	Diagnostic aid, cardiac imaging	IV solution	CardioTec

The CDs have obvious uses in parenteral formulations, including use as components of vehicles for peptides and other biologicals (ovine growth hormone, interleukin-2 and insulin). A special use of one γ-CD derivative, sugammadex, is discussed in Chapter 11 (section 11.6.1). Because it tightly binds the general anaesthetic rocuronium when injected IV it reverses its action and thus shortens the duration of anaesthesia at will.

Calixarenes

Research continues into other agents, apart from surfactants (which are discussed in Chapter 5), that can enhance the solubility of drugs. The calixarenes are another type of host, existing in a 'cup shape' in a rigid conformation. The 4-sulfonic calix[*n*]arenes can form host–guest-type interactions with drugs such as nifedipine, a poorly water-soluble agent,[17] seen in Fig. 4.9.

Table 4.13 Properties of α, β and γ cyclodextrins

Property	Alpha (α)	Beta (β)	Gamma (γ)
Molecular weight	973	1135	1297
Glucose monomers	6	7	8
Internal cavity diameters (nm)	0.5	0.6	0.8
Water solubility ($g\ 100\ cm^{-3}$; 25°C)	14.2	1.85	23.2
Surface tension ($mN\ m^{-1}$)	71	71	71
Melting range (°C)	255–260	255–260	240–245
Water of crystallisation (no. of molecules)	10.2	13–15	8–18
Water in cavity (no. of molecules)	6	11	17

Reproduced with permission from Brewster ME *et al*. Development of a non-surfactant formulation for alfaxalone through the use of chemically-modified cyclodextrins. *J Parenter Sci Technol* 1989;43:262.

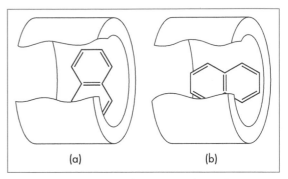

Figure 4.7 Two models of a complex of cyclodextrin with a lipophilic guest compound: (a) equatorial inclusion, (b) axial inclusion.

Reproduced with permission from Harata K, Uedaira H. *Bull Chem Soc Jpn* 1975;48:375.

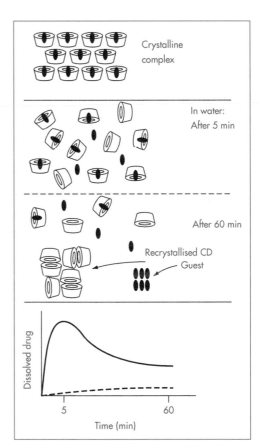

Figure 4.8 Schematic representation of the dissolution–dissociation–recrystallisation process of a cyclodextrin complex with a poorly soluble guest. The complex rapidly dissolves, and a metastable oversaturated solution is obtained. The anomalously high level of dissolved guest drops back but remains higher than the level that can be obtained with non-complexed drug. Solid curve = complexed drug; broken curve = non-complexed drug.

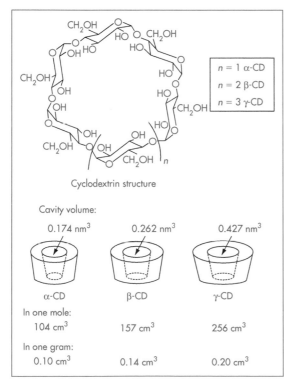

Cyclodextrin structure

$n = 1$ α-CD
$n = 2$ β-CD
$n = 3$ γ-CD

Cavity volume:

α-CD	β-CD	γ-CD
$0.174\ nm^3$	$0.262\ nm^3$	$0.427\ nm^3$

In one mole:

| 104 cm³ | 157 cm³ | 256 cm³ |

In one gram:

| 0.10 cm³ | 0.14 cm³ | 0.20 cm³ |

Figure 4.6 Structures of the α-, β- and γ-cyclodextrins.

Reproduced from Szejtli J. *Pharm Tech Int* 1991;3(2):15.

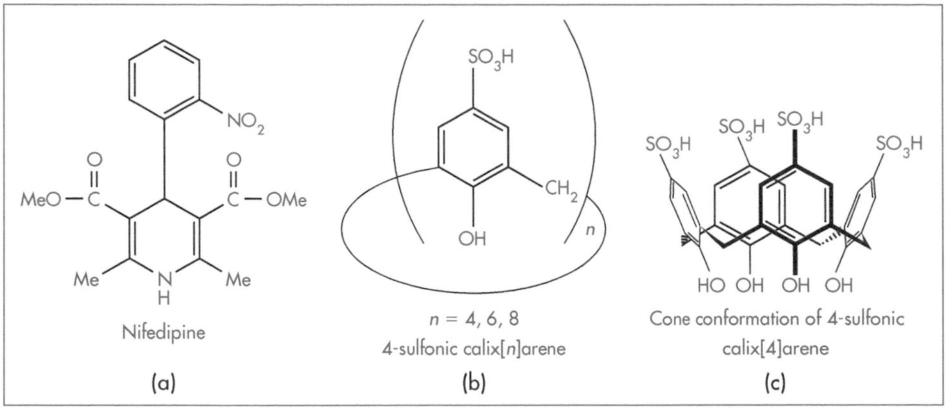

Figure 4.9 Molecular structures of (a) nifedipine and (b) 4-sulfonic calix[*n*]arenes. As *n* increases (4, 6, 8) the cavity size (see (c)) increases from 0.3 nm, through 0.76 nm to 1.16 nm. The solubility increase for nifedipine is greatest with calix[8]arene, being nearly 250% at a concentration of 0.008 mol dm^{-3} and pH of 5.

Reproduced with permission from Yang W, de Villiers MM. The solubilization of the poorly water soluble drug nifedipine by water soluble 4-sulphonic calix[n]arenes. *Eur J Pharm Biopharm* 2004;58:629–636. Copyright Elsevier 2004.

4.7 Solubility problems in formulation

4.7.1 Mixtures of acidic and basic compounds

Sometimes a combination formulation requires the admixture of acidic and basic drugs. One example (Septrin infusion) is discussed here.

Because sulfamethoxazole (**XVIII**) is a weakly acidic substance and trimethoprim (**XIX**) is a weakly basic one, for optimal solubility basic and acidic solutions, respectively, are required. In consequence, in an ordinary aqueous solution sulfamethoxazole and trimethoprim demonstrate a high degree of incompatibility and mutual precipitation occurs on mixing. To optimise mutual dissolution, an aqueous solution that includes 40% propylene glycol is used in the formulation of the infusion. This solution, which has a pH between 9.5 and 11.0, allows adequate amounts of both substances to coexist in solution to give the correct ratio of concentration for antibacterial action. On dilution, the infusion becomes less stable and at the recommended 1 in 25 dilution stability is about 7 h. Owing to incompatibility of the two constituents, their degrees of solubility are sensitive to changes in ionic composition, pH and any drug additives. If there is imbalance in pH or ionic composition, then precipitation of one or other of the components may well occur.

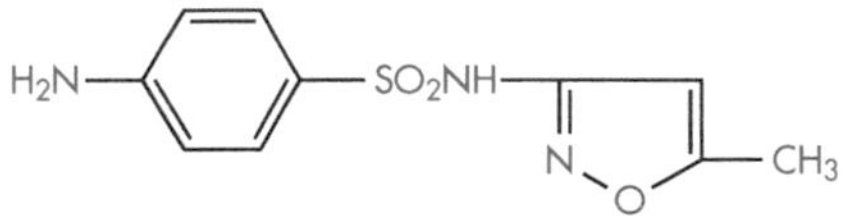

Structure XVIII Sulfamethoxazole, pK_a = 6.03

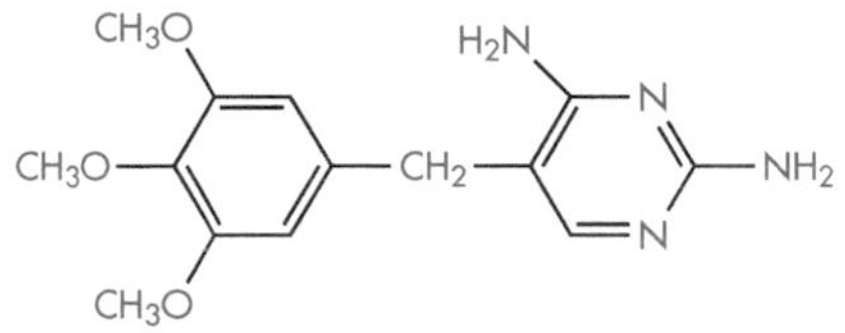

Structure XIX Trimethoprim, pK_a = 7.05

4.7.2 Choice of drug salt to optimise solubility

The choice of a particular salt of a drug for use in formulations may depend on several factors. The solubility of the drug in aqueous media may be markedly dependent on the salt form. The chemical stability rather than the solubility may be a criterion and in many cases this is dependent on the choice of salt, sometimes through a pH effect. Deliberate choice of an insoluble form for use in suspensions is an obvious ploy; the formation of water-soluble entities from poorly soluble acids or bases by the use of hydrophilic counterions is frequently attempted to produce injectable solutions of a drug. Table 4.14 gives some indication of the range of solubilities that can be obtained through the use of different salt forms, in this case of an experimental antimalarial drug (**XX**).

Table 4.14 Solubilities of salts of an antimalarial drug (XX)

Salt	Melting point (°C)[a]	Solubility (mg cm^{-3})	Saturated solution pH
Free base	215	7–8	–
Hydrochloride	331	32–15	5.8
dl-Lactate	172 (dec)	1800	3.8
l-Lactate	193 (dec)	900	–
2-Hydroxy-1-sulfonate	250 (dec)	620	2.4
Methanesulfonate	290 (dec)	300	5.1
Sulfate	270 (dec)	20	–

[a](dec) = with decomposition.
Reproduced from Agharkar S et al. Enhancement of solubility of drug salts by hydrophilic counterions: properties of organic salts of an antimalarial drug. *J Pharm Sci* 1976;65:747. Copyright Wiley-VCH Verlag GmbH & Co. KGaA. Reproduced with permission.

Structure XX Compound used in Table 4.14

The large hydrophobic compound **XX**, even as its hydrochloride salt, is poorly soluble and this is presumably the reason for its poor oral bioavailability. Similar conclusions were drawn several years ago for novobiocin. The acid salt administered to dogs at 12.5 mg kg^{-1} was not absorbed, but the monosodium salt, which is about 300 times as soluble in water, produced plasma levels of 22 µg cm^{-3} after 3 h. Unfortunately, the sodium salt is unstable in solution. An amorphous form of the acid produced even higher levels of drug than the sodium salt, illustrating the fact that choice of salt and crystalline form of a drug substance may be of critical importance.

Some of the solubility differences obviously arise from differences in the pH of the salt solutions, which in the case of compound **XX** ranged from 2.4 to 5.8 pH units. This is not atypical. The pH of solutions of salts of a 3-oxyl-1,4-benzodiazepine derivative at 5 mg cm^{-3} ranged from 2.3 for its dihydrochloride, to 4.3 for the maleate, and to 4.8 for the methanesulfonate.

Further examples of the solubility range in drug salts and derivatives are shown in Table 4.15. The increase in the solubility on the formation of the hydrochloride is readily attributable in the case of tetracycline to a lowering of the solution pH by the hydrochloride. The common ion effect (see section 4.2.3) can, however, produce an unexpected trend in the solubilities and dissolution rates (since these are proportional to the solubility in the diffusion layer at the surface of the solid) of bases in the presence of high concentrations of hydrochloric acid.[18] Increase in Cl$^-$ concentrations will cause the equilibrium between solid (s) and solution (aq) forms

$$BH^+Cl^-_s \overset{K_{sp}}{\rightleftharpoons} (BH^+)_{aq} + (Cl^-)_{aq}$$

to be pushed to the left-hand side, with a resultant decrease in solubility. The solubility of **XX** as the hydrochloride decreases from 24×10^{-5} mol dm^{-3} in 1.3 mmol dm^{-3} chloride ion, to 3×10^{-5} mol dm^{-3} in 40 mmol dm^{-3} chloride ion concentration. It should be noted that the stomach contents are rich in chloride ions. The common ion effect will be apparent in many infusion fluids to which drugs may be added, and therefore the effect of pH as well as electrolyte concentrations must be considered.

Consideration of Table 4.15 suggests that the hydrochloride salts of tetracyclines are always more

Table 4.15 Aqueous solubilities of tetracycline, erythromycin and chlorhexidine salts

Compound	Solubility in water (mg cm^{-3})
Tetracycline	1.7
Tetracycline hydrochloride	10.9
Tetracycline phosphate	15.9
Erythromycin	2.1
Erythromycin estolate[a]	0.16
Erythromycin stearate	0.33
Erythromycin lactobionate	20
Chlorhexidine	0.08
Chlorhexidine dihydrochloride	0.60
Chlorhexidine digluconate	>700

[a]Lauryl sulfate ester of erythromycin propionate

readily dissolved than the base. The situation is more complex than at first appears, however. In dilute HCl at pH 1.2, the free base dissolves more than the hydrochloride, probably owing to the differences in crystallinity. The amount of compound derived from the base in solution decreases with time as the drug is converted to the hydrochloride. At pH 1.6 the rate of solution of the two forms is identical, and at pH 2.1 the hydrochloride has a higher solubility owing to its effect on local pH around the dissolving particles.

Erythromycin (**XXI**) is labile at pH values below pH 4, and hence is unstable in the stomach contents. Erythromycin stearate (the salt of the tertiary aliphatic amine and stearic acid), being less soluble, is not as susceptible to degradation. The salt dissociates in the intestine to yield the free base, which is absorbed. There are differences in the absorption behaviour of the erythromycin salts and differences in toxicity, which may be related to their aqueous solubilities. Erythromycin ethylsuccinate was originally developed for paediatric use because its low water solubility and relative tastelessness were suited to paediatric formulations. The soluble lactobionate is used in IV infusions.

Structure XXI   Erythromycin

4.7.3 Drug solubility and biological activity

There should be a broad correlation between aqueous solubility and indices of biological activity. On the one hand, as drug solubility in aqueous media is inversely related to the solubility of the agent in biological lipid phases, there will be some relationship between pharmacodynamic activity and drug solubility. On the

other, we should expect that drug or drug salt solubility might influence the absorption phase; drugs of very low aqueous solubility will dissolve slowly in the gastrointestinal tract, and in many cases the rate of dissolution is the rate-controlling step in absorption.

With drugs of low aqueous solubility such as digoxin, chlorpropamide, indometacin, griseofulvin and many steroids, the physical properties of the drug can influence biological properties. At early stages in a drug's development, pharmacological and toxicological tests are frequently carried out on extemporaneously prepared suspensions whose physical characteristics are not always well defined. This is not good practice as the toxicity of some drugs given by gavage to rats is dependent on the drug species used[19] (Table 4.16). This has been shown to be true with polymorphic forms of the same drug, but in the cases discussed in Table 4.16 different salts of the drugs were used.

Table 4.16 The effect of solubility in water on the toxicity of drugs given by gavage to albino rats

Drug	Salt	Solubility	$LD_{50} \pm$ SEM
Benzylpenicillin	Ammonium	$<20\,mg\,cm^{-3}$	8.4 ± 0.13
Benzylpenicillin	Potassium	$>20\,mg\,cm^{-3}$	6.7 ± 0.1
Iron	Free metal	Insoluble	98.6 ± 26.7
Iron	Ferrous sulfate	Soluble	0.78
Spiramycin	Free base	Poorly soluble	9.4 ± 0.8
Spiramycin	Adipate	Soluble	4.9 ± 0.2

Modified from Boyd E. *Predictive Toxicometrics*. Bristol: Scientechnica; 1972.

There are other examples in which aqueous solubility acts as a rough and ready guide to absorption characteristics. The least soluble of the cardiotonic glycosides (digitoxin, digoxin and ouabain), being the most lipid soluble, are best absorbed. But because of the lipophilicity of digitoxin and digoxin, the rate-limiting step is the rate of solution, which is influenced directly by the solubility of the compounds.

High-molecular-weight quaternary salts such as bephenium hydroxynaphthoate (**XXII**) and pyrvinium embonate (**XXIII**), being quaternary, have low lipid solubility but also have low aqueous solubility. They are virtually unabsorbed from the gut and indeed are used in the treatment of worm infestation of the lower bowel.

Structure XXII Bephenium hydroxynaphthoate

Structure XXIII Pyrvinium embonate

Key points

- As predicted from a simple model of the processes involved in the dissolution of a solute, there is often a good correlation between the molecular surface area and the aqueous solubility; the solubility of simple non-polar hydrocarbons decreases with increase of surface area. With polar molecules and weak organic electrolytes, it is, however, necessary to consider the surface area of each portion of the molecule separately in predicting the overall effect; the greater the surface area of the hydrophilic portion relative to the hydrophobic portion, the greater will be the solubility.

- There is a trend for a decrease of solubility with increasing boiling point of liquids and increasing melting points of closely related series of solids.

- The influence of substituents on solubility can be due to their effect on the molecular cohesion of solids or liquids and/or their interaction with water molecules. Substituents can be classified as either hydrophobic or hydrophilic, depending on their polarity.

- The way in which solute molecules interact with water determines their affinity for the solvent; ionic substituents readily interact with the polar water molecules and confer solubility on the solute.

- Additives may either increase or decrease the solubility of a solute depending on the effect of the additive on water structure, and the interaction of the additive with the solute and the solvent. Addition of another compound with an identical ion to that of a poorly soluble salt will cause precipitation of the salt; this is known as the common ion effect. Additives that increase solubility are said to 'salt in' the solute, whereas those that decrease the solubility 'salt out' the solute. Very soluble salts such as sodium benzoate with large anions or cations can salt in other solutes and are known as hydrotropic salts; the increase in solubility caused by their addition is referred to as hydrotropy. The effect of an additive on solubility is given by the Setschenow equation.

- pH has a major influence on solubility of solutes with ionisable substituents: acidic drugs are less soluble in acidic solutions, whereas basic drugs are less soluble in alkaline solutions. Amphoteric drugs are least soluble at their isoelectric point where they exist as zwitterions. The solubility of each type of drug may be calculated at any given pH from a knowledge of the pK_a of the drug and its solubility in the un-ionised form.

- Solubility of acids and bases in buffers of different pH may be measured by 'shake flask' or turbidimetric methods.

- Drug solubility may be increased by the use of mixed solvents, for example glycerol–water, ethanol–water and ethanol–glycerol mixtures, or by choice of drug salt. CDs may be used to encapsulate the water-insoluble drug.

4.8 Partitioning

Here we discuss the topic of partitioning of a drug or solute between two immiscible phases. One phase might be blood or water and the other a biomembrane, or an oil or a plastic. As many processes (not least the absorption process) depend on the movement of molecules from one phase to another, it is vital that this topic is mastered. Here we will learn of the simple concepts of the partitioning of drugs and the calculation of partition coefficient (P) of the un-ionised form of the solute (and its logarithm, $\log P$), as well as the use of the $\log P$ concept in determining the relative activities or toxicities of drugs from a knowledge of $\log P$ between an oil, most commonly octanol, and water. Where P cannot be measured, calculations of $\log P$ can be accomplished.[20, 21] An outline of the methods available is given here.

Whether in formulations containing more than one phase or in the body, drugs move from one liquid phase to another in ways that depend on their relative concentrations (or chemical potentials) and their affinities for each phase. So a drug will move from the blood into extravascular tissues if it has the appropriate affinity for the cell membrane and the non-blood phase.

The movement of molecules from one phase to another is called *partitioning*. Examples of the process include:

- drugs partitioning between aqueous phases and lipid biophases
- preservative molecules in emulsions partitioning between the aqueous and oil phases
- antibiotics partitioning into microorganisms
- drugs and preservative molecules partitioning into the plastic of containers or giving sets.

Plasticisers will sometimes partition from plastic containers into formulations. It is, therefore, important that the process can be quantified and understood.

4.8.1 The partition coefficient

If two immiscible phases are placed in contact, one containing a solute soluble to some extent in both phases, the solute will distribute itself so that when equilibrium is attained no further net transfer of solute takes place, as then the chemical potential of the solute

in one phase is equal to its chemical potential in the other phase. If we think of an aqueous (w) and an organic (o) phase, we can write, according to equations (2.28) and (2.30),

$$\mu_{\mathrm{w}}^{\ominus} + RT \ln a_{\mathrm{w}} = \mu_{\mathrm{o}}^{\ominus} + RT \ln a_{\mathrm{o}} \tag{4.17}$$

Rearranging equation (4.17) we obtain

$$\frac{\mu_{\mathrm{o}}^{\ominus} - \mu_{\mathrm{w}}^{\ominus}}{RT} + \ln \frac{a_{\mathrm{w}}}{a_{\mathrm{o}}} \tag{4.18}$$

The term on the left-hand side of equation (4.18) is constant at a given temperature and pressure, so it follows that $a_{\mathrm{w}}/a_{\mathrm{o}} = \mathrm{constant}$ and, of course $a_{\mathrm{o}}/a_{\mathrm{w}} = \mathrm{constant}$. These constants are the *partition coefficients* or *distribution coefficients*, P. If the solute forms an ideal solution in both solvents, activities can be replaced by concentration, so that

$$P = \frac{C_{\mathrm{o}}}{C_{\mathrm{w}}} \tag{4.19}$$

P is therefore a measure of the relative affinities of the solute for an aqueous and a non-aqueous or lipid phase. Unless otherwise stated, P is calculated according to the convention in equation (4.19), where the concentration in the non-aqueous (oily) phase is divided by the concentration in the aqueous phase. The higher the value of P, the greater is the lipid solubility of the solute.

It has been shown for several systems that the partition coefficient can be approximated by the solubility of the agent in the organic phase divided by its solubility in the aqueous phase, a useful starting point for estimating relative affinities.

As early as 1891, Nernst stressed the fact that the partition coefficient as a function of concentration would be constant only if a single molecular species were involved. In some systems the association of the solute in one of the solvents complicates the calculation of partition coefficient; a simple example of the treatment of the partitioning of a dimerising compound gives the following equation for the partition coefficient (see Derivation Box 4D).

$$K' = \frac{\sqrt{C_2}}{C_1} \tag{4.20}$$

Table 4.17 illustrates the use of equations (4.19) and (4.20). Being weak electrolytes, many drugs will ionise in at least one phase, usually the aqueous phase. The partitioning of the drug between the organic and water phases depends on the ionic state of the drug and, as we have seen in section 2.5, this is determined by its pK_a and the pH of the aqueous phase. The partition coefficient refers to the distribution of one species, in this case the un-ionised drug, whereas the assay method will usually determine both the ionised and un-ionised drug in the aqueous phase. Because ionised species cannot, in general, partition into organic hydrophobic solvents, the ratio of drug concentrations in organic and aqueous phases determined from assay data will yield an *apparent partition coefficient*, P_{app}, which will vary with pH, rather than the true partition coefficient P. The relationship between the true thermodynamic P and P_{app} is given by the following equations, which have been derived in Derivation Box 4D:

For acids:

$$\log P = \log P_{app} - \log\left(\frac{1}{1 + 10^{pH - pK_a}}\right) \quad (4.21)$$

For bases:

$$\log P = \log P_{app} - \log\left(\frac{1}{1 + 10^{pK_a - pH}}\right) \quad (4.22)$$

Table 4.17 Distribution of two acids between immiscible phases at 25°C

C_1 (mol dm^{-3})^a	C_2 (mol dm^{-3})^b	C_2/C_1	$\sqrt{C_2}/C_1$
Succinic acid			
0.191	0.0248	0.130	
0.370	0.0488	0.132	
0.547	0.0736	0.135	
0.749	0.1010	0.135	
Benzoic acid			
4.88×10^{-3}	3.64×10^{-2}	7.46	39.06
8.00×10^{-3}	8.59×10^{-2}	10.75	36.63
16.00×10^{-3}	33.8×10^{-2}	21.13	36.36
23.7×10^{-3}	75.3×10^{-2}	31.77	36.63

Reproduced with permission from Glasstone S, Lewis D, *Elements of Physical Chemistry*, 2nd edn. London: Macmillan; 1964.
^{a}Aqueous-phase concentration.
^{b}Non-aqueous-phase concentration (succinic acid in ether; benzoic acid in benzene).

4.8.2 Free energies of transfer

The standard free energy of transfer of a solute between two phases is given by

$$\Delta G^{\ominus}_{trans} = \mu^{\ominus}_w - \mu^{\ominus}_o = RT \ln P \quad (4.23)$$

In a homogeneous series, P can be measured and the increase in its value observed for each substituent group (for example, $-CH_2-$). As the chain length of non-polar aliphatic compounds increases, it has been found that P increases by a factor of 2–4 per methylene group. The substituent contributions to P are additive, so a *substituent constant*, π_X, may be defined as

$$\pi_X = \log P_X - \log P_H \quad (4.24)$$

where P_X is the partition coefficient of the derivative of the parent compound whose partition coefficient is P_H and π_X is the logarithm of the partition coefficient of the function X. For example, π_{Cl} can be obtained by subtracting $\log P_{benzene}$ from $\log P_{chlorobenzene}$.

4.8.3 Octanol as a non-aqueous phase

Octanol is often used as the non-aqueous phase in experiments to measure the partition coefficient of drugs. Its polarity means that water is solubilised to some extent in the octanol phase and thus partitioning is more complex than with an anhydrous solvent, but perhaps its usefulness stems from the fact that biological membranes are also not simple anhydrous lipid phases. While octanol is favoured, other alcohols have also been used. For example, isobutanol has been used to show that the binding of many drugs to serum protein is determined by the hydrophobicity or lipophilicity of the drug, following the relationship

$$\log K = 0.9 \log P_{isobutanol} + constant \quad (4.25)$$

where K is an equilibrium constant measuring the binding of solute to protein. Transfer of a hydrophobic drug from an aqueous phase to a protein is, of course, a type of partitioning.

The correlation of lipophilicity and biological activity usually involves equations of the type

$$\log \frac{1}{C} = A \log P + constant \quad (4.26)$$

where C is the concentration required to produce a given pharmacological response.

4.9 Biological activity and partition coefficients: thermodynamic activity and Ferguson's principle

As the site of action of many biologically active species is in lipid components such as membranes, correlations between partition coefficients and biological activity were found early on by investigators of structure–action relationships. For example, a wide range of simple organic compounds can exert qualitatively identical depressant actions (narcosis) on many simple organisms. Lack of any chemical specificity in the compounds tested led to the suggestion that physical, rather than chemical, properties governed the activity of the compounds. Early work by Meyer (in 1899) and Overton (in 1895) related narcotic potency to the oil/water partition coefficient of the compounds concerned, and in a later reinterpretation of the data it was concluded that narcosis commences when any chemically non-specific substance has attained a certain molar concentration in the lipids of the cells.

In 1939 Ferguson[22] placed the Overton–Meyer theory on a more quantitative basis by applying thermodynamics to the problem of narcotic action. By expressing compound potency in terms of thermodynamic activity, rather than concentration, he avoided the problem of there being various distribution coefficients between the numerous different phases within the cell, any of which might be the phase in which the drug exerted its pharmacological effects (the biophase). The fact that the narcotic action of a drug remains at a constant level while a critical concentration of drug is applied, decreasing rapidly when administration of the drug is stopped, indicates that an equilibrium exists between some external phase and the biophase.

According to equation (2.28) the chemical potentials in two phases at equilibrium are equal. Thus, from equation (2.30),

$$\mu_A^\ominus + RT \ln a_A = \mu_B^\ominus + RT \ln a_B \qquad (4.27)$$

If the standard states are identical, the activities will consequently be equal in the two phases. The activity of a substance in the biophase at equilibrium is thus identical to the readily determined value in an external phase.

For narcotic agents applied as a vapour, the stand-ard state can be taken to be the saturated vapour, and thus activity $a = p_t/p_s$ where p_t is the partial pressure of the vapour and p_s is the saturated vapour pressure at the same temperature. When the narcotic agent was applied in solution and was also of limited solubility, activity was equated with the ratio S_t/S_0 where S_t is the molar concentration of the narcotic solution and S_0 its limiting solubility; the ratio S_t/S_0 therefore represents proportional saturation. This is in contrast to the normal procedure of taking the standard state as an infinitely dilute solution.

From recalculations of published data and also from measurements of the potency of many different compounds, Ferguson concluded that, within reasonable limits, substances present at approximately the same proportional saturation (that is, with the same thermodynamic activity) in a given medium have the same biological potency. For example, while the bactericidal concentrations of thymol and acetone against *Bacillus typhosus* vary widely (0.0022 and 3.89 mol L^{-1}, respectively), their thermodynamic activities are very similar (0.38 and 0.40, respectively).

However, there are often problems in applying the equations to real life. For example, if an attempt is made to correlate hydrophobicity with the rate of inhibition of local anaesthetic activity, the answers are complex, i.e. there is not necessarily a clear correlation because: (1) molecular size as well as hydrophobicity is a factor in kinetics; (2) membranes are non-homogeneous and if adsorption occurs at phospholipid head groups there is no way to mimic this with octanol and water; and (3) there is the problem of using equilibrium measurements for kinetic predictions.

4.10 Using log *P*

As we have seen, the value of log*P* is a measure of lipophilicity and, as so many pharmaceutical and biological events are dependent on lipophilic characteristics, the examples where correlations can be found between log*P* and biological indices are legion. A selection of applications of the log*P* concept is discussed here. Table 4.18 provides a sample of log*P* data for a range of pharmaceuticals. The relatively simple *in vitro* measurement of *P* can give an accurate prediction of activity in a complex biological system, provided that the obvious limitations of the simple system are recognised and that the biological activity of the drug depends on its lipophilic nature. Applications of P or $\log P$ come into their own particularly in homologous series or series of closely related compounds, where the influence of substituent groups can be accurately examined.

Table 4.18 Log P values for representative drugs

Drug	log P
Acetylsalicylic acid (aspirin)	1.19
Amiodarone	6.7
Benzocaine	1.89
Bupivacaine	3.4
Bromocriptine	6.6
Caffeine	0.01
Chlorpromazine	5.3
Cisapride	3.7
Ciprofloxacin	−1.12
Desipramine	4.0
β-Estradiol	2.69
Glutethimide	1.9
Haloperidol	1.53
Hydrocortisone	4.3
Hyoscine	1.90
Indometacin	3.1
Lidocaine	2.26
Methadone	3.9
Misoprostil	2.9
Nicotinamide	−0.37
Norfloxacin	−1.55
Ondansetron	3.2
Oxytetracycline	−1.12
Pergolide	3.8
Phenytoin	2.5
Physostigmine	2.2
Prednisone	1.46
Sulfadiazine	0.12
Sulfadimethoxine	1.56
Sulfafurazole	1.01

Sulfaguanidine	−1.22
Sulfamerazine	0.13
Sulfanilamide	−1.05
Sulfapyridine	0.90
Sulfathiazole	0.35
Tetracaine	3.56
Thiopental	2.8
Xamoterol	0.5
Zimeldine	2.7

Data from Herbert BJ, Dorsey JG. *Anal Chem* 1995;67:744; Butterworth JF, Strichartz GR. *Anaesthesiology* 1990;72:711; Jack DB. *Handbook of Clinical Pharmacokinetic Data*. London: Macmillan; 1992.

4.10.1 The relationship between lipophilicity and behaviour of tetracyclines

The lipid solubility of four tetracyclines (minocycline, doxycycline, tetracycline and oxytetracycline) correlates inversely with the mean concentration of antibiotic in plasma and with renal uptake and excretion. Only the more lipophilic minocycline and doxycycline pass across the blood–brain and blood–ocular barriers in detectable concentrations. Table 4.19 gives some of these characteristics of the tetracyclines. These analogues of tetracycline, while active *in vitro* against meningococci, are not of equal value in clinical use; oxytetracycline and doxycycline fail to change the state of 'carriers' of the disease, whereas minocycline has a significant effect. It is thought that the ability to enter the saliva and tears influences the clinical activity, for although saliva does not usually wet the nasopharynx, tears pass into the nasopharynx as the normal route of drainage from the conjunctival sac.

The pH dependence of partition coefficients of tetracyclines is more complex than for most drugs, as the tetracyclines are amphoteric.

For slightly simpler amphoteric compounds, such as p-aminobenzoic acid and sulfonamides, the apparent partition coefficient is maximal at the isoelectric point. Figure 4.10 illustrates the variation with pH of $\log P_{app}$ for p-aminobenzoic acid and for two sulfonamides.

The participation of the zwitterionic species in the partitioning can be excluded because of its low concentration, thus $K_t \rightarrow 0$ in Scheme 4.1. From this we obtain P and P_{app} as follows:

Table 4.19 Some characteristics of four tetracyclines

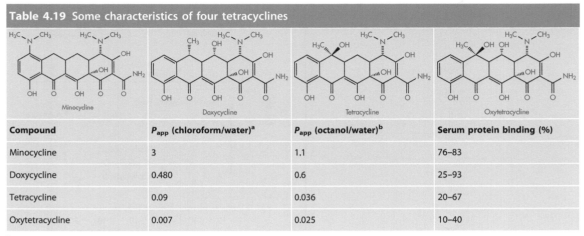

Compound	P_{app} (chloroform/water)[a]	P_{app} (octanol/water)[b]	Serum protein binding (%)
Minocycline	3	1.1	76–83
Doxycycline	0.480	0.6	25–93
Tetracycline	0.09	0.036	20–67
Oxytetracycline	0.007	0.025	10–40

[a]pH 7.4.
[b]pH 7.5.

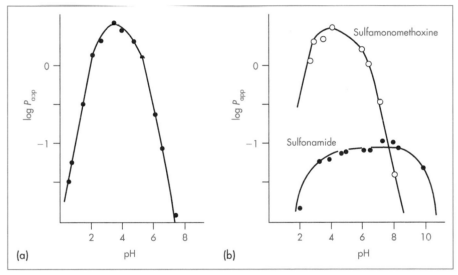

(a) pH

(b) pH

Figure 4.10 (a) Variation of $\log P_{app}$ with pH for p-aminobenzoic acid. (b) Variation of $\log P_{app}$ with pH for sulfamonomethoxine and sulfonamide.

Reproduced with permission from Terada H. *Chem Pharm Bull* 1972;20:765.

$$P = \frac{[I]_o}{[I]_w} \quad (4.28)$$

and

$$P_{app} + \frac{[I]_o}{[II]_w + [I]_w + [IV]_w + [III]_w}$$

$$= P \left[\frac{1}{\dfrac{[H^+]}{K_a} + \dfrac{K_c}{[H^+]} + K_t + 1} \right] \quad (4.29)$$

If $K_t \to 0$,

$$P_{app} \left[\frac{1}{\dfrac{[H^+]}{K_a} + \dfrac{K_c}{[H^+]} + 1} \right] \quad (4.30)$$

Passive diffusion of sulfonamides into human red cells is determined by plasma drug binding and lipid solubility. Apparent partition coefficients between chloroform and water at pH 7.4 show an almost linear relation with penetration constant for sulfonamides and a number of other acids. Penetration rates of sulfonamides into the aqueous humour and cerebrospinal fluid also correlate with partition coefficients (Fig. 4.11); moreover, the

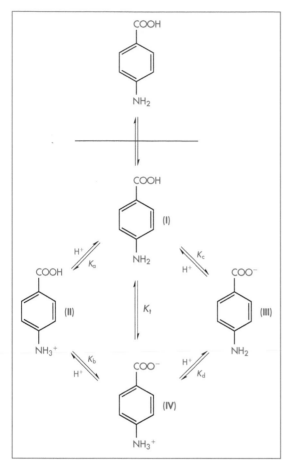

Scheme 4.1 Partitioning of *p*-aminobenzoic acid. K_a, K_b, K_c and K_d are microdissociation constants for each equilibrium and the relation between them is

$$K_1 = K_a + K_b$$

$$\frac{1}{K_2} = \frac{1}{K_c} + \frac{1}{K_d}$$

$$K_t = \frac{[\text{zwitterion}]}{[\text{neutral form}]} = \frac{K_b}{K_a} = \frac{K_c}{K_d}$$

where K_1 and K_2 are composite or macroscopic acid dissociation constants and K_t is the tautomeric constant between the zwitterionic and neutral forms.

Reproduced with permission from Terada H. Partition behavior of *p*-aminobenzoic acid and sulfonamides at various pH values. *Chem Pharm Bull* 1972;20:765.

antibacterial effects of a range of fatty acids and esters towards *B. subtilis* correlate with octanol/water partition coefficients.

There are many quantitative relationships between physiological action and $\log P$ or $\log P_{\text{app.}}$. A few examples are given in Box 4.1.

Local anaesthetic action on peripheral nerves is also proportional to P since the un-ionised form must diffuse

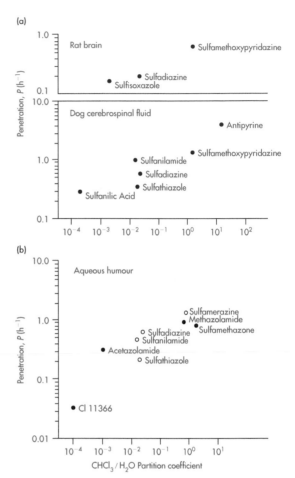

Figure 4.11 (a) Penetration rates of sulfonamides from plasma into rat brain and into canine cerebrospinal fluid. (b) Penetration rates of sulfonamides from plasma into aqueous humour for the rabbit (O) and for the rat (●) against partition coefficients (chloroform/water).

(a) Dog cerebrospinal fluid data from Rall DP. *J Pharm Exp Ther* 1959;125:185.

(b) Data from Wistrand PJ. *Acta Pharmacol Toxicol* 1960;17:337 and Sorsby A. *Br J Ophthalmol* 1949;33:347.

across the continuous cell layer of the perineurium. Once across the perineurium, the molecules ionise and they combine with the receptors in the nerve membrane in their ionised form.

The toxicity of some agents such as X-ray contrast media and penicillins has also been related to lipophilicity. Rates of entry into the brain of X-ray contrast agents used in cerebral angiography are proportional to P, and P correlates with clinical neurotoxicity. Figure 4.12 shows the positive relationship between toxicity of the penicillins and partition coefficient.

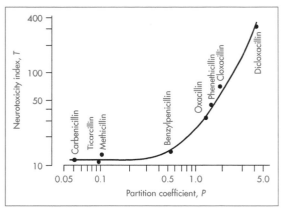

Figure 4.12 Relation of neurotoxicity to the hydrophobic character of various penicillins: the hydrophobic character is measured by the partition coefficient P and toxicity by a neurotoxicity index, T.

Reproduced from Weihrauch TR *et al*. Cerebral toxicity of penicillins in relation to their hydrophobic character. *Arch Pharmacol (NS)* 1975;289:55, with kind permission from Springer Science and Business Media.

4.10.2 Sorption

Figure 4.13 summarises the physicochemical problems in the use of preservative molecules in formulations. Solubility and partition coefficients of ionised species are determined, as we have seen, by the pH and ionic strength of the system. In this example, partitioning may occur from the aqueous phase to the oily phase of an emulsion, to the micellar phase of a surfactant, or to a closure. Adsorption may also occur on to container closures and suspended solid particles.

Permeation of antimicrobial agents into rubber stoppers and other closures is another example of partitioning. Although rubber is an amorphous solid, partitioning between the aqueous phase and rubber depends, as in liquid systems, on the relative affinities of the solute for each phase.

Glyceryl trinitrate, a volatile drug with a chloroform/water partition coefficient of 109, diffuses from simple tablet bases into the walls of plastic bottles and into plastic liners used in packaging tablets. This partitioning can be prevented if there is included in the tablet formulation an agent (such as polyoxyethylene glycol) that complexes with the drug substance, thereby increasing its affinity for the 'tablet phase' – in other words, reducing its escaping tendency or 'fugacity'. Significant losses of glyceryl trinitrate have been detected when the drug was given as an infusion

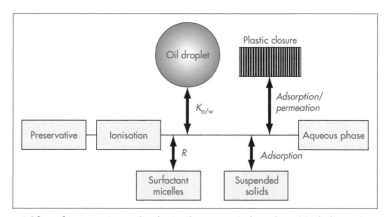

Figure 4.13 The potential fate of preservative molecules in pharmaceutical products. Much depends on the state of ionisation of the molecules. Partitioning into oil droplets or surfactant micelles can occur, as well as adsorption on to suspended solids. Adsorption, sorption or permeation of plastic closures can occur, leaving the less active form in the aqueous phase.

through plastic giving sets from a plastic reservoir, the absorption (of as much as 50% of the drug) resulting in the necessity to use unusually high doses of the drug.

Some relation has been found between the rate of sorption by poly(vinyl chloride) (PVC) bags of a series of drugs and their hexane/water partition coefficients.[23] Table 4.20 shows the data for sorption of 100 cm³ PVC infusion bags (equivalent to 11 g of PVC). In the table, P_{app} values have been calculated from

$$P_{app} = \left(\frac{1 - F_{\infty}}{F_{\infty}}\right)\frac{W_s}{W_p} \qquad (4.33)$$

where W_s is the weight of solution in contact with a given weight W_p of plastic and F_{∞} is the equilibrium fraction of drug remaining in solution. Only the unionised form of the drug is sorbed; the kinetics of the process can be accounted for by considering the diffusion of the molecules in the plastic matrix.

There are concerns over phthalates in medical devices, including diethylhexylphthalate (DEHP), used in medical products made of PVC such as IV bags, blood bags and tubing. DEHP can 'leach' out of PVC into liquids such as IV fluids, especially in the presence of formulations containing additives such as surfactants, as with Cremophor EL in Taxol. Figure 4.14 illustrates some of the problems that can occur in giving sets.

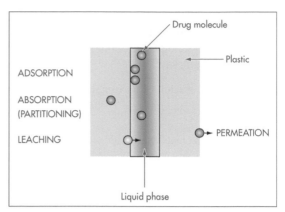

Figure 4.14 Diagram showing opportunities in plastic systems for adsorption of drug molecules, partitioning into (absorption) and eventually permeation through the plastic. Leaching of molecules from the plastic also may occur.

4.10.3 A chromatographic model for the biophase

Octanol/water partition coefficients, as we have seen, have been useful predictors of biological activity. In spite of this it has been suggested that bulk liquid phases may not be the most appropriate models for a structured biophase such as a biological membrane, and chromatographic stationary phases have been proposed as an alternative because of the structuring of the 'membranous' hydrophobic chains.

Table 4.20 Sorption into poly(vinyl chloride) and partitioning of drugs

Compound	Initial rate of sorption (10^{-2} h^{-1})	Extent of sorption at equilibrium (%)	log P_{app}	log P (hexane/water)
Medazepam	51	85	1.7	2.9
Diazepam	27	90	1.9	0.9
Warfarin (pH 2–4)	22	90	1.9	0.2
Glyceryl trinitrate	20	83	1.6	0.2
Thiopental (pH 4)	6	73	1.4	0.1
Oxazepam	4.6	46	0.9	−0.1
Nitrazepam	4.1	47	0.9	−0.1
Hydrocortisone acetate	0	0	–	−1.2
Pentobarbital (pH 4)	0	0	–	−1.3

Reproduced with permission from Illum L, Bundgaard H. Sorption of drugs by plastic infusion bags. *Int J Pharm* 1982;10:339–351. Copyright Elsevier 1982.

4.10.4 Calculating log P from molecular structures

The large number of methods used to calculate $\log P$ values have been elegantly reviewed by Leo *et al.*[21] The method proposed in 1964 by Fujita *et al.*[24] used values for the 'parent' molecule and values for substituents gathered by analysis of thousands of values of $\log P$ for homologous and other series. In this method of 'substituents', $\log P$ is considered to be an additive-constitutive free-energy-related property, where one can define Π for substituent X as the difference between the $\log P$ values for the parent solute and the compound with the substituent:

$$\Pi_{(X)} = \log P_{(R-X)} - \log P_{(R-H)} \qquad (4.34)$$

By definition $\Pi_{(H)} = 0$. For example,

$$\log P_{NO_2-C_6H_4CH_3} = \log P_{C_6H_6} + \Pi_{NO_2} + \Pi_{CH_3}$$
$$\log P = 2.13 - 0.28 + 0.56 = 2.41$$

compared with a measured value of 2.45.

The fragmental method developed by Rekker and Mannhold[25] uses the contributions of simple fragments. This may be illustrated by the example:

$$\log P_{C_6H_5OCH_2COOH} = f_{C_6H_5} \pm f_O + f_{CH_2}$$
$$+ f_{COOH} + PE1$$

where PE1 is a 'proximity effect', an adjusting fraction for polar fragments in non-polar surroundings. So

$$\log P_{C_6H_5OCH_2COOH} = 1.866 - 0.433$$
$$+ 0.53 - 0.954 + 0.861$$
$$= 1.87$$

compared with a measured value of 1.34.

A method based on the surface areas of molecules has also been proposed to obtain measures of $\log P$ in a manner analogous to the calculation of solubility.[26] Computer programs for calculation of $\log P$ are also in use and are described in detail in Leo *et al.*'s (1993) review.[21]

4.10.5 Drug distribution into human milk

The distribution of drugs into the milk of breastfeeding mothers is of obvious importance. Nearly all drugs find their way into milk and it is, therefore, useful to be able to predict which of them will achieve high concentrations in milk in relation to their plasma level, defined in one model[27] described below as the milk: plasma (M/P) ratio (Table 4.21). Three key parameters are the pK_a of the drug, plasma protein binding and the octanol/water partition coefficients of the drugs. Protein binding is the most important single predictor, an increase in M/P ratios generally being found as protein binding decreases. The equations used to calculate M/P ratios are shown in Box 4.2.

Table 4.21 Distribution of drugs into milk: the M/P ratio[b]

Drug	M/P
Acidic drugs	
Carbenicillin	0.02
Ethosuximide	0.78
Ibuprofen	0
Paracetamol	0.76
Valproic acid	0.05
Basic drugs	
Amitriptyline	0.83
Atenolol	0.32
Cimetidine	1.7
Clonazepam	0.33
Codeine	2.16
Lamotrigine	0.4–0.45
Morphine	2.46
Verapamil	0.6
Vigabatrin	0.01–0.05
Neutral drugs	
Alcohol	0.89
Digoxin	0.55
Medroxyprogesterone	0.72
Norethisterone	0.19
Prednisolone	0.13

[b] M/P = Milk : plasma drug concentration ratio.
Reproduced from Atkinson HC, Begg EJ. Prediction of drug distribution into human milk from physicochemical characteristics. *Clin Pharmacokinet* 1990;18:151–167, with kind permission from Springer Science and Business Media.

Box 4.2 The calculation of milk:plasma ratios

The two key equations, each with three independent variables, are as follows:

For basic drugs:

$$\ln\left(\frac{M}{P}\right) = 0.025 + 2.28\ln\left(\frac{M_u}{P_u}\right)$$
$$+ 0.89\ln f_{u,p}$$
$$+ 0.51\ln K \qquad (4.35)$$

For acidic drugs:

$$\ln\left(\frac{M}{P}\right) = -0.405$$
$$+ 9.36\ln\left(\frac{M_u}{P_u}\right) - 0.69\ln f_{u,p}$$
$$- 1.54\ln K \qquad (4.36)$$

where

M_u/P_u = milk:plasma unbound drug concentration ratio

$f_{u,p}$ = fraction of drug unbound in plasma

$f_{u,m}$ = fraction of drug unbound in milk

$K = (0.955/f_{u,m}) + [0.045 P_{app}(\text{milk/lipid})]$

P_{app} = apparent partition coefficient at pH 7.2

Few measurements of $f_{u,m}$ and P_{app}(milk/lipid) have been made, but these parameters can be predicted from $f_{u,p}$ and $\log P$.[28]

It is clear from equations (4.35) and (4.36) that there is a degree of empiricism about these equations, which arises in their derivation from the fitting of data sets based on the independent variables. The ratio M_u/P_u can be obtained from the modified Henderson–Hasselbalch equation.

For basic drugs,

$$\frac{M_u}{P_u} = \frac{1 + 10^{(pK_a - pH_m)}}{1 + 10^{(pK_a - pH_p)}} \qquad (4.37)$$

and for acidic drugs,

$$\frac{M_u}{P_u} = \frac{1 + 10^{(pH_m - pK_a)}}{1 + 10^{(pH_p - pK_a)}} \qquad (4.38)$$

where pH_m and pH_p are the pH values of milk and plasma, respectively. Milk has a mean pH of 7.2, slightly lower than that of plasma at 7.4. For neutral drugs the predicted M_u/P_u ratio would be unity, since the distribution of unbound un-ionised drugs would not be expected to be altered by pH gradients.

 Key points

- The partitioning of a drug or solute between two immiscible phases is quantified by the partition coefficient P (and its logarithm $\log P$). P is the ratio of concentration in the organic (or lipid) phase to that in the aqueous phase; the greater the value of P, the higher the lipid solubility.

- In the calculation of partition coefficient, consideration must be given to any aggregation or self-association of the drug in either of the solvents, and to changes of the ionisation of the drug with pH. In the case of ionisable drugs, the *true* partition coefficient refers to the distribution of the un-ionised form of the drug and this may be determined from measurements of the *apparent* partition coefficient as a function of pH.

- Ferguson's principle correlates the partition coefficient of a drug with its biological activity; it states that substances present at approximately the same proportional saturation (i.e. with the same thermodynamic activity) in a given medium have the same biological potency.

- Log P, usually measured using octanol as the non-aqueous solvent, is an indicator of the lipophilicity of a drug and can give a reasonably accurate prediction of *in vivo* activity if the biological activity of the drug depends on its lipophilic nature.

- Several methods are available for calculating $\log P$ from molecular structure.

Summary

Definitions of solubility, modes of expression of solubility and means of estimating solubility from the surface area of molecules were some of the key subjects discussed in this chapter. Molecular shape factors and substituents on molecules affect solubility, one of the key parameters of a drug substance. Effects such as solvation (or hydration in aqueous media) and the effects of additives on solubility are also dealt with, but perhaps the most important effect of all is that of pH on the solubility of ionisable drugs. This is treated in detail, and equations for acids, bases and zwitterions are considered. An understanding of pH–solubility relationships is vital to predicting the behaviour of ionic drugs in pharmaceutical formulations and in the body.

When additives, such as surfactants and CDs, do not achieve appropriate levels of practical solubility, we can resort to the use of cosolvents. The relative advantages and disadvantages of these different approaches to formulating a solution have to be considered, but in the last analysis other factors such as stability may determine which is the best approach to achieve a satisfactory solution formulation.

We have discussed the partitioning of a drug between immiscible phases and the importance of the partition coefficient (and its logarithm, log P) in defining the relative affinities of a solute for an aqueous and a non-aqueous or lipid phase, and as an important measure of the lipophilicity of a drug. Correlations between the partition coefficients and physiological action of several classes of drug have been examined. We have also seen the role of log P in quantifying a wide variety of diverse processes such as the extent to which a drug will adsorb on to container closures or distribute into human milk. Further examples of the importance of partitioning between aqueous and oily phases in, for example, emulsions and micellar systems will be examined in later chapters.

References

1. Amidon GL et al. Solubility of nonelectrolytes in polar solvents. II. Solubility of aliphatic alcohols in water. J Pharm Sci 1974;63:1858–1866.
2. Amidon GL. Theoretical calculation of heats of complexation in carbon tetrachloride. J Pharm Sci 1974;63:1520–1523.
3. Amidon GL et al. Solubility of nonelectrolytes in polar solvents. V. Estimation of the solubility of aliphatic monofunctional compounds in water using a molecular surface area approach. J Phys Chem 1975;79:2239–2246.
4. Hermann RB. Theory of hydrophobic bonding. II. Correlation of hydrocarbon solubility in water with solvent cavity surface area. J Phys Chem 1972;76:2754–2759.
5. Hermann RB. Theory of hydrophobic bonding. I. Solubility of hydrocarbons in water, within the context of the significant structure theory of liquids. J Phys Chem 1971;75:363–368.
6. Franks F. In: Duckworth RD (ed.) Water Relations of Foods. London: Academic Press; 1975.
7. Bergstrom CAS et al. Accuracy of calculated pH-dependent aqueous drug solubilities. Eur J Pharm Sci 2004;22:387–398.
8. Tse RL, Lee MW. pH of infusion fluids: a predisposing factor in thrombophlebitis. J Am Med Assoc, 1971; 215: 642.
9. Green AL. Ionisation constants and water solubilities of some aminoalkyl phenothiazine tranquillizers and related compounds. J Pharm Pharmacol 1967;19:10–16.
10. Bennett LJ, Miller KW. Application of regular solution theory to biomembranes. J Med Chem 1974;17:1124–1125.
11. Scott RS. Solutions of nonelectrolytes. Annu Rev Phys Chem 1956;7:43–66.
12. Krause GM, Cross JM, J Am Pharm Assoc, 1951; 40; 137.
13. Miyako Y et al. Solubility enhancement of hydrophobic compounds by cosolvents: role of solute hydrophobicity on the solubilisation effect. Int J Pharm 2010;393:48–54.
14. Mizuuchi H et al. Room temperature ionic liquids and their mixtures: potential pharmaceutical solvents. Eur J Pharm Sci 2008;33:326–331.
15. Loftsson T, Brewster ME. Pharmaceutical applications of cyclodextrins. 1. Drug solubilization and stabilization. J Pharm Sci 1996;85:1017–1025.
16. Kurkov SV, Loftsson T. Cyclodextrins. Int J Pharm 2013;453:167–180.
17. Yang W, de Villiers MM. The solubilization of the poorly water soluble drug nifedipine by water soluble 4-sulphonic calix[n]arenes. Eur J Pharm Biopharm 2004;586:29–36.
18. Serajuddin ATM. Salt formation to improve drug solubility. Adv Drug Del Rev 2007;59:603–616.
19. Boyd E. Predictive Toxicometrics. Bristol: Scientechnica; 1972.
20. Leo AJ et al. Partition coefficients and their uses. Chem Rev 1971;71:525–616.
21. Leo AJ et al. Calculating log P_{oct} from structures. Chem Rev 1993; 931:281–306.
22. Ferguson J. The use of chemical potentials as indices of toxicity. Proc R Soc Lond (Biol) 1939; 127:387–404.
23. Illum L, Bundgaard H. Sorption of drugs by plastic infusion bags. Int J Pharm 1982;10:339–351.
24. Fujita T et al. A new substituent constant, π, derived from partition coefficients. J Am Chem Soc 1964;86:5175–5180.
25. Rekker R, Mannhold R. Calculations of Drug Lipophilicity. Weinheim: VCH; 1992.
26. Broto P et al. Molecular structures: perception, autocorrelation descriptor and SAR studies. Perception of molecules: topological structure and 3-dimensional structure. Eur J Med Chem 1984;19:61–65.

27. Atkinson HC, Begg EJ. Prediction of drug distribution into human milk from physicochemical characteristics. *Clin Pharmacokinet* 1990;18:151–167.

28. Begg EJ *et al*. Prospective evaluation of a model for the prediction of milk: plasma drug concentrations from physicochemical characteristics. *Br J Clin Pharmacol* 1992; 33:501–505.

5

Surfactants

Certain compounds, because of their chemical structure, have a tendency to accumulate at the boundary between two phases. Such compounds are termed *amphiphiles, surface-active agents* or *surfactants*. Their adsorption at the various interfaces between solids, liquids and gases results in changes in the nature of the interface that are of considerable importance in pharmacy. For example, the lowering of the interfacial tension between oil and water phases facilitates emulsion formation; the adsorption of surfactants on insoluble particles enables these particles to be dispersed in the form of a suspension; and the incorporation of insoluble compounds within micelles of the surfactant can lead to the production of clear solutions.

In this chapter we will:

- see how the surface activity of a molecule is related to its molecular structure and look at the properties of some surfactants which are commonly used in pharmacy
- examine the nature and properties of films formed when water-soluble surfactants accumulate spontaneously at liquid–air interfaces and when insoluble surfactants are spread over the surface of a liquid to form a monolayer
- look at some of the factors that influence adsorption on to solid surfaces and how experimental data from adsorption experiments may be analysed to gain information on the process of adsorption
- examine why surfactants form aggregates or *micelles* in aqueous solutions when their concentration exceeds a critical concentration and some of the factors that influence micelle formation
- look at some of the properties of liquid crystals and surfactant vesicles and their potential as drug carriers
- see how micelles are able to solubilise water-insoluble drugs and discuss the pharmaceutical importance of this process.

5.1 Amphipathic compounds

Surface-active compounds are characterised by having two distinct regions in their chemical structure, termed *hydrophilic* ('water-liking') and *hydrophobic* ('water-hating') regions. The existence of two such moieties in a molecule is referred to as *amphipathy* and the molecules are consequently often referred to as *amphipathic* molecules.

The hydrophobic portions are usually saturated or unsaturated hydrocarbon chains or, less commonly, heterocyclic or aromatic ring systems. The hydrophilic regions can be anionic, cationic, zwitterionic or non-ionic. Surfactants are generally classified according to the nature of the hydrophilic group. Typical examples are given in Box 5.1.

The most commonly encountered *anionic* surfactants have carboxylate, sulfate, sulfonate and phosphate polar groups in combination with counterions such as sodium and potassium (for water solubility) or calcium and magnesium (for oil solubility). In the most common *cationic* surfactants the charge is carried on a nitrogen atom as, for example, with amine and quaternary ammonium surfactants. The quaternary ammonium compounds retain this charge over the whole pH range, whereas the amine-based compounds only function as surfactants in the protonated state and therefore cannot be used at high pH. By far the most common *non-ionic* surfactants are those with a poly(oxyethylene) chain as the hydrophilic group. In principle, it is possible to ethoxylate any material containing an active hydrogen, but the most commonly used starting materials are fatty alcohols, alkylphenols, fatty acids and fatty amines. *Zwitterionic* and *amphoteric* surfactants possess polar head groups which on ionisation may impart both positive and negative charges. The positive charge is almost always carried by an ammonium group and the negative charge is often a carboxylate. If the ammonium group is quaternary the molecule will exist as a zwitterion over a wide pH range since the quaternary ammonium group will be permanently charged. If not, the molecule will behave as a true amphoteric surfactant, that is, the molecule will change from net cationic to

---

Box 5.1 Classification of surfactants[a]

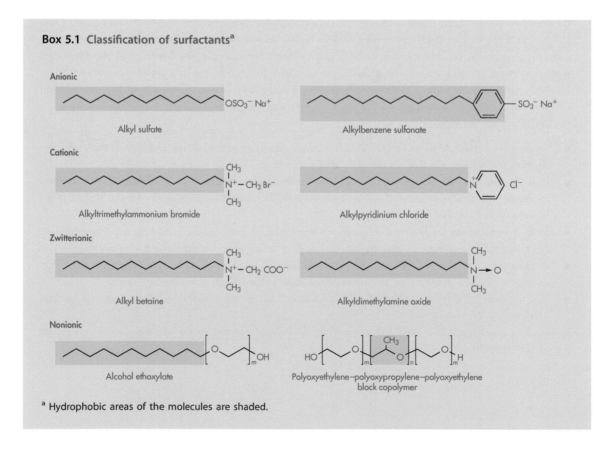

Anionic

Alkyl sulfate

Alkylbenzene sulfonate

Cationic

Alkyltrimethylammonium bromide

Alkylpyridinium chloride

Zwitterionic

Alkyl betaine

Alkyldimethylamine oxide

Nonionic

Alcohol ethoxylate

Polyoxyethylene–polyoxypropylene–polyoxyethylene block copolymer

[a] Hydrophobic areas of the molecules are shaded.

zwitterionic and finally to net anionic as the pH is increased; such surfactants will only therefore be zwitterionic over a certain range of pH that depends on the pK_a values of each charge group. At the isoelectric point both charged groups will be fully ionised and the molecule will have properties similar to those of non-ionic surfactants. As the pH shifts away from the isoelectric point, the molecule will gradually assume the properties of either a cationic or anionic surfactant. Common examples are N-alkyl derivatives of simple amino acids such as glycine (NH_2CH_2COOH), aminopropionic acid ($NH_2CH_2CH_2COOH$) and the alkyl betaines shown in Box 5.1.

The dual structure of amphipathic molecules is the unique feature that is responsible for the characteristic behaviour of compounds of this type. Thus their surface activity arises from adsorption at the solution–air interface – the means by which the hydrophobic region of the molecule 'escapes' from the hostile aqueous environment by protruding into the vapour phase above. Similarly, adsorption at the interface between non-aqueous solutions occurs in such a way that the hydrophobic group is in the solution in the non-aqueous phase, leaving the hydrophilic group in contact with the aqueous solution. Adsorption on hydrophobic particles such as carbon again represents a means of reduction of the contact between the hydrophobic groups and water and allows the consequent attainment of a minimum energy state. Perhaps the most striking consequence of the dual structure is micellisation – the formation in solution of aggregates in which the component molecules are usually arranged in a spheroidal structure with the hydrophobic cores shielded from the water by a mantle of hydrophilic groups.

Gemini surfactants (**I**) are a relatively new class of surfactant which self-assemble at concentrations much lower than conventional surfactants.[1] They comprise, as the name suggests, two surfactant molecules joined by a spacer, as shown. They have a design advantage in that two different surfactant molecules with different properties can be synthesised.

Magnetic surfactants are an exciting development in the field,[2] but may be a long way off from their use in medicinal products. They are based on typical cationic surfactants but utilise metallic complex anions. The resulting micellar solutions respond to

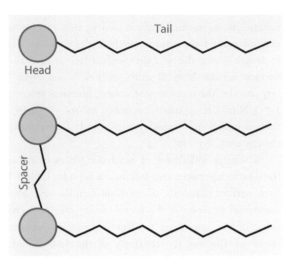

Structure I Gemini surfactant compared with a more conventional surfactant (top).

external magnetic fields which may have applications in drug targeting.

In the following sections we will examine in more detail the various characteristic properties of surfactants which arise as a consequence of their amphipathic nature.

5.2 Surface and interfacial properties of surfactants

5.2.1 Effects of amphiphiles on surface and interfacial tension

The molecules at the surface of a liquid are not completely surrounded by other molecules as they are in the bulk of the liquid. As a result there is a net inward force of attraction exerted on a molecule at the surface from the molecules in the bulk solution, which results in a tendency for the surface to contract.

The contraction of the surface is spontaneous; that is, it is accompanied by a decrease in free energy. The contracted surface thus represents a minimum free-energy state and any attempt to expand the surface must involve an increase in the free energy. The surface free energy of a liquid is defined as the work, w, required to increase the surface area A by 1 m²:

$$w = \gamma \Delta A \qquad (5.1)$$

where ΔA is the increase in surface area. γ is also referred to as *surface tension* and in this context is defined as the force acting at right angles to a line 1 m in length along the surface. Surface free energy and surface tension have SI units of $J\,m^{-2}$ and $N\,m^{-1}$ respectively (the units are, of course, identical since 1 $J = 1\,N\,m$). It is usual to quote values of surface tension in $mN\,m^{-1}$ (which is numerically equivalent to the cgs unit, $dyn\,cm^{-1}$).

A similar imbalance of attractive forces exists at the interface between two immiscible liquids. Table 5.1 lists surface tensions of various liquids and also interfacial tensions at the liquid–water interface. The value of the interfacial tension is generally between those of the surface tensions of the two liquids involved except where there is interaction between them. Table 5.1 includes several such examples. The interfacial tension at the octanol–water interface is considerably lower than the surface tension of octanol due to hydrogen bonding between these two liquids.

Amphiphilic molecules in aqueous solution have a tendency to seek out the surface and to orientate themselves in such a way as to remove the hydrophobic group from the aqueous environment and hence achieve a minimum free-energy state (Fig. 5.1). A consequence of the intrusion of surfactant molecules

into the surface or interfacial layer is that some of the water molecules are effectively replaced by hydrocarbon or other non-polar groups. Since the forces of intermolecular attraction between water molecules and non-polar groups are less than those existing between two water molecules, the contracting power of the surface is reduced and so therefore is the surface tension. In some cases the interfacial tension between two liquids may be reduced to such a low level (10^{-3} $mN\,m^{-1}$) that spontaneous emulsification of the two immiscible liquids is observed. These very low interfacial tensions are of relevance in understanding the formation and stabilisation of emulsions and are dealt with in more detail in Chapter 6.

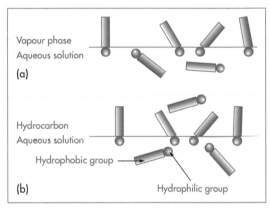

Figure 5.1 Orientation of amphiphiles at (a) solution–vapour interface, and (b) hydrocarbon–solution interface.

5.2.2 Change of surface tension with surfactant concentration: the critical micelle concentration

Figure 5.2 shows a typical plot of surface tension against the logarithm of concentration for a surfactant solution. Appreciable lowering of surface tension is evident even at low concentrations. As the surfactant concentration is increased, the surface tension continues to decrease as the concentration of surfactant molecules at the surface increases. At a certain concentration, characteristic of each surfactant, an alternative means of shielding the hydrophobic portion of the amphiphile from the aqueous environment occurs as the surfactant molecules form small spherical aggregates or *micelles* in the bulk of the solution. The hydrophobic groups of the surfactants form the core of these aggregates and are protected from contact with water by their hydrophilic groups, which form a shell

Table 5.1 Surface tensions of pure liquids and interfacial tensions against water at 20°C

Substance	Surface tension (mN m^{-1})	Interfacial tension (mN m^{-1})
Water	72	–
Glycerol	63	–
Oleic acid	33	16
Benzene	29	35
Chloroform	27	33
n-Octanol	27	8.5
Carbon tetrachloride	27	45
Castor oil	39	–
Olive oil	36	33
Cottonseed oil	35	–
n-Octane	22	51
Ethyl ether	17	11

around them. The concentration of surfactant molecules in the surface layer remains approximately constant in the presence of micelles and hence the γ–log(concentration) plot becomes almost horizontal. The concentration at which the micelles first form in solution is called the *critical micelle concentration* (cmc) and corresponds to the concentration at which there is an abrupt change of slope of the plot. It should be noted that the cmc is not dependent on the packing of molecules in the surface layer; the components of cetrimide (shown later in Table 5.6) have similar cross sectional areas but very different cmcs. We will consider the formation and properties of micelles in more detail in section 5.3. At the moment we will concentrate on the region of the γ–log(concentration) plot below the cmc and see how it is possible to calculate the area occupied by a surfactant molecule at the surface using the Gibbs equation.

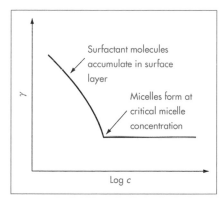

Figure 5.2 Typical plot of the surface tension, γ, against logarithm of surfactant concentration, *c*.

5.2.3 Gibbs adsorption equation

It is important to remember that an equilibrium is established between the surfactant molecules at the surface or interface and those remaining in the bulk of the solution. This equilibrium is expressed in terms of the Gibbs equation. In developing this expression it is necessary to imagine a definite boundary between the bulk of the solution and the interfacial layer (Fig. 5.3). The real system containing the interfacial layer is then compared with this reference system, in which it is assumed that the properties of the two bulk phases remain unchanged up to the dividing surface. A thermodynamic derivation of the Gibbs equation,

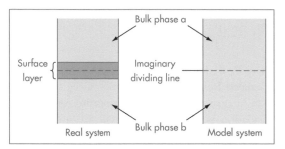

Figure 5.3 Diagrammatic representation of an interface between two bulk phases in the presence of an adsorbed layer.

$$\Gamma_2 = -\frac{1}{RT}\frac{d\gamma}{d\ln a_2} = -\frac{a_2}{RT}\frac{d\gamma}{da_2} \qquad (5.2)$$

is provided in Derivation Box 5A, where Γ_2 is the surface excess concentration.

The form of the Gibbs equation applicable to dilute solutions is

$$\Gamma_2 = -\frac{1}{RT}\frac{d\gamma}{d\ln c} = -\frac{c}{RT}\frac{d\gamma}{dc} \qquad (5.3)$$

where activity, a_2, in equation (5.2) has been replaced by concentration, *c*. Equation (5.3) is the form of the Gibbs equation applicable to the adsorption of nonionic surfactants at the surface of the solution. For ionic surfactants the derivation becomes more complex since consideration must be taken of the adsorption of both surfactant ion and counterion. The general form of the Gibbs equation is then written

$$\begin{aligned}
\Gamma_2 &= -\frac{1}{xRT}\frac{d\gamma}{d\ln c} \\
&= -\frac{1}{xRT}\frac{d\gamma}{2.303\,d\log c}
\end{aligned} \qquad (5.4)$$

where *x* has a numerical value varying from 1 (for ionic surfactants in dilute solution or in the presence of excess electrolyte) to 2 (in concentrated solution).

Application of the Gibbs equation to surfactant solutions

The slope of the plot of surface tension against log (concentration) reaches a limiting value at concentrations just below the cmc (Fig. 5.2). The surfactant molecules are closely packed in the surface over this narrow concentration range and we can calculate the area *A* that each molecule occupies at the surface from

$$A = \frac{1}{N_A \Gamma_2} \qquad (5.5)$$

where Γ_2 is the value of surface excess concentration calculated from the Gibbs equation using the limiting $d\gamma/(d \ln c)$ value and N_A is the Avogadro constant. The calculation is shown in Example 5.1 using surface tension data for the surface-active drug, diphenhydramine.

An interesting effect arises when the surfactant is contaminated with surface-active impurities. A pronounced minimum in the surface tension–log c plot is observed at the cmc, which would seem to be an apparent violation of the Gibbs equation, suggesting a desorption (positive $d\gamma/d$ [log c] value) in the vicinity of the cmc. The minimum in fact arises because of the release below the cmc of the surface-active impurities on the breakup of the surfactant micelles in which they were solubilised.

5.2.4 The influence of the surfactant structure on surface activity

The surface activity of a particular surfactant depends on the balance between its hydrophilic and hydrophobic properties. For the simplest case of a homologous series of surfactants, an increase in the length of the hydrocarbon chain as the series is ascended results in increased surface activity. Conversely, an increase in the hydrophilicity, which for polyoxyethylated non-ionic

Example 5.1 Calculation of area per molecule using the Gibbs equation

The limiting slope of a plot of γ against log c just below the cmc for the antihistamine diphenhydramine hydrochloride (Box 5.2) is -0.0115 N m^{-1} at 30°C. Calculate the area per molecule of this drug at the air–solution interface.

Answer

The surface excess concentration, Γ_2, may be calculated from equation (5.4), assuming a value of $x = 1$:

$$\Gamma_2 = \frac{0.0115}{8.314 \times 303 \times 2.303}$$
$$= 1.982 \times 10^{-6} \, \text{mol m}^{-2}$$

Substituting in equation (5.5),

$$A = 1/(6.023 \times 10^{23} \times 1.982 \times 10^{-6})$$
$$= 83.8 \times 10^{-20} \, \text{m}^2 \, \text{molecule}$$

The area per molecule of diphenhydramine = $0.84 \, \text{nm}^2$.

surfactants may be effected by increasing the length of the ethylene oxide chain, results in a decreased surface activity. This latter effect is demonstrated by Fig. 5.4,

Example 5.2 Use of Traube's rule

The surface tension lowering of an anionic surfactant (mol wt = 328 Da) with a hydrocarbon chain length of 16 carbon atoms is 15 mN m^{-1} at a concentration of 0.0276% w/v. For a surfactant with an identical hydrophilic group and a hydrocarbon chain length of 14 carbon atoms, estimate the percentage concentration that is required to produce an equal lowering of surface tension, assuming that both concentrations are below the cmc.

Answer

The molar concentration of the first surfactant = 8.415×10^{-4} mol dm^{-3}. Since the second surfactant has two CH_2 groups fewer than the first, the concentration required to produce an equal lowering of surface tension is, according to Traube's rule,

$$8.415 \times 10^{-4} \times 3 \times 3 = 75.74 \times 10^{-4} \, \text{mol dm}^{-3}$$

The molecular weight of the second surfactant = $328 - 28 = 300$ Da. Thus, the concentration required = 0.227% w/v.

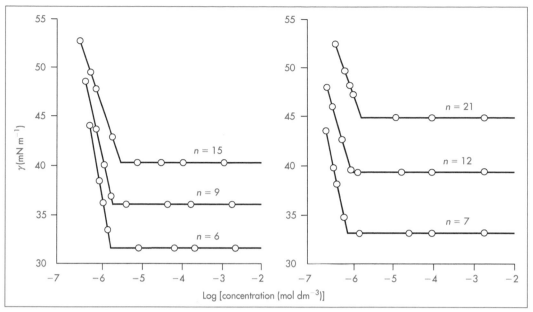

Figure 5.4 Surface tension versus log concentration plots for non-ionic surfactants with the general formula $CH_3(CH_2)_{15}(OCH_2CH_2)_nOH$ for a series of ethylene oxide chain lengths, n.

Reproduced from Elworthy PH, Macfarlane CB. Surface activity of a series of synthetic non-ionic detergents. *J Pharm Pharmacol* 1962;14:100T. Copyright Wiley-VCH Verlag GmbH & Co. KGaA. Reproduced with permission.

from which it is noted that lengthening the hydrophilic chain results in an increase in both the surface tension (decrease of surface activity) and the cmc.

The relationship between hydrocarbon chain length and surface activity is expressed by *Traube's rule*, which states that 'in dilute aqueous solutions of surfactants belonging to any one homologous series, the molar concentrations required to produce equal lowering of the surface tension of water decreases threefold for each additional CH_2 group in the hydrocarbon chain of the solute'. Traube's rule also applies to the interfacial tension at oil–water interfaces.

5.2.5 Surface activity of drugs

The surface activity at the air–solution interface has been reported for a wide variety of drugs.[3] This surface activity is a consequence of the amphiphilic nature of the drugs. The hydrophobic portions of the drug molecules are in general more complex than those of typical surfactants, often being composed of aromatic or heterocyclic ring systems. Examples of the types of drug that exhibit surface activity are illustrated in Box 5.2. They include the phenothiazine tranquillisers such as promazine, chlorpromazine, promethazine, and

antidepressants, such as imipramine, amitriptyline and nortriptyline, which have tricyclic hydrophobic moieties; the antihistamines (for example, chlorcyclizine and diphenhydramine) and the antiacetylcholine drugs such as orphenadrine, which are based on a diphenylmethane hydrophobic group; the local anaesthetics (tetracaine, for example); and several antihistamines, such as brompheniramine and mepyramine, which have a hydrophobic group consisting of a single phenyl ring. Many peptides also have amphiphilic structures and adsorb at the air–water interface.

As with typical surfactants, the surface activity depends on the nature of the hydrophobic and hydrophilic portions of the drug molecule. The presence of any substituents on the aromatic ring systems can have an appreciable effect on hydrophobicity. Figure 5.5 shows the decrease of cmc and increased surface activity that is associated with the Br substituent on the phenyl ring of an antihistaminic drug. Similarly, substitution on the phenothiazine ring systems increases surface activity in the order $CF_3 \gg Cl > H$.

The surface activity of drugs may have biological consequences because of their propensity to bind hydrophobically to proteins and to other biological macromolecules and to associate with other amphipathic

Box 5.2 Structures of some surface-active drugs[a]

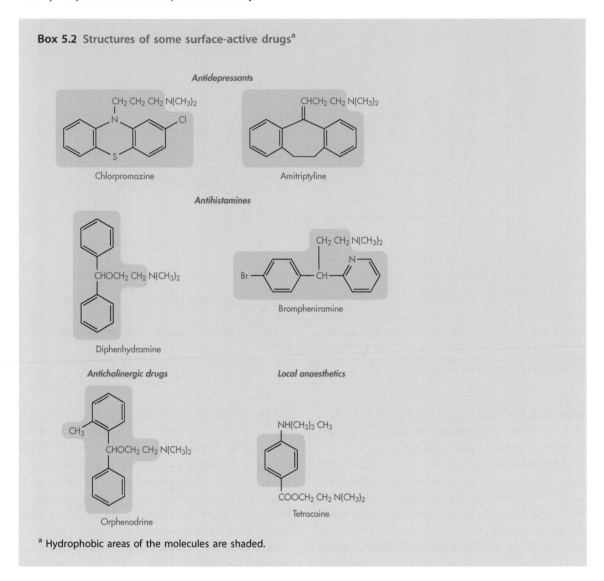

Antidepressants

Chlorpromazine

Amitriptyline

Antihistamines

Diphenhydramine

Brompheniramine

Anticholinergic drugs

Orphenadrine

Local anaesthetics

Tetracaine

[a] Hydrophobic areas of the molecules are shaded.

substances such as bile salts and, of course, with receptors.[3] The surface activity of drug solutions, whether caused by an excipient such as benzylkonium chloride or the drug itself, e.g. salbutamol sulfate, can have a direct effect on the spray pattern from nebulisers[4] (see Chapter 9).

5.2.6 Insoluble monolayers

In section 5.2.4 we examined the case in which the surface of a solution containing an amphiphile became covered with a monomolecular film as a result of spontaneous adsorption from solution. The molecules in such films are in equilibrium with those in the bulk of the solution, i.e. there is a continuous movement of molecules between the surface and the solution below it. If, however, a surfactant has a very long hydrocarbon chain it will be insufficiently water-soluble for a film to be formed in this way. In such cases we can spread a film on the surface of the solution by dissolving the surfactant in a suitable volatile solvent and carefully injecting the solution on to the surface. The *insoluble monolayer* formed by this process contains all of the molecules injected on the surface; there is no equilibrium with the bulk solution because of the low water solubility of the surfactant. Consequently, the number of molecules per unit area of surface is generally known directly.

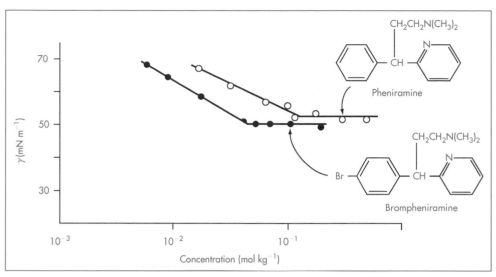

Figure 5.5 Surface tension, γ, as a function of log molal concentration at 30°C showing the increase of hydrophobicity associated with a Br substituent on the phenyl ring of an antihistamine.

Reproduced from Attwood D, Udeala OK. The surface activity of some antihistamines at the air–solution interface. *J Pharm Pharmacol* 1975;27:754. Copyright Wiley-VCH Verlag GmbH & Co. KGaA. Reproduced with permission.

Although the films are called insoluble films, this is not meant to imply that any insoluble substance will form a stable monolayer; in fact, only two classes of materials will do so. The simpler and larger of the two classes includes the water-insoluble amphiphiles, discussed above. Such structures orientate themselves at the water surface in the manner of typical surfactants, with the polar group acting as an anchor and the hydrocarbon chain protruding into the vapour phase. The other class of film-forming compounds includes a range of amphipathic polymeric materials such as proteins and synthetic polymers. With these compounds a high degree of water insolubility is not so essential and stable films will form, providing there is a favourable free energy of adsorption from the bulk solution.

Key points

- Surface and interfacial tensions arise because of an imbalance of attractive forces on the molecules of a liquid at these interfaces such that the surface or interface has a tendency to contract.
- Surfactant molecules are amphiphilic, i.e. they have both hydrophilic and hydrophobic regions. They are classified according to the nature of the hydrophilic group as anionic, cationic, non-ionic and zwitterionic surfactants. As a consequence of their amphiphilic nature they adsorb at interfaces in such a way that their hydrophobic regions are removed from the aqueous environment. The forces of attraction between surfactant and water molecules in the interface are weaker than those between two water molecules and hence the surface tension is reduced as a result of adsorption.
- The extent of adsorption at the interface can be calculated using the Gibbs equation. The lowering of surface tension increases with increase of surfactant concentration until the cmc is reached, i.e. until the surfactant forms micelles; at higher concentrations the surface tension remains effectively constant.
- The surface activity of a surfactant depends on the balance between its hydrophilic and hydrophobic properties. An increase in the overall hydrophobicity of the surfactant molecule, by for example increasing the length of the hydrocarbon chain, results in increased surface activity. Conversely, an increase in the hydrophilicity of the molecule, by for example increasing the length of the ethylene oxide chain of a polyoxyethylated non-ionic surfactant, results in a decreased surface activity.

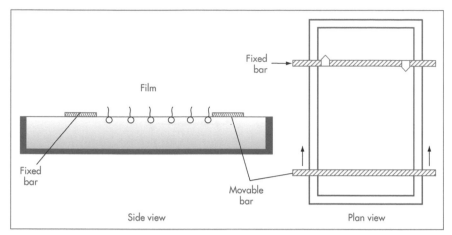

Figure 5.6 Langmuir trough for monolayer studies (not to scale). A Wilhelmy plate or other device is used to measure surface tension as the surface is compressed or expanded.

Experimental study of insoluble films

One of the earliest studies of insoluble films was conducted by Benjamin Franklin in 1765 on a pond in Clapham Common in London. Surprisingly, Franklin's experiment was sufficiently controlled to establish that olive oil formed a film of monolayer thickness (quoted as one ten-millionth of an inch: approximately 2.5 nm). Figure 5.6 illustrates an apparatus – the Langmuir trough – commonly used to study monolayers on a laboratory scale.

In its simplest form the apparatus consists of a shallow trough with waxed or Teflon sides (non-wetting), along which a non-wetting barrier may be mechanically moved. In use, the trough is filled completely so as to build up a meniscus above the level of the sides. The surface is swept clean with the moveable barrier and any surface impurities are sucked away using a water pump. The film-forming material is dissolved in a suitable volatile solvent and an accurately measured amount, usually about 0.01 cm^3, of this solution is carefully distributed on to the surface. The solvent evaporates and leaves a uniformly spread film entirely contained in the well-defined surface area between the two barriers. The film is compressed by moving the moveable barrier towards the fixed barrier in a series of steps. At each position of the two barriers the surface tension of the film-covered surface is measured directly using a Wilhelmy plate (thin glass or platinum plate) partially immersed in the subphase and attached to a sensitive electrobalance. The surface pressure, π, of the film is then calculated from the difference between the surface tension of the clean surface γ_0 and that of the film-covered surface, γ_m:

$$\pi = \gamma_0 - \gamma_m \tag{5.6}$$

There have been steady improvements in the design of Langmuir troughs over recent years and, in modern instruments, operation and data collection are under computer control.

The results are generally presented as graphs of π against the surface area per molecule, A, which is readily calculated from the number of molecules added to the surface and the area enclosed between the two barriers, as shown by Example 5.3.

Monolayer states

The surface film acts as a two-dimensional analogue to normal matter in that it may exist in different physical states, which in some ways resemble solids, liquids and gases. In this section we shall consider the three

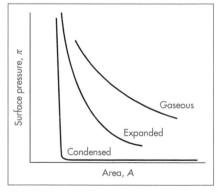

Figure 5.7 Surface pressure, π, versus area per molecule, A, for the three main types of monolayer.

Example 5.3 Calculation of the area per molecule in an insoluble monolayer

When 1 cm³ of a solution containing 8.5 mg per 100 cm³ of stearic acid (mol wt = 284.3 Da) dissolved in a volatile organic solvent is placed on the surface of water in a Langmuir trough, the solvent evaporates off, leaving the stearic acid spread over the surface as an insoluble monomolecular film. If the surface area occupied by the film is 400 cm², calculate the area occupied by each molecule of stearic acid in the film.

Answer

1 cm³ of the solution contains 8.5×10^{-5} g of stearic acid = 2.99×10^{-7} mol.

Since 1 mol contains 6×10^{23} (Avogadro constant) molecules, the solution contains

$$2.99 \times 10^{-7} \times 6 \times 10^{23} = 1.79 \times 10^{17} \text{ molecules}$$

Therefore, the area per molecule of stearic acid in the film is

$$\frac{400 \times 10^{-4}}{1.79 \times 10^{17}} = 2.23 \times 10^{-19} \text{ m}^2$$
$$= 0.22 \text{ nm}^2$$

different states of monolayers of simple amphiphiles, referred to as solid (or condensed), liquid (or expanded) and gaseous monolayers (Fig. 5.7).

Solid or condensed monolayers

Figure 5.8 shows the π–A curve for cholesterol, which produces a typical condensed film on an aqueous substrate. The film pressure remains very low at high film areas and rises abruptly when the molecules become tightly packed on compression. Simultaneous electron microscopy of the film-covered surface has shown cholesterol clusters or islands which gradually pack more tightly at greater pressures. The film becomes continuous as the pressure is further increased and at such high pressures the molecules are in contact and oriented as depicted in Fig. 5.8. The extrapolated limiting surface area of 0.39 nm² is very

close to the cross-sectional area of a cholesterol ring system calculated from molecular models, confirming a vertical orientation.

Similar films are formed by long-chain fatty acids such as stearic and palmitic acid, for which a limiting surface area of about 0.20 nm² is found. This value is very close to the cross-sectional area of the compounds in the bulk crystal, as determined by X-ray diffraction techniques.

Gaseous monolayers

These films represent the opposite extreme in behaviour to the condensed film. They resemble the gaseous state of three-dimensional matter in that the molecules move around in the film, remaining a sufficiently large distance apart so as to exert very little force on each other. Upon compression, there is a gradual change in the surface pressure, in marked contrast to the behaviour of solid films. It is thought that the molecules in these types of monolayer lie along the surface and this is certainly so with those dibasic esters with terminal polar groups that anchor the molecules flat on the surface. Those steroids in which the polar groups are distributed about the molecule tend to form gaseous films for similar reasons.

Expanded monolayers

Variously named liquid-expanded (LE), expanded or liquid, these monolayers represent intermediate states between gaseous and condensed films. The π–A plots are quite steeply curved and extrapolation to a limiting surface area yields a value that is usually several times greater than the cross-sectional area from molecular models. Films of this type tend to be formed by molecules in which close packing into condensed films is prohibited by bulky side-chains or, as in the case of oleyl alcohol (Fig. 5.9), by a *cis* configuration of the molecule.

Factors influencing monolayer state

Many factors, including both external factors such as temperature and also modifications to the molecular structure, influence the type of monolayer formed. Many simple molecules, rather than exhibiting behaviour exclusively characteristic of one monolayer state, show transitions between one state and another as the film is compressed. Estradiol diacetate, for example (Fig. 5.10), shows typical gaseous behaviour at a large area per molecule, and in this state the molecules are

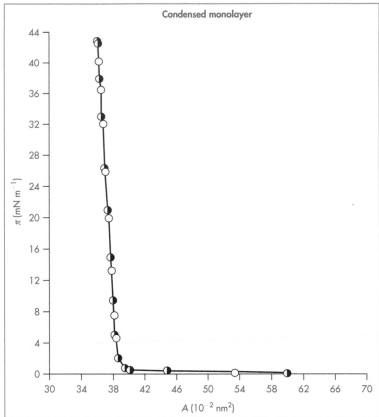

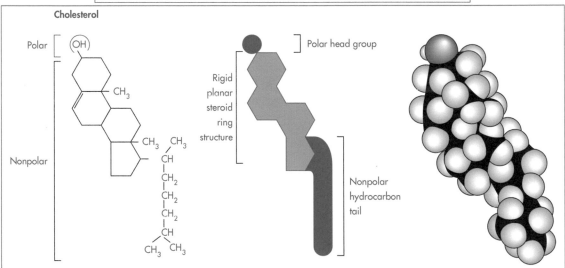

Figure 5.8 Surface pressure, π, versus area per molecule, A, for cholesterol, which shows a typical condensed monolayer, and schematic drawings of the oriented molecule, including a space-filling model.

Reproduced from Riess HE *et al*. Electron micrographs of cholesterol monolayers. *J Colloid Interface Sci* 1976;57:396. Copyright Elsevier 1976.

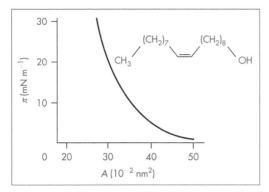

Figure 5.9 Surface pressure, π, versus area per molecule, A, for oleyl alcohol, which forms a typical expanded monolayer.

Reproduced from Crisp DJ. In: Danielli JF *et al.* (eds) *Surface Phenomena in Chemistry and Biology.* Oxford: Pergamon Press; 1958: 23. Copyright Wiley-VCH Verlag GmbH & Co. KGaA. Reproduced with permission.

thought to be lying along the surface, as might be expected from the location of the hydrophilic groups on the molecule. As compression is applied, the molecules are gradually pressed closer together until at a molecular surface area of approximately 0.96 nm^2 the molecules begin to stand upright. The film now undergoes a gradual transition to a condensed film as the proportion of upright molecules increases with further compression, until at approximately 0.38 nm^2 the film is wholly in the condensed form.

In some compounds, notably myristic acid, the extent of the gaseous, expanded and condensed regions varies with temperature (Fig. 5.11). There is an analogy between the π–A curves of such compounds and the pressure–volume isotherms of three-dimensional gases.

Figure 5.12 shows changes in monolayer type as the length of the alkyl chain is increased from lauric acid (*n*-dodecanoic acid) to stearic acid (*n*-octadecanoic acid). Lauric acid represents the minimum alkyl chain length for the formation of monolayers; shorter-chain-length compounds have sufficient aqueous solubility to cause loss of molecules from monolayer and resultant decrease of monolayer area. Lauric acid forms slightly soluble, gaseous monolayers; the addition of two more carbon atoms causes myristic acid (*n*-tetradecanoic acid) to exhibit a condensed gaseous phase region as well as an expanded phase, and further increase in the hydrocarbon chain length results in the additional formation of the solid phase. Replacement of the hydrogen atoms of the alkyl chain with a halogen such as fluorine also affects the type of monolayer.

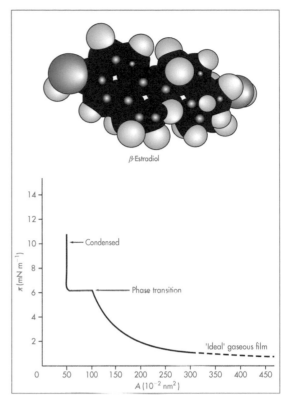

Figure 5.10 Surface pressure, π, versus area per molecule, A, for β-estradiol diacetate showing a transition from a gaseous to a condensed film on compression.

Reproduced from Cadenhead DA, Philips MC. Monolayers of some naturally occurring polycyclic compounds. *J Colloid Interface Sci* 1967;24:491. Copyright Elsevier 1967.

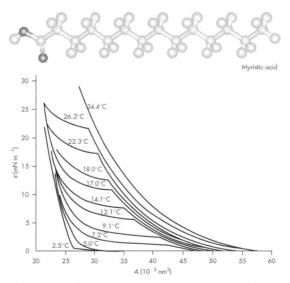

Figure 5.11 Surface pressure, π, versus area per molecule for myristic acid spread on 0.01 mol dm^{-3} HCl at different temperatures, showing a transition from condensed to an expanded film with temperature increase.

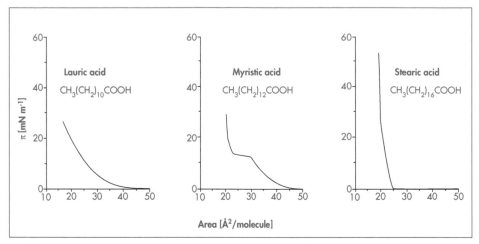

Figure 5.12 Surface pressure, π, versus area per molecule, A, for lauric acid, myristic acid and stearic acid spread on 0.001 mol dm^{-3} HCl aqueous subphase at 20 °C, showing changes in the nature of the isotherm caused by increasing the length of the hydrophobic chain.

Reprinted from Dynarowicztka P *et al. Modern Physicochemical Research on Langmuir Monolayers. Advances in Colloid and Interface Science 91.* New York: Elsevier; 2001: 221–293. Copyright Elsevier 2001.

Monolayers containing fluorocarbon chains are more stable than those formed from their hydrocarbon counterparts and, because the fluorocarbon chain is more hydrophobic than a hydrocarbon chain, compounds with shorter chains are able to form insoluble monolayers. Similarly, changes in the polarity, size and shape of the head group can influence the arrangements of the hydrocarbon chains and hence the monolayer structure, as illustrated by early studies with alcohols, esters, amides, amines and nitriles.

Visualisation of monolayer structures

There has been considerable interest in probing the structure of films transferred from the water surface on to solid substrates, the *Langmuir–Blodgett (LB) films*. The usual method of depositing a LB monolayer on to a hydrophilic substrate is to raise the substrate upward slowly through the monolayer-covered surface. A wide range of imaging techniques, including X-ray diffraction, neutron reflection, infrared and Raman spectroscopy, fluorescence microscopy and atomic force microscopy, have recently been used to study the structures formed in monolayers both *in situ* on the water surface and after deposition on to solid surfaces as LB films (see reviews by Peng *et al.*[5] and Dynarowicz-Łatka *et al.*[6]). Flanders and co-workers[7] used atomic force microscopy to visualise the disorder induced in a monolayer of palmitic acid when increasing amounts of a peptide (the 25-peptide amino terminus of lung surfactant protein B, SP-B$_{1-25}$) were

added. Elliptically shaped LE domains roughly 10 μm in diameter were shown to coexist with liquid-condensed phase in monolayers containing 5 wt% peptide. When the peptide content was increased to 10 wt%, the LE phase existed as a sheet-like region that covered more than one-third of the area of the image and contained clover-shaped liquid-condensed domains roughly 5 μm in dimension. Atomic force microscopy images at peptide contents of 15 and 20 wt% showed the existence of a broad, sheet-like region of LE phase containing circular (approximately 20 μm diameter) liquid-condensed regions with uniformly smooth boundaries.

Polymer monolayers

Monolayers of polymers and proteins lack the characteristic features described in the previous section. Most produce smooth curves, typical of those for gaseous monolayers of amphiphiles.

Lung surfactant monolayers

Lung surfactant is a lipid–protein complex secreted as vesicles or other aggregates by type II pneumocytes into the thin aqueous layer that covers the alveoli; it spontaneously adsorbs from the aggregates to form a film at the air–water interface, which acts to control surface tension during breathing.[8] Lung surfactant is a complex mixture of lipids and proteins consisting of 78–90% phospholipid, 5–10% protein and 4–10% neutral lipid. Phosphatidylcholine is by far the most abundant component of lung surfactant, accounting for 70–80% of total lipid. About 50–70% of the phosphatidylcholine is dipalmitoylphosphatidylcholine (DPPC), but other saturated and unsaturated phosphatidylcholines are present as well as other phospholipid classes. The neutral lipids are mainly accounted for by cholesterol. There are four specific surfactant-associated proteins, SP-A, SP-B, SP-C and SP-D, which are closely associated with the membrane and play varied roles in modifying its physical properties.

The different components of lung surfactant interact to determine the overall behaviour of the surfactant film. Maintenance of a stable surface film requires efficient transfer of phospholipids between the extracellular large aggregate surfactant pool and the air–liquid interface. This process involves rapid insertion of phospholipids into the expanding film during inhalation followed by tight phospholipid packing and partial exclusion from the compressed film during exhalation. Rigid monolayers formed by DPPC alone can provide the necessary low surface tension (less than 5 mN m^{-1}) on compression of the alveolar interface that accompanies exhalation. However, pure DPPC is not able to spread rapidly enough to cover the greatly enlarged interface that is formed when the lungs expand during inhalation. The re-spreading of the film is greatly enhanced by the presence of the neutral lipids and the surfactant proteins. In particular, the presence of SP-B has been correlated to the high compressibility and reversible re-spreading properties required for proper functioning of the membrane. SP-B is a relatively small (mol wt $\approx$ 8700 Da), very hydrophobic amphipathic protein which is found in mammalian lung surfactant as a disulfide-linked dimer consisting of alpha-helices. Studies on model lung surfactant systems have led to the view that SP-B readily penetrates and fluidises the lipid membrane so that the LE phase survives at higher degrees of compression. The effect of synthetic SP-B-derived peptides on the surface pressure–area plots of monolayers formed from mixtures of DPPC and palmitoyloleoylphosphatidylglycerol is shown in Fig. 5.13; increasing amounts of the SP-B peptides result in a more LE film.[9]

There are several *animal-derived* pulmonary surfactants[*]:

- poractant alfa (Curosurf), from porcine lungs
- calfactant (Infasurf), from calf lungs
- beractant (Survanta) from bovine lungs.

The first *synthetic* peptide-containing surfactant is lucinactant (Surfaxin), which has been approved by the US Food and Drug Administration and by the European Medicines Agency. Lucinactant contains two phospholipids and a high concentration of sinapultide (also known as KL-4), a synthetic peptide designed to have similar activity to SP-B. Any advantages of synthetic over natural surfactant are still under debate and scrutiny by specialists in the field.

 Clinical point

The lung surfactant membrane comprises a complex mixture of lipids and proteins that act to lower the surface tension of the alveolar air–water interface, thus facilitating the large surface-area changes that occur during the successive compression–expansion cycles that accompany the breathing process. When formation of this membrane is incomplete, as may occur for example in prematurely born infants suffering from respiratory distress syndrome, breathing is laboured and there is insufficient transport of oxygen into the blood stream. In the early 1990s the US Food and Drug Administration approved surfactant replacement therapy for clinical use in prematurely born infants. Several types of surfactant have come to the market for use in this therapy, including bovine- and pig-derived surfactants, which have helped significantly in reducing the morbidity and mortality of prematurely born infants suffering from respiratory distress syndrome.

5.2.7 Pharmaceutical applications of surface film studies

Study of polymers used as packaging materials and film coatings

Packaging materials must protect the drug without altering in any way the composition of the product.

---

[*] Beractant and poractant alfa are in the *British National Formulary* 68 (Sept 2014–March 2015).

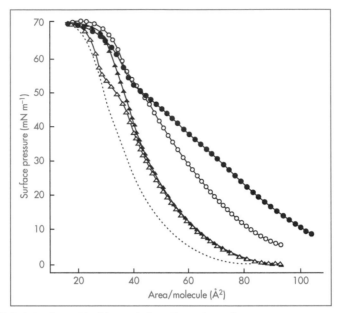

Figure 5.13 Effect of SP-B-derived peptide (N-term helix 1,2) on the surface pressure versus area per molecule plots of monolayers of 7:3 dipalmitoylphosphatidylcholine–palmitoyloleoylphosphatidylglycerol showing a more expanded monolayer with increasing amount of added peptide. Key: ⋯, 0; ▲, 1.3; △, 6.5; ○, 13; ●, 26% peptide. Note: 1 Å² = 0.01 nm².

Redrawn from Serrano AG et al. Critical structure–function determinants within the N-terminal region of pulmonary surfactant protein SP-B. *Biophys J* 2006;90:238–249. Copyright Elsevier 2006.

One problem is that of adsorption of constituents, for example preservatives, from the drug product (see section 5.2.8). The permeability of the packing material to gases or liquids should also be considered, since this may result in deterioration of the product due to oxidation, hydrolysis or loss of volatile ingredients. Monolayers are useful models by which the properties of polymers used as packaging materials can be investigated.

Several methods have been employed in the determination of the resistance of monolayers to evaporation. The evaporation rate may be determined from the increase in mass of a desiccant suspended over the monolayer, or from the loss of weight of a Petri dish containing solution and spread monolayer, under carefully controlled conditions. Such experiments are useful in determining the effect on permeability of incorporation of a plasticiser into the polymer structure.[10]

Polymer monolayers have been used as models to assess the suitability of new polymers and of polymer mixtures as potential enteric and film coatings for solid-dosage forms. The effects of substrate pH on the properties of three esters of cellulose, namely, cellulose acetate phthalate (cellacefate), cellulose acetate buty-rate and cellulose acetate stearate have been examined. Monolayers of the butyrate and stearate esters were virtually unaffected by changes of pH of the substrate from 3 to 6.5. Condensed films were formed at both pH values, indicating that disintegration in either the stomach or small intestine would be prevented. Neither of these cellulose esters would therefore be of use as enteric coatings. The phthalate ester, on the other hand, formed a much more condensed monolayer at pH 3 than at pH 6.5 (Fig. 5.14). The conformational changes of this ester suggested its suitability as an enteric coating: the more tightly packed film at low pH would restrict dissolution in the stomach, whereas the more expanded film at higher pH would allow penetration of water and tablet disintegration in the small intestine where the environmental pH is approximately 6.

Cell membrane models

Phospholipid monolayers provide useful models for studying drug–lipid interactions, as we can see from the following example,[11] which explores the interaction of the phenothiazine drugs trifluoperazine and chlorpromazine with the anionic glycerophospholipid dipalmitoylphosphatidylglycerol (DPPG). The surface pressure isotherms of Fig. 5.15 show interesting differ-

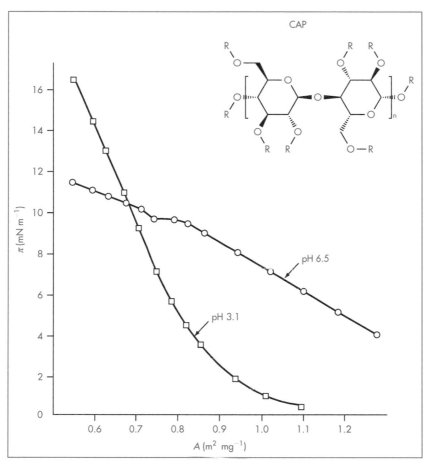

Figure 5.14 Surface pressure, π, versus area per molecule, A, for cellulose acetate phthalate (CAP) spread on an aqueous substrate, showing a more condensed monolayer at a substrate pH of 3 than at pH 6.5.

Reproduced with permission from Zatz JL, Knowles B. Monomolecular film properties of some cellulose esters. *J Pharm Sci* 1970;59:1188. Copyright Wiley-VCH Verlag GmbH & Co. KGaA. Reproduced with permission.

ences in the interaction of the two drugs with this phospholipid. Incorporation of chlorpromazine expands the monolayer and an additional phase transition appears at higher drug concentrations; at high surface pressures there is little increase in area, suggesting that this drug is being excluded from the interface. Trifluoperazine also expands the monolayer, although there is no appearance of an additional phase transition; the increase of area per molecule is noted even at high surface pressures, indicating that this drug remains in the monolayer. The considerable expansion of the monolayer observed even at relatively low drug/phospholipid ratios for both systems suggests that phospholipid molecules not in immediate contact with the drug are affected by incorporation of the drug into the monolayer. This 'cooperative effect', which is thought to be a consequence of either a

significant reorientation and different packing of the DPPG molecules or a change in their hydration state, may explain why drugs such as these with relatively non-specific effects on the membrane are highly effective at very low concentrations.

Cholesterol monolayers are also used to model drug–membrane interactions. Figure 5.16 shows the surface pressure–area isotherms for equimolar mixtures of valinomycin (a cyclic peptide), which orientates horizontally at the air–solution interface to give an expanded film, and cholesterol, which orients vertically, giving a solid film. The shape of the mixed isotherm at low and intermediate pressures is similar to that of valinomycin, while the behaviour at high surface pressures is similar to that of cholesterol, suggesting that the valinomycin has been squeezed out of the mixed film. The position of the mixed

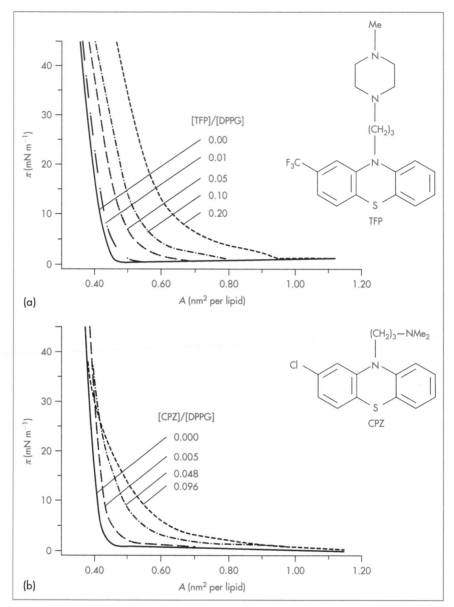

Figure 5.15 Surface pressure isotherms for mixed monolayers of dipalmitoylphosphatidylglycerol (DPPG) and (a) trifluoperazine (TFP) and (b) chlorpromazine (CPZ) for a range of drug/phospholipid molar ratios.

Reproduced from Hidalgo AA *et al.* Interaction of two phenothiazine derivatives with phospholipid monolayers. *Biophys Chem* 2004;109:85. Copyright Elsevier 2004.

curve to the left of the calculated average curve suggests some form of interaction between the components that condenses the mixed film.

5.2.8 Adsorption at the solid–liquid interface

The term *adsorption* is used to describe the process of accumulation at an interface. Adsorption is essentially a surface effect and should be distinguished from *absorption*, which implies the penetration of one component throughout the bulk of a second. The distinction between the two processes is not always clear-cut, however, and in such cases the non-committal word *sorption* is sometimes used.

There are two general types of adsorption: physical adsorption, in which the adsorbate is bound to the surface through weak van der Waals forces, and

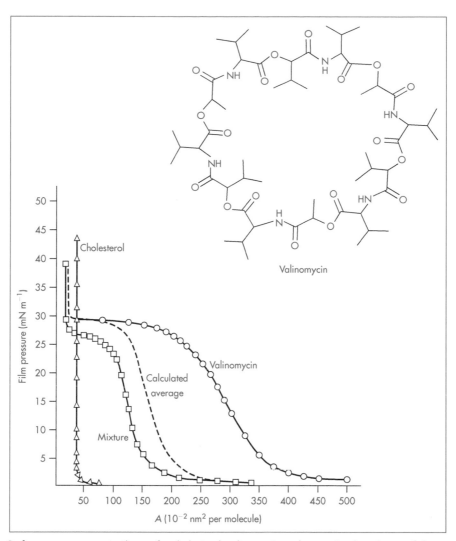

Figure 5.16 Surface pressure–area isotherms for cholesterol, valinomycin and an equimolar mixture of the two.

Reproduced from Riess HE, Swift HS. Monolayers of valinomycin and its equimolar mixtures with cholesterol and with stearic acid. *J Colloid Interface Sci* 1978;64:111. Copyright Elsevier 1978.

chemical adsorption or *chemisorption*, which involves the stronger valence forces. Of the two processes, chemisorption is the more specific, and usually involves an ion-exchange process. Frequently both physical and chemical adsorption may be involved in a particular adsorption process. This is the case with the adsorption of toxins in the stomach by attapulgite and kaolin: there is both chemisorption involving cation exchange with the basic groups of the toxins and physical adsorption of the remainder of the molecule.

Adsorption isotherms

The study of adsorption from solution is experimentally straightforward. A known mass of the adsorbent material is shaken with a solution of known concentration at a fixed temperature. The concentration of the supernatant solution is determined by either physical or chemical means and the experiment is continued until no further change in the concentration of the supernatant is observed, that is, until equilibrium conditions have been established. Equations originally derived for the adsorption of gases on solids are generally used in the interpretation of the data, the Langmuir and Freundlich equations being the most commonly used.

Key points

- Insoluble amphiphilic compounds may form films when injected on to water surfaces using volatile solvents. An important difference between these insoluble monolayers and the films produced when surfactant molecules accumulate spontaneously at the surface of surfactant solutions is that the molecules of the insoluble monolayers remain in the surface film and are not in equilibrium with surfactant molecules in the bulk of the solution as they are in surfactant solutions.
- Insoluble films may be tightly packed, as in solid (or condensed) films, or more loosely packed, as in liquid (or expanded) and gaseous films. The three types of film are identified from plots of surface pressure against area per molecule derived from measurements using a Langmuir trough. Many factors, including external factors such as temperature and also modifications to the molecular structure, influence the type of monolayer formed.
- Films formed by lung surfactants at the alveolar air–water interface facilitate the large surface area changes that occur during the successive compression–expansion cycles that accompany the breathing process.
- Surface film studies are useful when selecting polymers for use as packaging materials and as film coatings, and in the study of models of the cell membrane.

Langmuir equation

When applied to adsorption from solution, the Langmuir equation becomes

$$\frac{x}{m} = \frac{abc}{1 + bc} \tag{5.7}$$

where x is the amount of solute adsorbed by a weight, m, of adsorbent, c is the concentration of solution at equilibrium, b is a constant related to the enthalpy of

adsorption, and a is related to the surface area of the solid. Figure 5.17 shows a typical Langmuir isotherm for the adsorption of the antidepressant drug amitriptyline on carbon black.

Equation (5.7) can be arranged into the linear form

$$\frac{c}{x/m} = \frac{1}{ab} + \frac{c}{a} \tag{5.8}$$

Values of a and b may be determined from the intercept and slope of plots of $c/(x/m)$ against concentration, as shown in Example 5.4.

The value of a is a measure of the adsorptive capacity of the adsorbent for the particular adsorbate under examination. Table 5.2 gives the adsorptive capacity of carbon black for a series of antidepressant and phenothiazine drugs, arranged in order of decreasing degree of adsorption.

Deviations from the typical Langmuir plot can occur at high concentrations and are then usually attributed to the formation of multilayers.

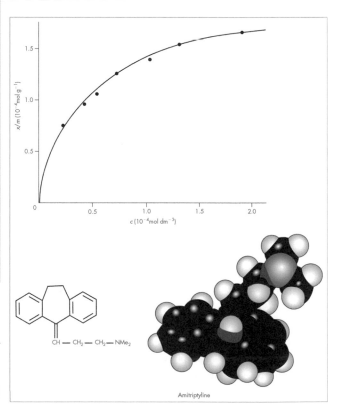

Figure 5.17 Langmuir adsorption isotherm of amitriptyline on carbon black from aqueous solution at 30°C.

Example 5.4 Use of the Langmuir equation

Calculate the Langmuir constants for the adsorption of amitriptyline on carbon black using the following data (taken from Fig. 5.17):

$10^3\ x/m$ (mol g^{-1})	0.75	0.95	1.10	1.25	1.40	1.55	1.65
$10^4 c$ (mol dm^{-3})	0.25	0.40	0.60	0.70	1.10	1.35	1.95
$10^2 c/(x/m)$ (g dm^{-3})	3.33	4.21	5.45	5.60	7.86	8.71	11.82

Answer

The gradient of the plot of $c/(x/m)$ against c (Fig. 5.18) = 4.88×10^2 g mol^{-1} = $1/a$. Therefore,

$$a = 1/\text{gradient} = 2.05 \times 10^{-3}\ \text{mol g}^{-1}$$

Intercept = $2.35 \times 10^{-2} = 1/ab$. Therefore,

$$b = 1/2.35 \times 10^{-2} \times 2.05 \times 10^{-3}$$
$$= 2.07 \times 10^4\ \text{dm}^3\ \text{mol}^{-1}$$

Freundlich equation

The Freundlich equation is generally written in the form:

$$\frac{x}{m} = ac^{1/n} \tag{5.9}$$

where a and n are constants, the form $1/n$ being used to emphasise that c is raised to a power less than unity. $1/n$ is a dimensionless parameter and is related to the intensity of drug adsorption. Equation (5.9) can be

Table 5.2 Langmuir constants a and b in the adsorption of antidepressants and phenothiazines on carbon black

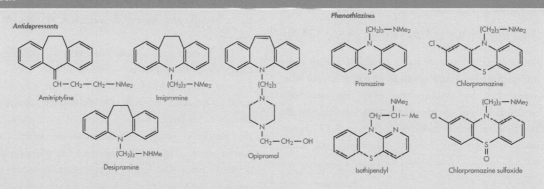

Drug	a (10^3 mol kg^{-1})	b (10^{-4} dm^3 mol^{-1})
Antidepressants		
Amitriptyline	2.05	2.07
Imipramine	1.80	1.48
Opipramol	1.51	1.77
Desipramine	1.36	4.70
Phenothiazines		
Promazine	1.70	3.36
Chlorpromazine	1.70	4.37
Isothipendyl	1.30	2.23
Chlorpromazine sulfoxide	1.13	3.18

Reproduced from Nambu N et al. *Chem Pharm Bull* 1975;23:1404.

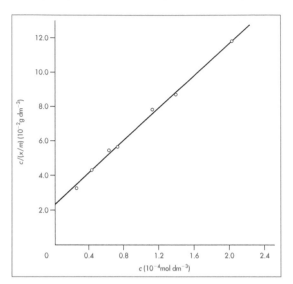

Figure 5.18 Adsorption of amitriptyline on carbon black plotted according to equation (5.8) using the data from Fig. 5.17.

written in a linear form by taking logarithms of both sides, giving

$$\log(x/m) = \log a + (1/n)\log c \qquad (5.10)$$

A plot of $\log(x/m)$ against $\log c$ should be linear, with an intercept of $\log a$ and gradient of $1/n$; it is generally assumed that, for systems that obey this equation, adsorption results in the formation of multilayers rather than a single monolayer. Figure 5.19 shows Freundlich isotherms for the adsorption of local

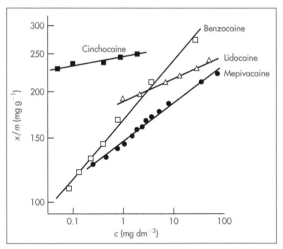

Figure 5.19 Freundlich adsorption isotherms of local anaesthetics on activated carbon at pH 7.0 and 25°C.

Reproduced from Abe I et al. Adsorption of local anesthetics on activated carbon: Freundlich adsorption isotherms. J Pharm Sci 1990;79:354. Copyright Wiley-VCH Verlag GmbH & Co. KGaA. Reproduced with permission.

anaesthetics on activated carbon; the method of calculating the constants a and $1/n$ from these plots is given in Example 5.5.

Factors affecting adsorption

Solubility of the adsorbate

Solubility is an important factor affecting adsorption. In general, the extent of adsorption of a solute is inversely proportional to its solubility in the solvent from which adsorption occurs. This empirical rule is termed *Lundelius's rule*. There are numerous examples of the applicability of this rule; for example, in Lundelius's original work it was noted that the adsorption of iodine on to carbon from CCl_4, $CHCl_3$ and CS_2 was $1 : 2 : 4.5$, respectively. These ratios are close to the inverse ratios for the solubilities of iodine in the respective solvents. The effect of solubility on adsorption might be expected since, in order for adsorption to occur, solute–solvent bonds must first be broken. The greater the solubility, the stronger are these bonds and hence the smaller the extent of adsorption.

For homologous series, adsorption from solution increases as the series is ascended and the molecules become more hydrophobic. There is, for example, a good correlation between the Freundlich adsorption constant, $1/n$ (related to the extent of adsorption) and the molecular weight of the local anaesthetics discussed above (Fig. 5.20). The data for phenobarbital deviated from this linear relationship, possibly as a result of the difficulty of adhesion of the phenobarbital molecules to the carbon surface, because the barbiturate ring and benzene ring are not aligned in the same plane.

pH

pH affects adsorption for a variety of reasons, the most important from a pharmaceutical viewpoint being its effect on the ionisation and solubility of the adsorbate drug molecule. In general, for simple molecules adsorption increases as the ionisation of the drug is suppressed, the extent of adsorption reaching a maximum when the drug is completely un-ionised. Figure 5.21 shows that the pH profile for the sorption (this is not a true adsorption process) of benzocaine by nylon 6 powder is indeed almost superimposable on the drug dissociation curve. For amphoteric compounds, adsorption is at a maximum at the isoelectric point,

Example 5.5 Use of the Freundlich equation

The following data refer to the adsorption of tetracaine from aqueous solution at 25°C on to a sample of activated charcoal:

Equilibrium conc. (mg dm^{-3})	0.155	0.468	1.259	2.510	5.370
Amount adsorbed (mg g^{-1})	202.8	217.8	232.0	243.2	254.7

Show that these data can be represented by the Freundlich isotherm and calculate the constants a and $1/n$.

Answer

Plot a graph of $\log(x/m)$ against $\log c$, noting that the data for the amount adsorbed are given per gram of carbon (x/m). This graph is linear, showing that the data can be represented by the Freundlich equation. At $\log c = 0$, the value of $\log(x/m)$ interpolated from this graph is 2.359. Therefore,

$$a = 229 \, \text{mg g}^{-1}$$

The gradient of this plot = 0.065. Therefore,

$$1/n = 0.065$$

---

that is, when the compound bears a net charge of zero. In general, pH and solubility effects act in concert, since the un-ionised form of most drugs in aqueous solution has low solubility. Of the two effects, the solubility effect is usually the stronger. Thus, in the adsorption of hyoscine and atropine on magnesium trisilicate it was noted[12] that hyoscine, although in its completely un-ionised form, was less strongly adsorbed than atropine, which at the pH of the experiment was 50% ionised. The reason for this apparently anomalous result is clear when the solubilities of the two bases are considered. Hyoscine base is freely soluble (1 in 9.5 parts of water at 15°C) compared with atropine base (1 in 400 at 20°C). Even when 50% ionised, atropine is less soluble than hyoscine and consequently more strongly adsorbed.

Nature of the adsorbent

The physicochemical nature of the adsorbent can have profound effects on the rate and capacity for adsorption. The most important property affecting adsorption is the surface area of the adsorbent; the extent of adsorption is proportional to the specific surface area. Thus, the more finely divided or the more porous the solid, the greater will be its adsorption capacity. Indeed, adsorption studies are frequently used to calculate the surface area of a solid.

Adsorbent–adsorbate interactions are of a complex nature and beyond the scope of this book. Particular adsorbents have affinities for particular adsorbates for a wide variety of reasons. The surfaces of adsorbent clays such as bentonite, attapulgite and kaolin carry cation-exchange sites, and such clays have strong

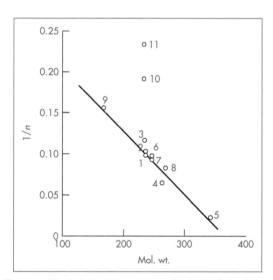

Figure 5.20 Relationship between the Freundlich adsorption constant, $1/n$, and the molecular weight for (1) procaine, pH 7; (2) procaine, pH 11; (3) lidocaine, pH 7; (4) tetracaine, pH 7; (5) cinchocaine, pH 7; (6) mepivacaine, pH 6.6; (7) mepivacaine, pH 8.6; (8) chloroprocaine, pH 7; (9) benzocaine, pH 7; (10) phenobarbital, pH 7; (11) phenobarbital, pH 9.

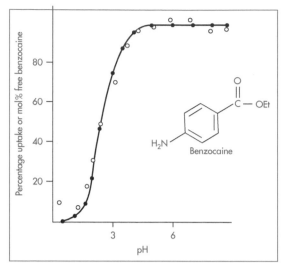

Figure 5.21 pH profile for the sorption of benzocaine by nylon 6 powder from buffered solutions at 30°C and ionic strength 0.5 mol dm^{-3} (○) and the corresponding drug dissociation curve (●).

Reproduced from Richards NE, Meakin BJ. The sorption of benzocaine from aqueous solution by nylon 6 powder. *J Pharm Pharmacol* 1974;26:166. Copyright Wiley-VCH Verlag GmbH & Co. KGaA. Reproduced with permission.

affinities for protonated compounds, which they adsorb by an ion-exchange process. In many cases, different parts of the surface of the same adsorbent have different affinities for different types of adsor-

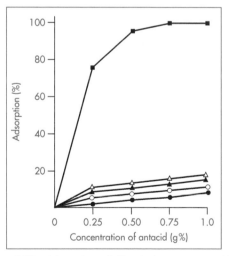

Figure 5.22 Adsorption of digoxin by some antacids at 37 ± 0.1°C. (■) Magnesium trisilicate; (△) aluminium hydroxide gel BP (Aludrox was used in the concentration range 2.5–10%v/v); (▲) light magnesium oxide; (○) light magnesium carbonate; (●) calcium carbonate. Initial concentration of the glycoside: 0.25 mg%.

Reproduced from Khalil SAH. The uptake of digoxin and digitoxin by some antacids. *J Pharm Pharmacol* 1974;26:961. Copyright Wiley-VCH Verlag GmbH & Co. KGaA. Reproduced with permission.

bents. There is evidence, for example, that anionic materials are adsorbed on the cationic edge of kaolin particles, while cationics are adsorbed on the cleavage surface of the particles, which are negatively charged. An example of the differing affinities of a series of adsorbents used in antacids is shown in Fig. 5.22. The adsorptive capacity of a particular adsorbent often depends on the source from which it was prepared and also on its pretreatment.

Temperature

Since adsorption is generally an exothermic process, an increase in temperature normally leads to a decrease in the amount adsorbed. The changes in enthalpy of adsorption are usually of the order of those for condensation or crystallisation. Thus small variations in temperature tend not to alter the adsorption process to a significant extent.

Some medical and pharmaceutical applications and consequences of adsorption

Adsorption at the solid–liquid interface plays a crucial role in preparative and analytical chromatography, and in heterogeneous catalysis, water purification and solvent recovery. These applications are, however, outside the scope of this book and we will be concerned with examples of the involvement of adsorption in more medical and pharmaceutical situations.

 Clinical point

The 'universal antidote' for use in reducing the effects of poisoning by the oral route is composed of activated charcoal, magnesium oxide and tannic acid. A more recent use of adsorbents has been in dialysis to reduce toxic concentrations of drugs by passing blood through a haemodialysis membrane over charcoal and other adsorbents. Several drugs are adsorbed effectively by activated charcoal. These include chlorphenamine, dextropropoxyphene hydrochloride, colchicine, diphenylhydantoin and aspirin. Some of these are easily recognisable as surface-active molecules (chlorphenamine, dextropropoxyphene) and will be expected to adsorb on to solids. Highly ionised substances of low molecular weight are not well adsorbed, neither are drugs such as tolbutamide that are poorly soluble in acidic media. The formation of a monolayer of drug molecules covering the surface of the charcoal particles through non-polar interactions is indicated.

Adsorption of poisons/toxins

The direct application of *in vitro* data for estimating doses of activated charcoal for antidotal purposes may lead to use of inadequate amounts of adsorbent.[13] In an animal study, charcoal:drug ratios of 1 : 1, 2 : 1, 4 : 1 and 8 : 1 reduced absorption of drugs as follows: pentobarbital sodium, 7%, 38%, 62% and 89%; chloroquine phosphate 20%, 30%, 70% and 96%; isoniazid 1.2%, 7.2%, 35% and 80%. Activated charcoal, of course, is not effective in binding all poisons. Biological factors such as gastrointestinal motility, secretions and pH may influence charcoal adsorption. While 5 g of activated charcoal has been said to be capable of binding 8 g of aspirin *in vitro*,[14] 30 g of charcoal *in vivo* was reported to inhibit the gastrointestinal absorption of 3 g of aspirin by only 50%.[15] The surface area of the charcoal is a factor in its effectiveness; charcoal tablets have been found to be approximately half as effective as powdered material.

Taste masking

The intentional adsorption of drugs such as diazepam on to solid substrates should be mentioned, the object being to minimise taste problems. Desorption of the drug *in vivo* is essential but should not occur during the shelf-life of the preparation. Desorption may be a rate-limiting step in absorption. Diazepam adsorbed on to an inorganic colloidal magnesium aluminium silicate (Veegum) had the same potency in experimental animals as a solution of the drug, but when adsorbed on to microcrystalline cellulose (Avicel), its efficacy was much reduced. Flocculation of the cellulose in the acidic environment of the stomach probably retards the desorption process.

Haemoperfusion

Carbon haemoperfusion is an extracorporeal method of treating cases of severe drug overdoses, and originally involved perfusion of the blood directly over charcoal granules. Although activated charcoal granules were very effective in adsorbing many toxic materials, they were found to give off embolising particles and also to lead to removal of blood platelets. Microencapsulation of activated charcoal granules by coating with biocompatible membranes such as acrylic hydrogels was found to be a successful means of eliminating charcoal embolism and to lead to a much reduced effect on platelet count. *In vitro* tests showed that the coated granules had a reduced adsorption rate, although the adsorptive capacity was unchanged.[16] A large proportion of drug overdoses in Great Britain at one time involved barbiturates, and the applicability of carbon haemoperfusion in the treatment of such cases was demonstrated.[17] Many other drugs taken as overdoses are also present in the plasma at sufficiently high concentration to allow removal by this technique.

Adsorption in drug formulation

Examples of the adsorption of drugs and excipients on to solid surfaces are found in many aspects of drug formulation, some of which, for example the adsorption of surfactants and polymers in the stabilisation of suspensions, are considered elsewhere in this book (see section 6.7). An interesting approach to the improvement of the dissolution rate of poorly water-soluble drugs is to adsorb very small amounts of surfactant on to the drug surface. For example, the adsorption of Pluronic F127 on to the surface of the hydrophobic drug phenylbutazone significantly increased its dissolution rate when compared with untreated material.[18]

In addition to the beneficial use of surfactants in the preparation of formulations, we should be aware of problems that can arise as a result of inadvertent adsorption occurring both in the manufacture and storage of the product and in its subsequent usage. Problems arising from the adsorption of medicaments on adsorbents such as antacids which may be taken simultaneously by the patient, or which may be present in the same formulation, are discussed in section 11.7. Problems also arise from the adsorption of medicaments on to the container walls. Containers for medicaments, whether glass or plastic, may adsorb a significant quantity of the drug or bacteriostatic or fungistatic agents present in the formulation and thereby affect the potency and possibly the stability of the product. The problem is particularly significant where the drug is highly surface active and present in low concentration. With plastic containers the process is often referred to as sorption rather than adsorption, since it often involves significant penetration of the drug into the polymer matrix. Plastics are a large and varied group of materials and their properties are often modified by various additives, such as plasticisers, fillers and stabilisers (see Chapter 7). Such additives may have a pronounced effect on the sorption characteristics of the plastics. The sorption of the fungistatic agent sorbic acid from aqueous solution by plastic cellulose acetate and cellulose triacetate shows an appreciable pH dependence; the sorption declines to zero in the vicinity of the point of maximum ionisation of the sorbic acid. The sorption of local anaesthetics by polyamide and polyethylene depends on the kind of plastic, the reaction conditions and the chemical structure of the drugs. As with sorbic acid, significant sorption was observed only when the drugs were in their un-ionised forms.

Key points

- Adsorption of solutes on to solid surfaces from solution can occur by physical adsorption, involving weak van der Waals forces, or by a chemical process. Adsorption data can be analysed using the Langmuir equation or, if multilayer adsorption occurs, by the Freundlich equation.

- The extent of adsorption is influenced by pH, mainly through its effect on ionisation of the solute; adsorption increases as the ionisation of the solute decreases and is at a maximum for an un-ionised compound. The greater the solubility of a solute in a particular solvent, the lower is the extent of its adsorption. The extent of adsorption is proportional to the surface area of the adsorbent; the more finely divided or the more porous the solid, the greater will be its adsorption capacity. An increase of temperature normally leads to a decrease in the amount adsorbed.

- The adsorption processes can be used advantageously, as in the removal of toxic drugs in the case of overdosing, or can cause problems, as in the unintentional

adsorption of drugs by antacids from the gastrointestinal tract, or the adsorption of drugs on to the walls of the container.

5.3 Micellisation

As the concentration of aqueous solutions of many amphiphilic substances increases, there is a pronounced change in the physical properties of the solution. For example, we have seen in section 5.2.2 that an inflection appears in surface tension plots of surfactant solutions at a critical concentration (the cmc) which is attributable to the self-association of the amphiphile into small aggregates called *micelles*. Similar inflection points are observed when other physical properties such as solubility, conductivity, osmotic pressure and light-scattering intensity are plotted as a function of concentration (Fig. 5.23).

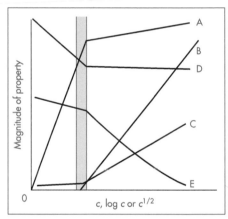

Figure 5.23 Solution properties of an ionic surfactant as a function of concentration, c. A, Osmotic pressure (against c); B, solubility of a water-insoluble solubilisate (against c); C, intensity of light scattered by the solution (against c); D, surface tension (against log c); E, molar conductivity (against $c^{1/2}$).

The idea that molecules should come together at a critical concentration to form aggregates in solution was quite controversial when first proposed by McBain in 1913, but the concept of micellisation has long gained universal acceptance. The micelles are in dynamic equilibrium with free molecules (monomers) in solution; that is, the micelles are continuously breaking down and reforming. It is this fact that distinguishes micellar solutions from other types of colloidal solution and this difference is emphasised by referring to micelle-forming compounds as *association colloids*.

The primary reason for micelle formation is the attainment of a state of minimum free energy. At low concentration, amphiphiles can achieve an adequate decrease in the overall free energy of the system by accumulation at the surface or interface, in such a way as to remove the hydrophobic group from the aqueous environment. As the concentration is increased, this method of free-energy reduction becomes inadequate and the monomers form into micelles. The hydrophobic groups form the core of the micelle and so are shielded from the water.

The free-energy change of a system is dependent on changes in both the entropy and the enthalpy; that is, $\Delta G = \Delta H - T\Delta S$. For a micellar system at normal temperatures the entropy term is by far the most important in determining the free-energy changes ($T \Delta S$ constitutes approximately 90–95% of the ΔG value). Micelle formation entails the transfer of a hydrocarbon chain from an aqueous to a non-aqueous environment (the interior of the micelle). To understand the changes in enthalpy and entropy that accompany this process, we must first consider the structure of water itself.

5.3.1 Water structure and hydrophobic bonding

Water possesses many unique features that distinguish it from other liquids. These arise from the unusual structure of the molecule in which the O and H atoms are arranged at the apices of a triangle (Fig. 5.24).

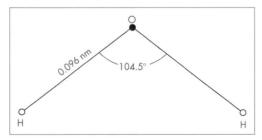

Figure 5.24 Diagram of the water molecule showing bond angle and length.

Each of the covalent bonds between a hydrogen atom and the oxygen atom of the water molecule involves the pairing of the electron of the hydrogen atom with

an electron in the oxygen atom's outer shell of six electrons. This pairing leaves two lone pairs of electrons in the outer shell, the orbitals of which point to the vertices of an approximately regular tetrahedron formed by the lone pairs and the OH bonds. The resulting tetrahedral structure has two positively charged sites at one side and two negatively charged sites at the other. It will readily attach itself by hydrogen bonds to four neighbouring molecules, two at the negatively charged sites and two at the positively charged sites. In its usual form, ice demonstrates an almost perfect tetrahedral arrangement of bonds with a distance of about 0.276 nm between neighbouring oxygen atoms. There is much unfilled space in the crystal, which accounts for the low density of ice.

When ice melts, a high degree of hydrogen bonding persists in the resulting liquid. In spite of extensive investigation by a variety of techniques such as X-ray diffraction, thermochemical determination, infrared and Raman spectroscopy, the structural nature of liquid water is still to be completely resolved. There are, broadly speaking, two distinct types of model: those that involve distortion but not breaking of hydrogen bonds, and a second type in which unbonded detached water molecules exist in addition to the hydrogen-bonded structures. Of the former type, the model that is considered to be the most acceptable is one in which all the water molecules continue to be hydrogen-bonded to their four neighbours, but the intermolecular links are bent or stretched to give an irregular framework. Such distorted networks are known to exist in some of the denser forms of ice.

Many proposed structures for water involve mixtures of structured material and free water molecules. One of the most highly developed theories encompasses the so-called 'flickering cluster' concept of water structure. The model is based on the cooperative nature of hydrogen bonding. The formation of one hydrogen bond on a water molecule leaves the molecule more susceptible to further hydrogen bonding, and similarly, when one bond breaks there is a tendency for large groups of bonds to break. As a result, clusters of ice-like hydrogen-bonded material are imagined to be suspended in a fluid of unbonded water (Fig. 5.25). Because of the continual formation and rupture of hydrogen bonds throughout the liquid, these clusters have only a temporary existence, and are aptly described by the term 'flickering'.

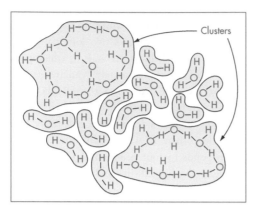

Figure 5.25 Water clusters with unassociated water molecules around them.

Most of the models proposed for the structure of water, only two of which have been considered here, can account for some, but not all, of the physical and thermodynamic anomalies that have been observed with water.

The flickering cluster model can be used to describe possible structural changes that occur when non-polar and polar solutes are dissolved in water. A non-polar molecule or portion of a molecule tends to seek out the more ice-like regions within the water. Such regions, as we have seen, contain open structures into which the non-polar molecules may fit without breaking hydrogen bonds or otherwise disturbing the surrounding ice-like material. In solution, therefore, hydrophobic molecules tend always to be surrounded by structured water. This concept is important in discussing interactions between non-polar molecules in aqueous solution, such as those that occur in micelle formation. The interaction of hydrocarbons in aqueous solution was first thought to arise simply as a consequence of the van der Waals forces between the hydrocarbon molecules. It was later realised, however, that changes in the water structure around the non-polar groups must play an important role in the formation of bonds between the non-polar molecules – the so-called *hydrophobic bonds*. In fact the contribution from the van der Waals forces is only about 45% of the total free energy of formation of a hydrophobic bond. When the non-polar groups approach each other until they are in contact, there will be a decrease in the total number of water molecules in contact with the non-polar groups. The formation of the hydrophobic bond in this way is thus equivalent to the partial removal of hydrocarbon from an aqueous environment and a consequent loss of the ice-like structuring that always surrounds the hydrophobic molecules. The increase in entropy and decrease in free energy that accompany the loss of structuring make the formation of the hydrophobic bond an energetically favourable process.

There is much experimental evidence to support this explanation for the decrease in ΔG. Thus the enthalpy of micelle formation becomes more negative as the temperature is increased, a fact which was attributed to a reduction in water structure as temperature is increased. Nuclear magnetic resonance measurements indicate an increase in the mobility of water protons at the onset of micellisation. The addition of urea, a water-structure-breaking compound, to surfactant solutions leads to an increase of cmc, again indicating the role of water structure in the micellisation process. An alternative explanation of the free-energy decrease emphasises the increase in internal freedom of the hydrocarbon chains that occurs when these chains are transferred from the aqueous environment, where their motion is restrained by the hydrogen-bonded water molecules, to the interior of the micelle. It has been suggested that the increased mobility of the hydrocarbon chains, and of course their mutual attraction, constitute the principal hydrophobic factor in micellisation.

5.3.2 Theories of micelle formation

Two general approaches have been employed in attempting to describe the process of micellisation. In one of these, the phase separation model, the cmc is assumed to represent the saturation concentration of the unassociated molecules and the micelles are regarded as a distinct phase that separates out at the cmc. In the alternative approach, the micelle and associated monomers are assumed to be in an association–dissociation equilibrium to which the law of mass action may be applied. Neither of these models is rigorously correct, although the mass action approach seems to give a more realistic description of micellisation, and thus will be considered in more detail.

The aggregation process may in its simplest form be described by

$$ND^+ + (N - p)X^- \rightleftharpoons M^{p+} \qquad (5.11)$$

Equation (5.11) represents the formation of a cationic micelle M^{p+} from N surfactant ions D^+ and $(N - p)$ firmly held counterions X^-. Whenever the thermodynamics of a process is under consideration, it is important to define the standard states of the species. In this example, the standard states are such that the mole fractions of the ionic species are unity and the solution properties are those of the infinitely dilute solutions. The equilibrium constant K_m may be written in the usual way,

$$K_m = \frac{[M^{p+}]}{[D^+]^N [X^-]^{N-p}} \qquad (5.12)$$

where activity coefficients have been neglected. The analogous equation for non-ionic micelles is of a simpler form since counterion terms and charges need not be considered.

$$K_m = \frac{[M]}{[D]^N} \qquad (5.13)$$

Equations (5.12) and (5.13) are important in that they can be used to predict the variation of both monomers and micelles with total solution concentration.

Figure 5.26 shows the result of such a calculation for a model system. It illustrates several important points about the micellisation process. According to the mass action treatment, the monomer concentration decreases very slightly above the cmc: this is a very small effect (although it can be detected experimentally from very precise surface-tension measurements) and for most purposes it is reasonable to assume that the monomer concentration remains constant at the cmc

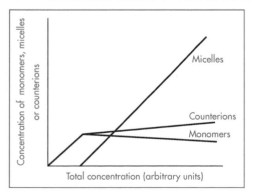

Figure 5.26 Concentration of micelles, monomers and counterions against total concentration (arbitrary units) calculated from equation (5.12) for an aggregation number (N) of 100, micellar equilibrium constant (K_m) of 1, and with 85% of the counterions bound to the micelle.

value. A second point of interest illustrated by the mass action treatment concerns the predicted sharpness of the cmc. It is readily shown by calculations that combinations of low values of N and K_m lead to gradual changes of slope of the cmc region, while larger values for both of these parameters give sharp inflections. The cmc, rather than being an exact concentration, is often a range of concentration over which the solution properties exhibit a gradual change and hence is often difficult to locate exactly.

5.3.3 Micellar structure

Critical packing parameter

The shape of the micelle formed by a particular surfactant is influenced to a large extent by the geometry of the surfactant molecule, as can be seen if we consider the packing of space-filling models of the surfactants. The dimensionless parameter of use in these considerations is called the *critical packing parameter* (CPP) and is defined as

$$CPP = \frac{v}{l_c a} \qquad (5.14)$$

where v is the volume of one chain, a is the cross-sectional area of the surfactant head group and l_c is the extended length of the surfactant alkyl chain (Fig. 5.27). This parameter provides a simple geometric characterisation of the surfactant molecule, which is useful when we consider the structure of the aggregate that will be formed in solution. Consideration of the packing of molecules into spheres shows that, when CPP ≤ 1/3, which is the case for surfactants having a single hydrophobic chain and a simple ionic or large non-ionic head group, a spherical micelle will be formed. Most surfactants of pharmaceutical interest fall into this category. It is easily seen that if we double v by adding a second alkyl chain, then the value of CPP will exceed 1/3 and non-spherical structures such as bilayers (CPP ≈ 1) will form in solution, from which vesicles are formed (see section 5.4.2). One important factor not considered in this simple geometrical model is the interaction between the head groups in the aggregate. The 'effective' cross-sectional area of the surfactant molecule is strongly influenced by the interaction forces between adjacent head groups in the micelle surface. These forces are decreased by addition of electrolyte, leading to a decrease of a, an increase of

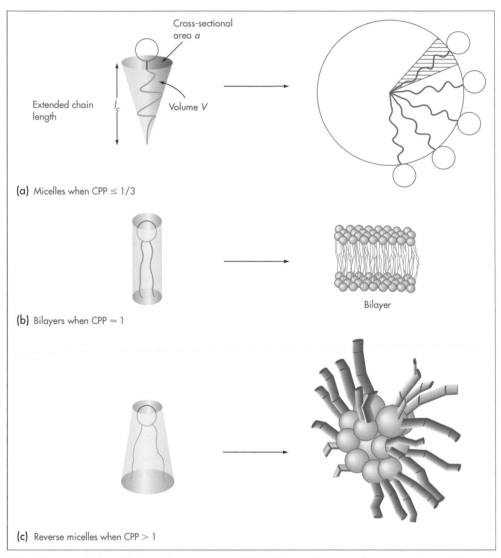

Figure 5.27 Influence of the critical packing parameter, CPP (v/l_ca), on the type of aggregate formed by surfactants in solution.

the CPP and a change of shape of the aggregate, as discussed below.

In non-aqueous media, reverse (or inverted) micelles may form, in which the hydrophilic charge groups form the micellar core shielded from the non-aqueous environment by the hydrophobic chains; such structures are generally formed when CPP > 1 (Fig. 5.27).

Ionic micelles

As we have seen from consideration of the simple geometrical packing model, charged micelles of low aggregation number have a CPP < 1/3 and conse-

quently adopt a spherical or near-spherical shape at concentrations not too far removed from the cmc. The hydrophobic part of the amphiphile is located in the core of the micelle. Around this core is a concentric shell of hydrophilic head groups with $(1-\alpha)N$ counterions, where α is the degree of ionisation. This compact region is termed the *Stern layer* (Fig. 5.28). For most ionic micelles the degree of ionisation α is between 0.2 and 0.3; that is, 70–80% of the counterions may be considered to be bound to the micelles.

The outer surface of the Stern layer is the shear surface of the micelle. The core and the Stern layer together constitute what is termed the *kinetic micelle*.

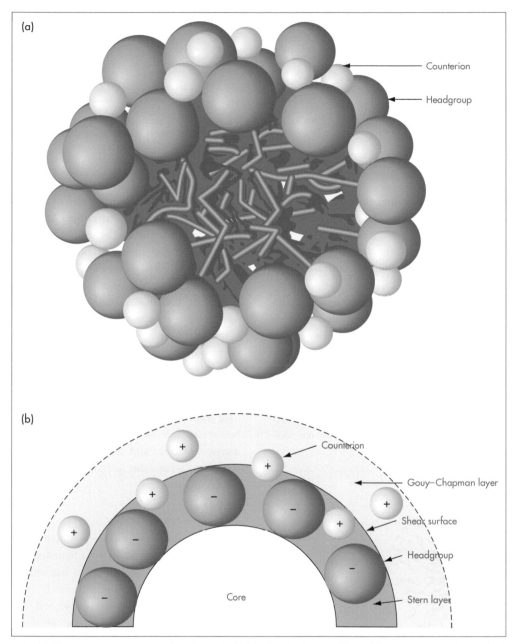

Figure 5.28 (a) Diagrammatic representation of a spherical ionic micelle and (b) partial cross-section of an anionic micelle showing charged layers.

Surrounding the Stern layer is a diffuse layer called the *Gouy–Chapman electrical double layer*, which contains the αN counterions required to neutralise the charge on the kinetic micelle. The thickness of the double layer is dependent on the ionic strength of the solution and is greatly compressed in the presence of electrolyte.

In highly concentrated solution, a gradual change in micellar shape is thought to occur with many ionic systems, the micelles elongating to form cylindrical structures (Fig. 5.29).

Non-ionic micelles

In general, non-ionic surfactants form larger micelles than their ionic counterparts. The reason for this is clearly attributable to the removal of electrical work that must be done when a monomer of an ionic

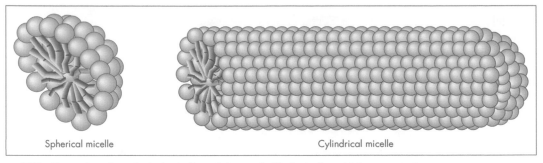

Figure 5.29 Elongation of a spherical micelle to form a cylindrical micelle at high concentration.

surfactant is added to an existing charged micelle. As a consequence of the larger size, the non-ionic micelles are frequently asymmetric. The micelles of Cetomacrogol 1000 ($C_{16}H_{33}(OCH_2CH_2)_{21}OH$, abbreviated to $C_{16}E_{21}$), for example, are thought to be ellipsoidal with an axial ratio not exceeding 2 : 1.

Non-ionic micelles have a hydrophobic core surrounded by a shell of oxyethylene chains, which is often termed the *palisade layer* (Fig. 5.30). This layer is capable of mechanically entrapping a considerable number of water molecules, as well as those that are hydrogen-bonded to the oxyethylene chains. Micelles of non-ionic surfactants tend, as a consequence, to be highly hydrated. The outer surface of the palisade layer forms the shear surface; that is, the hydrating molecules form part of the kinetic micelle.

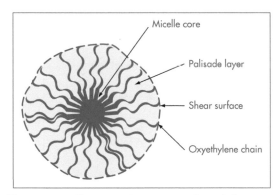

Figure 5.30 Diagrammatic representation of the cross-section of a non-ionic micelle.

5.3.4 Factors affecting the critical micelle concentration and micellar size

Structure of the hydrophobic group

The hydrophobic group plays an important role in determining the type of association of the amphiphile.

Compounds with rigid aromatic or heteroaromatic ring structures (many dyes, purines and pyrimidines, for example) associate by a non-micellar process involving the face-to-face stacking of molecules one on top of the other, rather than by micellisation. Such systems do not exhibit cmcs. Association usually commences at very low concentrations and growth of aggregates may occur by the stepwise addition of monomers. Consequently, the aggregates continuously increase in size rather than attain an equilibrium size as in micellisation. Some drugs are thought to associate in this manner.[3,19]

Micellar amphiphiles of the most common type have hydrophobic groups constructed from hydrocarbon chains. Increase in length of this chain results in a decrease in cmc, and for compounds with identical polar head groups this relationship is expressed by the linear equation

$$\log[\text{cmc}] = A - Bm \qquad (5.15)$$

where m is the number of carbon atoms in the chain and A and B are constants for a homologous series. A corresponding increase in micellar size with increase in hydrocarbon chain length is also noted.

Many drugs are surface active and form small micelles in aqueous solution. For these and other amphiphiles with more complex hydrophobic regions, the effect of substituents on hydrophobicity can be roughly estimated from Table 4.4, in Chapter 4. In the series of micellar diphenylmethane drugs shown in Table 5.3 there is an increased hydrophobicity (as evidenced by a decrease in cmc and increase in aggregation number) following the introduction of —CH_3, —Br and —Cl substituents to the hydrophobic ring systems.

Table 5.3 Effect of substituents on the micellar properties of some diphenylmethane drugs

Drug	R^1	R^2	R^3	Critical micellar concentration (mol kg^{-1})	Micellar aggregation number
Diphenhydramine	H	H	H	0.132	3
Orphenadrine	H	CH_3	H	0.096	7
Bromodiphenhydramine	Br	H	H	0.053	11
Chlorphenoxamine	Cl	H	CH_3	0.045	13

Reproduced from Attwood D. *J Pharm Pharmacol* 1972;24:751; 1976;28:407.

Nature of the hydrophilic group

The most important point to be noted here is the pronounced difference in properties between amphiphiles with ionic hydrophilic groups and those in which this group is uncharged. In general, non-ionic surfactants have very much lower cmc values and higher aggregation numbers than their ionic counterparts with similar hydrocarbon chains, mainly because the micellisation process for such compounds does not involve any electrical work.

The properties of the polyoxyethylated non-ionic surfactants show a pronounced dependence on the length of the polyoxyethylene chain. An increase in the chain length confers a greater hydrophilicity to the molecule and the cmc increases, as shown in Table 5.4.

Nature of the counterion

The counterion associated with the charged group of ionic surfactants has a significant effect on the micellar properties. There is an increase in micellar size for a particular cationic surfactant as the counterion is changed according to the series $Cl^- < Br^- < I^-$, and for a particular anionic surfactant according to $Na^+ < K^+ < Cs^+$. Generally, the more weakly hydrated a counterion, the larger the micelles formed by the surfactant. This is because the weakly hydrated ions can be adsorbed more readily in the micellar surface and so decrease the charge repulsion between the polar groups. A greater depression of cmc and a greater increase in micellar size are noted with organic counterions such as maleates, than with inorganic ions.

Addition of electrolytes

Addition of electrolytes to ionic surfactants decreases the cmc and increases the micellar size. The effect is simply explained in terms of a reduction in the magnitude of the forces of repulsion between the charged head groups in the micelle and a consequent decrease in the electrical work of micellisation. At sufficiently high electrolyte concentration the reduction of head group interaction is sufficient to increase CPP to such an extent that spherical micelles can no longer form. Table 5.5 shows the effect of sodium chloride addition on the micellar properties of the cationic surfactant

Table 5.4 Values of cmc and micellar weights of hexadecyl polyoxyethylene ethers $CH_3(CH_3)_{15}(CH_2CH_2)_nOH$

Property	n =					
	6	7	9	12	15	21
10^6 cmc (mol kg^{-1})	1.7	1.7	2.1	2.3	3.1	3.9
10^{-5} Micellar weight	12.3	3.27	1.4	1.17	–	0.82
Aggregation number	2430	590	220	150	–	70

Reproduced from Elworthy PH, Macfarlane CB. *J Chem Soc* 1963;907; 1962;537.

Table 5.5 Effect of electrolyte on the micellar properties of dodecyltrimethylammonium bromide $CH_3(CH_2)_{11}\,N^+(CH_3)_3Br^-$

NaCl concentration (mol dm^{-3})	Critical micellar concentration (mol dm^{-3})	Aggregation number
0.00	0.014 6	61
0.10	0.004 28	74
0.50	0.001 71	90

Reproduced from Anacker EW. In: Jungermann E (ed.) *Cationic Surfactants.* New York: Marcel Dekker; 1970.

dodecyltrimethylammonium bromide. The micellar properties of non-ionic surfactants, in contrast, are little affected by electrolyte addition.

Effect of temperature

If aqueous solutions of many non-ionic surfactants are heated, they become turbid at a characteristic temperature called the *cloud point* (see Fig. 5.33 in section 5.4.1). Other non-ionic surfactants have cloud points above 100°C. The process is reversible; that is, cooling the solution restores clarity. The turbidity at the cloud point is due to separation of the solution into two phases. At temperatures up to the cloud point, an

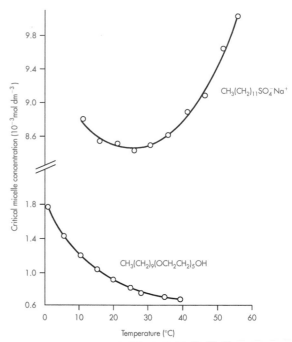

Figure 5.31 Variation of cmc with temperature for sodium dodecyl sulfate ($CH_3(CH_2)_{11}SO_4^- \; Na^+$) and pentaoxyethylene glycol monodecyl ether ($CH_3(CH_2)_9(OCH_2CH_2)_5OH$).

Modified from Goddard ED, Benson GC. Conductivity of aqueous solutions of some paraffin salts. *Can J Chem* 1957;35:986. © 1957 Canadian Science Publishing or its licensors. Reproduced with permission.

Key points

- Micelles form at the cmc, which has a characteristic value for a particular surfactant under a given set of conditions. Micelles are in dynamic equilibrium with free molecules of surfactant in solution; that is, they are continuously breaking down and reforming. The main driving force for the formation of micelles is the increase of entropy that occurs when the hydrophobic regions of the surfactant are removed from water and the ordered structure of the water molecules around this region of the molecule is lost.
- An increase in hydrophobic chain length causes a decrease in the cmc and increase of size of ionic and non-ionic micelles; an increase of polyoxyethylene chain length has the opposite effect on these properties in non-ionic micelles. Electrolyte addition to micellar solutions of ionic surfactants reduces the cmc and increases the micellar size, sometimes causing a change of shape from sphere to ellipsoids. Solutions of some non-ionic surfactants become cloudy on heating and separate reversibly into two phases at the cloud point.
- The core of the micelle contains the hydrophobic region of the surfactant. The core of ionic micelles is surrounded by a concentric shell (the Stern layer) that encloses the charged head groups and about 70–80% of the counterions. Surrounding the Stern layer is a diffuse layer (the Gouy–Chapman layer) that contains the remaining counterions. The core of non-ionic micelles is surrounded by a shell of oxyethylene chains (the palisade layer), which contains entrapped water.

increase in micellar size and a corresponding decrease in cmc are noted for many non-ionic surfactants (Fig. 5.31). The cloud point is very sensitive to additives in the system, which can increase or decrease the clouding temperature.

Temperature has a comparatively small effect on the micellar properties of ionic surfactants. The temperature dependence of the cmc of sodium lauryl (dodecyl) sulfate shown in Fig. 5.31 is typical of the effect observed.

5.4 Liquid crystals and surfactant vesicles

5.4.1 Liquid crystals

Lyotropic liquid crystals

Surfactant solutions at concentrations close to the cmc are clear and isotropic; that is, the magnitudes of physical properties such as viscosity and refractive index do not depend on the direction in which these properties are measured. As the concentration is increased, there is frequently a transition from the typical spherical micellar structure to a more elongated or rod-like micelle. Further increase in concentration may cause the orientation and close packing of the elongated micelles into hexagonal arrays. A new phase containing these ordered arrays separates out from the remainder of the solution, which contains randomly orientated rods, but remains in equilibrium with it. This new phase is a liquid crystalline state termed the *middle phase* or *hexagonal phase*. With some surfactants, further increase of concentration results in the separation of a second liquid crystalline state, the *neat phase* or *lamellar phase*. In some surfactant systems another liquid crystalline state, the *cubic phase*, occurs

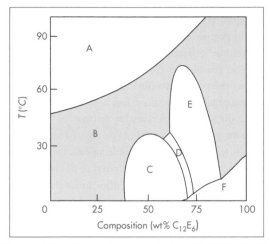

Figure 5.33 Phase diagram of the $CH_3(CH_2)_{11}(OCH_2CH_2)_6OH$ ($C_{12}E_6$)–H_2O system: A, two isotropic liquid phases; B, micellar solution; C, middle or hexagonal phase; D, cubic phase; E, neat or lamellar phase; F, solid phase. The boundary between phases A and B is the cloud point.

Modified from Clunie JS *et al*. Phase equilibria of dodecylhexaoxyethylene glycol monoether in water. *Trans Farad Soc* 1969;65:287, with permission of the Royal Society of Chemistry.

between the middle and neat phases. The most common type of cubic phase is the micellar cubic phase formed by the close packing of spherical micelles; a more complex cubic phase, the bicontinuous cubic phase, occurs with some amphiphilic lipids such as glyceryl monooleate (see section 5.4.2). Finally, in all systems, surfactant separates out of solution. The liquid crystalline phases that occur on increasing the concentration of surfactant solutions are referred to as *lyotropic* liquid crystals; their structure is shown diagrammatically in Fig. 5.32. The phase diagram in Fig. 5.33 shows the transition from micellar solution to liquid crystalline phase and finally to pure amphiphile for the polyoxyethylated non-ionic surfactant $C_{12}E_6$ [$CH_3(CH_2)_{11}(OCH_2CH_2)_6OH$].

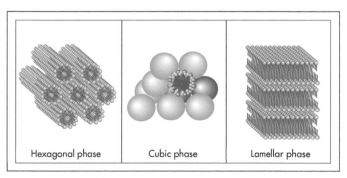

| Hexagonal phase | Cubic phase | Lamellar phase |

Figure 5.32 Diagrammatic representation of forms of lyotropic liquid crystals.

Liquid crystals are anisotropic; that is, their physical properties vary with direction of measurement. The middle phase, for example, will flow only in a direction parallel to the long axis of the arrays. It is rigid in the other two directions. On the other hand, the neat phase is more fluid and behaves as a solid only in the direction perpendicular to that of the layers. Similarly, plane-polarised light is rotated when travelling along any axis except the long axis in the middle phase and a direction perpendicular to the layers in the neat phase. Because of this ability to rotate polarised light, the liquid crystals are visible when placed between crossed polarisers, and this provides a useful means of detecting the liquid crystalline state.

Thermotropic liquid crystals

A second category of liquid crystals is the type produced when certain substances, notably the esters of cholesterol, are heated. These systems are referred to as *thermotropic* liquid crystals and, although not formed by surfactants, their properties will be described here for purposes of comparison. The for-mation of a cloudy liquid when cholesteryl benzoate is heated to temperatures between 145 and 179°C was first noted in 1888 by the Austrian botanist, Reinitzer. The name 'liquid crystal' was applied to this cloudy intermediate phase because of the presence of areas with crystal-like molecular structure within this solution.

Although the compounds that form thermotropic liquid crystalline phases are of a variety of chemical types, such as azo compounds, azoxy compounds or esters, the molecular geometries of the molecule have some characteristic features in that they are generally elongated, flat and rigid along their axes. The presence of easily polarisable groups often enhances liquid crystal formation.

The arrangement of the elongated molecules in thermotropic liquid crystals is generally recognisable as one of three principal types: namely, *smectic* (soap-like), *nematic* (thread-like) and *cholesteric*. The molecular arrays are illustrated diagrammatically in Fig. 5.34.

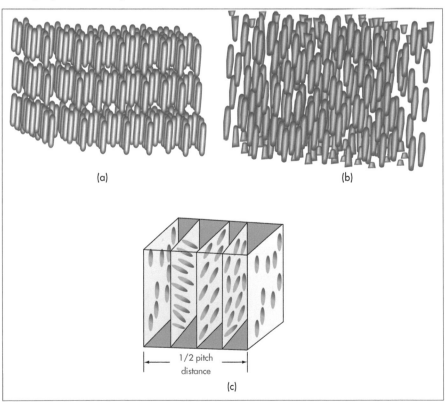

Figure 5.34 Diagrammatic representation of forms of thermotropic liquid crystals: (a) smectic; (b) nematic; and (c) a stylised diagram of cholesteric liquid crystals.

In the nematic liquid crystalline state, groups of molecules orientate spontaneously with their long axes parallel, but they are not ordered into layers. Because the molecules have freedom of rotation about their long axis, the nematic liquid crystals are quite mobile and are readily oriented by electric or magnetic fields. Nematic liquid crystals are formed, for example, when p-azoxyanisole is heated.

The molecules in smectic liquid crystals are more ordered than the nematic since not only are they arranged with their long axes parallel but they are also arranged into distinct layers. As a result of this two-dimensional order, the smectic liquid crystals are viscous and are not oriented by magnetic fields. Examples of compounds forming smectic liquid crystals are octyl p-azoxycinnamate and ethyl p-azoxybenzoate.

If a nematic liquid crystal is made of chiral molecules, i.e. the molecules differ from their mirror image, a cholesteric (or chiral nematic) liquid crystal is obtained. The cholesteric phase is formed by several cholesteryl esters and can be visualised as a stack of very thin two-dimensional nematic-like layers in which the elongated molecules lie parallel to each other in the plane of the layer. The orientation of the long axes in each layer is displaced from that in the adjacent layer and this displacement is cumulative through successive layers so that the overall displacement traces out a helical path through the layers. The helical path causes very pronounced rotation of polarised light, which can be as much as 50 rotations per millimetre. The pitch of the helix (the distance required for one complete rotation) is very sensitive to small changes in temperature and pressure and dramatic colour changes can result from variations in these properties. When non-polarised light is passed through the cholesteric material, the light is separated into two components, one with the electric vector rotating clockwise and the other with the electric vector rotating anticlockwise. One of these components is transmitted and the other reflected, depending on the material involved. This process is called *circular dichroism* and it gives the cholesteric phase a characteristic iridescent appearance when illuminated by white light.

5.4.2 Liposomes, niosomes and surfactant vesicles

Phospholipids and other surfactants having two hydrophobic chains have CPP values of approximately 1 (see section 5.3.3) and tend to form lamellar phases. When equilibrated with excess water, these lamellar phases may form vesicles that can entrap drug and these have potential use as drug carriers. In this section we will consider several types of vesicular structures; Box 5.3 shows some of the amphiphiles that form such structures.

Liposomes

Liposomes are formed by naturally occurring phospholipids such as lecithin (phosphatidylcholine). When first formed in solution they are usually composed of several bimolecular lipid lamellae separated by aqueous layers (*multilamellar liposomes*). Sonication of these units can give rise to *unilamellar liposomes*. The net charge of the liposome can be varied by incorporation of, for example, a long-chain amine such as stearylamine (to give positively charged vesicles) or dicetyl phosphate (to give negatively charged species). Positively charged vesicles are being used experimentally as carriers for DNA: the anionic DNA condenses around the cationic vesicles to provide compact units for cell delivery. Water-soluble drugs can be entrapped in liposomes by intercalation in the aqueous layers, while lipid-soluble drugs can be solubilised within the hydrocarbon interiors of the lipid bilayers. The use of liposomes as drug carriers has been reviewed.[20] Since liposomes can encapsulate drugs, proteins and enzymes, the systems can be administered intravenously, orally or intramuscularly in order to decrease toxicity, to increase specificity of uptake of drug and in some cases to control release. Liposomes have several disadvantages as carriers for delivery of drugs, however; for example, phospholipids are liable to oxidative degradation and must be stored and handled in a nitrogen atmosphere.

Surfactant vesicles and niosomes

Surfactants having two alkyl chains can pack in a similar manner to the phospholipids (see Box 5.3 for examples). Vesicle formation by the dialkyldimethylammonium cationic surfactants has been studied extensively. As with liposomes, sonication of the turbid solution formed when the surfactant is dispersed in

Box 5.3 Some vesicle-forming amphiphiles

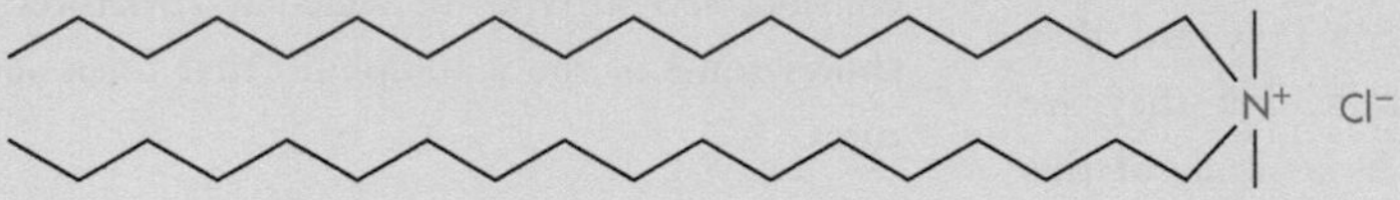

Dioctadecyldimethylammonium chloride

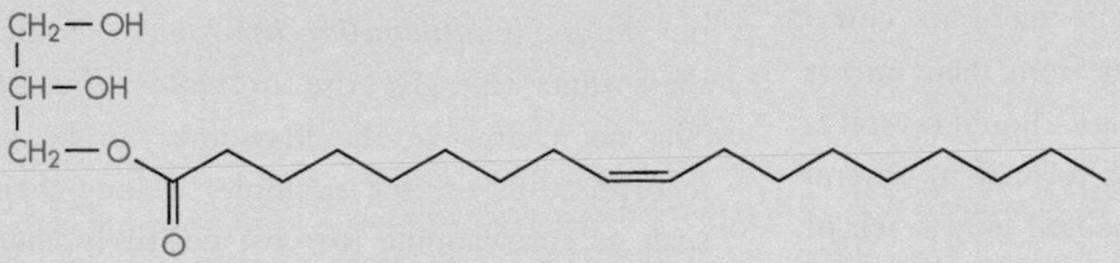

Glyceryl monooleate

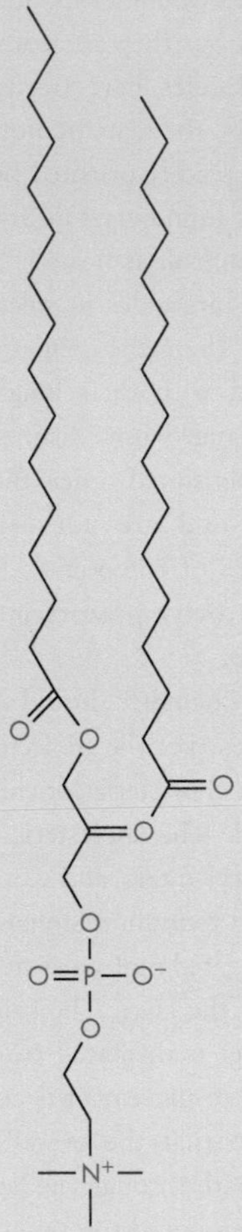

Lecithin

water leads ultimately to the formation of optically transparent solutions that may contain single-compartment vesicles. For example, sonication of dioctadecyl-dimethylammonium chloride for 30 seconds gives a turbid solution containing bilayer vesicles of 250–450 nm diameter, while sonication for 15 minutes produces a clear solution containing monolayer vesicles of diameter 100–150 nm. The main use of such systems has been as membrane models rather than as drug delivery vehicles because of the toxicity of ionic surfactants.

Some dialkyl polyoxyethylene ether non-ionic surfactants also form vesicles, as do mixtures of cholesterol and a single alkyl-chain non-ionic surfactant with a glyceryl head group. The resultant vesicles have been termed *niosomes*. These vesicles behave *in vivo* like liposomes, prolonging the circulation of entrapped drug and altering its organ distribution and metabolic stability. As with liposomes, the properties of niosomes depend both on the composition of the bilayer and on the method of production; Fig. 5.35 shows a freeze-fracture electron micrograph of a multilamellar niosome. Being non-ionic, niosomes are likely to be less toxic than vesicles produced from ionic surfactants and represent promising vehicles for drug delivery.[21,22]

Monoolein vesicles

Polar amphiphilic lipids such as glyceryl monooleate (monoolein) also form bilayers, the nature of which depends on the temperature and concentration. An interesting phase formed at monoolein concentrations

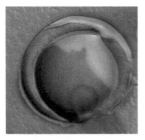

Figure 5.35 Freeze-fracture electron micrograph of a multilamellar niosome.

of 60–80% w/w is the bicontinuous cubic phase. The structure of this phase is unique and consists of a curved bicontinuous lipid bilayer extending in three dimensions, separating two networks of water channels with pores of about 5 nm diameter (Fig. 5.36). On dilution, these structures coexist with excess water and there is the formation of dispersed cubic phase vesicles or *cubosomes*. Cubic phases have been shown to incorporate and deliver small-molecule drugs and large proteins by oral and parenteral routes, in addition to local delivery in vaginal and periodontal cavities.[23]

5.5 Properties of some commonly used surfactants

5.5.1 Anionic surfactants

Sodium Lauryl Sulfate BP is a mixture of sodium alkyl sulfates, the chief of which is sodium dodecyl sulfate, $C_{12}H_{25}SO_4^-Na^+$. It is very soluble in water and is used pharmaceutically as a preoperative skin cleaner, having bacteriostatic action against Gram-positive bacteria,

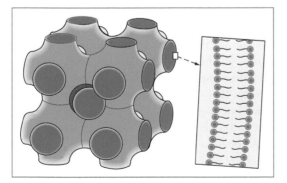

Figure 5.36 Structure of glyceryl monooleate–water cubic phase with inset showing the lipid bilayer.

Redrawn from Shah JC *et al*. Cubic phase gels as drug delivery systems. *Adv Drug Deliv Rev* 2001;47:229. Copyright Elsevier 2001.

Key points

- There are two main categories of liquid crystal: lyotropic liquid crystals, which are observed in highly concentrated surfactant solutions; and thermotropic liquid crystals, which are produced when certain substances, notably cholesterol esters, are heated.
- Phase diagrams of surfactants may show transitions from micellar solutions to hexagonal (or middle), cubic and lamellar (or neat) liquid crystalline phases as the surfactant concentration is increased.
- There are three main types of thermotropic liquid crystals: nematic, in which the groups of molecules are ordered with their long axes parallel; smectic, which are similar to nematic but are also arranged into distinct layers; and cholesteric, which are stacks of nematic-like layers in which the orientation of the long axes traces out a helical path through the layers.

and also in medicated shampoos. It is a component of Emulsifying Wax BP.

Sodium dodecyl sulfate has been studied in depth. The cmc at 25°C is 8.2×10^{-3} mol dm^{-3} (0.23% w/v). The effect of temperature on the cmc is shown in Fig. 5.31.

5.5.2 Cationic surfactants

The quaternary ammonium and pyridinium cationic surfactants are important pharmaceutically because of their bactericidal activity against a wide range of Gram-positive and some Gram-negative organisms. They may be used on the skin, especially in the cleaning of wounds. Aqueous solutions are used for cleaning contaminated utensils.

Cetrimide BP consists mainly of tetradecyltrimethylammonium bromide together with smaller amounts of dodecyl- and hexadecyltrimethylammonium bromides. The properties of the individual components have been studied in detail and are summarised in Table 5.6. Solutions containing

Table 5.6 Micellar properties of a commercial sample of cetrimide and its main constituents at 25°C

Constituent	Percentage (calculated on dry-weight basis)	Critical micellar concentration (mmol dm^{-3})	Micellar molecular weight (×10^{-4})
Tetradecyltrimethylammonium bromide	68	3.3	2.7
Dodecyltrimethylammonium bromide	22	5.3	2.1
Hexadecyltrimethylammonium bromide	7	0.82	3.3
Cetrimide	–	2.9	2.5

Data from Barry BW *et al. J Colloid Interface Sci* 1970;33:554; 1972;40:174.

0.1–1% of cetrimide are used for cleaning the skin, wounds and burns, for cleaning contaminated vessels, polythene tubing and catheters, and for storage of sterilised surgical instruments. Solutions of cetrimide are also used in shampoos to remove scales in seborrhoea. In the form of Cetrimide Emulsifying Wax BP, it is used as an emulsifying agent for producing oil-in-water creams suitable for the incorporation of cationic and non-ionic medicaments (anionic medicaments would, of course, be incompatible with this cationic surfactant).

Benzalkonium chloride is a mixture of alkylbenzyldimethylammonium chlorides of the general formula $[C_6H_5CH_2N(CH_3)_2R]Cl$, where R represents a mixture of the alkyls from C_8H_{17} to $C_{18}H_{37}$. In dilute solution (1 in 1000 to 1 in 2000) it may be used for the preoperative disinfection of skin and mucous membranes, for application to burns and wounds, and for cleaning polythene and nylon tubing and catheters. Benzalkonium chloride is also used as a preservative for eye drops and as a permitted vehicle for the preparation of certain eye drops.

5.5.3 Non-ionic surfactants

The amphiphilic nature of non-ionic surfactants is often expressed in terms of the balance between the hydrophobic and hydrophilic portions of the molecule. An empirical scale of hydrophile–lipophile balance (HLB) numbers has been devised (see Chapter 6, section 6.4.2). The lower the HLB number, the more lipophilic is the compound, and vice versa. HLB values for a series of commercial non-ionic surfactants are quoted in Tables 5.7 and 5.8. The choice of surfactant for medicinal use involves a consideration of the toxicity of the substance, which may be ingested in large amounts. The following surfactants are widely used in pharmaceutical formulations.

Sorbitan esters (Spans)

The commercial products are mixtures of the partial esters of sorbitol and its mono- and dianhydrides with oleic acid. They are generally insoluble in water and are used as water-in-oil emulsifiers and as wetting agents. The main sorbitan esters are listed in Table 5.7 together with a space-filling model of sorbitan palmitate.

Polysorbates (Tweens)

Commercial products are complex mixtures of partial esters of sorbitol and its mono- and dianhydrides condensed with approximately 20 moles (usually) of ethylene oxide for each mole of sorbitol and its anhydride. The space-filling model of polysorbate 20 is shown in Table 5.8. The polysorbates are miscible with water, as reflected in their higher HLB values (Table 5.8), and are used as emulsifying agents for oil-in-water emulsions.

Polyoxyethylene alkyl ethers

The polyoxyethylene alkyl ethers are glycol ethers of *n*-alcohols, also known as macrogol ethers (macrogol being the non-proprietary name for polyethylene glycol (PEG)). They tend to be mixtures of polymers of slightly varying molecular weights, and the numbers used to describe their chain lengths are average values.

A widely used example is *Cetomacrogol 1000 BP* (Macrogol Cetostearyl Ether), which is a water-soluble substance with the general structure $CH_3(CH_2)_m(OCH_2CH_2)_nOH$, where *m* may be 15 or 17 and the number of oxyethylene groups, *n*, is between 20 and 24. It is used in the form of Cetoma-

Table 5.7 HLB values of sorbitan esters

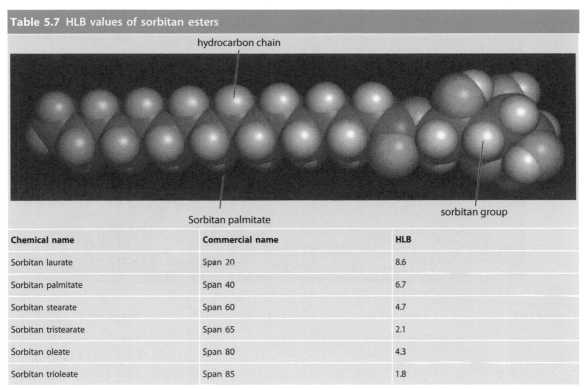

hydrocarbon chain

Sorbitan palmitate

sorbitan group

Chemical name	Commercial name	HLB
Sorbitan laurate	Span 20	8.6
Sorbitan palmitate	Span 40	6.7
Sorbitan stearate	Span 60	4.7
Sorbitan tristearate	Span 65	2.1
Sorbitan oleate	Span 80	4.3
Sorbitan trioleate	Span 85	1.8

crogol Emulsifying Wax BP in the preparation of oil-in-water emulsions and also as a solubilising agent for volatile oils. The cmc and micellar molecular weight in aqueous solution are 6×10^{-2} g dm^{-3} and 1.01×10^5 Da, respectively.

Other macrogol ethers are commercially available as the *Brij* series – for example, Brij 30 (polyoxyethylene (4) lauryl ether, $C_{12}H_{35}(OCH_2CH_2)_4OH$), Brij 72 (polyoxyethylene (2) stearyl ether, $C_{18}H_{37}(OCH_2CH_2)_2OH$) and Brij 97 (polyoxyethylene (10) oleyl ether, $C_{18}H_{35}(OCH_2CH_2)_{10}OH$).

Polyoxyethylene castor oil derivatives

Polyoxyethylene castor oil derivatives are a series of non-ionic surfactants synthesised by reacting either castor oil or hydrogenated castor oil with varying amounts of ethylene oxide. The most widely used are the Cremophor series (BASF Corporation).

Cremophor EL (Polyol 35 Castor Oil USP, Macrogolglycerol Ricinoleate Ph Eur) is a mixture of 83% relatively hydrophobic components (mainly glycerol polyoxyethylene glycol ricinoleate) and 17% relatively hydrophilic components (mixture of PEGs and glycerol ethoxylates). Cremophor EL solubilises the fat-soluble vitamins in aqueous solutions for oral and topical

administration, and is also used as a solubilising agent in the preparation of intravenous anaesthetics and other products, although care should be taken when Cremophor is used in injection formulations because of the possibility of an anaphylactic response to this surfactant. However, in this respect it should be noted that other non-ionic surfactants, including polysorbate 80, also can cause adverse reactions in some patients.

Cremophor RH40 (Polyol 40 Hydrogenated Castor Oil USP/NF, Macrogolglycerol Hydroxystearate Ph Eur) is a mixture of approximately 75% relatively hydrophobic components, mainly fatty-acid esters of glycerol PEG and fatty-acid esters of PEG and 25% relatively hydrophilic components consisting of PEGs and glycerol ethoxylates. Cremophor RH40 is also used as a solubilising agent for fat-soluble vitamins and may be used in preference to Cremophor EL in oral preparations, since it is almost tasteless.

Polyglycolysed glycerides

There are several commercially available polyglycolysed glycerides used as micellar solubilising agents, including Labrafil M-1944CS, Labrafil M-2125CS, Labrasol and Gelucire 44/14. They are produced by the partial pegylation of glycerides (fatty-acid esters of glycerol)

Table 5.8 HLB and cmc values of polysorbates

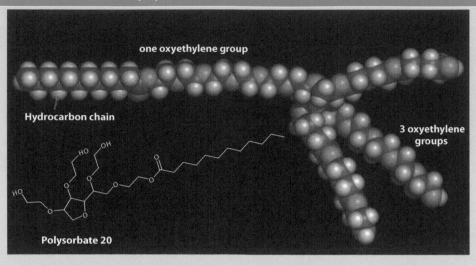

Chemical name	Commercial name	HLB	cmc[a] (g dm^{-3})
Polyoxyethylene (20) sorbitan laurate	Polysorbate (Tween) 20	16.7	0.060
Polyoxyethylene (20) sorbitan palmitate	Polysorbate (Tween) 40	15.6	0.031
Polyoxyethylene (20) sorbitan stearate	Polysorbate (Tween) 60	14.9	0.028
Polyoxyethylene (20) sorbitan tristearate	Polysorbate (Tween) 65	10.5	0.050
Polyoxyethylene (20) sorbitan oleate	Polysorbate (Tween) 80	15.0	0.014
Polyoxyethylene (20) sorbitan trioleate	Polysorbate (Tween) 85	11.0	0.023

[a]Data from Wan LS, Lee PFS. *J Pharm Sci* 1974;63:136.

derived from fixed oils of vegetable origin – apricot kernel oil in the case of Labrafil M-1944CS, corn oil for Labrafil M-2125CS, coconut oil for Labrasol and palm kernel oil for Gelucire 44/14. Glycerides are fatty-acid esters of glycerol and may be triglycerides, in which all three hydroxyl groups of glycerol are esterified; diglycerides, in which two are esterified; or monoglycerides, in which only one hydroxyl is esterified. The fatty acids vary depending on the source of the vegetable oil. The main fatty acid of apricot kernel oil is oleic acid and hence Labrafil M-1944CS consists of mixtures of tri-, di- and monoglycerides of oleic acid (C18), although of course other fatty-acid esters are also present in smaller amounts. Corn oil, from which Labrafil M-2125CS is produced, consists mainly of

linoleic acid (unsaturated C18); coconut oil from which Labrasol is produced contains mainly caprylic (C8) and capric (C10) acids; and palm kernel oil consists mainly of lauric (C12) and myristic (C14) acids. The polyoxyethylene glycol also varies between these commercial products – both Labrafil M-1944CS and Labrafil M-2125CS are esters of PEG 300, Labrasol is an ester of PEG 400, and Gelucire 44/14 an ester of PEG 1500. Summarising the average composition of these polyglycolysed glycerides, we may write:

- PEG 300 oleic glycerides (Labrofil M-1944CS)
- PEG 300 linoleic glycerides (Labrofil M-2125CS)
- PEG 400 caprylic/capric glycerides (Labrosol)
- PEG 1500 lauric/myristic glycerides (Gelucire 44/14).

Polyoxyethylene esters

Vitamin E TPGS (D-α-tocopheryl polyethylene glycol 1000 succinate)

Vitamin E TPGS (**II**) is prepared by the esterification of the acid group of crystalline D-α-tocopheryl acid succinate by PEG 1000.

$n = 20–22$

Structure II Vitamin E TPGS

It is used as an emulsifier, micellar solubilising agent, an absorption enhancer and as a vehicle for lipid-based drug delivery formulations. It is also a water-soluble source of the water-insoluble oil vitamin E (D-α-tocopherol).

Solutol HS-15 (polyoxyethylene 660 hydroxystearate)

Solutol HS-15 (**III**) is also known as polyoxyethylene 660 hydroxystearate or macrogol 660. It is a mixture of ~70% polyglycol mono- and diesters of 12-hydroxystearic acid (lipophilic) and ~30% of free PEG (hydrophilic). Structure **III** shows the general formula of the monoesters of Solutol HS-15.

$n = \sim 15$

Structure III Solutol HS-15

Solutol HS 15 is a water-soluble, micelle-forming, solubilising agent used commercially in oral and parenteral formulations with lipophilic drugs and vitamins.

Poloxamers

Poloxamers are synthetic block copolymers of hydrophilic poly(oxyethylene) and hydrophobic poly(oxypropylene) with the general formula $E_mP_nE_m$, where E = oxyethylene (OCH_2CH_2) and P = oxypropylene (OCH_2CHCH_3) and the subscripts m and n denote chain lengths. Properties such as viscosity, HLB and physical state (liquid, paste or solid) are dependent on the relative chain lengths of the hydrophilic and hydrophobic blocks. The convention for naming these

compounds is to use a number, the first two digits of which, when multiplied by 100, correspond to the approximate average molecular weight of the poly(oxypropylene) block and the third digit, when multiplied by 10, corresponds to the percentage by weight of the poly(oxyethylene) block. For example, the poly(oxypropylene) block of poloxamer 188 has a molecular weight of approximately 1800 Da and about 80% by weight of the molecule is poly(oxypropylene). These copolymers were introduced to the market in 1951 by the Wyandotte Chemical Corporation (now BASF-Wyandotte) under the trade name Pluronic. The nomenclature adopted by this company indicates the physical state by a letter (F, P or L, denoting solid, paste or liquid, respectively) followed by a two- or three-digit number. The last digit of this number is the same as that for the equivalent poloxamer and is approximately one-tenth of the weight percentage of poly(oxyethylene); the first digit (or two digits in a three-digit number) multiplied by 300 gives a rough estimate of the molecular weight of the hydrophobe. So, for example, Pluronic F68 is a solid, the molecular weight of the hydrophobe is approximately 1800 Da, and the poly(oxyethylene) content is approximately 80% of the molecule by weight. A grid was developed by BASF to interrelate the properties of the Pluronics (Fig. 5.37a). The BASF nomenclature has been adopted by the other major supplier of poloxamers, Uniqema, which markets the copolymers as the Synperonic series. The relationship between the Pluronic (and Synperonic) and poloxamer nomenclatures is shown in Table 5.9, which also gives the composition of each copolymer.

Included in Table 5.9 are examples of block copolymers of poly(oxyethylene) and poly(oxypropylene) with the general formula $P_nE_mP_n$ (meroxapols). The nomenclature for these 'reverse' block copolymers uses three digits, the first two (approximately one-hundredth of the molecular weight of the poly-(oxypropylene) block) separated from the third (approximately one-tenth of the weight percentage of poly(oxyethylene) in the molecule) by the letter R. For example, 25R4 contains 40% by weight of poly(oxyethylene), and the total molecular weight of the poly(oxypropylene) blocks is approximately 2500 Da. The properties of the members of the Pluronic R series are interrelated using the grid shown in Fig. 5.37b.

Table 5.9 Nomenclature of $E_mP_nE_m$ and $P_nE_mP_n$ block copolymers

Poloxamer	Pluronic	Mol. wt of P block	Chain length, n	Weight % of E block	Chain length, m	Mol. wt of copolymer
188	F68	1 750	30	80	80	8 750
217	F77	2 050	35	70	54	6 835
237	F87	2 250	39	70	60	7 500
238	F88	2 250	39	80	102	11 250
288	F98	2 750	47	80	125	13 750
338	F108	3 250	56	80	148	16 250
407	F127	4 000	69	70	106	13 335
105	L35	5 950	103	50	68	11 900
123	L43	1 200	21	30	6	1 715
124	L44	1 200	21	40	9	2 000
181	L61	1 750	30	10	2	1 945
182	L62	1 750	30	20	5	2 190
183	L63	1 750	30	30	9	2 500
184	L64	1 750	30	40	13	2 915
212	L72	2 050	35	20	6	2 565
231	L81	2 250	39	10	3	2 500
282	L92	2 750	47	20	8	3 440
331	L101	3 250	56	10	4	3 610
401	L121	4 000	69	10	5	4 445
402	L122	4 000	69	20	11	5 000
185	P65	1 750	30	50	20	3 500
333	P103	3 250	56	30	16	4 645
334	P104	3 250	56	40	25	5 415
335	P105	3 250	56	50	37	6 500
403	P123	4 000	69	30	19	5 715
171*	17R1	1 410	–	10	–	1 565
252*	25R2	2 100	–	20	–	2 625
258*	25R8	2 100	–	80	–	10 500
311*	31R1	2 450	–	10	–	2 720

Modified from Edens MW. In: Nace VM (ed.) *Nonionic Surfactants. Polyoxyalkylene Block Copolymers.* Surfactant Science Series 60. New York: Marcel Dekker; 1996: 185–210.
*$P_nE_mP_n$ block copolymers.

The poloxamers are water-soluble and, as might be expected from their amphiphilic structure, are also surface active. Many of the series form micelles, the properties of which have been reviewed by several authors.[24,25]

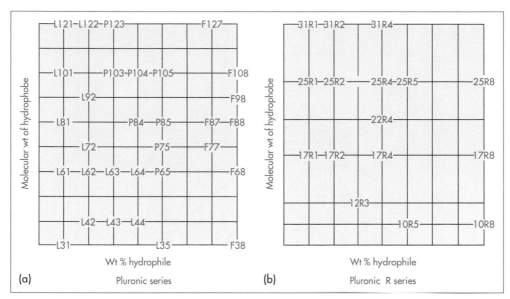

Figure 5.37 The Pluronic grid for (a) the poly(oxyethylene)–poly(oxypropylene)–poly(oxyethylene) (Pluronic) series and (b) the poly(oxypropylene)–poly(oxyethylene)–poly(oxypropylene) (Pluronic R) series of block copolymers.

Poloxamers are used as emulsifying agents for intravenous fat emulsions, as solubilising agents to maintain clarity in elixirs and syrups and as wetting agents for antibacterials. They may also be used in ointment or suppository bases and as tablet binders or coaters.

5.6 Solubilisation

As we have seen in section 5.3, the micellar core is essentially a paraffin-like region and as such is capable of dissolving oil-soluble molecules. This process, whereby water-insoluble substances are brought into solution by incorporation into micelles, is termed *solubilisation* and the incorporated substance is referred to as the *solubilisate*. The subject of solubilisation has been reviewed extensively[3,26] and it is only possible in this book to give an outline of this phenomenon.

5.6.1 Determination of maximum additive concentration

The maximum amount of solubilisate that can be incorporated into a given system at a fixed concentration is termed the *maximum additive concentration*. The simplest method of determining the maximum additive concentration is to prepare a series of vials containing surfactant solution of known concentra-

tion. Increasing concentrations of solubilisate are added and the vials are then sealed and agitated until equilibrium conditions are established. The maximum concentration of solubilisate forming a clear solution can be determined by visual inspection or from extinction or turbidity measurement on the solutions.

Solubility data are expressed as solubility–concentration curves or as phase diagrams. The latter are preferable since a three-component phase diagram completely describes the effect of varying all three components of the system – namely, the solubilisate, the solubiliser and the solvent. The axes of the phase diagram form an equilateral triangle (Fig. 5.38), each side of which is divided into 100 parts to correspond to percentage composition.

A typical phase diagram of a solubilised system is shown in Fig. 5.39. In solutions of high water content the oil is solubilised in the micelles of the non-ionic surfactant Brij 97 ($C_{18}H_{35}(OCH_2CH_2)_{10}OH$), forming an isotropic micellar solution (often referred to as the L_1 region). When the concentration of the oil is increased, stable oil-in-water emulsions may be formed, while an increase in the surfactant concentration results in the formation of the liquid-crystalline regions, labelled middle and neat phases (see section 5.4). It is important in formulation to avoid boundary regions, as otherwise there is a danger of unwanted phase transitions.

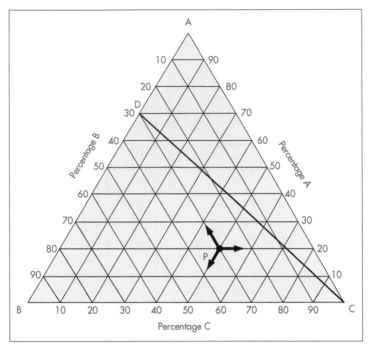

Figure 5.38 Three-component phase diagram. Point P represents a system of composition 20% A, 30% B and 50% C. Line CD represents the dilution of a mixture, originally containing 70% A and 30% B, with component C.

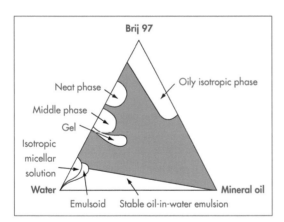

Figure 5.39 Partial phase diagram for the Brij 97 ($C_{18}H_{35}(OCH_2CH_2)_{10}OH$)–water–mineral oil solubilised system.

Redrawn with permission from Lachampt R, Vila RM. A contribution to the study of emulsions. *Am Perfum Cosmet* 1967;82:29.

5.6.2 Location of the solubilisate

The site of solubilisation within the micelle is closely related to the chemical nature of the solubilisate (Fig. 5.40). It is generally accepted that non-polar solubilisates (aliphatic hydrocarbons, for example) are dissolved in the hydrocarbon core of ionic and non-ionic micelles. Water-insoluble compounds containing polar groups are oriented with the polar group at the core–surface interface of the micelle and the hydrophobic group buried inside the hydrocarbon core of the micelle. In addition, solubilisation in non-ionic polyoxyethylated surfactants can occur in the polyoxyethylene shell (palisade layer) that surrounds the core. *p*-Hydroxybenzoic acid, for example, is solubilised entirely within this region of the cetomacrogol micelle, while esters of *p*-hydroxybenzoic acid are located at the palisade–core junction, with the ester group just within the core.

Solubilisates that are located within the micellar core increase the size of the micelles in two ways. Micelles become larger not only because their core is enlarged by the solubilisate but also because the number of surfactant molecules per micelle (the aggregation number) increases in an attempt to cover the swollen core. Solubilisation within the palisade layer, on the other hand, tends not to alter the aggregation number, the increase in micellar size resulting solely from the incorporation of solubilisate molecules.

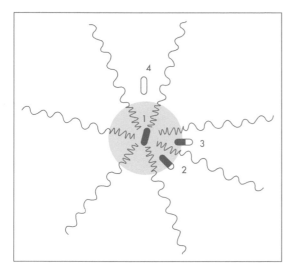

Figure 5.40 Schematic representation of sites of solubilisation depending on the hydrophobicity of the solubilisate. Completely water-insoluble hydrophobic molecules are incorporated in the micelle core (case 1); water-soluble molecules may be solubilised in the polyoxyethylene shell of a non-ionic micelle (case 4); solubilisates with intermediate hydrophobicities (cases 2 and 3) are incorporated in the micelle with the hydrophobic region (black) in the core and the hydrophilic region (white) at the micelle–water interface.

Redrawn from Torchilin V. Structure and design of polymeric surfactant-based drug delivery systems. *J Control Release* 2001;73:137. Copyright Elsevier 2001.

5.6.3 Factors affecting solubilisation

Nature of the surfactant

Chain length of hydrophobe

It is difficult to generalise about the way in which the structural characteristics of a surfactant affect its solubilising capacity because this is influenced by the solubilisation site within the micelle. In cases where the solubilisate is located within the core or deep within the micelle structure, the solubilisation capacity increases with increase in alkyl chain length, as might be expected. Table 5.10 clearly shows an increase of solubilising capacity of a series of polysorbates for selected barbiturates as the alkyl chain length is increased from C_{12} (polysorbate 20) to C_{18} (polysorbate 80). Similar effects have been noted for the solubilisation of barbiturates in polyoxyethylene surfactants with the general structure $CH_3(CH_2)_m$ $(OCH_2CH_2)_nOH$ with increasing alkyl chain length, m. There is a limit, however, to the improvement of solubilising capacity caused by increase of alkyl chain length in this way: an increase of m from 16 to 22,

Table 5.10 Solubilising capacity of polysorbates for the barbiturates at 30°C

Drug	Surfactant	Solubility (mg drug per g surfactant)
Phenobarbital	Polysorbate 20	55
	Polysorbate 40	61
	Polysorbate 60	63
	Polysorbate 80	66
Amobarbital	Polysorbate 20	32
	Polysorbate 40	38
	Polysorbate 80	40
Secobarbital	Polysorbate 20	111
	Polysorbate 80	144

Reproduced from Ismail AA *et al. J Pharm Sci* 1970;59:220.

although producing larger micelles, does not result in a corresponding increase of solubilisation.[27]

Ethylene oxide chain length

The effect of an increase in the ethylene oxide chain length of a polyoxyethylated non-ionic surfactant on its solubilising capacity is again dependent on the location of the solubilisate within the micelle and is complicated by corresponding changes in the micellar size. Table 5.11 shows the solubilisation capacity of a series of polyoxyethylated non-ionic surfactants with a hydrocarbon chain length of 16 (C_{16}) and an increasing number of ethylene oxide units (E) in the polyoxyethylene chain. As seen from this table, the aggregation number decreases with increase in the hydrophilic chain length so, although the number of steroid molecules solubilised per micelle also decreases, the total amount solubilised per mole of surfactant (number of steroid molecules per micelle × number of micelles per mole) actually increases because of the increasing number of micelles.

Similar results were observed in a study of the solubilisation of the poorly water-soluble mydriatic drug tropicamide by a series of poloxamers.[28] Figure 5.41 shows an increase of solubilisation (expressed as moles of tropicamide per mole of poloxamer) with increase of the oxyethylene content of the poloxamer. When the data were expressed as the moles of drug solubilised per ethylene oxide unit of the poloxamer, however, the solubilisation capacity decreased with

Table 5.11 Micellar solubilisation parameters for steroids in *n*-alkyl polyoxyethylene surfactants C_nE_m (where *n* = alkyl (C) chain length and *m* = polyoxyethylene (E) chain length) at 25°C

Steroid molecules per micelle

Surfactant	Aggregation number	Micelles per mole ($\times 10^{-21}$)	Hydrocortisone	Dexamethasone	Testosterone	Progesterone
$C_{16}E_{17}$	99	6.1	9.1	6.7	6.0	5.6
$C_{16}E_{32}$	56	10.8	7.6	5.3	4.6	4.3
$C_{16}E_{44}$	39	15.4	5.8	4.2	3.6	3.3
$C_{16}E_{63}$	25	24.1	4.0	3.3	2.4	2.3

Reproduced from Barry BW, El Eini DID. *J Pharm Pharmacol* 1976;28:210.

increasing ethylene oxide chain length. Again, the reason for this decrease is that the micellar size per ethylene oxide equivalent decreases with increasing length of the ethylene oxide chain.

Nature of the solubilisate

Although many possible relationships between the amount solubilised and various physical properties of the solubilisate molecule (for example, molar volume, polarity, polarisability and chain length) have been

explored, it has not been possible to establish simple correlations between them. In general, a decrease in solubility in a surfactant solution occurs when the alkyl chain length of a homologous series is increased. Unsaturated compounds are generally more soluble than their saturated counterparts. Branching of the hydrocarbon chain of the solubilisate has little effect, but increased solubilisation is often noted following cyclisation. Unfortunately, these generalisations apply only to very simple solubilisates.

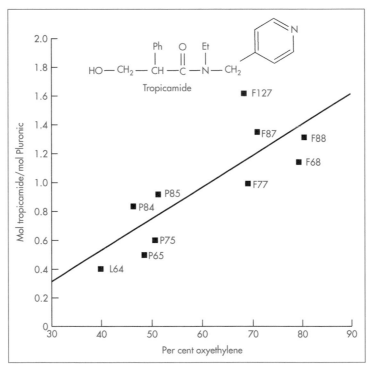

Figure 5.41 Moles of tropicamide solubilised per mole of Pluronic plotted against the oxyethylene content of the poloxamer (see Table 5.9 for details of the Pluronics).

Reproduced from Saettone MF *et al*. Solubilisation of tropicamide by poloxamers: physicochemical data and activity data in rabbits and humans. *Int J Pharm* 1988;43:67. Copyright Elsevier 1988.

More specific rules can be formulated for particular series of solubilisates. For example, it is clear from studies of the effect of steroid structure on solubilisation by a series of surfactants that the more hydrophilic is the substituent in position 17 of the ring structure, the lower the quantity of surfactant required to effect solubilisation of the hormone. Thus the extent of solubilisation of hormones in sodium lauryl sulfate follows the series progesterone <testosterone<deoxycorticosterone, the C_{17} substituents, being $-COCH_3$, $-OH$ and $-COCH_2OH$, respectively (Box 5.4).

Box 5.4 Structures of some steroid solubilisates

Progesterone	R $= -COCH_0$
Testosterone	R $= -OH$
Deoxycorticosterone	R $= -COCH_2OH$

A relationship between the lipophilicity of the solubilisate, expressed by the partition coefficient between octanol and water, $P_{octanol}$ (see Chapter 4), and its extent of solubilisation has been noted for the solubilisation of substituted barbituric acids by polyoxyethylene stearates, of substituted benzoic acids by polysorbate 20 and of several steroids by polyoxyethylene non-ionic surfactants. An exhaustive survey of data for the solubilisation of some 64 drugs by bile salt micelles revealed linear relationships between $\log P_m$ and $\log P_{octanol}$ for each of seven bile salts examined.[29]

Effect of temperature

In most systems the amount solubilised increases as temperature increases. The effect is particularly pronounced with some non-ionic surfactants where it is a consequence of an increase in the micellar size with temperature increase. Table 5.12 shows an increased solubilisation of two drugs by aqueous micellar solutions of bile salts as temperature is increased over the range 27–45°C.

A complicating factor when considering the effect of temperature on the amount solubilised is the change in the aqueous solubility of the solubilisate with temperature increase. In some cases, although the amount of drug that can be taken up by a surfactant solution increases with temperature increase, this may simply reflect an increase in the amount of drug dissolved in the aqueous phase rather than an increased solubilisation by the micelles. This point is illustrated by a study of the solubilisation of benzoic acid by a series of polyoxyethylated non-ionic surfactants, details of which are given in Table 5.13. Although the extent of solubilisation of benzoic acid increases with temperature, the data when plotted reveal a minimum micelle/water distribution coefficient, P_m, at about 27°C. The decrease in P_m (and therefore the amount of drug solubilised in the micelles) with temperature increase up to this temperature is possibly due to the increase in aqueous solubility of benzoic acid; the subsequent increase of P_m at higher temperatures is due to a rapid increase of micellar size as the cloud point is approached and a consequent ability of the micelles to incorporate more solubilisate.

Methods of preparation of solubilised systems

The method of preparation of the solubilised system can have a significant influence on the solubilisation capacity.[30] The simplest and most commonly used method of incorporation of the drug is the so-called 'shake flask' method in which excess solid drug is equilibrated with the micellar solution and unsolubilised drug is subsequently removed by filtration or centrifugation. Larger amounts of drug can often be solubilised by co-mixing the drug and copolymer at elevated temperature (typically about 60°C) and adding the resultant intimate mixture to water or buffer to form the solubilised micellar solution – a method often referred to as 'melt loading'. Other methods, including dialysis, solvent evaporation and cosolvent evaporation methods, involve the use of non-aqueous solvents to dissolve the drug and copolymer. In the dialysis method drug and copolymer are dissolved in a water-miscible organic solvent followed by dialysis against water until the organic phase is replaced with water. In the solvent evaporation method, the drug and copolymer are dissolved in volatile organic solvents that are

Table 5.12 The effect of temperature on the maximum additive concentrations (MAC) of griseofulvin and hexestrol in bile salts

Solubilisate	Bile salt	10^3 MAC (moles solubilisate/mole surfactant)		
		27°C	37°C	45°C
Griseofulvin	Sodium cholate	5.36	6.18	6.80
	Sodium deoxycholate	4.68	6.18	7.54
	Sodium taurocholate	3.77	4.90	6.15
	Sodium glycocholate	3.85	5.13	5.29
Hexestrol	Sodium cholate	187	195	197
	Sodium deoxycholate	164	167	179
	Sodium taurocholate	220	225	223
	Sodium glycocholate	221	231	251

Reproduced from Wiedmann TS, Kamel L. *J Pharm Sci* 2002;91:1743.

allowed to evaporate at room temperature; the resultant dried drug–copolymer film is then pulverised and dispersed in water. Alternatively, a micellar solution is formed by adding water slowly to a solution of drug and polymer in a water-miscible organic solvent (cosolvent) and removing the organic solvent by evaporation (cosolvent evaporation method). In a variation of this method, an oil-in-water emulsion is formed by mixing the organic solvent containing dissolved drug with an aqueous solution of the copolymer; the volatile solvent is then allowed to evaporate, leaving the solubilised micellar solution.

5.6.4 Pharmaceutical applications of solubilisation

A wide range of insoluble drugs has been formulated using the principle of solubilisation. Only a few representative examples will be discussed in this section.

Non-ionic surfactants are efficient solubilisers of iodine, and will incorporate up to 30% iodine by weight, of which three-quarters is released as available iodine on dilution. Such iodine–surfactant systems (referred to as *iodophors*) are more stable than iodine–iodide systems. They are preferable in instrument sterilisation since corrosion problems are reduced. Loss of iodine by sublimation from iodophor solutions is significantly less than from simple iodine solutions such as Iodine Solution NF. There is also evidence of an ability of the iodophor solution to penetrate hair follicles of the skin, so enhancing activity.

The low solubility of steroids in water presents a problem in their formulation for ophthalmic use. The requirements of optical clarity preclude the use of oily solutions or suspensions and there are many examples of the use of non-ionic surfactants as a means of producing clear solutions that are stable to sterilisation.

Table 5.13 Micelle/water distribution coefficients, P_m, for the solubilisation of benzoic acid by *n*-alkyl polyoxyethylene surfactants C_nE_m (where n = alkyl (C) chain length and m = polyoxyethylene (E) chain length) as a function of temperature

Surfactant formula	18°C	25°C	31°C	37°C	45°C
$C_{16}E_{16}$	59.51	50.07	43.75	44.11	–[a]
$C_{16}E_{30}$	47.80	45.55	35.42	38.23	38.66
$C_{16}E_{40}$	37.07	32.72	28.76	29.90	37.06
$C_{16}E_{96}$	31.22	27.43	25.43	27.46	32.35

Reproduced from Humphries KJ, Rhodes CT. *J Pharm Sci* 1968;57:79.
[a] No P_m value determined at this temperature for $C_{16}E_{16}$ because the cloud point temperature was exceeded.

| Table 5.14 Solubilisation of vitamins by 10% polysorbate solutions |||||
Polysorbate	Vitamin D_2 (IU cm^{-3})	Vitamin E (mg cm^{-3})	Vitamin K_3 (mg cm^{-3})	Vitamin A alcohol (IU cm^{-3})
20	20 000	5.7	4.7	80 000
40	16 000	3.8	4.0	60 000
60	15 000	3.2	3.7	60 000
80	20 000	4.5	4.5	80 000

Reproduced from Gstirner F, Tata PS. *Mitt dt Pharm Ges* 1958;28:191.

In most formulations, solubilisation has been achieved using polysorbates or polyoxyethylene sorbitan esters of fatty acids.

Essential oils are extensively solubilised by surfactants, polysorbates 60 and 80 being particularly well suited to this purpose.

The polysorbate non-ionics have also been employed in the preparation of aqueous injections of the water-insoluble vitamins A, D, E and K. Table 5.14 shows the solubility of these vitamins in 10% polysorbate solutions, polysorbate 20 and 80 being the best two solubilisers.

One of the problems encountered with the use of non-ionic surfactants as solubilisers is that they are prone to clouding on heating (see section 5.3.4). Moreover the presence of solubilisate can reduce the cloud point. For this reason, sucrose esters may be more suitable as alternative solubilisers for the vitamins, although they do have the disadvantage of a slightly higher haemolytic activity.

It has been possible to give only a brief description of the types of drugs that have been formulated using solubilisation. Many other drugs have been formulated in this way, including the analgesics, sedatives, sulfonamides and antibiotics. The reader is referred to reference 3 for a more complete survey of this topic and for a discussion of the effects of solubilisation on drug activity and absorption characteristics. The use of surfactants and surfactant mixtures for the solubilisation of poorly water-soluble drugs in marketed oral and injectable formulations has been comprehensively reviewed by Strickley.[31]

Solubilisation may play an important role *in vivo* in the absorption of drugs from the gastrointestinal tract, as discussed in the Clinical Point below and discussed further in section 8.2.3.

 Clinical point

The absorption of drugs dissolved in triglyceride oils, such as soybean oil, and administered orally in soft gel capsules, may be enhanced by mixed micelle formation in the gastrointestinal tract, particularly if the absorption is normally dissolution rate-limited. The lipid triglycerides are acted upon by pancreatic lipase in the intestine to form monoglycerides and fatty acids, which interact with bile salts to form small droplets or vesicles in which the drug is solubilised. Progressive breakdown of these vesicles leads eventually to the formation of mixed micelles with an approximate size of 3–10 nm. The mixed micelles can play an important role in the absorption process, transporting high concentrations of the hydrophobic drug across the aqueous boundary layer which separates the absorptive membrane from the intestinal lumen. The disruption of the micelles at the intestinal membrane, as a consequence of the lower pH at this location, releases the solubilised drug, which can then be readily absorbed across the cell membrane by passive diffusion.

The mixed micelles comprising bile salts and lipolytic products formed in the intestine have a much higher solubilising capacity for hydrophobic drugs than simple bile salt micelles. For example, the solubility of cinnarizine in mixed micelles is 44 μg mL^{-1} under physiological conditions, compared to only 4 μg mL^{-1} in simple bile salt micelles.

Key points

- An important property of surfactant micelles is their ability to solubilise water-insoluble compounds. The location of solubilisates in the micelles is closely related to the chemical nature of the solubilisate.
- In general, non-polar solubilisates are dissolved in the micelle core and water-insoluble compounds having polar groups are oriented with the polar group at the surface and the hydrophobic group in the core. Solubilisation in non-ionic surfactants can also occur in the palisade layer.
- The extent of solubilisation is influenced by the volume of the micelle core, the ethylene oxide chain length of non-ionic surfactants, the lipophilicity of the solubilisate and the temperature.
- Some pharmaceutical applications of solubilisation have been discussed.

Summary

In this chapter we have seen that molecules having distinct hydrophilic and hydrophobic regions (so-called amphiphiles or surfactants) will accumulate at air–water and oil–water interfaces and in so doing will reduce respectively the surface and interfacial tension. This process is spontaneous and leads to the removal of the hydrophobic regions from solution by their protruding into the air or lipophilic phase. At concentrations above a critical value (the cmc), such molecules will form small spherical aggregates or micelles in solution, the cores of which are formed from the hydrophobic region of the surfactant and protected from the aqueous environment by a shell of polar groups or polyoxyethylene chains. Micelles are transient structures composed of typically 60–100 molecules that are in equilibrium with free surfactant molecules in solution, the concentration of which effectively remains at the cmc value as the solution concentration is increased. Micelles are useful in pharmaceutical formulation because of their ability to incorporate poorly water-soluble drugs. The balance between the hydrophobic and hydrophilic regions of the surfactant determines the degree of lowering of surface or interfacial tension, the cmc and the micellar properties. The tendency for accumulation at surfaces also leads to the adsorption of amphiphilic molecules on to solid surfaces; this process can lead to removal of active ingredients from solution, which is advantageous when this material is a poison or toxin but problematic when the active ingredient is a drug or preservative.

As the surfactant concentration is increased there is frequently a transition from the typical spherical micellar structure to a more elongated or rod-like micelle. Further increase in concentration may lead to the formation of a liquid crystalline state, termed the *middle phase* or *hexagonal phase* in which the elongated micelles are arranged into hexagonal arrays. With some surfactants, further increase of concentration results in the formation of a cubic phase and eventually at very high concentrations a further liquid crystalline state, the *neat phase* or *lamellar phase* may be observed.

Water-insoluble amphiphilic molecules will form films or monolayers when spread over the water surface. Depending on the molecular structure of the amphiphile, these may be tightly packed as in solid or condensed films, or more loosely packed as in liquid or expanded films and gaseous films. Lung surfactants form films at the alveolar air–water interface that facilitate the large surface area changes that occur during the successive compression–expansion cycles accompanying the breathing process.

References

1. Diamant H, Andelman D. In Zana R, Xia J (eds) *Gemini Surfactants: Interfacial and Solution Behaviour.* New York: Marcel Dekker; 2003.
2. Brown P *et al.* Properties of new magnetic surfactants. *Langmuir* 2013;29:3246–3251.
3. Attwood D, Florence AT. *Surfactant Systems.* London: Chapman and Hall; 1983.
4. Arzhavitina A, Steckel H. Surface active drugs significantly alter the drug output rate from medical nebulizers. *Int J Pharm* 2010;384:128–136.
5. Peng JB *et al.* The structures of Langmuir–Blodgett films of fatty acids and their salts. *Adv Colloid Interface Sci* 2001;91:163–219.

6. Dynarowicz-Łatka P *et al* (2001). Modern physicochemical research on Langmuir monolayers. *Adv Colloid Interface Sci* 2001;91:221–293.

7. Flanders BN *et al*. Imaging of monolayers composed of palmitic acid and lung surfactant protein B. *J Microsc* 2001;202:379–385.

8. Notter RH. Lung surfactants. Basic science and clinical applications. In: Lenfant C (ed.) *Lung Biology in Health and Disease, 149*. New York: Marcel Dekker; 2000: 1–444.

9. Serrano AG *et al*. Critical structure–function determinants within the N-terminal region of pulmonary surfactant protein SP-B. *Biophys J* 2006;90:238–249.

10. Zatz JL *et al*. Monomolecular film properties of protective and enteric film formers. II. Evaporation resistance and interactions with plasticizers of poly (methyl vinyl ether-maleic anhydride). *J Pharm Sci* 1969;58:1493–1496.

11. Hidalgo AA *et al*. Interaction of two phenothiazine derivatives with phospholipid monolayers. *Biophys Chem* 2004;109:85–104.

12. El-Masry S, Khalil SAH. Adsorption of atropine and hyoscine on magnesium trisilicate. *J Pharm Pharmacol* 1974;26:243–248.

13. Chin L *et al*. Optimal antidotal dose of activated charcoal. *Toxicol Appl Pharmacol* 1973;26:103–108.

14. Decker WJ *et al*. Absorption of drugs and poisons by activated charcoal. *Toxicol Appl Pharmacol* 1968;13:454–460.

15. Decker WJ *et al*. Inhibition of aspirin absorption by activated charcoal and apomorphine. *Clin Pharm Ther* 1969;10:710–713.

16. Kolthammer J. In vitro adsorption of drugs from horse serum onto carbon coated with an acrylic hydrogel. *J Pharm Pharmacol* 1975;27:801–805.

17. Vale JA *et al*. Use of charcoal haemoperfusion in the management of severely poisoned patients. *Br Med J* 1975;1:5–9.

18. Rouchotas C *et al*. Comparison of surface modification and solid dispersion techniques for drug dissolution. *Int J Pharm* 2000;195:1–6.

19. Attwood D. The mode of association of amphiphilic drugs in aqueous solution. *Adv Colloid Interface Sci* 1995;55:271–303.

20. Crommelin DJA, Schreier H. Liposomes. In: Kreuter J (ed.) *Colloidal Drug Delivery Systems*. New York: Marcel Dekker; 1994, Chapter 3.

21. Bouwstra JA, Hofland HEJ. Niosomes. In: Kreuter J (ed.) *Colloidal Drug Delivery Systems*. New York: Marcel Dekker; 1994, Chapter 4.

22. Uchegbu IF, Florence AT. Nonionic surfactant vesicles (niosomes): physical and pharmaceutical chemistry. *Adv Colloid Interface Sci* 1995;58:1–55.

23. Shah JC *et al*. Cubic phase gels as drug delivery systems. *Adv Drug Del Rev* 2001;47:229–250.

24. Booth C, Attwood D. Effect of block copolymer architecture and composition on the association properties of poly (oxyalkylene) copolymers in aqueous solution. *Macromol Rapid Commun* 2000;21:501–527.

25. Nace VM. *Nonionic Surfactants. Polyoxyalkylene Block Copolymers*. Surfactant Science Series 60. New York: Marcel Dekker; 1996: 185–210.

26. Hurter PN *et al*. Solubilisation in amphiphilic copolymer solutions. In: Christian SD, Scamehorn JF (eds) *Solubilisation in Surfactant Aggregates*. Surfactant Science Series 55. New York: Marcel Dekker; 1995: 191–235.

27. Arnarson T, Elworthy PH. Effects of structural variations of nonionic surfactants on micellar properties and solubilisation: surfactants based on erucyl and behenyl (C_{22}) alcohols. *J Pharm Pharmacol* 1980;32:381–385.

28. Saettone MF *et al*. Solubilisation of tropicamide by poloxamers: physicochemical data and activity data in rabbits and humans. *Int J Pharm* 1988;43:67–76.

29. Wiedmann TS, Kamel L. Examination of the solubilisation of drugs by bile salt micelles. *J Pharm Sci* 2002;91:1743–1764.

30. Aliabadi HM, Lavasanifar A. Polymeric micelles for drug delivery. *Expert Opin Drug Deliv* 2006;31:39–162.

31. Strickley RG. Solubilizing excipients in oral and injectable formulations. *Pharm Res* 2004;21:201–229.

6

Emulsions, suspensions and related colloidal systems

Emulsions and suspensions are 'disperse' systems, that is, they comprise respectively a liquid or solid phase dispersed in an external liquid phase. Aerosols are either liquids or solids dispersed in a gas. While emulsions have been formulated from oily drugs or nutrient oils, they also provide vehicles for drug delivery with the drug dissolved in the oil or water phase. Suspensions, on the other hand, are usually prepared from water-insoluble drugs for delivery orally or by injection, usually by the intramuscular route. An increasing number of modern delivery systems are suspensions – of liposomes or of polymer or protein microspheres, nanospheres or dendrimers – hence the need to understand the formulation and stabilisation of these systems. Pharmaceutical emulsions and suspensions are in the colloidal state, that is, where the particles range from the nanometre size to visible or 'coarse' dispersions several micrometres in diameter.

In this chapter we will:

- examine the properties of colloidal systems (disperse systems with particles below about 1µm in diameter), and in particular the forces of interaction between the colloidal particles which are responsible for the stability of the colloidal dispersion
- introduce the main types of emulsions, including oil-in-water (o/w), water-in-oil (w/o), non-aqueous systems (o₁/o₂), multiple emulsions (w/o/w; o/w/o), microemulsions and self-emulsifying delivery systems (SEDDS), and for each type examine the factors leading to emulsion stability and physical instability, including flocculation and coalescence
- discuss approaches to the formulation of emulsions to provide vehicles for drug delivery and parenteral nutrition
- consider aqueous and non-aqueous pharmaceutical suspensions, their formulation and forms of instability, which are principally sedimentation, flocculation and caking

- examine some aspects of the physicochemical behaviour of concentrated suspensions which are used in a variety of pharmaceutical processes
- see how colloidal stability theory may be applied to a variety of other colloidal systems such as blood and other cell suspensions.

6.1 Colloids and their classification

The word 'colloid' derives from the Greek *kolla* (glue) and was coined with the impression that colloidal substances were amorphous or glue-like rather than crystalline forms of matter. The colloidal state was recognised by Thomas Graham in 1861 and described poetically by Wolfgang Ostwald some 50 years later as the 'world of neglected dimensions', a reference both to the fact that colloid science had somehow remained a Cinderella topic, and to the special world of systems in which the particles are extremely small. Colloid chemistry is important in pharmacy because of the growing number of nanoparticles and other colloidal systems used in drug delivery and targeting (Chapter 14).

Colloids can be broadly classified as those that are *lyophobic* (solvent hating) or more specifically, in aqueous systems, *hydrophobic* (water hating) and those that are *lyophilic* or *hydrophilic*. Surfactant molecules, because of their dual affinity for water and oil and their consequent tendency to associate into micelles, form hydrophilic colloidal dispersions in water. Proteins and gums also form lyophilic colloidal systems. Water-insoluble drugs in fine dispersion or clays and oily phases will form lyophobic dispersions. While lyophilic dispersions (such as phospholipid vesicles and micelles) are inherently stable, lyophobic colloidal dispersions have a tendency to coalesce because they are thermodynamically unstable as a result of their high surface energy in their native state.

Pharmaceutical colloids such as emulsions and suspensions (Fig. 6.1) and aerosols are readily identified (Table 6.1). The *disperse phase* is the phase that is subdivided. The *continuous phase* is the phase in which the disperse phase is distributed. Many colloidal systems that exist in nature, including suspensions of microorganisms, blood, platelets and isolated cells in culture, are also in effect colloidal dispersions. Colloid science is interdisciplinary, for although it deals with complex systems it is nevertheless a unifying discipline

as it bridges the physical and biological sciences. The concepts of the stability of colloidal systems can be applied with little modification to our understanding of interactions between living cells, for example (see section 6.5).

It is because of the subdivision of matter in colloidal systems that they have special properties. The large surface-to-volume ratio of the particles dispersed in a liquid medium results in a tendency for

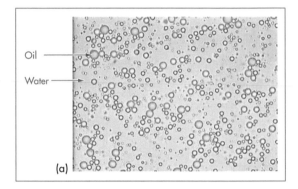

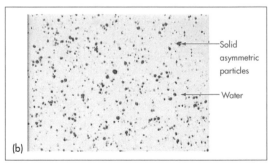

Figure 6.1 Photomicrographs of (a) an oil-in-water emulsion and (b) a suspension.

Table 6.1 Main types of colloidal systems		
Type	**Disperse phase**	**Continuous phase**
o/w emulsion	Oil	Water
w/o emulsion	Water	Oil
Suspension	Solid	Water or oil
Aerosol	Solid or liquid	Air

particles to associate to reduce their surface area, so reducing their contact with the medium. Emulsions and aerosols are thermodynamically unstable two-phase systems that reach equilibrium only when the globules have coalesced to form one phase, for which the surface area is at a minimum. Many pharmaceutical problems revolve around the stabilisation of colloidal systems.

Some biological phenomena can be understood in terms of the association of cells with other cells or with inanimate or other substrates. This chapter describes various colloidal systems, deals with the theoretical approaches to colloid stability and discusses the pharmaceutical problems encountered with colloidal dosage forms. At the close of the chapter some of the biological implications of the subject are indicated, which include the increasing use of particles in the nanometre (nm) size range (*nanoparticles*) and particles in the micrometre (μm) size range (*microparticles*) as carriers for drugs for targeting and for modifying the disposition of drug molecules contained within them. The dividing line between the colloidal and non-colloidal systems in terms of the nature of the dispersing medium and the dispersed material is not one that can be defined exactly.

6.2 Colloid stability

In dispersions of fine particles in a liquid or of particles in a gas, frequent encounters between the particles occur owing to:

- Brownian movement
- creaming or sedimentation
- convection.

Creaming of emulsions occurs when the oil droplets of an o/w emulsion migrate to the emulsion surface or the water droplets in a w/o emulsion move toward the bottom of the container. The rate of creaming depends on the difference in density between the dispersed particles and the dispersion medium, the particle radius, *a*, and the viscosity of the dispersion medium, *η*. According to Stokes' law the rate of sedimentation (or creaming) of a spherical particle, *v*, in a fluid medium, is given by

$$v = \frac{2ga^2(\rho_1 - \rho_2)}{9\eta} \qquad (6.1)$$

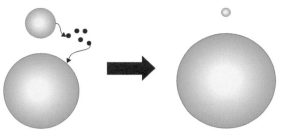

Figure 6.2. Representation of the process of Ostwald ripening: a small particle partially dissolves in the continuous phase and the molecules are taken up by the larger particle, until the smaller particle disappears completely.

where ρ_1 is the density of the particles, ρ_2 is the density of the medium and *g* is the gravitational constant.

Creaming of an emulsion or sedimentation of a given suspension can be reduced in several ways:

- by forming smaller particles
- by increasing the viscosity of the continuous phase
- by decreasing the density difference between the two phases.

Particles will still collide, but the frequency or the impact of the collisions can be minimised. What is the fate of particles when they come into close contact? The encounters may lead to permanent contact of solid particles or to coalescence of liquid droplets. If they are allowed to continue unchecked, the colloidal system destroys itself through growth of the disperse phase and excessive creaming or sedimentation of the large particles; with emulsions this process is often referred to as the *cracking* of the emulsion. Whether these collisions result in permanent contact or whether the particles rebound and remain free depends on the balance of the attractive and repulsive forces of interaction between the particles and on the nature of the surface of the particles.

An additional cause of emulsion instability is the tendency for the growth of the larger droplets at the expense of smaller droplets in a process known as *Ostwald ripening*. Molecules diffuse from the smaller droplets to the larger ones through the continuous phase, with a resultant increase of the mean droplet size, driven by the fact that large particles are energetically more favoured than smaller ones (Fig. 6.2).

6.2.1 Forces of interaction between colloidal particles

There are five possible forces between colloidal particles:

1. electrostatic forces of repulsion
2. van der Waals forces, or electromagnetic forces of attraction
3. Born forces – essentially short-range and repulsive
4. steric forces, which are dependent on the geometry and conformation of molecules (particularly macromolecules) at the particle interface
5. solvation forces due to changes in quantities of adsorbed solvent on the very close approach of neighbouring particles.

Independent consideration of the electrostatic repulsion and van der Waals forces of attraction by Derjaguin and Landau (in 1941) and by Verwey and Overbeek (in 1948) produced a quantitative approach to the stability of hydrophobic suspensions, known as the DLVO theory of colloid stability.

Van der Waals forces between particles of the same kind are always attractive. The multiplicity of interactions between pairs of atoms or molecules on neighbouring particles must be taken into account in the calculation of attractive forces. Hamaker (in 1937) first determined equations for these forces on the basis of the additivity of van der Waals energies between neighbouring molecules, assuming that the energies of attraction varied with the inverse sixth power of the distance between them. At greater separations of the particles, the power law changes to the inverse seventh power. The model considers two spherical particles of radius a at a distance H, R being $2a + H$ (Fig. 6.3).

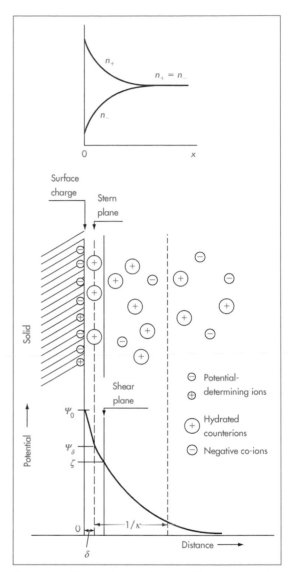

Figure 6.4 Representation of the conditions at a negative surface, with a layer of adsorbed positive ions in the Stern plane. The number of negative ions increases and the number of positive ions decreases (see upper diagram) as one moves away from the surface, the electrical potential becoming zero when the concentrations are equal. The surface potential, ψ_0, and the potential at the Stern plane, ψ_δ, are shown. As the particle moves, the effective surface is defined as the surface of shear, which is a little further out from the Stern plane, and would be dependent on surface roughness and adsorbed macromolecules. It is at the surface of shear that the zeta potential, ζ, is located. The thickness of double layer is given by $1/\kappa$.

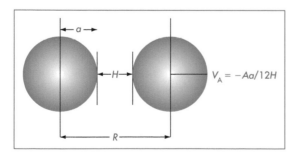

Figure 6.3 Diagram of the interaction between two spheres of radius a at a distance of separation H with a centre-to-centre distance of ($R = H + 2a$) used in calculating energies of interaction.

Hamaker calculated the energy of attraction, V_A, to be

$$V_A = -\frac{A}{6}\left(\frac{2a^2}{R^2 - 4a^2} + \frac{2a^2}{R^2} + \frac{R^2 - 4a^2}{R^2}\right) \quad (6.2)$$

The Hamaker constant, A, depends on the properties of the particles and of the medium in which they are dispersed. When H/a is small, that is, when the particles are large relative to the distance of separation, equation (6.2) reduces to the simpler form:

$$V_A = -\frac{Aa}{12H} \quad (6.3)$$

The electrical charge on particles is due either to ionisation of surface groups or to adsorption of ions that confer their charge to the surface. A particle surface with a negative charge is shown in Fig. 6.4 along with the layer of positive ions that are attracted to the surface in the Stern layer, and the diffuse or electrical double layer that accumulates and contains both positive and negative ions.

Electrostatic forces arise from the interaction of the electrical double layers surrounding particles in suspension (Fig. 6.4). This interaction leads to repulsion if the particles have surface charges and surface potentials of the same sign and magnitude. When the surface charge is produced by the adsorption of potential-determining ions, the surface potential, ψ_0, is determined by the activity of these ions and remains constant during interaction with other particles, if the extent of adsorption does not change. The interaction therefore takes place at *constant surface potential*. In emulsion systems where the adsorbed layers can desorb, or in conditions of low availability of potential-determining ions, the interaction takes place not at constant surface potential but at *constant surface charge* (or at some intermediate state). The electrostatic repulsive force decays as an exponential function of the distance and has a range of the order of the thickness of the electrical double layer, equal to the Debye–Hückel length, $1/\kappa$:

$$1/\kappa = \left(\frac{\varepsilon\varepsilon_0 RT}{F^2 \Sigma c_i z_i^2}\right)^{1/2} \quad (6.4)$$

where ε_0 is the permittivity of the vacuum, ε is the dielectric constant (or relative permittivity) of the dispersion medium, R is the gas constant, T is temperature, F is the Faraday constant and c_i and z_i are the concentration and the charge number of the ions of

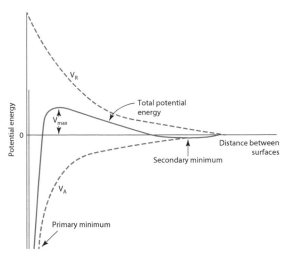

Figure 6.5 Schematic form of the curve of total potential energy (V_{total}) against distance of surface separation (H) for interaction between two particles, with $V_{\text{total}} = V_A + V_R$.

type i in the dispersion medium. For monovalent ions in water, $c = 10^{-15}\kappa^2$ (with c in mol dm^{-3} and κ in cm^{-1}). No simple equations can be given for the repulsive interactions. However, for small surface potentials and low values of κ (that is, when the double layer extends beyond the particle radius) and at constant ψ_0, the repulsive energy is

$$V_R = 2\pi\varepsilon\varepsilon_0 a\psi_\delta^2 \frac{\exp(-\kappa H)}{1 + H/2a} \quad (6.5)$$

For small values of ψ_δ and exp $(-\kappa H)$ this simplifies to

$$V_R = 2\pi\varepsilon\varepsilon_0 a\psi_\delta^2 \exp(-\kappa H) \quad (6.6)$$

The equations do not take into account the finite size of the ions; the potential to be used is ψ_δ, the potential at the Stern plane (the plane of closest approach of ions to the surface), which is difficult to measure. The nearest experimental approximation to ψ_δ is often the zeta potential (ζ) measured by electrophoresis.

In the DLVO theory the combination of the electrostatic repulsive energy V_R with the attractive potential energy V_A gives the total potential energy of interaction: $V_{\text{total}} = V_A + V_R$.

V_{total} plotted against the distance of separation H gives a potential energy curve showing certain characteristic features, illustrated in Fig. 6.5. The maximum and minimum energy states are shown. If the maximum is too small, two interacting particles may reach the primary minimum and in this state of close approach the depth of the energy minimum can mean that escape is improbable. Subsequent irreversible changes in the system may then occur, such as sintering and recrystallisation in suspensions or coalescence in emulsions forming irreversible structures. When the maximum in V_{total} is sufficiently high, the two particles do not reach the stage of being in close contact. The depth of the secondary minimum is important in determining events in a hydrophobic dispersion. If the secondary minimum is smaller than the thermal energy, kT (where k is the Boltzmann constant), the particles will always repel each other, but when the particles are large enough the secondary minimum can trap particles for some time as there is no energy barrier to overcome. At intermediate distances the energy of repulsion may be the larger of the two.

Effect of electrolytes on stability

Pharmaceutical colloids are rarely simple systems. Suspensions, except for some nanosuspensions, rarely comprise only particles of a single size; they usually also contain additives. The influence of these, including electrolytes, has to be considered. Electrolyte concentration and valence (z) are accounted for in the term ($\Sigma c_i z_i^2$) in equation (6.4) and thus in equations (6.5) and (6.6). Figure 6.6 gives an example of the influence of electrolyte concentration on the electrostatic repulsive force. As the electrolyte concentration is increased, κ increases due to compression of the double layer with consequent decrease in $1/\kappa$.

At low electrolyte concentrations (low κ) the double layer is diffuse and V_R extends to large distances around the particles. Summation of V_R and V_A gives a total energy curve having a high primary maximum but no secondary minimum. The decrease of the double layer when more electrolyte is added produces a more rapid decay in V_R and the resultant total-energy curve now has a small primary maximum but, more importantly, a secondary minimum. This concentration of electrolyte would produce a stable suspension, since flocculation could occur in the secondary minimum and the small primary maximum would be sufficient to prevent coagulation in the primary minimum. At high concentrations of added electrolyte, the range of V_R would be so small that the van der Waals attractive forces would dictate the shape of the total energy curve. As a consequence, this curve has no primary maximum, so the dispersion would be unstable with no energy barrier to prevent coagulation

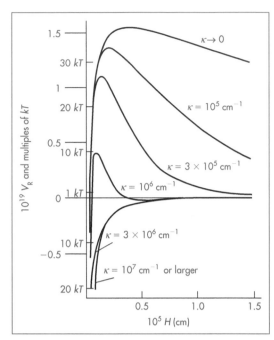

Figure 6.6 The energy of interaction of two spherical particles as a function of the distance, H, between the surfaces. For monovalent ions c (mol dm^{-3}) = $10^{-15}\kappa^2$ (cm^{-1}). In this example, $a = 10^{-5}$ cm, $A = 10^{-19}$ J and ψ_0 = RT/F = 26.5 mV.

Reproduced from Overbeek J Th. Recent developments in the understanding of colloid stability. *J Colloid Interface Sci* 1977;58:408. Copyright Elsevier 1977.

of the particles in the primary minimum. The practical importance of this can be seen when nanoparticles are dispersed in cell culture media with high levels of electrolyte and flocculate as a result.

We can see from equation (6.4) that the magnitude of the effect of an electrolyte of a given concentration on V_R also depends on the valence of the ion of opposite charge to that of the particles (the counterion): the greater the valence of the added counterion, the greater its effect on V_R. These generalisations are known as the Schulze–Hardy rule. Note that it does not matter which particular counterion of a given valence is added.

Effect of surface potential on stability

A second parameter that influences the shape of the total energy curve is the surface potential of the particles. We can see from equation (6.5) that V_R will increase with an increase in ψ_0; the changes that occur in the total curve are seen in Fig. 6.7. There is a decrease in the primary maximum as the surface potential decreases and you should note the appear-

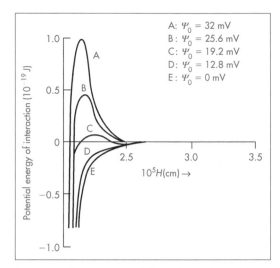

Figure 6.7 The influence of the surface potential (ψ_0) on the total potential energy of interaction of two spherical particles.

ance of a secondary minimum at the intermediate value of ψ_0 (see curve C).

6.2.2 Repulsion between surfaces with macromolecular stabilisers

The increasing use of non-ionic macromolecules as stabilisers, which has occurred since the origins of the DLVO theory, has led to the awareness of other stabilising forces. The approach of particles with hydrated macromolecules adsorbed to their surfaces leads, on the interaction of these layers, to repulsion

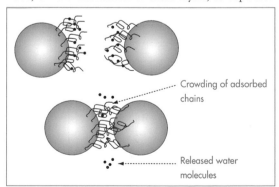

Figure 6.8 Enthalpic stabilisation: representation of enthalpic stabilisation of particles with adsorbed hydrophilic chains. The hydrated chains of the polyoxyethylene molecules —$(OCH_2CH_2)_n$OH protrude into the aqueous dispersing medium. On close approach of the particles to within 2δ (twice the length of the stabilising chains), hydrating water is released, resulting in a positive enthalpy change which is energetically unfavourable.

(Fig. 6.8), because of the consequent positive enthalpy change ($+\Delta H$) that ensues. In more general terms, the approach of two particles with adsorbed stabilising chains leads to a steric interaction when the chains interact. The repulsive forces may not always be enthalpic in origin. Loss of conformational freedom leads to a negative entropy change ($-\Delta S$). Each chain loses some of its conformational freedom and its contribution to the free energy of the system is increased, leading to repulsion. This volume restriction is compounded by an 'osmotic effect' that arises as the macromolecular chains on neighbouring particles crowd into each other's space, increasing the concentration of chains in the overlap region. The repulsion that arises is due to the osmotic pressure of the solvent attempting to dilute out the concentrated region: this can only be achieved by the particles moving apart.

Quantitative assessment of the steric effect depends on three parameters:

1. the hydrophilic polymer chain length, δ
2. the interaction of the solvent with the chains
3. the number of chains per unit area of interacting surface.

The steric effect does not come into play until $H = 2\delta$, so the interaction increases suddenly with decreasing distance. There are many problems in applying such equations in practice, the main ones being the lack of an accurate knowledge of δ, and the difficulty in taking account of desorption and changes in chain conformation or solvation during interaction. When the steric contribution is combined with the electrostatic and van der Waals interactions, a minimum in the energy at large separations still obtains, but repulsion is generally evident at all shorter distances, provided that the adsorbed macromolecules or surfactants do not desorb into the continuous phase or otherwise move away from the points of interaction (Fig. 6.9).

For particles with a hydrated stabilising layer of thickness δ, the volume of the overlapping region (V_{ov}) is as derived as described in Fig. 6.10:

$$V_{ov} = \frac{2\pi}{3}\left(\delta - \frac{H}{2}\right)^2\left(3a + 2\delta + \frac{H}{2}\right) \qquad (6.7)$$

The difference between chemical potential in the overlap volume and the potential when the particles are at an infinite distance apart is a measure of the repulsive force, an osmotic force, caused by the increased

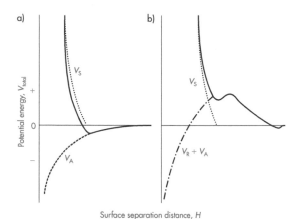

Figure 6.9. Entropic (steric) stabilisation: the potential energy–distance plots for (a) particles with no electrostatic repulsion, $V_{total} = V_S + V_A$ and (b) with electrostatic repulsion, $V_{total} = V_S + V_A + V_R$.

concentration of the polymer chains in the region of overlap. This can be written in terms of free energy as

$$\Delta G_m = 2\pi_E \frac{2\pi}{3}\left(\delta - \frac{H}{2}\right)^2\left(3a + 2\delta + \frac{H}{2}\right) \quad (6.8)$$

Substituting for π_E (where $\pi_E = RTBc^2$) and using $R = kN_A$, where k is the Boltzmann constant and B the second virial coefficient, we obtain

$$\frac{\Delta G_m}{kT} = \frac{4\pi}{3}BN_Ac^2\left(\delta - \frac{H}{2}\right)^2\left(3a + 2\delta + \frac{H}{2}\right) \quad (6.9)$$

where c is the concentration of surfactant in the interfacial layer and N_A is the Avogadro constant.

This equation probably appears more complex than it is. Apart from telling us the effect of increasing or decreasing δ, for example, by using different polymers of different length (δ), we can find out the effect of temperature and additives, as B is proportional to $(1 - \theta/T)$, where θ is the temperature (the theta temperature) at which the polymer and solvent have no affinity for each other. Thus when $T = \theta$, B tends to zero, and the stabilising influence of the hydrated layer disappears, as hydration is lost. Heating reduces ΔG_m in this case. Additives that salt out the macromolecules from solution will have the same effect.

The requirement for the strict applicability of the equations is that the particles are monosized, which is rarely the case with pharmaceutical emulsions and suspensions. Where particles of two radii, a_1 and a_2, interact, equation (6.3) is modified to:

$$V_A = \frac{Aa_1a_2}{6(a_1 + a_2)H} \quad (6.10)$$

Similarly, V_R is expressed by an analogue of equation (6.5), namely,

$$V_R = \frac{\varepsilon}{4}\frac{a_1a_2}{(a_1 + a_2)}(\psi_1 + \psi_2)^2\ln[1 + \exp(-kH)]$$
$$+ (\psi_1 - \psi_2)^2\ln[1 - \exp(-kH)] \quad (6.11)$$

where ψ_1 and ψ_2 are the surface potentials of particles 1 and 2.

These equations have been applied not only to the study of suspensions but to the reversible interaction of

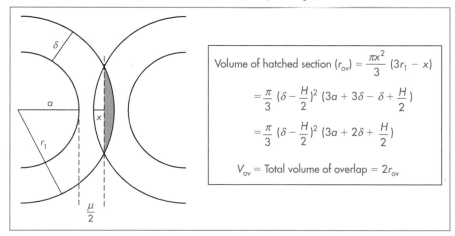

Figure 6.10 The model used in the derivation of equation (6.7): particles of radius a with adsorbed layer of thickness δ approach to a distance H between the particle surfaces; $r_1 = (a + \delta)$ and x is the distance between the surface and the line bisecting the volume of overlap.

microbial cells with a solid substrate such as glass before permanent adhesion occurs due to the formation of polymeric bridges between cell and glass.

 Key points

- Colloids can be broadly classified as
  - *lyophobic* (solvent hating) (= *hydrophobic* in aqueous systems) or
  - *lyophilic* (= *hydrophilic* in aqueous systems).
- Emulsions and suspensions are 'disperse' systems: a liquid or solid phase dispersed in an external liquid phase.
  - The *disperse phase* is the phase that is subdivided/dispersed.
  - The *continuous phase* is the phase in which the disperse phase is distributed.
- Emulsions and suspensions are intrinsically unstable systems. Creaming of an emulsion or sedimentation of a suspension can be minimised by reducing particle size, increasing the viscosity of the continuous phase or decreasing the density difference between the continuous and disperse phases. If growth of the dispersed particles is unchecked, the colloidal system will be destroyed, for example, an emulsion will separate into two phases (that is, they *crack*).
- Colloidal particles can interact by electrostatic forces of repulsion, van der Waals forces of attraction, short-range repulsive Born forces, steric forces and solvation forces. In the DLVO theory, the electrostatic repulsive energy, V_R, is combined with the attractive potential energy, V_A, to give the total potential energy of interaction, V_{total}. DLVO plots show the variation of V_{total} with distance of separation of the particles.
- Electrolyte addition affects the width of the double layer around the dispersed particles and hence the value of V_R. At low electrolyte concentration, DLVO plots have a high primary maximum but no secondary minimum; addition of more electrolyte compresses the double layer, producing plots with a small primary maximum but, more importantly, a secondary minimum (conditions for a stable suspension); at high electrolyte concentrations there is no primary maximum and the dispersion is unstable.
- Colloids can be stabilised by the repulsive forces that arise from adsorption of macromolecules and surfactants to their surfaces. Stabilisation arises because of loss of freedom of movement of the chains of the adsorbed molecules (negative entropy change), an osmotic effect and release of hydrating water (positive enthalpy change).

6.3 Disperse system flow

Colloidal systems, whether suspensions or emulsion, have flow and viscous properties which are important in a number of pharmaceutical processes. Figure 6.11 links some of these together: blood is a suspension and mixing nanoparticles with blood results in more complex flow patterns; aerosol formation and the related spray drying and spray coating of solid-dosage forms with solutions or suspensions, as well as the spreading of these systems on solid surfaces are topics which arise in many pharmaceutical domains (see e.g. Chapter 1). The movement of particles *in vivo* in tissues, and their escape from the circulation after intravenous (IV) injection, are important features in determining their ability to arrive at biological targets (see Chapter 14). Liquid droplets in emulsions which are spherical but also deformable can often negotiate capillaries and tracks which suspensions cannot. So the opportunity for emulsions to jam is reduced compared to suspensions, where particle asymmetry may also be a determinant in flow characteristics. Surface/interfacial tension has a key role in determining emulsion behaviour.

In this section we will examine the various types of flow, commencing with the simplest type of flow, Newtonian flow, which may be exhibited by dilute colloidal solutions and then considering the various

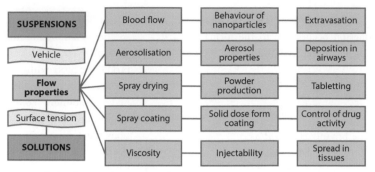

Figure 6.11 Varied aspects of the flow and viscosity of solutions and disperse systems (suspension or emulsion), which pervade many processes *in vitro* and *in vivo*, are listed here. Flow properties of suspensions are important factors in successful spray coating and spray drying, as well as the spreading of liquid dispersions on surfaces, as in the film coating of tablets (discussed in Chapter 1). Aerosol properties will also be determined by the behaviour of the primary suspension or solution. The high viscosity of concentrated drug suspensions (or solutions, for example of proteins) can lead to problems with injectability and the spread of any depot after intramuscular injection.

types of non-Newtonian flow, which are exhibited by the more complex colloidal systems.

Newtonian flow

We can imagine the flow of a liquid as the movement of imaginary planes within the liquid, over each other. The internal resistance offered to the relative motion of these planes causes a retardation of flow. Figure 6.12 shows the flow of a liquid through a narrow tube as the movement of a series of concentric annuli. As you can see, the flow rate is highest in the centre of the tube and gradually decreases across the tube, reaching a minimum value at the tube walls. The gradient of velocity, u, in a direction, x, at right angles to the wall, i.e. du/dx, is the *shear rate*, D. The external force which is required to overcome the internal friction and to cause movement is called the shear force, F, or when it refers to unit surface area, A, is called the *shear stress*, τ.

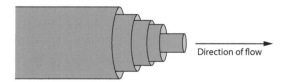

Direction of flow

Figure 6.12 Diagrammatic representation of the flow of a liquid through a narrow tube as the movement of a series of concentric annuli.

In a Newtonian liquid, the velocity gradient or shear rate is directly proportional to the shear stress, and the proportionality constant is the *coefficient of viscosity*, or more simply the *viscosity*, η, i.e. $\tau = \eta D$. Viscosity has units of N m^{-2} s. This unit replaces the former

unit, the poise P, and the two units can be interconverted using

$$1 \text{ P} = 0.1 \text{ Nm}^{-2} \text{ s or } 1 \text{ cP} = 1 \text{ mN m}^{-2} \text{ s}$$

The centipoise, cP, is still widely used and is a convenient measure of viscosity since water has a viscosity of 1 cP at 20°C.

The viscosity may be combined with the density, ρ, using the *kinematic viscosity*, $\upsilon = \eta/\rho$. Kinematic viscosity has units of m^2 s^{-1} which are related to the former unit, the stokes, St, by

$$1 \text{ St} = 10^{-4} \text{ m}^2 \text{ s}^{-1} \text{ or } 1 \text{ cSt} = 10^{-6} \text{ m}^2 \text{ s}^{-1}$$

Although not an SI unit, centistokes, cSt, retain their use in describing the viscosity grade of several polymers, for example the silicones (see section 7.5.3).

The flow behaviour of a colloidal solution may be represented by plots of shear stress, τ, against shear rate, D, as shown in Fig. 6.13. In Newtonian flow, the viscosity is independent of the shear rate and this is characterised by linear plots of τ against D. The gradient of these plots is η (Example 6.1).

In deriving an equation for the viscosity of a colloidal dispersion of spherical particles, Einstein considered particles that were far enough apart to be treated independently. The particle volume fraction is defined by

$$\phi = \frac{\text{volume occupied by the particles}}{\text{total volume of the suspension}} \quad (6.12)$$

The dispersion is assigned an effective viscosity, η_*, given by

$$\eta_* = \eta_0(1 + 2.5\phi) \quad (6.13)$$

Example 6.1 Calculation of viscosity from shear stress vs shear strain plots for a Newtonian dispersion

The following data were obtained in a study of the shear stress, τ, of a dilute emulsion as a function of shear rate, D.

D (s^{-1})	1.0	2.4	3.6	4.6	6.0	7.1
τ (mN m^{-2})	2.6	6.3	9.4	12.0	15.7	18.6

Show that the emulsion exhibits Newtonian flow properties and determine its viscosity.

Answer

The plot of τ (as ordinate) against D (as abscissa) is linear and hence the dilute emulsion exhibits Newtonian flow. The gradient, $\tau / D = 2.6$ mN m^{-2} s, is equal to the viscosity, η.

where η_0 is the viscosity of the suspending fluid. Various terms may be used to describe the viscosity characteristics:

- the *relative viscosity*, η_{rel}, is the ratio η_*/η_0

- the *specific viscosity*, η_{sp}, is $\eta_{rel} - 1$
- the *reduced viscosity* is the ratio $\eta_{sp}/\varnothing$
- the *intrinsic viscosity*, $[\eta]$ is the value of $\eta_{sp}/\varnothing$ extrapolated to zero volume fraction.

Hence from equation (6.13), the intrinsic viscosity in an ideal dispersion should equal 2.5. As we have seen, the assumptions involved in the derivation of the Einstein equation do not hold for colloidal systems subject to Brownian forces, electrical interactions and van der Waals forces. Brownian forces result from 'the random jostling of particles by the molecules of the suspending fluid due to thermal agitation and fluctuation on a very short time scale'. The coefficient 2.5 in Einstein's equation (6.13) applies only to spheres; asymmetric particles will produce coefficients greater than 2.5, as shown in Example 6.2.

Other problems in deriving *a priori* equations result from the polydisperse nature of pharmaceutical dispersions. The particle size distribution will determine η. A polydisperse dispersion of spheres has a lower viscosity than its monodisperse equivalent. Structure formation during flow is an additional complication and results in non-Newtonian flow properties, as illustrated below. Examples of non-Newtonian

Example 6.2 Determination of intrinsic viscosity of a colloidal dispersion

The viscosity of a colloidal dispersion was measured as a function of concentration, c, with the following results.

η_* (mN m^{-2} s)	2.34	4.18	5.97	7.68	9.87	12.76
c (% $^w/_v$)	0.5	1.10	1.65	2.15	2.75	3.50

If the viscosity of the continuous phase was 0.903 mN m^{-2} s, determine the intrinsic viscosity of the dispersed particles assuming Newtonian flow properties and assuming that the volume fraction can be equated to the concentration.

Answer

At each concentration, calculate values of

- $\eta_{rel} = \eta_*/\eta_0$
- $\eta_{sp} = \eta_{rel} - 1$
- η_{sp}/c

A plot of η_{sp}/c against c should be linear with an intercept equal to the intrinsic viscosity, which for spherical, non-interacting colloidal particles should have a value of 2.5 according to equation (6.13). The intercept of the plot from the data given above is 3.1, suggesting that the colloidal particles do not conform to the exacting requirements of the Einstein equation, probably because of interparticle interactions and/or particle asymmetry.

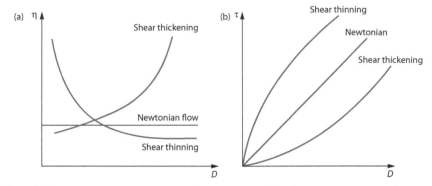

Figure 6.13 Plots of (a) apparent viscosity η against shear rate D and (b) shear stress τ against shear rate D, comparing Newtonian and non-Newtonian flow characteristics.

flow in emulsions and suspensions will be considered in sections 6.4.12 and 6.7.3, respectively.

Non-Newtonian flow

When shear stress and shear rate are not linearly related the flow is described as non-Newtonian. There are several types of flow behaviour.

Shear thinning (pseudoplastic flow)

When the apparent viscosity decreases with increasing shear rate, we say that the fluid exhibits shear thinning or pseudoplastic flow. This type of flow is compared with Newtonian flow in Fig. 6.13a. Since the apparent viscosity is derived by drawing tangents to this plot, it will generate the type of rheogram shown in Fig. 6.13b. Shear thinning is particularly common to colloidal dispersions containing asymmetric particles such as methyl cellulose or tragacanth. These particles provide the greatest resistance to flow when they are randomly oriented at low-velocity gradients. As the shear rate is gradually increased, they begin to align themselves with the flow lines and their resistance to flow is greatly reduced. Eventually, at high rates of shear, alignment is complete and the viscosity becomes constant. This type of flow is also characteristic of systems in which particle aggregation occurs. Under shear, these aggregates break down, releasing some of the solvent which they have immobilised, thus lowering the viscosity of the system.

There are several mathematical relationships describing pseudoplastic flow; we will consider only the equation proposed by Ostwald:

$$\tau = KD^n \tag{6.14}$$

where K is a constant, often called the consistency index, and n is a number less than 1, referred to as the flow behaviour index. When $n = 1$, equation (6.14) represents Newtonian flow and K is the viscosity.

We can show that a system exhibits pseudoplastic flow by plotting rheological data using equation (6.14) in its logarithmic form

$$\log \tau = \log K + n \log D \tag{6.15}$$

Linearity of plots of log shear stress, τ, as a function of log shear rate D, demonstrates shear-thinning behaviour; values of flow behaviour index and consistency index may be obtained from the gradient and intercept of the plot, respectively, as shown in Example 6.3.

Shear thickening (dilatancy)

In this type of flow the apparent viscosity increases with increasing shear rate (see Fig. 6.13a). Dilatant systems obey equation (6.14) with a value of $n > 1$.

A well-known example of the dilatant effect is the drying out of wet sand when it is walked upon. As the shear rate is increased when the sand is compressed, the dense packing is broken down to allow the particles to flow past each other. The resulting expansion leaves insufficient liquid to fill the voids and the system apparently 'dries out'. The dry footprint soon becomes wet again as the pressure is released. Similarly, starch paste stirs easily if you stir it slowly but soon thickens up and resists stirring if you try to stir it quickly.

Plastic flow

This type of flow is similar to shear thinning except that the system does not flow noticeably until the shear stress exceeds a certain minimum value, called the *critical shear stress*, τ_0. At high shear stresses the rheogram may become linear (Fig. 6.14), in which

Example 6.3 Calculation of the consistency index and the flow behaviour index for a colloidal dispersion exhibiting shear-thinning behaviour

The following data were obtained in a study of the shear stress, τ, as a function of shear rate, D, for a colloidal dispersion.

D (s^{-1})	2	4	6	8	10
τ (Pa)	140	181	210	234	253

Show graphically that the dispersion exhibits shear-thinning behaviour and determine values for the consistency index and the flow behaviour index.

Answer

A plot of log τ (as ordinate) against log D (as abscissa) should be linear, showing that the dispersion exhibits shear-thinning behaviour.

The flow behaviour index n determined from the gradient = 0.36.

The intercept = 2.04 = log K, hence the consistency index = 109.6

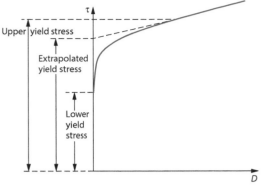

Figure 6.14 A plot of shear stress τ against shear rate D for a colloidal dispersion exhibiting plastic flow properties.

at the point where the plot becomes linear is called the *upper yield stress*, extrapolation of the linear portion of the rheogram to zero shear rate gives the *extrapolated yield stress* and the shear stress at which flow is first observed (i.e. τ_0) is the *lower yield stress* (Example 6.4) Some substances show a non-linear relationship between shear rate and shear stress after yielding and these are called *Casson bodies*.

Thixotropy and rheopexy

Both of these terms refer to time-dependent phenomena. In a *thixotropic* system the apparent viscosity decreases as a continuous shear stress is applied at a constant rate of shear. If this system is allowed to stand for a while it regains its structure and its shear stress returns to its original value when shearing is recommenced at the same shear rate. A consequence of

case we say that the system exhibits *Bingham flow*. Several characteristics describing the flow properties may be obtained from the rheogram – the shear stress

Example 6.4 Determination of the parameters describing the plastic flow of a colloidal dispersion

The shear stress τ of a concentrated emulsion was determined at a series of shear rates, D, with the following results.

τ (N m^{-2})	103	112	120	127	136	146	157	166	176
D (s^{-1})	0.50	1.0	1.5	2.0	3.0	4.0	5.0	6.0	7.0

Describe the flow characteristics of this emulsion, giving values of rheological parameters which characterise the flow properties.

Answer

A plot of τ against D yields the following values:

Lower yield stress = 80 N m^{-2}

Extrapolated yield stress = 107 N m^{-2}

Upper yield stress = 122 N m^{-2}

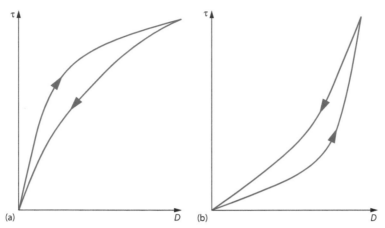

Figure 6.15 Plots of shear stress τ against shear rate *D* for colloidal dispersions exhibiting (a) thixotropic and (b) rheopectic flow properties showing hysteresis loops resulting from time-dependent flow.

this time-dependent effect is that the rheogram exhibits a hysteresis loop, as seen in Fig. 6.15a, when the shear rate is first increased and then decreased. Solutions of high-molecular-weight polymers are generally thixotropic because of chain entanglements, which are gradually reduced on shearing and then reform on standing due to Brownian motion.

The apparent viscosity of *rheopectic* substances increases as continuous shear stress is applied at a constant rate of shear and then returns to its initial value after a regeneration period. This type of flow results in a hysteresis loop of the type shown in Fig. 6.15b.

Viscoelasticity

Many dispersed systems exhibit the properties of both solids and liquids when a constant small shear stress is applied, i.e. they flow but they also show elasticity. When such dispersions are stressed they deform and the increase in deformation (strain) as a function of time is called creep. Creep compliance is the ratio of the strain to the applied constant stress. In the creep testing of a colloidal dispersion, the stress is applied for a given time and then removed and the recovery with time is studied. Figure 6.16 shows a typical plot of creep compliance against time curve. As soon as a stress is applied there is an immediate strain, which is represented by AB. This is called the instantaneous elastic compliance, J_0, and is the region in which the bonds between the primary structural units in the system stretch elastically. The curvature in the region BC gradually decreases and eventually the increase of creep compliance with time becomes linear over the

region CD. The region BC represents the retarded elastic compliance, J_R, and CD is the region of Newtonian compliance J_N. When the stress at D is removed there is an instantaneous elastic recovery over the region DE, followed by a retarded elastic recovery over the region EF and then an eventual flattening of the curve beyond F. The vertical distance, FG, to the

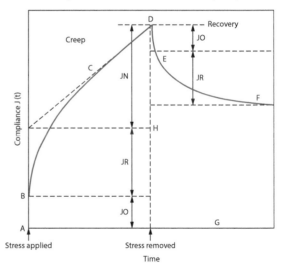

Figure 6.16 Model plot of creep compliance against time. A–B is the region of instantaneous elastic modulus (compliance) in which the bonds between the primary structure units in the system stretch elastically. B–C is a time-dependent region. C–D is a region of Newtonian compliance; here some bonds rupture but do not reform in the period of the test. On removal of the stress the recovery curve is given by DF. An instantaneous elastic recovery (D–E) of the same magnitude as (A–B) is followed by retarded elastic recovery to E–F. As bonds were irreversibly broken during the period of applied stress, this part of the structure is not recovered; hence F–G is equal to D–H.

time abscissa represents the non-recoverable strain per unit stress and this is related to the degree of structural alteration which has occurred during the test.

6.4 Emulsions

Emulsions – liquid dispersions usually of an oil/lipid phase and an aqueous phase – are a traditional pharmaceutical dosage form. Oil-in-water (o/w) systems have enjoyed a renaissance as vehicles for the delivery of lipid-soluble drugs (as with the anaesthetic propofol). Their use as a delivery system necessitates an understanding of the factors governing the formu-

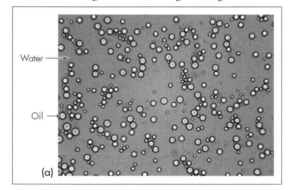

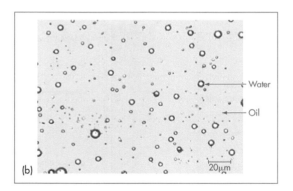

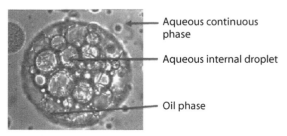

Figure 6.17 Photomicrograph of emulsions: (a) an oil-in-water (o/w) emulsion, (b) a water-in-oil (w/o) system, (c, bottom figure) a water-in-oil-in-water emulsion, in which the internal water droplets can be seen in the larger oil droplets.

lation and stability of o/w and w/o emulsions, multiple emulsions (w/o/w or o/w/o) and microemulsions, which occupy a position between swollen micelles and emulsions with very small globule sizes. Photomicrographs of o/w, w/o systems and multiple emulsions are shown in Fig. 6.17. It is also possible to formulate emulsions without water. Non-aqueous or anhydrous emulsions can also be formulated as o_1/o_2 systems or as oil in a polar solvent emulsions, as well as multiple oil-in-oil-in-oil systems or variants.

6.4.1 Stability of o/w and w/o emulsions

Adsorption of a surfactant at the oil–water interface, by lowering interfacial tension during manufacture, aids the dispersal of the oil into droplets of a small size and maintains the particles in a dispersed state (Fig. 6.18). Unless the interfacial tension is zero, there is a natural tendency for the oil droplets to coalesce to

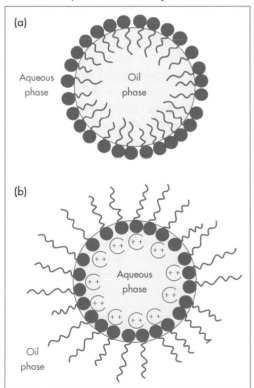

Figure 6.18 Surfactant films at the water–oil interface in o/w and w/o emulsions: (a) formation of a monomolecular film at the oil–water interface for the stabilisation of o/w emulsions; (b) stabilisation of w/o emulsions by the oriented adsorption of divalent soap salts (not to scale).

reduce the area of oil–water contact, but the presence of the surfactant monolayer at the surface of the droplet reduces the possibility of collisions leading to coalescence. Charged surfactants will lead to an increase in negative or positive zeta potential and will thus help to maintain stability by increasing V_R. Non-ionic surfactants such as the alkyl or aryl polyoxyethylene ethers, sorbitan polyoxyethylene derivatives, sorbitan esters and polyoxyethylene–polyoxypropylene–polyoxyethylene ABA block copolymers are widely used in pharmaceutical emulsions because of their lack of toxicity and their relatively low sensitivity to additives. These non-ionic stabilisers adsorb on to the emulsion droplets and, although they generally reduce zeta potentials, they maintain stability by creating a hydrated layer on the hydrophobic particle in o/w emulsions. They effectively convert a hydrophobic colloidal dispersion into a hydrophilic dispersion.

In w/o emulsions the hydrocarbon chains of the adsorbed molecules protrude into the oily continuous phase. Stabilisation arises from steric and enthalpic forces, as described in section 6.2.2; there is also a barrier to coalescence that is due to the presence of surfactant or polymer molecules and their effect on the elasticity of the interface. Emulsions are more complex than suspensions, because of the possibility (a) of movement of the surfactant into either the continuous or disperse phase; (b) of micelle formation in both phases; and (c) of formation of liquid crystalline phases between the disperse droplets.

It is usually observed that mixtures of surfactants form more stable emulsions than do single surfactants. This may be because complex formation at the interface results in a more 'rigid' stabilising film. Certainly where complex films can be formed, such as between sodium lauryl sulfate and cetyl alcohol, the stability of emulsions prepared with such mixtures is high. Theory has not developed to an extent that it can readily cope with mixtures of stabiliser molecules. Complex formation between surfactant and cosurfactants in the bulk phase of emulsion systems is dealt with in section 6.4.7, as this frequently leads to semisolid systems of high intrinsic stability.

6.4.2 HLB system

In spite of many advances in the theory of stability of lyophobic colloids, resort has still to be made to an empirical and practical approach to the choice of an optimal emulsifier, that was devised in 1949 by Griffin. In this system a hydrophile–lipophile balance (HLB) can be calculated for each surfactant. This number is a measure of the relative contributions of the hydrophilic and lipophilic regions of the molecule. The method allows the effective HLB of surfactant mixtures to be calculated.

The HLB number of a surfactant is calculated according to an empirical formula. For non-ionic surfactants the values range from 0 to 20 on an arbitrary scale (Fig. 6.19). At the higher end of the scale the surfactants are hydrophilic and act as solubilising agents, detergents and o/w emulsifiers. To maintain stability, an excess of surfactant is required in the continuous phase; hence, in general, water-soluble surfactants stabilise o/w emulsions and water-insoluble (oil-soluble) surfactants stabilise w/o emulsions. In the stabilisation of oil globules it is essential that there is a degree of surfactant hydrophilicity to confer an enthalpic stabilising force and a degree of hydrophobicity to secure adsorption at the o/w interface. The balance between the two will depend on the nature of the oil and the mixture of surfactants; hence the need to apply the HLB system.

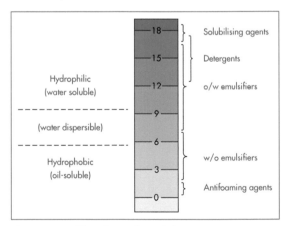

Figure 6.19 The HLB scale and the approximate ranges into which solubilising agents, detergents, emulsifiers and antifoaming agents fall, based on the method devised by Griffin (Griffin WC. Classification of surface active agents by HLB. *J Soc Cosmet Chemists* 1949; 1:311–326).

The HLB of polyhydric alcohol fatty acid esters such as glyceryl monostearate may be obtained from

$$\text{HLB} = 20\left(1 - \frac{S}{A}\right) \qquad (6.16)$$

where S is the saponification number of the ester and A is the acid number of the fatty acid. The HLB of polysorbate 20 (Tween 20) calculated using this formula is 16.7, with $S = 45.5$ and $A = 276$.

Typically, the polysorbate (Tween) surfactants have HLB values in the range 9.6–16.7; the sorbitan ester (Span) surfactants have HLBs in the lower range of 1.8–8.6.

For those materials for which it is not possible to obtain saponification numbers, for example, beeswax and lanolin derivatives, the HLB is calculated from

$$HLB = (E + P)/5 \qquad (6.17)$$

where E is the percentage by weight of oxyethylene chains, and P is the percentage by weight of polyhydric alcohol groups (glycerol or sorbitol) in the molecule.

If the hydrophile consists only of oxyethylene groups ([—CH_2CH_2O—], mol wt = 44 Da), a simpler version of the equation is

$$HLB = E/5 \qquad (6.18)$$

giving the upper end of the scale (20) for the polyoxyethylene glycol molecule itself. Some HLB values of typical surfactants used in pharmacy are given in Table 6.2. A more detailed list is given in Tables 5.7 and 5.8 in Chapter 5. Example 6.5 shows the application of equations (6.17) and (6.18) in the calculation of the HLB of two typical non-ionic surfactants.

Example 6.5 Calculation of the HLB of a non-ionic surfactant

Calculate HLB values for (a) Polysorbate 20 and (b) $C_{10}H_{21}(CH_2\ CH_2O)_8OH$

Answer

a) Polysorbate 20 has a molecular weight of approximately 1300 Da and contains 20 oxyethylene groups and two sorbitan rings. Thus, from equation (6.17)

$$E = \frac{20 \times 44 \times 100}{1300} = 68$$

$$P = \frac{182 \times 100}{1300} = 14$$

Hence,

$$HLB = 82/5 = 16.4$$

b) The hydrophobic portion of $C_{10}H_{21}(CH_2 CH_2O)_8OH$ is $C_{10}H_{21}OH$ with a molecular weight = 158 Da

The polyoxyethylene hydrophilic portion is $(CH_2\ CH_2O)_8$ with a molecular weight = 352 Da

Therefore, the weight fraction of polyoxyethylene = $352/(158 + 352) = 0.69$

Applying equation (6.18),

HLB of $C_{10}H_{21}(CH_2\ CH_2O)_8OH = 0.69 \times 100/5 = 13.8$

Table 6.2 Typical HLB numbers of some surfactants

Compound	HLB
Glyceryl monostearate	3.8
Sorbitan monooleate (Span 80)	4.3
Sorbitan monolaurate (Span 20)	8.6
Triethanolamine oleate	12.0
Polyoxyethylene sorbitan monooleate (Tween 80)	15.0
Polyoxyethylene sorbitan monolaurate (Tween 20)	16.7
Sodium oleate	18.0
Sodium lauryl sulfate[a]	40.0

[a]Although applied mainly to non-ionic surfactants, it is possible to obtain numbers for ionic surfactants.

Group contribution

The HLB system has been put on a more quantitative basis by calculating group contributions or group numbers to the HLB number such that an HLB was obtained from

$$HLB = \Sigma(\text{hydrophilic group numbers}) + \Sigma(\text{lipophilic group numbers}) + 7 \qquad (6.19)$$

Some group numbers are given in Table 6.3. Equation 6.19 should be applied with caution to non-ionic surfactants, particularly those with a polyoxyethylene chain as the only hydrophilic moiety, where considerable deviation from experimental values is noted.[1] Example 6.6 shows the calculation of the HLB for an anionic surfactant using the group contribution method.

Example 6.6 Calculation of the HLB using group contributions

Calculate the HLB value for sodium dodecyl sulfate (SDS) using the group contribution method.

Answer

The HLB of $CH_3(CH_2)_{11}SO_4Na$ is calculated from equation (6.19) using the group contributions of Table 6.3 as follows:

HLB = Σ(hydrophilic group numbers) + Σ(lipophilic group numbers) + 7

= 38.7 + (12 × −0.475) + 7 = 40.0

The calculated HLB of SDS is 40.0, which agrees with the experimental value in Table 6.2.

Table 6.3 Group contributions to HLB numbers[a]

Group	Group number
Hydrophilic groups	
—SO₄Na	38.7
—COONa	19.1
—SO₃Na	11
—COOH	2.1
Ester (free)	2.4
Hydroxyl (free)	1.9
Hydroxyl (sorbitan)	0.5
—CH₂CH₂O-	0.33
Lipophilic groups	
—CH—;—CH₂—; =CH and —CH₃	-0.475
Phenyl	-1.66

[a] Values from reference 1.

Choice of emulsifier or emulsifier mixture

Regardless of any theories, the appropriate choice of emulsifier or emulsifier mixture is usually made by preparing a series of emulsions with a range of surfactants of varying HLB values. It is assumed that the HLB of a mixture of two surfactants containing fraction f of A and $(1 - f)$ of B is the algebraic mean of the two HLB numbers:

$$\text{HLB}_{\text{mixture}} = f\text{HLB}_A + (1 - f)\text{HLB}_B \qquad (6.20)$$

Example 6.7 shows how equation (6.20) may be used to calculate the quantities of a surfactant mixture required to emulsify a mixture of two oils. For reasons not explained by the HLB system, mixtures of high HLB and low HLB give more stable emulsions than do single surfactants. Apart from the possibility of complex formation at the interface, the solubility of surfactant components in both the disperse and the continuous phase maintains the stability of the surfactant film at the interface. Creaming of emulsions (a function of particle size) is observed and is taken as an index of stability. The system with the minimum creaming or separation of phases is deemed to have an optimal HLB. It is therefore possible to determine optimum HLB numbers required to produce stable emulsions of a variety of oils. Table 6.4 shows the required HLB of surfactants to achieve stability of five oils. A more sensitive method would be to determine the mean globule size in emulsions using techniques such as laser diffraction methods to produce data such as those in Fig. 6.20. For a mineral o/w emulsion stabilised by a mixture of two non-ionic surfactants, an optimal HLB of between 7.5 and 8 is identified.

Table 6.4 Required HLB for different oils for o/w emulsion formation

Oil	HLB
Caprylic/capric triglycerides (medium-chain-length triglycerides)	5
Cottonseed oil	6
Soybean oil	6
Olive oil	7
Hydrogenated castor oil	8
Corn oil	8
Vaseline oil	8.5
Dodecane	9–9.5
Mineral oil	10–12
Cyclohexane	12
Isopropyl myristate	12
Castor oil	14

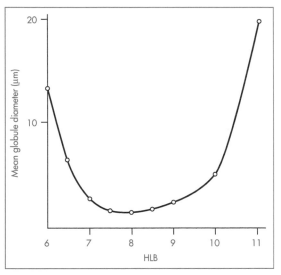

Figure 6.20 Variation of mean globule size in a mineral oil-in-water emulsion as a function of the HLB of the surfactant mixtures present at a level of 2.5%. Surfactants: Brij 92–Brij 96 mixtures.

Source: P. Depraetre, M. Seiller, A. T. Florence and F. Puisieux (unpublished material).

Example 6.7 **Calculation of the quantities of a surfactant mixture required to emulsify a mixture of two oils**

Calculate the relative amounts of Tween 80 (HLB 15.0) and Span 80 (HLB 4.3) required to emulsify 100 g of an o/w emulsion containing 35 g olive oil and 5 g isopropyl myristate using a total emulsifier concentration of 4 g.

Answer

An equation similar to equation (6.20) can be used to calculate the required HLB of the oil mixture:

$$HLB_{mixture} = f_O \, HLB_O + (1 - f_O) \, HLB_{IM}$$

where subscripts O and IM refer to olive oil and isopropyl myristate respectively.

The weight percentages of olive oil and isopropyl myristate in the 40 g of the oil mixture are 0.875 and 0.125 respectively, hence, using the required HLB values of olive oil (7) and isopropyl myristate (12) from Table 6.4 gives

$$HLB_{mixture} = 0.875 \times 7 + 0.125 \times 12 = 7.6$$

Using equation (6.20) to calculate the proportions of the two surfactants required to produce this required HLB gives

$$HLB_{mixture} = f_T \, HLB_T + (1 - f_T) \, HLB_S$$

where subscripts T and S refer to Tween 80 and Span 80 respectively.

$$7.6 = f_T \times 15.0 + (1 - f_T) \times 4.3$$
$$10.7 \, f_T = 3.3$$

Hence, $f_T = 0.31$ and $f_S = 0.69$. The total weight of emulsifier in the formulation is 4 g, therefore,

weight of Tween 80 = $0.31 \times 4 = 1.24$ g and the weight of Span 80 = $0.69 \times 4 = 2.76$ g

At the optimum HLB the mean particle size of the emulsion is at a minimum (Fig. 6.20) and this factor would explain to a large extent the stability of the system (see equations 6.1 and 6.2, for example).

Although the optimum HLB values for forming o/w emulsions are obtained in this way, it is possible to formulate stable systems with mixtures of surfactants well below the optimum. This is sometimes because of the formation of a viscous network of surfactant in the continuous phase. The high viscosity of the medium surrounding the droplets prevents their collision and this overrides the influence of the interfacial layer and barrier forces due to the presence of the adsorbed layer.

The HLB system has several drawbacks. The calculated HLB, of course, cannot take account of the effect of temperature or that of additives. The presence in emulsions of agents that salt in or salt out surfactants will respectively increase and decrease the effective (as opposed to the calculated) HLB values. Salting out the surfactant (for example, with NaCl) will make the molecules less hydrophilic and one can thus expect a higher optimal calculated HLB value for the stabilising surfactant for o/w emulsions containing sodium chloride. Examples are shown in Fig. 6.21, in which the effects of NaCl and NaI are compared.

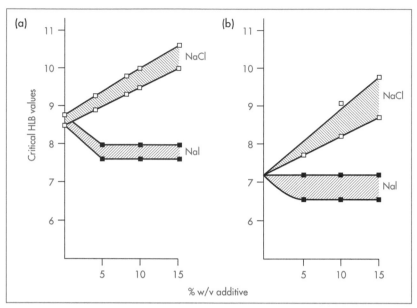

Figure 6.21 The change in critical HLB values as a function of added salt concentration, where the salt is either NaCl or NaI. Results were obtained from measurements of particle size, stability, viscosity and emulsion type as a function of HLB for liquid paraffin-in-water emulsions stabilised by Brij 92–Brij 96 mixtures. Data from different experiments showed different critical values; hence, on each diagram hatching represents the critical regions while data points actually recorded are shown. Results in (a) show particle size and stability data; those in (b) show the HLB at transition from pseudoplastic to Newtonian flow properties (see section 6.4.12) and emulsion type (o/w → w/o transitions).

Reproduced from Florence AT *et al.* Emulsion stabilization by non-ionic surfactants: the relevance of surfactant cloud point. *J Pharm Pharmacol* 1975;27:385. Copyright Wiley-VCH Verlag GmbH & Co. KGaA. Reproduced with permission.

6.4.3 Multiple emulsions

Multiple emulsions are emulsions whose disperse phase contains droplets of another phase (Fig. 6.17). Water-in-oil-in-water (w/o/w) or o/w/o emulsions may be prepared, both forms being of interest as drug delivery systems. w/o emulsions, in which a water-soluble drug is dissolved in the aqueous phase, may be injected by the subcutaneous or intramuscular routes to produce a delayed-action preparation. To escape, the drug has to diffuse through the oil to reach the tissue fluids. The main disadvantage of a w/o emulsion is generally its high viscosity, brought about through the influence of the oil on the bulk viscosity. Emulsifying a w/o emulsion using surfactants that stabilise an oily disperse phase can produce w/o/w emulsions with an external aqueous phase and lower viscosity than the primary emulsion. On injection, into muscle, for example, the external aqueous phase dissipates rapidly, leaving behind the w/o emulsion. Nevertheless, biopharmaceutical differences have been observed between w/o and multiple emulsion systems (Fig. 6.22).

Physical degradation of w/o/w emulsions can arise by several routes (Fig. 6.23a):

- coalescence of the internal water droplets
- coalescence of the oil droplets
- rupture of the oil film separating the internal and external aqueous phases
- osmotic flux of water to and from the internal droplets, possibly associated with inverse micellar species in the oil phase.

The external oil particles may coalesce with others (which may or may not contain internal aqueous droplets), as in route (a); the internal aqueous droplets may be expelled individually (routes b, c, d, e) or more than one may be expelled (route f), or less frequently they may be expelled in one step (route g); the internal droplets may coalesce before being expelled (routes h, i, j, k); or water may pass by diffusion through the oil phase, gradually resulting in shrinkage of the internal droplets (routes l, m, n). Figure 6.23 is of course oversimplified; in practice the number of possible combinations is large. Several factors will determine the breakdown mechanisms in a particular system, but

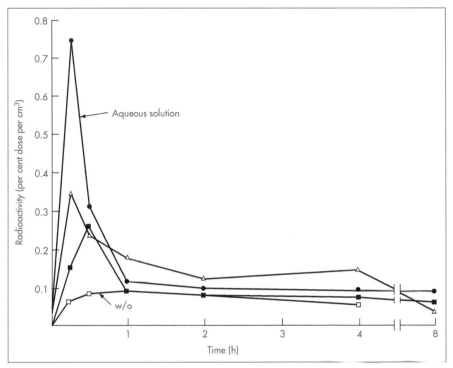

Figure 6.22 Blood levels of 5-fluoro(^{3}H)uracil (5-FU) following intramuscular injection of (●) an aqueous solution, (□) a w/o emulsion prepared with hexadecane, and a w/o/w emulsion prepared with (△) isopropyl myristate or (■) hexadecane as the oil phase.

one of the main driving forces behind each step will be the reduction in the free energy of the system brought about by the reduction in the interfacial area.

Mechanisms of drug release from multiple emulsion systems include diffusion of the drug molecules from the internal droplets (1), from the medium of the 'external' droplets (2), or by mass transfer due to the coalescence of the internal droplets (3), as shown in Fig. 6.23b.

6.4.4 Non-aqueous emulsions

Relatively few studies have been carried out on non-aqueous emulsions, but these can be useful as topical vehicles or reservoirs for the delivery of hydrolytically unstable drugs.[2] Systems such as castor oil or propylene glycol in silicone oil can be formulated using silicone surfactants; the HLB number clearly does not help in formulation in these cases, especially if the continuous phase has low polarity. For hydrocarbon–formamide emulsions, surfactants that stabilise aqueous systems can be used, taking into account the change in effective HLB number of the replacement for the aqueous phase. The key to stabilisation lies in

the sufficient solubility of the emulsifier in the continuous phase.

6.4.5 Microemulsions

Microemulsions consist of apparently homogeneous transparent systems of low viscosity that contain high concentrations (15–25%) of emulsifier mixture. They were first described by J. T. Schulman[3] as disperse systems with spherical or cylindrical droplets in the size range 8–80 nm. They are essentially swollen micellar systems, but obviously the distinction between a swollen micelle and small emulsion droplet is difficult to assess.

Microemulsions form spontaneously when the components are mixed in the appropriate ratios and are thermodynamically stable. In their simplest form, microemulsions are small droplets (diameter 5–140 nm) of one liquid dispersed throughout another by virtue of the presence of a fairly large concentration of a suitable combination of surfactants. They can be dispersions of oil droplets in water (o/w) or water droplets in oil (w/o). An essential requirement for their formation and stability is the attainment of a very low

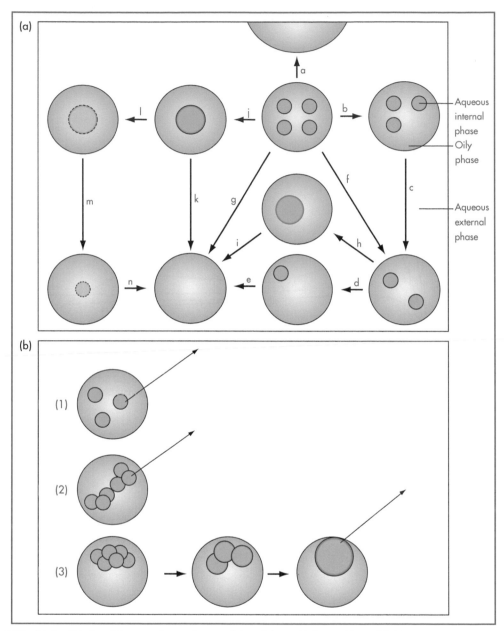

Figure 6.23 (a) Possible breakdown pathways (see text) in w/o/w multiple emulsions. (b) Diagrammatic representation of mechanisms of drug release. See text for explanation.

(a) Reproduced from Whitehill D, Florence AT. Some features of breakdown in water-in-oil-in-water multiple emulsions. *J Colloid Interface Sci* 1981;79:243–256. Copyright Elsevier 1981.

(b) After Davis SS. *J Clin Pharm* 1976;1:11.

interfacial tension, γ. Since microemulsions have a very large interface between oil and water (because of the small droplet size), they can only be thermodynamically stable if the interfacial tension is so low that the positive interfacial energy (given by γ*A*, where *A* is the interfacial area) can be compensated by the negative free energy of mixing ΔG_m. We can calculate a rough measure of the limiting value required as follows: ΔG_m is given by $-T\,\Delta S_m$ (where T is the temperature), and the entropy of mixing (ΔS_m) is of the order of the Boltzmann constant. Hence $k_B T = 4\pi r^2 \gamma$. Therefore, for a droplet radius r of about 10 nm, an interfacial tension of 0.03 mN m^{-1} would be required. The role of the surfactants in the system is thus to reduce the interfacial tension between oil and water (typically about 50 mN m^{-1}) to this low level.

Cosurfactants

With the possible exception of double-alkyl chain surfactants and a few non-ionic surfactants, it is generally not possible to achieve the required interfacial area with the use of a single surfactant. If, however, a second amphiphile (cosurfactant) is added to the system, the effects of the two surfactants can be additive provided that the adsorption of one does not adversely affect that of the other and that mixed micelle formation does not reduce the available concentration of surfactant molecules.

The importance of the cosurfactant is illustrated in the following example. The interfacial tension between cyclohexane and water is approximately 42 mN m^{-1} in the absence of any added surfactant. The addition of the ionic surfactant SDS (sodium dodecyl sulfate) in increasing amounts causes a gradual reduction of γ to a value of about 2 mN m^{-1} at an SDS concentration of 10^{-4} g cm^{-3}. Addition of 20% pentanol to the cyclohexane–water system in the absence of SDS reduces the interfacial tension to 10 mN m^{-1}. It is then theoretically possible by the addition of SDS to achieve a negative interfacial tension at SDS concentrations below the level at which it forms micelles (the critical micelle concentration). The changes in interfacial tension occurring in this system are illustrated in Fig. 6.24. Although pentanol is not generally regarded as a

surfactant, it has the ability to reduce interfacial tension by virtue of its amphiphilic nature (a short hydrophobic chain and a terminal hydrophilic hydroxyl group) and functions as the cosurfactant in this system. Its presence means that, in order to produce a microemulsion, the SDS is now required to produce a much smaller lowering of the interfacial tension (10 mN m^{-1} rather than 42 mN m^1 in its absence).

The simplest representation of the structure of microemulsions is the droplet model, in which microemulsion droplets are surrounded by an interfacial film consisting of both surfactant and cosurfactant molecules, as illustrated in Fig. 6.25. The orientation of the amphiphiles at the interface will, of course, differ in o/w and w/o microemulsions. As shown in Fig. 6.25, the hydrophobic portions of these molecules will be in the dispersed oil droplets of o/w systems, with the hydrophilic groups protruding in the continuous phase, while the opposite situation will be true of w/o microemulsions.

Whether the systems form o/w or w/o microemulsions is determined to a large extent by the nature of the surfactant. The geometry of the surfactant molecule is important. If the volume of the surfactant molecule is

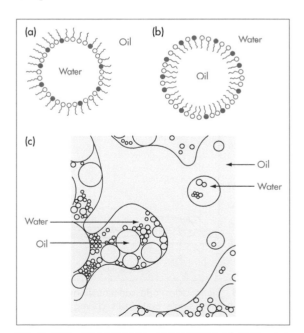

Figure 6.25 Diagrammatic representation of microemulsion structures: (a) a water-in-oil microemulsion droplet; (b) an oil-in-water microemulsion droplet; and (c) an irregular bicontinuous structure.

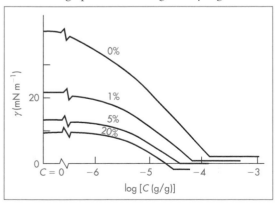

Figure 6.24 Interfacial tension, γ, between solutions of sodium dodecyl sulfate (SDS) of concentration C in aqueous 0.30 mol dm^{-3} NaCl and solutions of 1-pentanol in cyclohexane with the percentage concentrations indicated.

v, the cross-sectional area of its head group is a, and its length is l, then when the *critical packing parameter* v/al (see section 5.3.3) has values between 0 and 1, o/w systems are likely to form; but when v/al is greater than 1, w/o microemulsions are favoured. Values of the critical packing parameter close to unity can result in the formation of a bicontinuous structure in which areas of water can be imagined to be separated by a connected amphiphile-rich interfacial layer, as depicted in Fig. 6.25c. Values of the parameters v, a and l can readily be estimated, but it should be noted that the critical packing parameter is based purely on geometric considerations. Penetration of oil and cosurfactant into the surfactant interface and hydration of the surfactant head groups will also influence the packing of the molecules in the interfacial film around the droplets. In many systems, inversion from w/o to o/w microemulsions can occur as a result of changing the composition or the temperature. In general, o/w microemulsions are favoured when small amounts of oil are present and w/o systems form in the presence of small amounts of water. Under such conditions the droplet model is a reasonable representation of the system. The structure of microemulsions containing almost equal amounts of oil and water is best represented by a bicontinuous structure.

Reviews of parenteral microemulsions as drug delivery systems have been published.[4,5]

6.4.6 Self-emulsifying drug delivery systems

Microemulsions carrying a variety of anticancer drugs such as paclitaxel and vincristine, and an antimalarial, artemether, amongst other drugs have been prepared and studied experimentally.[5] Utilisation of microemulsions and emulsions in therapy is aided by the development of self-emulsifying drug delivery systems (SEDDS) and the analogous self-microemulsifying delivery systems (SMEDDS), systems which disperse *in vivo* to form emulsions or microemulsions.

Simple formulations comprising a solution of a lipophilic drug in an oil (for example, a medium-chain-length triglyceride or vegetable oil) loaded into a gelatin capsule rely on the surfactants present in the gastrointestinal tract (bile salts and lecithin) to solubilise the lipophilic drug in a colloidal dispersion in the intestine from which the drug may be absorbed. The bioavailability of drugs from such formulations can vary considerably, mainly because the efficiency of solubilisation depends to a large extent on the bile salt concentration in the gastrointestinal tract, which can show a wide interpatient variability. More reliable bioavailability is achieved from formulations in which suitable surfactants (and cosurfactants, if required) are added to the oil/drug solution; on contact with water in the gastrointestinal tract these spontaneously form emulsions (SEDDS) or microemulsions (SMEDDS) depending on the formulation.

The extent of absorption of poorly water-soluble drugs from o/w dispersions is influenced by droplet size: the smaller the droplet, the more rapid the breakdown of the triglycerides in which the drug is dissolved and hence the more rapidly the drug is released from the vehicle. The reason for this is that, before the drug can be released from the oil droplets, it

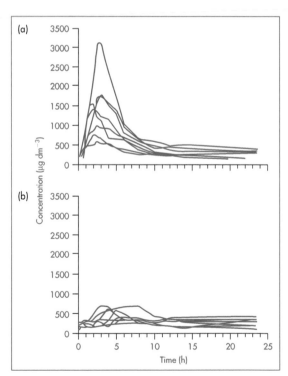

Figure 6.26 Blood ciclosporin concentration–time curves obtained following single oral doses (10 mg kg^{-1}) of (a) microemulsion and (b) conventional formulations in eight liver transplant recipients with external biliary diversion.

Reproduced from Trull AK *et al. Absorption of cyclosporin from conventional and new microemulsion oral formulations in liver transplant recipients with external biliary diversion. Br J Clin Pharmacol* 1995;39:627. Copyright Wiley-VCH Verlag GmbH & Co. KGaA. Reproduced with permission.

is first necessary to hydrolyse the oil. The pancreatic lipase which is responsible for this hydrolysis acts only at the interface of the oil droplets; the smaller the droplet size, the larger the interface exposed to the enzyme and hence the more rapid the breakdown of the triglycerides (oil) in which the drug is dissolved. As a consequence, the release of drug into the aqueous environment, which is an essential first step in its absorption, is more rapid when the droplet size is reduced and the interfacial area so increased. As a consequence of their much smaller droplet size, SMEDDS formulations have the potential to achieve higher, less variable bioavailability than SEDDS. An illustration of this is seen from the development of the Neoral formulation for the delivery of ciclosporin (see clinical points box).

Clinical point: A self-microemulsifying drug delivery formulation

A formulation of ciclosporin (Neoral, Novartis) incorporates the drug in a preconcentrate that forms a microemulsion on dilution in aqueous fluids.[6,7] The original formulation (Sandimmun) was an emulsion preconcentrate (SEDDS) comprising a solution of ciclosporin in a vegetable oil (olive oil or corn oil) and ethanol, and containing a polyglycolysed glyceride (Labrafil M-1944CS) as a surfactant. When administered orally as a liquid formulation, this mixture was stirred with several millilitres of a non-carbonated liquid (e.g. water, milk or orange juice) to form a coarse o/w dispersion before drinking. Alternatively, when the preconcentrate was delivered in a gelatin capsule, the emulsification occurred on release of the capsule contents in the aqueous environment of the gastrointestinal tract. The bioavailability characteristics were improved by the addition of the surfactants polyoxyl 40 hydrogenated castor oil (Cremophor RH40) and a polyglycolysed glyceride (Labrafil M-2125CS), together with a cosolvent (propylene glycol) to form the microemulsion preconcentrate (SMEDDS) Neoral. The residence time of ciclosporin in the gastro-

intestinal tract is shorter and the rate of absorption is faster with this microemulsion formulation. Some data can be found in Fig. 6.26.

6.4.7 Structured (semisolid) emulsions

So far we have considered only relatively simple dilute emulsions. Many pharmaceutical preparations, lotions or creams are, in fact, complex semisolid or structured systems that contain excess emulsifier over that required to form a stabilising monolayer at the oil–water interface. The excess surfactant can interact with other components either at the droplet interface or in the bulk (continuous) phase to produce complex semisolid multiphase systems. Theories derived to explain the stability of dilute colloidal systems cannot be applied directly. In many cases the formation of stable interfacial films at the oil–water interface cannot be considered to play the dominant role in maintaining stability. Rather it is the structure of the bulk phase that maintains the disperse phase at a distance. Even very complex emulsions are often mobile at some point in their lifetime, e.g. during manufacture at elevated temperatures, or may become so during application of high shear rates in use. Under these conditions globules previously unable to interact become free to do so.

Stable o/w creams prepared with ionic or non-ionic emulsifying waxes are composed of (at least) four phases (Fig. 6.27): (1) dispersed oil phase; (2) crystalline gel phase; (3) crystalline hydrate phase; and (4) bulk aqueous phase containing a dilute solution of surfactant. The interaction of the surfactant and fatty alcohol components of emulsifying mixtures to form these structures (body) is critical. It is also time-dependent, giving the name 'self-bodying' to these emulsions. The overall stability of a cream is dependent on the stability of the crystalline gel phase.

Emulsion stability is increased by the presence of liquid crystalline phases, as they form multilayers at the oil–water interface. These multilayers thus protect against coalescence by reducing the van der Waals forces of attraction and by retarding film thinning between approaching droplets, the viscosity of the liquid crystalline phases being at least 100 times that of the continuous phase in the absence of these structures. Guidelines have been devised for the formulation

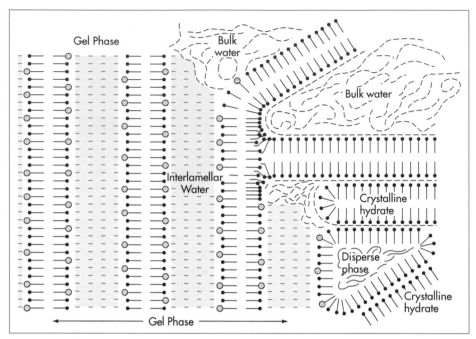

Figure 6.27 Schematic diagram of a typical semisolid cream prepared with cetostearyl alcohol and ionic surfactant. Note the four phases: (1) the dispersed oil phase; (2) the crystalline gel phase containing interlamellar fixed water; (3) phase composed of crystalline hydrates of cetostearyl alcohol; (4) bulk water phase.

Reproduced with permission from Eccleston GM. The microstructure of semisolid creams. *Pharm Int* 1986;7:63.

of self-bodied emulsions, the main ones of which are as follows[8]:

- The *lipophilic component* should be an amphiphile that promotes the formation of w/o emulsions and is capable of complexing with the hydrophilic surfactant at the o/w interface.
- The *hydrophilic component* should be a surfactant that promotes the formation of o/w systems and is capable of complexing with the lipophilic component at the o/w interface.

The rigidity and strength of networks prepared with cetostearyl alcohol and alkyltrimethylammonium bromides (C_{12}–C_{18}) increase as the alkyl chain length increases. The rheological stability of ternary systems is markedly dependent on the alcohol chain length; networks prepared with ionic or non-ionic surfactants and pure cetyl or pure stearyl alcohol are weaker than those prepared with cetostearyl alcohol.

6.4.8 Biopharmaceutical aspects of emulsions

Where traditionally emulsions have been used to deliver oils (castor oil, liquid paraffin) in a palatable form, a major use now is in IV nutrition. Lipid o/w emulsions are used as vehicles for lipophilic drugs (diazepam, propofol) for IV use. Griseofulvin, presented as an emulsion, exhibits enhanced oral absorption; an emulsion of indoxole has superior bioavailability over other oral forms. Medium-chain triglycerides and mono- and diglycerides promote the absorption of ceftriaxone and cefoxitin as well as ciclosporin.

In the case of griseofulvin, administration in a fatty medium enhances absorption. Fat is emulsified by the bile salts, and the administration of a pre-emulsified form increases the opportunity for solubilisation and hence transport across the microvilli by fat absorption pathways. The influence of the emulsifier on membrane permeability is one factor that must be considered. Knowledge that nanoparticles may be absorbed albeit in low amounts from the gut by the gut-associated lymphoid tissue suggests that we may have to revise our views on the nature of absorption of many drugs from the gastrointestinal tract.

Drug release from emulsions is related to the partition coefficient of the drug and the volume of the disperse phase, as well as to the concentration of

Table 6.5 Drugs formulated as emulsions

Drug	Product	Company	Route
Ciclosporin A	Gengraf	Abbot	Oral
Ciclosporin A	Restasis	Allergan	Ocular topical use
Dexamethasone palmitate	Lipotalon/Limethason	Merckle	Intra-articular
Diazepam	Diazepam	Braun Melsungen	IV
Diazepam	Stesolid	Dumex	IV
Etomidate	Etomidate-Lipuro	Braun Melsungen	IV
Propofol	Diprivan	AstraZeneca	IV
Ritonavir	Norvir	Abbott	Oral

Modified from Tamilvanan S *et al.* Formulation of multifunctional oil-in-water nanosized emulsions for active and passive targeting of drugs to otherwise inaccessible internal organs of the human body. *Int J Pharm* 2009;381:62–72. Copyright Elsevier 2009.

surfactant that might solubilise the drug in the aqueous phase. Table 6.5 lists some drugs currently marketed as emulsions; Scheme 6.1 shows their structures and partition coefficients.

There are suggestions of cross-allergy[12] of the soybean oil present in all the emulsion formulations discussed here to peanut oil and hence adverse events in those with peanut allergies. Bioequivalence, antimicrobial preservatives and difference in lipid loads and lipid types are aspects which complicate comparison of propofol formulations. The propofol prodrug fospropofol (Lusedra) (Scheme 6.2) is available as an aqueous solution, and may be one route to avoid some of the problems encountered with more elaborate formulations.

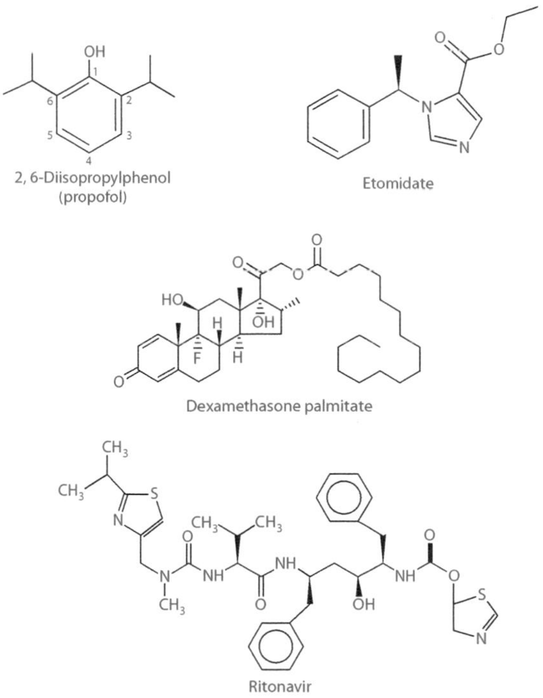

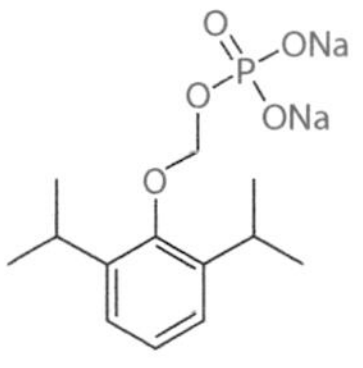

Scheme 6.2 Fospropofol sodium, which is metabolised to propofol and can be formulated as a solution

Prostaglandin E₁ (PGE₁) formulations

Lipid emulsion formulations of PGE₁ have been used in the treatment of vascular disorders. They exhibit a reduced incidence of side-effects at the site of injection. A soybean emulsion stabilised by egg-yolk lecithin[13] releases the PGE₁ over a period of 4–16 h depending on pH (Fig. 6.28). The partition coefficients of PGE₁ between soybean emulsion and aqueous buffers at 20°C are shown in Fig. 6.29, explaining why the release profiles have the pH dependency shown in Fig. 6.28. The release profile follows the expected pH trend, but a more detailed analysis shows that the majority of the drug is associated with the phospholipid.

Scheme 6.1 Structures of propofol, etomidate, dexamethasone palmitate and ritonavir. Their log *P* values (range reported) as follows: for propofol = 3.81–4.16; for etomidate = 2.5–2.66; for dexamethasone palmitate = 9.8; and for ritonavir = 3.9–4.3 (N.B.: water solubility 400 µg mL^{-1} in 0.1 N HCl).

Clinical issues: the search for clinically optimal formulations

Etomidate and propofol are both IV anaesthetics. Etomidate was first formulated as a racemic mixture but the dextrorotatory form (the structure having R chirality) is substantially more active than its enantiomer, hence its reformulation as the single potent enantiomer.

Etomidate is available in two formulations:

- a clear colourless solution for injection of 2 mg mL^{-1} of etomidate in an aqueous solvent containing 35% propylene glycol (Hypnomidate).
- a lipid emulsion preparation (Etomidate Lipuro).

The hypnotic effects and onset of activity of both formulations are virtually identical.

It has been found that propylene glycol-based formulations cause pain on injection, not least in paediatric subjects, and some patients also develop phlebitis and signs of an allergic reaction.

Three papers on the topic explain progress in identifying the overall better formulation:

- Nyman et al.[9] conclude, as stated in the title of their paper: 'Etomidate-Lipuro is associated with considerably less injection pain in children compared with propofol with added lidocaine'.
- Kam et al.[10] in a comparison of propofol-Lipuro with a non-emulsion form, propofol plus lidocaine 10 mg, found that injection pain was reduced when using the emulsion formulation.
- Suttmann et al.[11] found that, with the then-new formulation of etomidate as a lipid emulsion, neither venous sequelae nor allergic reactions were observed in any of the eight volunteers studied.

The *British National Formulary* 68 lists only emulsion formulations of propofol:

- Diprivan (long-chain triglyceride-only emulsion).
- Propoven® (long- and medium-chain triglyceride emulsion).
- Propofol-Lipuro® (long- and medium-chain triglyceride emulsion).

but as one commentary emphasises, 'Not all propofols are equal'.

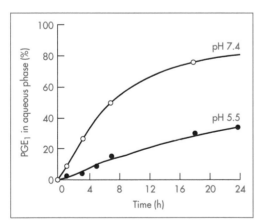

Figure 6.28 Release profiles of PGE$_1$ from particles in Lipo-PGE$_1$ diluted 10-fold with buffer solutions at 5°C: (●), pH 5.5; (○), pH 7.4.

Reproduced from Yamaguchi T *et al*. Distribution of prostaglandin E$_1$ in lipid emulsion in relation to release rate from lipid particles. *Chem Pharm Bull* 1994;42:446–450. Copyright Wiley-VCH Verlag GmbH & Co. KGaA. Reproduced with permission.

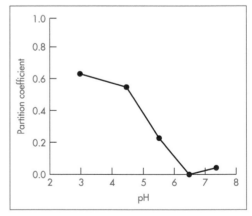

Figure 6.29 The pH–partition profiles of PGE$_1$ between soybean oil and water at 20°C, explaining why the release profiles have the pH dependency shown in Fig. 6.28.

Reproduced from Yamaguchi T *et al*. Distribution of prostaglandin E$_1$ in lipid emulsion in relation to release rate from lipid particles. *Chem Pharm Bull* 1994;42:446–450. Copyright Wiley-VCH Verlag GmbH & Co. KGaA. Reproduced with permission.

Intravenous lipid emulsions in detoxification

An interesting and valuable use of lipid emulsions is as a means of reducing high levels of drugs and other toxic materials from the circulation. IV administration of a lipid emulsion can reduce the levels of very lipophilic drugs which have accumulated at toxic amounts.[14] The lipid particles act as a 'sink' for lipophilic drugs which will partition into the particles.

Drugs that have been reported to be taken up in this way in animal work and in some human studies include:

- amiodorone
- mepivacaine
- bupivacaine
- verapamil.

Calculated log P values for these molecules are 7.57, 1.95, 3.4 and 3.79, respectively. Success will be related to log P, the amount of drug in the blood and the concentration of lipid particles administered. L-type calcium channel blocker drugs are used as cardiac antiarrhythmics or antihypertensives, depending on whether the drugs have higher affinity for the heart (such as verapamil: Fig. 6.30) or for the vessels (e.g. nifedipine). The IV administration of Intralipid is seen to return the disturbed Ca^{2+} currents to nearly normal as a result of the free drug partitioning into the lipid droplets.

6.4.9 Preservative availability in emulsified systems

Microbial spoilage of emulsified products is avoided by the inclusion of appropriate amounts of a preservative in the formulation. Infected topical emulsions have

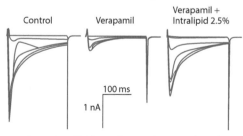

| Control | Verapamil | Verapamil + Intralipid 2.5% |

100 ms

1 nA

Figure 6.30 Intralipid emulsion administred IV decreases free verapamil concentrations and reverses verapamil-induced Ca^{2+} channel block. Graph depicts L-type Ca^{2+} currents in (from left to right) the control, verapamil and verapamil plus Intralipid. Kryshtal D *et al.* (*Circulation* 2010; 122:A18810) state that 'rapid intravenous administration of Intralipid may be an effective antidote for hypotension caused by acute verapamil poisoning'.

been the cause of outbreaks of pseudomonal and other bacterial skin infections. The incorporation of preservatives into pharmaceutical emulsions is not without problems as most agents partition to the oily or micellar phases of complex systems; some are inactivated by surfactants.

The amount of preservative remaining in the aqueous phase (C_w) is related to the total amount (C) of preservative with a partition coefficient P in an emulsion with an oil/water phase ratio of Φ by equation (6.21):

$$C_w = \frac{C(\Phi + 1)}{R(P\Phi + 1)} \qquad (6.21)$$

where R is the preservative/emulsifier ratio or interaction ratio. P and R need to be determined experimentally.

The presence of surfactant micelles alters the native partition coefficient of the preservative molecule because the micellar phase offers an alternative site for preservative molecules. The partitioning then occurs between the oil globule and the aqueous micellar phases.

For preservatives that are less soluble in the oily phase $(P < 1)$, the concentration in all phases increases when the proportion of the oil phase is increased. In contrast, for those preservatives that are more soluble in oil than in water $(P > 1)$, the concentration in all phases decreases when the proportion of the oil phase is increased. This is the case with phenol and chlorocresol (see data given in Table 6.6).

In an emulsion containing 60% arachis oil (Φ = 1.5) and 1% polysorbate, 9.6% of the phenol but only 0.3% of the more lipophilic chlorocresol is free in the water phase. As much as 93% of the phenol and 99.9% of chlorocresol are locked up in the oily phase or the micellar phases in emulsions containing 10% polysorbate 80.

The use of these equations can be criticised because of the simple manner in which R has been measured and defined, but they are useful to estimate effects of changing parameters. When the emulsified system is very complex, containing not one but at least two emulsifying agents (as most do), the determination of the parameters of the equation is a lengthy process, and a direct experimental approach to the determination of free aqueous concentration, such as a dialysis technique, may be the only approach.

Table 6.6 Percentage (W) of phenol and chlorocresol partitioned to various sites in arachis oil emulsions

Arachis oil in water Φ (phase ratio)	Phenol				Chlorocresol			
	Oil W_o	Aqueous phase W_a	Micelles W_m	Water W_w	Oil W_o	Aqueous phase W_a	Micelles W_m	Water W_w
0.18	38	62	15.6	46.4	74.8	25.2	21.3	3.9
0.25	46.8	53.2	13.6	39.6	80.5	19.5	17	2.5
0.5	64	36	10.4	25.6	89.3	10.7	9.5	1.2
1.0	78.2	21.8	7.7	14.1	94.4	5.6	5.1	0.5
1.5	84.2	15.8	6.2	9.6	96.2	3.8	3.5	0.3

Reproduced from Konning GK. *Can J Pharm Sci* 1974;9:103.
Note that $W_a = W_m + W_w$. Phenol and chlorocresol are present in 2.5% concentration.
Stabiliser: 1% polysorbate 80.

6.4.10 Mass transport in oil-in-water emulsions

Not only preservative molecules partition from the phases in emulsions: drug molecules and flavouring and colouring agents also do. Interest in the extent and rate of flavour release on ingestion of a food emulsion has resulted in quantitative studies of the topic. The model used is equally applicable to drug release in the gastrointestinal tract as in the mouth, since dilution of the emulsion system occurs in both instances.

The concentration of the solute in the aqueous phase immediately after dilution C_w^0 and on re-establishing equilibrium C_w^e depends on the various properties of the solutes, such as the partition coefficient.

Usually, drugs dissolved in oils are absorbed mainly via the aqueous phase. Transport from one phase to the other and partitioning are therefore important. In the absorption of drugs from o/w emulsions when the drug partition coefficient is greater than 1, the *amount* of drug in the aqueous phase (rather than the concentration) is a critical factor for absorption. In the absorption of poorly oil-soluble drugs, drug absorption from emulsions is greater than from aqueous solution. In an emulsion of volume ratio, Φ, the drug concentration in the aqueous phase (C_w) is related to the overall concentration of the drug (C) by the expression:

$$C_w = C \frac{(\Phi + 1)}{(P\Phi + 1)} \qquad (6.22)$$

where P is the oil/water partition coefficient of the drug or other agent.

6.4.11 Intravenous fat emulsions

Clinical point

Fat emulsions are used to supply a large amount of energy in a small volume of isotonic liquid; they supply the body with essential fatty acids and triglycerides. Fat emulsions for IV nutrition contain vegetable oil and phospholipid emulsifier. Several commercial fat emulsions are available, such as Intralipid, Lipiphysan, Lipofundin and Lipofundin S. They contain either cottonseed oil or soybean oil. In Intralipid, for example, purified egg-yolk phospholipids are used as the emulsifiers, and isotonicity is obtained by the addition of sorbitol, xylitol or glycerol.

Intralipid has also been used as the basis of an IV drug carrier, for example for diazepam (Diazemuls) and propofol (Diprivan), as an alternative to solubilisation in non-ionic micellar systems such as Cremophor EL.

To avoid adverse effects on injection it is important that the particle size of the emulsions is small and remains so on storage. After storage of Intralipid for 2 years at 4°C, more than 99% of the particles visible by light microscopy had a diameter of less than 1 µm; that is, there was practically no change in mean diameter.

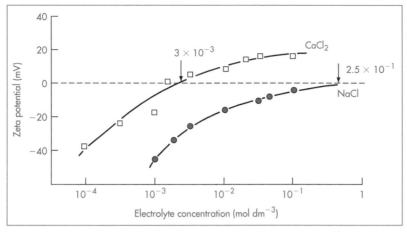

Figure 6.31 Zeta potential of Intralipid 20% diluted into varying concentrations (mol dm^{-3}) of (●) NaCl, (□) CaCl$_2$.
Reproduced with permission from Whateley TL *et al*. Particle size stability of Intralipid and mixed total parenteral nutrition mixtures. *J Clin Hosp Pharm* 1984;91:13–26.

Chylomicrons

Fat that finds its natural way into plasma occurs in three forms: as lipoprotein complexes, as free fatty acids bound to albumin, or as an emulsion of particles in the size range 0.4–3.0μm. These natural emulsion globules are *chylomicrons* (from the Greek *chylo*, meaning *juice* or *milky fluid*, and *micron*, meaning *small particle*). There are pronounced physical similarities between chylomicrons and the fat particles of the Intralipid emulsion. Chylomicrons are lipoprotein particles that consist of triglycerides (85–92%), phospholipids (6–12%), cholesterol (1–3%) and proteins (1–2%). They transport dietary lipids from the intestines to other locations in the body. Chylomicrons are one of the five major groups of lipoproteins (chylomicrons, very-low-density lipoproteins, intermediate-density lipoprotein, low-density lipoproteins, high-density lipoproteins) that enable fats and cholesterol to move within the water-based solution of the blood stream.

Clinical point

The addition of electrolyte or drugs to IV fat emulsions is generally contraindicated because of the risk of destabilising the emulsion. Addition of cationic local anaesthetics reduces the electrophoretic mobility of the dispersed fat globules, and this contributes to instability.[15]

Minimum stability (and a minimum value of zeta potential) is caused by addition to Intralipid of 3×10^{-3} mol dm^{-3} CaCl$_2$ and 2.5×10^{-1} mol dm^{-3} NaCl, which are thus recommended as the maximum additive levels (Fig. 6.31).

6.4.12 Emulsion rheology

Most emulsions, unless very dilute, display both plastic and pseudoplastic flow behaviour rather than simple Newtonian flow (see section 6.3). An attempt has been made[16] to calculate the shear conditions for simple pharmaceutical operations such as the spreading of an ointment or cream on the skin, ointment milling and the flow of liquid through a hypodermic needle. The flow properties of fluid emulsions should have little influence on their biological behaviour, although the rheological characteristics of semisolid emulsions may affect their performance. The 'pourability', 'spreadability' and 'syringeability' of an emulsion will, however, be directly determined by its rheological properties. The high viscosity of w/o emulsions leads to problems with intramuscular administration of injectable formulations. Conversion to a multiple emulsion (w/o/w), in which the external oil phase is replaced by an aqueous phase, leads to a dramatic decrease in viscosity and consequent improved ease of injection.

The influence of phase volume on the flow properties of an emulsion is shown in Fig. 6.32. In this diagram the relative viscosity (η_{rel}) of the system increases with increasing ϕ, and at any given phase volume increases with decreasing mean particle size, D_m. These and

Key points

- Emulsions can exist as o/w and w/o emulsions, multiple emulsions (w/o/w or o/w/o), non-aqueous emulsions, microemulsions and semisolid emulsions.

- Adsorption of surfactant at the oil/water interface lowers the interfacial tension and aids the dispersal of the oil into droplets of a small size. Charged surfactants in the interfacial layer lead to an increase in zeta potential and will thus help to maintain stability by increasing V_R; non-ionic surfactants maintain stability by creating a hydrated layer on the hydrophobic particle in o/w emulsions and by steric and enthalpic forces in w/o emulsions.

- Mixtures of surfactants usually form more stable emulsions than do single surfactants, possibly because complex formation at the interface results in a more rigid stabilising film.

- Surfactants may be selected as emulsifiers on the basis of their HLB value (an empirical measure of the balance between hydrophobic and hydrophilic regions of the surfactant molecule). HLB values may be calculated from simple empirical equations or from summation of contributions from groups present in the molecule. Surfactants with a high HLB are water-soluble and are useful in the formation of o/w emulsions; those with low HLB are insoluble in water and are used in the formation of w/o emulsions. Mixtures of high- and low-HLB surfactants produce more stable emulsions than do single surfactants; the HLB of a mixture of two surfactants is the algebraic mean of the two HLB values. Optimum HLB values have been determined for a variety of oils used in o/w emulsions.

- Multiple emulsions are emulsions whose disperse phase contains droplets of another phase. They are made by emulsifying a w/o emulsion with a hydrophilic surfactant to produce a w/o/w system, or an o/w system with a low HLB surfactant to produce an o/w/o system. They are of interest in drug delivery as delayed-action formulations.

- Microemulsions are homogeneous transparent systems of low viscosity that form spontaneously when the components are mixed in the appropriate ratios and are thermodynamically stable. They can be dispersions of oil droplets in water (o/w) or water droplets in oil (w/o) with a mean droplet diameter of 5–140 nm. An essential requirement for their formation and stability is the attainment of a very low interfacial tension, which is achieved using a cosurfactant.

- SEDDS and SMEDDS are preconcentrates comprising drug, oil (e.g. medium-chain triglyceride) and surfactant which form emulsions or microemulsions on contact with water in the gastrointestinal tract.

- Semisolid emulsions contain more emulsifier than is required to form a stabilising monolayer at the oil–water interface. Stable o/w creams prepared with ionic or non-ionic emulsifying waxes are composed of (at least) four phases: a dispersed oil phase, a crystalline gel phase, a crystalline hydrate phase and a bulk aqueous phase containing a dilute solution of surfactant. The overall stability of a cream is dependent on the stability of the crystalline gel phase.

- Emulsions are of interest as vehicles for drug delivery in which the drug is dissolved in the disperse phase. For example, lipid o/w emulsions are used as vehicles for lipophilic drugs (diazepam, propofol) for IV use. IV fat emulsions such as Intralipid, Lipiphysan, Lipofundin and Lipofundin S are used to supply a large amount of energy in a small volume of isotonic liquid; they supply the body with essential fatty acids and triglycerides.

other factors that affect emulsion viscosity are listed in Table 6.7.

As most emulsions are polydisperse, the influence of particle size and, in particular, of particle size distribution on viscosity is important. Figure 6.32 shows the viscosity of w/o emulsions varying in mean particle size (D_m) stabilised with sorbitan trioleate.

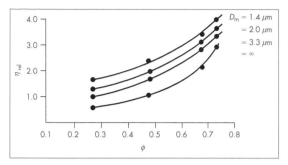

Figure 6.32 The relative viscosities of w/o emulsions stabilised with sorbitan trioleate; as a function of volume fraction and globule diameters D_m.

Reproduced from Sherman P. The flow properties of emulsions. *J Pharm Pharmacol* 1964;16:1. Copyright Wiley-VCH Verlag GmbH & Co. KGaA. Reproduced with permission.

Several equations for the viscosity of emulsion systems take the form

$$\eta_{rel} - 1 = \eta_{sp} = \frac{\alpha\phi}{1 - h\phi} \tag{6.23}$$

where $\alpha = 2.5$, and h is a measure of the fluid immobilised between the particles in concentrated emulsions and dispersions, which therefore reduces the total volume of liquid available for the particles to move around in. Immobilised liquid attached to solvated macromolecular stabilisers effectively increases the concentration of the particles and increases viscosity.

Table 6.7 Factors that influence emulsion viscosity
Internal (disperse) phase
Volume fraction (ϕ)
Viscosity
Particle size and size distribution
Chemical nature
Continuous phase
Viscosity
Chemical constitution and polarity
Emulsifier
Chemical constitution and concentration
Solubility in the continuous and internal (disperse) phase
Physical properties of the interfacial film
Electroviscous effects
Presence of additional stabilisers, pigments, hydrocolloids, etc.

In emulsions in which ϕ does not exceed 0.65, an equation of the form

$$\eta_{rel} = 1 + \frac{2.5\phi}{6(1 - h\phi)} \tag{6.24}$$

may be used, while for emulsions in which η_{rel} becomes infinite when $\phi \to 0.74$, the appropriate equation is

$$\eta_{rel} = 1 + \frac{2.5\phi}{2(1 - h\phi)} \tag{6.25}$$

where h has a value of 1.28–1.35.

When an emulsion is aged, its mean globule size increases. The ensuing changes in D_m and globule size distribution cause a fall in emulsion viscosity at high rates of shear. Provided no other changes have occurred in the system, the viscosity at any given time should be predictable from viscosity–D_m relationships derived from fresh emulsions of the same formulation. Viscosity changes at low rates of shear are more difficult to predict because of the complication of particle aggregation, which may change with time. Creep compliance tests show viscoelastic behaviour for concentrated o/w emulsions stabilised by mixtures of non-ionic emulsifiers and fatty alcohols. The rheological characteristics of these emulsions change with time as a result of interactions between the components of the system and they are termed 'self-bodying' emulsions.

6.5 Suspensions

Suspensions are dispersions of an insoluble drug or other substance in an aqueous or non-aqueous continuous phase. Pharmaceutical suspensions tend to be coarse dispersions rather than true colloids, although there are many sub-micrometre polymer dispersions available as drug carriers. There are also suspensions of drug nanocrystals, as discussed in Chapter 14. Drugs in suspension are prepared mainly for oral, intramuscular or subcutaneous use, but suspensions of drugs are also used as reservoirs in transdermal patch preparations and in conventional topical formulations. Many therapeutic aerosols are suspensions of drugs in a volatile propellant.

Problems can arise when a drug is dispersed in a liquid. Sedimentation, caking (leading to difficulty in resuspension), flocculation and particle growth (through dissolution and recrystallisation) are all possible. In practice we wish to avoid the problems of aggregation of particles in suspensions and in many lyophilised preparations and to ensure their efficient redispersion on reconstitution with water or other media. Adhesion of suspension particles to container walls has also been identified as a problem, particularly with low-dose drugs.

Formulation of pharmaceutical suspensions to minimise caking can be achieved by the production of flocculated systems. A flocculate, or floc, is a cluster of particles held together in a loose open structure; a suspension consisting of particles in this state is termed *flocculated* (Fig. 6.33). There are various states of flocculation and deflocculation. Unfortunately, flocculated systems clear rapidly and the preparation often appears unsightly, so a partially deflocculated formulation is the ideal pharmaceutical.

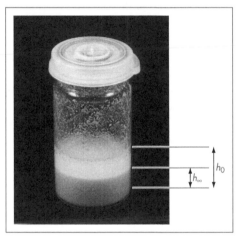

Figure 6.33 A flocculated suspension that has rapidly settled, clearly identifying the sedimentation layer, from which can be calculated the ratio R (equation 6.26) as R = h_∞/h_0.

Suspensions of liposomes, microspheres and microcapsules, and nanospheres and nanocapsules formed from a variety of polymers or proteins form a relatively new class of pharmaceutical suspension in which physical stability is still paramount. It is important that on injection these carrier systems do not aggregate, as this will change the effective size and the fate of the particles. One exception to this would be the deliberate flocculation of latex particles administered to the eye, where aggregation leads to agglomerated particles that do not easily pass through the drainage ducts of the eye.

6.5.1 Stability of suspensions

In order to quantify the sedimentation of suspended particles, the ratio R of sedimentation layer volume (V_s) to total suspension volume (V_t) may be used. A measure of sedimentation may also be obtained from the height of the sedimented layer (h_∞) in relation to the initial height of the suspension (h_0).

$$R = \frac{V_s}{V_t} \approx \frac{h_\infty}{h_0} \qquad (6.26)$$

In a completely deflocculated system the particles are not associated; pressure on the individual particles can lead in this layer to close packing of the particles to such an extent that the secondary energy barriers are overcome and the particles become irreversibly bound together. In flocculated systems (where the repulsive barriers have been reduced) particles settle as flocs and not as individual particles. The supernatant clears but, because of the random arrangement of the particles in the flocs, the sediment is not closely packed and caking does not readily occur.

In flocculated or concentrated suspensions, zone settling occurs (Fig. 6.34a). In the region A–B of Fig. 6.34b there is hindered settling of the particle interface at a constant rate; at B–C a transitional settling occurs; from C to D consolidation of the sediment occurs.

Suspension stability is governed by the same forces as in other disperse systems such as emulsions. There are differences, however, as coalescence obviously cannot occur in suspensions; the adsorption of stabilising polymers and surfactants may also occur in a different fashion. Flocculation, unlike coalescence, can be a reversible process and partial or controlled flocculation is attempted in formulation, as discussed above.

Caking of the suspension, which arises on close packing of the sedimented particles, cannot be eliminated by reduction of particle size or by increasing the viscosity of the continuous phase. Fine particles in a viscous medium settle more slowly than coarse particles but, after settling, they form a more closely packed sediment that may be difficult to re-disperse. Particles in a close-packed condition brought about by settling and by the pressure of particles above thus experience greater forces of attraction. Flocculating agents can prevent caking; deflocculating agents increase the tendency to cake. The addition of floccu-

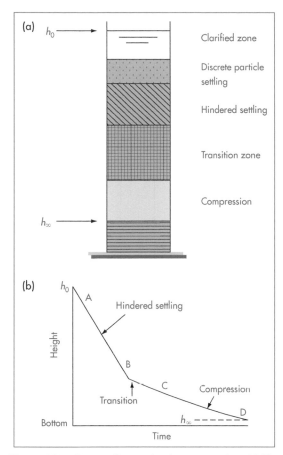

(a)

h_0

Clarified zone

Discrete particle settling

Hindered settling

Transition zone

Compression

h_∞

(b)

h_0

A

Hindered settling

Height

B

C

Compression

Transition

D

Bottom

h_∞

Time

Figure 6.34 Zone sedimentation in a suspension. (a) The various zones are delineated, showing the clear layer at the top of the suspension and the sedimented layer at the bottom; immediately above this layer is a region in which the particles are crowded and begin to be compressed to form sediment. (b) The height of the interface between the clarified zone and the suspension as a function of time.

lating and deflocculating agents is often monitored by measurement of the zeta potential of the particles in a suspension.

Zeta potential and its relationship to stability

Most suspension particles dispersed in water have a charge acquired by specific adsorption of ions or by ionisation of ionisable surface groups, if present. If the charge arises from ionisation, the charge on the particle will depend on the pH of the environment. As with other colloidal particles, repulsive forces arise because of the interaction of the electrical double layers on adjacent particles. The magnitude of the charge can be determined by measurement of the electrophoretic mobility of the particles in an applied electric field. A microelectrophoresis apparatus in which this mobility may be measured is shown schematically in Fig. 6.35.

The velocity of migration of the particles (μ_E) under unit applied potential can be determined microscopically with a timing device and an eyepiece graticule. For non-conducting particles, the Henry equation is used to obtain ζ from μ_E. This equation can be written in the form

$$\mu_E = \frac{\zeta \varepsilon}{4\pi\eta} f(\kappa a) \qquad (6.27)$$

where $f(\kappa a)$ varies between 1 for small κa and 1.5 for large κa; ε is the dielectric constant of the continuous phase and η its viscosity. In systems with low values of κa, the equation can be written in the form

$$\mu_E = \frac{\zeta \varepsilon}{4\pi\eta} \qquad (6.28)$$

The zeta potential (ζ) is not the surface potential (ψ_0) discussed earlier but is related to it. Therefore ζ can be used as a reliable guide to the magnitude of electric repulsive forces between particles. Changes in ζ on the addition of flocculating agents, surfactants and other additives can then be used to predict the stability of the system.

The changes in a bismuth subnitrate suspension system on addition of dibasic potassium phosphate as flocculating agent are shown in Fig. 6.36. Bismuth subnitrate has a positive zeta potential; addition of phosphate reduces the charge and the zeta potential falls to a point where maximum flocculation is observed. In this zone there is no caking. Further addition of phosphate leads to a negative zeta potential and a propensity towards caking. Flocculation can therefore be controlled by the use of ionic species with a charge opposite to the charge of the particles dispersed in the medium.

The rapid clearance of the supernatant in a flocculated system is undesirable in a pharmaceutical suspension. The use of thickeners such as sodium carboxymethylcellulose hinders the movement of the particles by increasing the viscosity of the medium, slowing down sedimentation. The incompatibility of any anionic agents with cationic flocculating agents has to be considered. A technique to overcome the problem is the conversion of the particle surfaces into

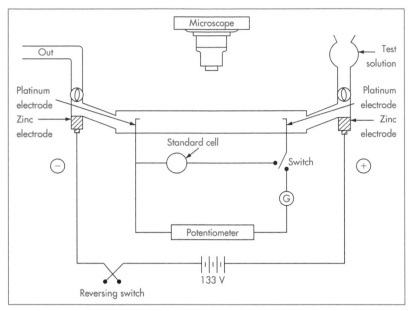

Figure 6.35 Schematic drawing of a microelectrophoresis apparatus showing the positioning of the anode and cathode and the capillary in which the velocity of particulates is monitored to allow calculation of zeta potential.

positive surfaces so that they require anions and not cations to flocculate them. Negatively charged or neutral particles can be converted into positively charged particles by addition of a surface-active amine. Such a suspension can then be treated with phosphate ions to induce flocculation.

It is perhaps not surprising that with some complex systems the interpretation of behaviour is open to debate. Consider the system shown in Fig. 6.37. One starts with a clumped suspension of sulfamerazine, a flocculated system that produces non-caking sediments. Addition of the surfactant sodium dioctyl sulfosuccinate (docusate sodium) confers a greater

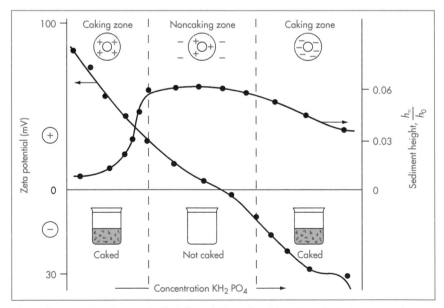

Figure 6.36 Caking diagram showing controlled flocculation of a bismuth subnitrate suspension employing dibasic potassium phosphate as the flocculating agent.

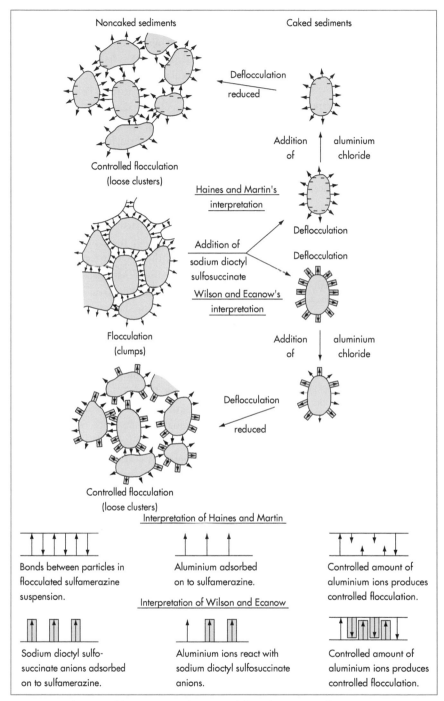

Figure 6.37 Diagrammatic drawing of flocculation and controlled flocculation in a sulfamerazine suspension: the effect of the addition of sodium dioctyl sulfosuccinate (docusate sodium) and aluminium chloride is shown and two interpretations of the results are outlined.

Reproduced from Woodford R, *Pharmacy Digest*, 1966; 29: 17.

negative charge on the suspension particles and deflocculation results. Addition of aluminium chloride as a flocculating agent reduces the negative charge in a controlled way to produce the loose clusters illustrated in the diagram. These are the observable results of these procedures. The different interpretations of the effects are diagrammatically realised, the difference lying in the manner in which the aluminium ions adsorb on to the sulfamerazine particles; in one view they adsorb directly, and in the other view they interact with the surfactant ions on the surface.

 Clinical point Barium sulfate as an X-ray contrast medium

The formulation of barium sulfate ($BaSO_4$) suspensions as a radiopaque material has to be carefully controlled for use. Flocculation of the suspended particles, which can be caused by the mucin in the gastrointestinal tract, causes artefacts to be seen in radiography. Factors such as particle size, zeta potential, pH dependence of the properties of adjuvants and the whole suspension, and the film-forming characteristics of the formulation must be taken into account. The preparation must flow readily over the mucosal surface, penetrate into folds and coat the surface evenly with a thin radiopaque layer. A film 2 μm thick will absorb twice as much radiation as a layer 1 μm thick if the average $BaSO_4$ particle size and concentration are the same in both cases. The adhesion of wet films of barium sulfate suspensions to surfaces and their thickness have been assessed *in vitro* by a simple method in which a clean microscope slide is dipped into the suspension and allowed to drain for 30 seconds. The gross appearance displays evidence of irregular coating caused by foaming, bubble formation or coagulation of particles. Commercially available suspensions preferred by radiologists are strongly negative at low pH, presumably resisting flocculation because of strong interparticle repulsion.

Polymers as flocculating agents

In many applications, such as water purification, suspended particles have to be removed by filtration. Flocculated particles are more readily removed than deflocculated particles. Polymers have been widely used as flocculating agents. Polymers used as flocculating or destabilising agents frequently act by adsorption and interparticle bridging. To be effective, the polymer must contain chemical groups that can interact with the surface of the colloidal particles. A particle–polymer complex is then formed, with polymer emerging into the aqueous phase. This free end will attach itself to another particle ('bridging') and thus promote flocculation. If there are no particles with which to interact, the polymer can coat the particle, leading to restabilisation. As can be seen in Fig. 6.38, however, the action of polymeric agents that can anchor at the particle surface is very concentration-dependent.

Polyacrylamide (30% hydrolysed) is an anionic polymer that can induce flocculation in kaolinite at very low concentrations. Restabilisation occurs by 'overdosing', probably by the mechanism outlined in Fig. 6.38. Dosages of polymer that are sufficiently large to saturate the colloidal surfaces produce a stable colloidal system, since no sites are available for the formation of interparticle bridges. Under certain conditions, physical agitation of the system can lead to breaking of polymer–suspension bonds and to a change in the state of the system.

6.5.2 Extemporaneous suspensions

Extemporaneous preparation of suspensions of drugs is still widely practised in hospital pharmacies, particularly to prepare dose forms for paediatric use when either a commercial product is unavailable or the dose has to be adjusted or the child cannot swallow tablets or capsules, as discussed in Chapter 10. Drugs such as acetazolamide, amiodarone and mercaptopurine are examples. In such formulations, alternatives to traditional suspending agents are required. The ideal suspending agent should:

- be readily and uniformly incorporated in the formulation
- be readily dissolved or dispersed in water without resort to special techniques

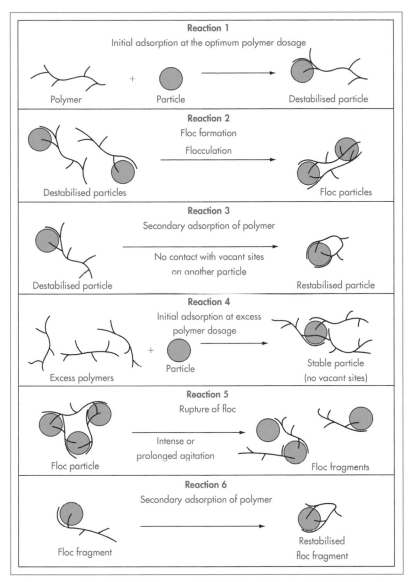

Figure 6.38 Schematic representation of the bridging model for the destabilisation of colloids by polymers: the concentration dependence of the process is illustrated.

Reproduced from Weber WJ. *Physicochemical Processes for Water Quality Control*. New York: Wiley; 1972. Copyright Wiley-VCH Verlag GmbH & Co. KGaA. Reproduced with permission.

- ensure the formation of a loosely packed system that does not cake
- not influence the dissolution rate or absorption rate of the drug
- be inert, non-toxic and free from incompatibilities.

Among the alternative suspending agents are sodium carboxymethylcellulose, microcrystalline cellulose, aluminium magnesium silicate (Veegum), sodium alginate (Manucol) and sodium starch (Primojel). Pregelatinised starches, Primojel and Veegum, are promising alternatives to compound tragacanth powder. Paediatric formulations demand special care because of the potential toxicities of formulation additives. Some issues are discussed in the text *Paediatric Drug Handling*,[17] and in Chapter 10.

6.5.3 Suspension rheology

Dilute *flocculated* suspensions exhibit pseudoplastic flow; more concentrated flocculated suspensions tend to exhibit plastic flow as a consequence of the closer

Key points

- Suspensions are coarse dispersions of an insoluble drug or other substance in an aqueous or non-aqueous continuous phase.
- They are inherently unstable due to sedimentation, caking (leading to difficulty in resuspension), flocculation and particle growth (through dissolution and recrystallisation).
- In a *deflocculated* system the particles settle separately and caking occurs because of close packing and irreversible binding of the sedimented particles. In *flocculated systems* particles settle as flocs, the sediment is not closely packed and caking does not occur; clearance of the supernatant is, however, too rapid for an acceptable pharmaceutical formulation. The aim in the formulation of suspensions is, therefore, to achieve *partial or controlled flocculation* by the addition of flocculating agents, for example, ions with opposite charge to that of the dispersed particles. Suspension stability may be assessed by measurement of the zeta potential of the particles and by the ratio of the height or volume of the sediment to that of the suspension.

packing of their particles at higher concentrations. At shear stresses below τ_0 in concentrated suspensions, the three-dimensional structure of the flocculated suspension is maintained, the apparent viscosity is relatively high and very little flow occurs. As the shear stress is increased between the lower and upper yield stresses, the floccules are progressively broken down and eventually, at shear stresses above the upper yield stress, the flow appears to become Newtonian. The effect is shown schematically in Fig. 6.39. As a consequence, the viscosity (gradient of the plot of shear stress vs shear rate) of both pseudoplastic and plastic suspensions decreases with increasing shear rate, as illustrated in Fig. 6.40.

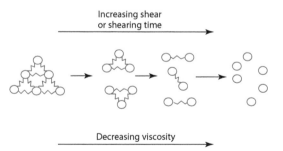

Figure 6.39 Schematic showing the viscosity decrease with increasing shear in a flocculated suspension caused by the breakdown of floccules.

Shear thickening (dilatancy) is shown by concentrated suspensions of densely packed *deflocculated* particles in which there is only sufficient liquid to fill the void spaces in between the particles. The apparent viscosity is low at low shearing stress, but increases as the

applied stress increases. This effect is due to the increase of electrostatic repulsion that occurs when the charged particles are forced close together (as seen from the DLVO plot of Fig. 6.5), causing the particles to rebound, creating voids into which liquid flows, leaving other parts of the dispersion 'dry'.

6.5.4 Non-aqueous suspensions

Many pharmaceutical aerosols consist of solids dispersed in a non-aqueous propellant. Few studies have been published on the behaviour of such systems, although their sensitivity to water is well established. Low amounts of water adsorb at the particle surface and can lead to aggregation of the particles with each other or to deposition on the walls of the container, which adversely affects the product performance.

6.5.5 Electrostatics in aerosols

Aerosol particles can become electrostatically charged as they are projected from the aerosol canister. The net charge is sufficient to affect deposition in the respiratory tract. Positive charges have been found on particles below 0.6 μm and negative charges above that size in Intal Forte, Tilade and Flixotide aerosols, which are suspension formulations with plastic valves. The number of charges on the particles ranged from zero to several thousands!

As Schein[18] has written in an article on continuing puzzles in electrostatics, charging of solid surfaces 'remains one of the most poorly understood areas of

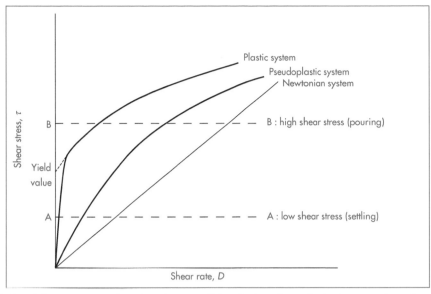

Figure 6.40 A plot of shear stress $\tau = \eta D$ against shear rate D for plastic and pseudoplastic suspensions. As $\eta = \tau/D$, the slope of the line represents the viscosity at each rate of shear; in both the plastic and pseudoplastic systems the viscosity at level A is greater than that at level B.

Modified from Samyn JC, An industrial approach to suspension formulation. *J Pharm Sci*, 1961; 50: 517. Copyright Wiley-VCH Verlag GmbH & Co. KGaA. Reproduced with permission.

solid-state physics'. It would be an advance to have charge correlated with the properties of the powders that experience this effect, but the issue in pharmaceuticals is often the presence of excipients. Particle adhesion, say to plastic components as in spacers, has been thought to be due to electrostatic interactions between the charges on the particles and the resultant induced charges on any surface (Fig. 6.41). But the physical picture is more complex, and appears to be related to the discreteness of the charge, which produces strong electrostatic forces.[19]

6.5.6 Adhesion of suspension particles to containers

When the walls of a container are wetted repeatedly, an adhering layer of suspension particles may build up, and this subsequently dries to a hard and thick layer. In Fig. 6.42 three types of wetting are shown. Where the suspension is in constant contact with the container wall, *immersional wetting* occurs, in which particles are pressed up to the wall and may or may not adhere. Above the liquid line, *spreading wetting* of the suspension during shaking or pouring may also lead to adhesion of the particles contained in the spreading liquid. *Adhesional wetting* occurs when a liquid drop remains suspended, like a drop of water on a clothes

line. Evidently the surface tension of the suspension plays a part in the spreading and wetting processes. Adhesion increases with increase in suspension

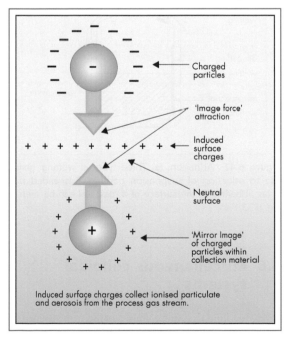

Figure 6.41. Schematic of induced positive charges on surfaces close to a negatively charged aerosol particle, which leads to particle adhesion.

Redrawn from www.verantis.com.

concentration, and with the number of contacts the suspension makes with the surfaces in question. Additives, especially surfactants, will modify the adhesion of suspension particles. They will act in two ways: (a) by decreasing the surface tension; and (b) by adsorption modifying the forces of interaction between particle and container. The example illustrated in Figs 6.43 and 6.44 refers to the addition of benzethonium chloride to chloramphenicol suspensions. Benzethonium chloride converts both the glass surface and the particles into positively charged entities (Fig. 6.43). Adhesion in the presence of this cationic surfactant is concentration-dependent, the process being akin to flocculation. At low concentrations the surfactant adsorbs by its cationic head to the negative glass and to the suspension particle. The glass is thus made hydrophobic. At higher concentrations hydrophobic interactions occur between coated particle and surface (Fig. 6.44). Further increase in concentration results in multilayer formation of surfactant, rendering the surfaces hydrophilic. In this condition the particles repel, reducing adhesion.

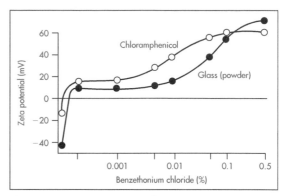

Figure 6.43 Zeta potential of glass (powder) and chloramphenicol in aqueous benzethonium chloride solutions.

Reproduced from Uno H, Tanaka S. Adhesion of suspension particles on the wall surface of a container. Mechanism of particle adhesion. *Kolloid Z Z Polym* 1972;250:238, with kind permission from Springer Science and Business Media.

theme include microsphere-in-water-in-oil systems (s/w/o) and vesicle-in-water-in-oil (v/w/o) formulations. Figure 6.45 shows (a) the appearance of a vesicle-based system and (b) the modes of release of drug encapsulated in the system.

6.7 Applications of colloid stability theory to other systems

There are several colloidal systems other than synthetically produced emulsions and suspensions that are of relevance – blood and other cell suspensions, for example – whose behaviour can now be better understood by application of colloid stability theory. The adhesion of cells to surfaces, the aggregation of platelets, the spontaneous sorting out of mixed-cell aggregates and other such phenomena depend to a large extent on interaction between the surfaces of the objects in question, although the surfaces are frequently more labile and less homogeneous than those encountered in model colloids. The extended circulation in the blood of 'long-life' or 'stealth' liposomes whose surfaces are modified by protruding long surface-bonded hydrophilic chains (usually polyoxyethylene glycols) may also be ascribed to their modified interactions *in vivo* with opsonins and with scavenging cells of the reticuloendothelial system.

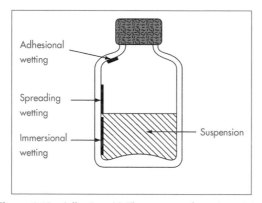

Figure 6.42 Adhesion. (a) Three types of wetting, giving rise to adhesion of suspension particles. Suspended particles adhering to the surface of a glass vial can be seen in Fig. 6.33.

6.6 Miscellaneous colloidal systems

Several colloidal systems have not been mentioned in this chapter because they are dealt with elsewhere. These include nanoparticle suspensions used in drug delivery and targeting, and vesicular dispersions (liposomes, niosomes, etc.). Variations on the emulsion

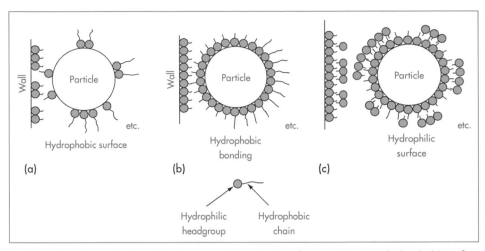

Figure 6.44 Adsorption of benzethonium chloride on particle and wall surfaces creating in (a) hydrophobic surfaces and in (b) hydrophobic bonding between the adsorbed molecules. In (c) further additions of the benzethonium chloride result in the conversion to hydrophilic surfaces.

Modified from Uno H, Tanaka S. *Kolloid Z Z Polym* 1972;250:238.

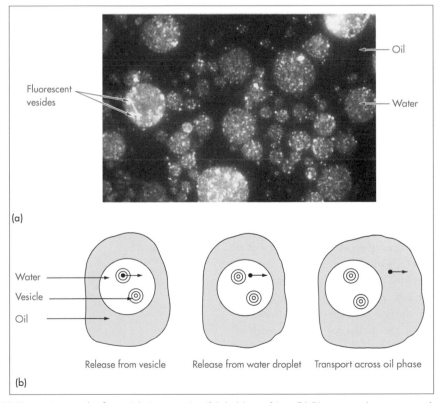

Figure 6.45 (a) Photomicrograph of a vesicle-in-water-in-oil (v/w/o) emulsion. (b) Diagrammatic representation of the modes of release of solutes from the formulation (● = drug).

6.7.1 Cell–cell interactions

A simple way of considering interactions between free-floating cells is to treat the cells as spheres. Adhesion between cells in contact is, however, best considered as interaction between planar surfaces (Fig. 6.46). Cell adhesion and separation occur during the interaction of sperm and egg, in cell fusion and in parasitism; phagocytosis may also have an adhesive component. Cell adhesion can occur with a variety of non-living materials such as implanted prosthetic devices.

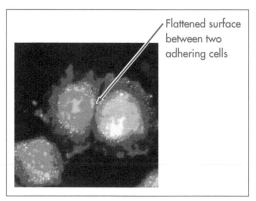

Flattened surface between two adhering cells

Figure 6.46 Interacting cells with a planar interface formed between them.
Photograph: J. Ivaska, Centre for Biotech, Finland.

Adhesion is primarily a surface phenomenon. The main factors that act to produce adhesion are:

- bridging mechanisms
- electrostatic interactions
- interactions involving long-range forces.

As in suspension flocculation, the bridging agent will be a molecule that combines in some way with both surfaces and thus links them together. Macromolecules may adsorb on to the surface of the particle and, if the length of the molecule is greater than twice the range of the electrostatic forces of repulsion, the other end of the molecule may adsorb on to a second surface. Flexible molecules may adsorb on to the same cell or particle. Alternatively, polyvalent ions may bind to charged groups on the two adjacent surfaces. Brownian motion may provide the means for close approach of the particles, or the polyvalent ion and may so reduce the electrostatic repulsion that the cells can approach each other.

Electrostatic forces of attraction will come into play when the surfaces have opposite sign or charge or

when the surfaces possess mosaics of charges such that interaction can occur. The long-range forces are those discussed earlier in the chapter. Low pH, high ionic strength and the presence of covalent cations all favour cell–cell adhesion.

It is not possible to discuss all cell–cell interactions rigorously from a purely physical point of view. Often adhesion results in the secretion of complex chemicals that further induce interaction that cannot be treated by any physicochemical model.

6.7.2 Adsorption of microbial cells to surfaces

The contamination of pharmaceutical suspensions for oral use can be a problem. Under some conditions, bacteria may be strongly adsorbed and therefore more resistant to the effects of preservatives. In other cases, the bacteria may be free in the liquid phase of the suspension.

Two distinct phases of bacterial adsorption on to glass have been observed[20]; the first, reversible, phase may be interpreted in terms of DLVO theory. Reversible sorption of a non-mobile strain (*Achromobacter*) decreased to zero as the electrolyte concentration of the medium was increased, as would be expected. The second, irreversible, phase is probably the result of polymeric bridging between bacterial cell and the surface in contact with it. It is obviously not easy to apply colloid theory directly, but the influence of factors such as surface potential, pH and additives can usually be predicted and experimentally confirmed.

In the agglutination of erythrocytes and the adsorption of erythrocytes to virus-infected cells,

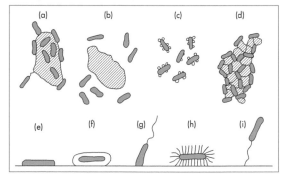

Figure 6.47 Various types of bacterial sorption on solid surfaces (see text).
Reproduced with permission from Zvyagintsev D. *Interaction between Micro-organisms and Solid Surfaces*. Moscow: Moscow University Press; 1973.

projections of small radius of curvature have been observed and could well account for the local penetration of the energy barrier and strong adhesion at the primary minimum. The various modes of cell sorption are shown diagrammatically in Fig. 6.47.

Sorption of microbial cells is selective but there is no obvious relation between Gram-staining characteristics and attachment. In Fig. 6.47, bacterial cells are shown adsorbing on to larger solid particles (a) or free in suspension (b); (c) illustrates the opposite effect – small particles are shown adsorbed on to bacterial cells. The bacterial cells are adsorbed on to flocculated particles in (d), on to solid surfaces in (e); (f)–(i) show the more complicated behaviour of bacterial forms with coats, cilia and flagella. The adsorption affects growth partly by masking the cell surface and partly by altering the release of metabolites from the cell.

In addition to the van der Waals and electrical forces, steric forces resulting from protruding polysaccharide and protein molecules affect interactions; specific interactions between charged groups on the cell surface and on the solid surface, hydrogen bonding or the formation of cellular bridges may all occur to complicate the picture.

6.7.3 Blood as a colloidal system

Blood is a non-Newtonian suspension showing a shear-dependent viscosity. At low rates of shear, erythrocytes form cylindrical aggregates (rouleaux), which break up when the rate of shear is increased. Calculations show that the shear rate (D) associated with blood flow in large vessels such as the aorta is about $100\ s^{-1}$, but for flow in capillaries it rises to about $1000\ s^{-1}$. The flow characteristics of blood are similar to those of emulsions except that, while shear deformation of oil globules can occur with a consequent change in surface tension, no change in membrane tension occurs on cell deformation.

Velocity gradients in blood vessels are reduced in cases of retarded peripheral circulation, especially in shock. Under these conditions erythrocytes may aggregate and the discovery of agents that are capable of reducing this structural viscosity is thus of great clinical value. Dextrans and polyvinylpyrrolidones diminish attraction between individual cells in blood and improve flow properties.

Aggregation of platelets involves a contact phase and an adhesive phase, shown diagrammatically in Fig. 6.48. Shearing effects of blood may dislodge platelets. Interest in platelet interaction with simpler surfaces has been stimulated by the increasing use of plastic prosthetic devices which come into contact with blood.

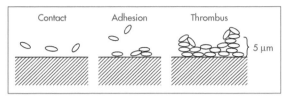

Figure 6.48 Sequence in the formation of a thrombus at a surface, involving three stages: contact, adhesion and thrombus growth.

While we do not have a clear idea of the physical and chemical properties of surfaces that are responsible for the attraction of platelets, a relationship between adhesion and the critical surface tension of uncharged hydrophobic surfaces has been demonstrated. The number of platelets adsorbed increases as the critical surface tension increases. There is other evidence that platelets adhere readily to high-energy hydrophilic surfaces and less readily to low-energy hydrophobic surfaces. Thus platelet adhesion to glass is reduced following coating of the latter with dimethylsiloxane.

6.8 Foams

Aqueous foams are formed from a three-dimensional network of surfactant films in air. They are disperse systems with a high surface area. Consequently, foams tend to collapse spontaneously. They can, however, if suitably stabilised, be used as formulations for the delivery of enemas and topical products. There are several parameters that contribute to the stability of foams:

- foam viscosity
- foam drainage rates
- foam deformation
- foam density
- foam structure.

There is a European Pharmacopoeia monograph on medicated foams. Relative foam density is an indication of foam 'firmness' and foam 'expansion time' which relates to the foamability of a formulation. The

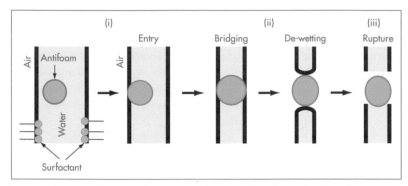

Figure 6.49 A schematic drawing of the antifoaming mechanism of antifoam droplets: (i) entering a foam lamella; (ii) bridging–de-wetting; and (iii) rupturing the foam wall.
Reproduced from Perry D *et al. Foam Control in Aqueous Coatings.* Midland, MI, USA: Dow Corning Corporation; 2001.

density of foams (FD) is measured by weighing a volume of foam compared to the same volume of water,

$$FD = [m(\text{foam}/m(\text{water})]$$

Foams that develop in production of liquids or in ampoules are troublesome, hence there is an interest in breaking foams and preventing foam formation. The breaking and prevention of liquid foams are less well understood than the stabilisation of foams. It is recognised, however, that small quantities of specific agents can reduce foam stability markedly. There are two types of such agent:

1. *foam breakers*, which are thought to act as small droplets forming in the foam lamellae (Fig. 6.49)
2. *foam preventatives*, which are thought to adsorb at the air–water interface in preference to the surfactants that stabilise the thin films. Once adsorbed they do not have the capacity to stabilise the foam.

It is well established that pure liquids do not foam. Transient foams are obtained with solutes such as short-chain aliphatic alcohols or acids that lower the surface tension moderately; really persistent foams arise only with solutes that lower the surface tension strongly in dilute solution – the highly surface-active materials such as detergents and proteins. The physical chemistry of the surface layers of the solutions is what determines the stability of the system.

Ordinarily, three-dimensional foams of surfactant solutes persist for a matter of hours in closed vessels. Gas slowly diffuses from the small bubbles to the large ones (since the pressure and hence thermodynamic activity of the gas within the bubbles are inversely proportional to bubble radius). Diffusion of gas leads to a rearrangement of the foam structures and this is often sufficient to rupture the thin lamellae in a well-drained film.

The most important action of an antifoam agent is to eliminate surface elasticity – the property that is responsible for the durability of foams. To do this it must displace foam stabiliser. It must therefore have a low interfacial tension in the pure state to allow it to spread when applied to the foam, and it must be present in sufficient quantity to maintain a high surface concentration. Many foams can be made to collapse by applying drops of liquids such as ether, or long-chain alcohols such as octanol. Addition of ether, which has a low surface tension, to an aqueous foam will locally produce regions with a low surface tension. These regions are rapidly pulled out by surrounding regions of higher tension. The foam breaks because the ethereal region cannot stretch. Long-chain alcohols also break foams because the surface is swamped by rapidly diffusing molecules so that changes in surface tension are rapidly reversed (that is, elasticity disappears).

Generally more effective and more versatile than any soluble antifoams are the silicone fluids, which have surface tensions as low as 20 mN m^{-1}. Quantities of the order of 1–60 ppm prevent foaming in fermentation vats, sewage tanks and dyebaths. Antifoam droplets are seen in Fig. 6.49 entering the foam lamella, bridging between the surfaces, de-wetting and then rupturing the foam wall.

Clinical point

X-ray studies have clearly shown the presence of foam in the upper gastrointestinal tract in humans. Silicone antifoaming agents derive their value from their ability to change the surface tension of the mucus-covered gas bubbles in the gut and thus to cause the bubbles to coalesce. A range of polydimethylsiloxanes is available commercially, including Dimethicone 20, 200, 350, 500 and 1000 (the numbers refer to the viscosity of the oil in centistokes). In simple *in vitro* tests, polydimethylsiloxane of molecular weight used in pharmaceutical formulations (Dimethicone 1000) has poor antifoaming properties. The addition of a small percentage (2–8%) of hydrophobic silica, which on its own is a weak defoamer, increases the antifoaming effect, the finely divided silica particles being suspended in the silicone fluid. The product is a simple physical mixture of silica and polydimethylsiloxane.

Some *in vivo* results are listed in Table 6.8. The incorporation of these materials into antacid tablets is widespread; certain antacids have been found, however, to adsorb the polydimethylsiloxane and reduce its antifoaming potential.[21]

Summary

This chapter has covered the topic of pharmaceutical colloids, with a special emphasis on emulsions and suspensions. These have been rather traditional pharmaceutical forms, but they are attracting increasing interest because of increased knowledge of the biodistribution and fate of colloidal particles in the body, and the need to deliver highly lipophilic and often very potent drugs in carriers. Emulsions, microemulsions and solid suspensions are all, therefore, important in modern drug delivery.

The chapter has dealt with the stability and stabilisation of colloidal systems and covered topics such as their formation and aggregation. If the particle size of a colloidal particle determines its properties (such as its viscosity or its fate in the body), then maintenance of that particle size throughout the lifetime of the product is important. The emphasis in the section on stability is therefore understandable. Various forms of emulsions, microemulsions and multiple emulsions have also been discussed, while other chapters deal with other important colloidal systems, such as protein and polymer micro- and nanospheres and phospholipid and surfactant vesicles. Suspensions also feature in processing technologies, as in the formation of granules and spherules where a powder–liquid mass is the basis for further processing. Some aspects of these systems are discussed and should be read in the light of

Table 6.8 *In vivo* effects of polydimethylsiloxane (PDMS)				
Treatment by mouth	**Volume (cm³)**	**Dose (mg/rat)**		**Mean percentage reduction[a] in foam height (± SEM)**
		PDMS	**Silica**	
PDMS	0.25	250		19 ± 4
	0.50	500		29 ± 6
	1.00	1000		56 ± 6
	2.00	2000		84 ± 3
PDMS containing 65 w/v silica	0.005	4.7	0.2	45 ± 6
	0.01	9.4	0.6	58 ± 5
	0.02	18.9	1.1	61 ± 5
	0.04	37.7	2.0	87 ± 2

Reproduced from Birtley RDN *et al. J Pharm Pharmacol* 1973;25:859.
[a] Ten rats in each group; foam induced by saponin.

an understanding of contact angles and solid-surface hydrophobicities.

Towards the end of the chapter we point out the biological importance of an understanding of colloid chemistry and several examples of biological importance are covered. Pharmaceutical and biological colloids are often very complex systems, but even so the fundamental principles can be applied to obtain an appreciation of the behaviour of systems such as blood, platelets and microorganisms when they come in contact with inert or biological surfaces. In simplifying the concepts here, we do not pretend that there are no other forces at work. It is nonetheless useful to think of complex systems in a straightforward physicochemical manner, as pointed out in the introduction to the book.

References

1. Gao X *et al*. Calculation of hydrophile–lipophile balance for polyethoxylated surfactants by group contribution method. *J Colloid Interface Sci* 2006;298:441–450.
2. Suitthimeathegorn O *et al*. Novel anhydrous emulsions: formulation as controlled release vehicles. *Int J Pharm* 2005;298:367–371.
3. Hoar TP, Schulman JT. Transparent water-in-oil dispersions: the oleopathic hydro-micelle. *Nature* 1943; 152:102–103.
4. Date AA, Nagarsenker MS. Parenteral microemulsions: an overview. *Int J Pharm* 2008;355:19–30.
5. Ansari MJ *et al*. Microemulsions as potential delivery systems: a review. *PDA J Pharm Sci Technol* 2008;62:66–79.
6. Kovarik JM *et al*. Cyclosporine pharmacokinetics and variability from a microemulsion formulation – a multicenter investigation in kidney transplant patients. *Transplantation* 1994;58:658–663.
7. Mueller EA *et al*. Improved dose linearity of cyclosporine pharmacokinetics from a microemulsion formulation. *Pharm Res* 1994;11:301–304.
8. Barry BW. Structure and rheology of emulsions stabilized by mixed emulsifiers. *Rheol Acta* 1971;10:96–105.
9. Nyman Y *et al*. Etomidate-Lipuro is associated with considerably less injection pain in children compared with propofol with added lidocaine. *Br J Anaesth* 2006;97:536–539.
10. Kam E *et al*. Comparison of propofol-Lipuro with propofol mixed with lidocaine 10 mg on propofol injection pain. *Anaesthesia* 2004;59:1167–1169.
11. Suttmann H *et al*, A new formulation of etomidate in lipid emulsion. Bioavailability and venous irritation. *Anaesthesist* 1989;38:421–423.
12. Gangineni K *et al*. Propofol and peanut allergy (letter). *Anaesthesia* 2007;62:1191.
13. Yamaguchi T *et al*. Distribution of prostaglandin E_1 in lipid emulsion in relation to release rate from lipid particles. *Chem Pharm Bull* 1994;42:446–450.
14. Kaplan A, Whelan M. (2012) The use of IV lipid emulsion for lipophilic drug toxicities. *J Am Anim Hosp Assoc* 2012;48:221–227.
15. Whateley TL *et al*. Particle size stability of Intralipid and mixed total parenteral nutrition mixtures. *J Clin Hosp Pharm* 1984;91:13–26.
16. Henderson NL *et al*. Approximate rates of shear encountered in some pharmaceutical processes. *J Pharm Sci* 1961;50:788–791.
17. Costello I *et al*. *Paediatric Drug Handling*. London: Pharmaceutical Press; 2007.
18. Schein LB. Recent progress and continuing puzzles in electrostatics. *Science* 2007;316:1572–1573.
19. Kwok PCL *et al*. Electrostatic charge characteristics of aerosols produced from metered dose inhalers. *J Pharm Sci* 2005;94:2789–2799.
20. Marshall KC *et al*. Mechanism of the initial events in the sorption of marine bacteria to surfaces. *J Gen Microbiol* 1971;68:337–348.
21. Rezak MJ. *In vitro* determination of deforming inactivation of silicone antacid tablets. *J Pharm Sci* 1966;55:538–539.

7

Polymers and macromolecules

This survey of the pharmaceutical aspects of polymers, copolymers and macromolecules emphasises their use in formulation but also deals with the uses of some polymers such as dextran in therapeutics. It stresses the key features of polymers – their molecular weight distribution and their versatility in terms of their molecular weight, morphology, crystallinity, solubility and performance.

It is convenient to think of polymeric systems as either water-soluble or water-insoluble. This division, while not rigid because some polymers are water-dispersible, is useful in that it separates the two main areas of use that form the basis of this chapter. Water-soluble materials can be used to modify the viscosity of aqueous solutions and to maintain the stability of suspensions, or to form the basis of film coatings and water-soluble matrices. The higher-molecular-weight polyoxyethylene glycols, for example, are used as suppository bases. Water-soluble polymers can be crosslinked electrostatically or covalently to give hydrogels. Crosslinked hydrogels absorb water but do not dissolve so possess intermediate properties. The differences in release of drugs from water-insoluble matrices and from swelling hydrogels should be appreciated.

Bioadhesives are usually water-soluble, while pressure-sensitive adhesives used in transdermal patches tend to be insoluble polyacrylates and polysiloxanes. Water-insoluble materials form membranes and matrices which form the basis of many sustained-release dosage forms. The factors affecting the transport of drugs in these systems should be understood: that is to say, the thickness of the membrane, the solubility of the drug in the membrane and the relationship of this to its lipophilicity generally, copolymer ratios, porosity and the heterogeneity of the mix caused by fillers or plasticisers.

A number of clinical applications of polymer solutions, gels and structures are also discussed as examples of the versatility of polymers, including the formulation of artificial tears, artificial saliva and synovial fluid supplements. This illustrates the relationship between the physical properties of polymers and their uses and performance in various roles as solutions, gels or solids.

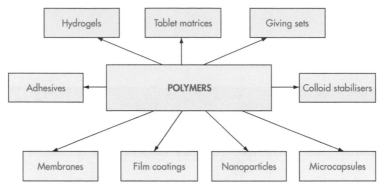

Scheme 7.1 The spectrum of uses for polymers in pharmaceutics

7.1 Pharmaceutical polymers

Natural polymers such as acacia and tragacanth have been used in pharmacy for many years. Mostly they have been replaced by synthetic polymers whose properties are more readily characterised and controlled.

A wide spectrum of polymers are used widely in pharmaceutical systems as suspending and emulsifying agents, flocculating agents, adhesives, packaging and coating materials, and increasingly as components of controlled and site-specific drug delivery systems (Scheme 7.1). The synthesis of polymers with specific properties (e.g. pH-dependent solubility or viscosity, biodegradability, membrane-forming character) offers exciting possibilities, especially as it holds out the hope of obtaining new polymers for drug delivery devices, so essential for the efficient use of many of today's potent and toxic drugs. Polymer biodegradability is an issue in some applications.

7.1.1 Definitions

Polymers are substances of high molecular weight made up of repeating *monomer* units. Substances with short chains containing relatively few monomers are called *oligomers*. Polymers owe their unique properties to their size, their three-dimensional shape and sometimes to their flexibility and asymmetry. The chemical reactivity of polymers depends on the chemistry of their monomer units, but their properties depend to a large extent on the way the monomers are assembled; it is this fact that leads to the versatility of synthetic polymers. Polymer molecules may be linear or branched, and separate linear or branched chains may be joined by crosslinks. Extensive crosslinking leads to a three-dimensional and often insol-

uble polymer network. Polymers in which all the monomeric units are identical are referred to as *homopolymers*; those formed from more than one monomer type are called *copolymers*. Various arrangements of the monomers A and B in the copolymer molecules (Fig. 7.1) can be produced with consequent

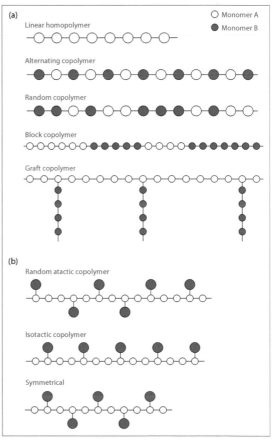

Figure 7.1 (a) Varieties of copolymer molecular structures attainable though the polymerisation of two different monomers represented by A and B. (b) Representations of random atactic, isotactic and symmetrical copolymers.

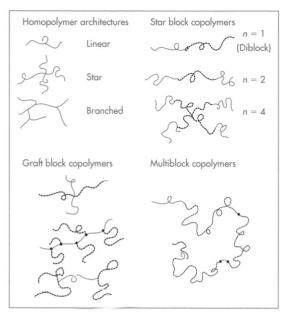

Figure 7.2 The range of structures of homopolymers and star block, graft block and multiblock copolymers.

effects on the physical properties of the resulting polymer. Synthetic polymers may have their main chains substituted in different ways, depending on the conditions of the reaction, such that atactic (random), isotactic or syndiotactic forms are produced, as diagrammatically represented in Fig. 7.1.

Copolymers may be described as alternating copolymers, block copolymers or graft copolymers. The molecular architecture of copolymers may, however, be more complicated than represented in Fig. 7.1. Block copolymers such as the polyoxyethylene–polyoxypropylene–polyoxyethylene (ABA) systems have both hydrophobic (A) and hydrophilic regions (B); they form an interesting group of surfactants and are discussed in Chapter 5. Homopolymers can be linear, star or branched (Fig. 7.2), giving rise to so-called star block copolymers defined by the number of arms (n).

Polymers that have fairly symmetrical chains and strong interchain forces can be drawn into fibres. *Plastics* are polymers with lower degrees of crystallinity that can be moulded. Further down the rigidity scale are *rubbers* and *elastomers*, whose properties are well known.

It is apparent that polymer molecules will have a much wider range of physical properties than small chemical entities. Even when considering one chemical type (for example, polyethylene), its properties may be altered by increasing or decreasing the molecular weight (Fig. 7.3). There is a degree of control over properties that is not present with small organic materials. It is because of this that synthetic polymers also have an advantage over many variable natural polymers, although many natural derivatives such as cellulosic derivatives are used extensively. Natural materials can be modified chemically, and this approach can lead to useful new products, as with those derived from cellulose or dextran. The structural formulae of some common macromolecules are given in Table 7.1.

Dendrimers are highly branched polymer constructs formed from a central core that defines their initial geometry.[1] Their branch-like structure (Fig. 7.4) leads to spheres, which in higher generations appear to be the size of micelles, and ultimately nanospheres of small dimensions. They can be functionalised and in this way 'layered' systems can be formed by using different monomers for succeeding reactions (generations); such chemical architecture has virtually no bounds.[2] Dendrons are partial dendrimers, usually having a branched structure coupled to a linear chain.

7.1.2 Polydispersity

Nearly all synthetic polymers, possibly with the exception of dendrimers and some low-molecular-weight systems, and naturally occurring macromolecular substances exist with a range of molecular weights; exceptions to this are proteins and natural polypeptides, each of which occurs with a single well-defined molecular weight. The molecular weight of a polymer

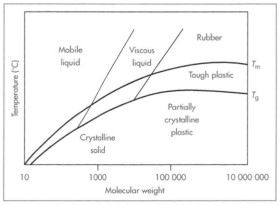

Figure 7.3 Approximate relation between molecular weight, glass transition temperature (T_g), melting point (T_m) and polymer properties.

Reproduced from Billmeyer FW. *Textbook of Polymer Science*, 2nd edn. New York: Wiley; 1971.

Table 7.1 Structural formulae of some macromolecular compounds

Name	Chain structure	Monomer
Polymers with a carbon chain backbone		
Polyethylene	$-CH_2-CH_2-CH_2-CH_2-CH_2-$	$CH_2=CH_2$
Polypropylene	$-CH_2-CH-CH_2-CH-CH_2-CH-CH_2-$ with CH_3 substituents	$CH_2=CH-CH_3$
Polystyrene	$-CH_2-CH-CH_2-CH-CH_2-CH-CH_2-$ with phenyl substituents	$CH=CH_2$ with phenyl
Poly(vinyl chloride)	$-CH_2-CH-CH_2-CH-CH_2-CH-CH_2-$ with Cl substituents	$CH_2=CH-Cl$
Polytetrafluoroethylene	$-C-C-C-C-C-C-$ with F substituents	$F_2C=CF_2$
Polyacrylonitrile	$-CH_2-CH-CH_2-CH-CH_2-CH-CH_2-$ with CN substituents	$CH_2=CH-CN$
Poly(vinyl alcohol)	$-CH_2-CH-CH_2-CH-CH_2-CH-CH_2-$ with HO substituents	$CH_2=CH-OH$
Poly(vinyl acetate)	$-CH_2-CH-CH_2-CH-CH_2-CH-CH_2-$ with $O-C=O-CH_3$ substituents	$CH_2=CH-O-C=O-CH_3$
Polyacrylamide	$-CH_2-CH-CH_2-CH-CH_2-CH-CH_2-$ with $CONH_2$ substituents	$CH_2=CH-O=C-NH_2$
Poly(methyl methacrylate)	$-CH_2-C-CH_2-C-CH_2-C-CH_2-$ with CH_3 and $COOCH_3$ substituents	$CH_2=C-CH_3-COOCH_3$
Polyvinylpyrrolidone	$-CH_2-CH-CH_2-CH-CH_2-CH-CH_2-$ with pyrrolidone substituents	$CH_2=CH$ with pyrrolidone
Polymers with a heterochain backbone		
Poly(ethylene oxide)	$-O-CH_2-CH_2-O-CH_2-CH_2-O-CH_2-CH_2-O-$	CH_2-CH_2 epoxide (with O)

Table 7.1 *(continued)*

Name	Chain structure	Monomer
Poly(propylene oxide)		
Cellulose (polyglucoside, β → 1,4)		Glucose
Chitosan		
Amylose (polyglucoside, α → 1,4) (component of starch)		Glucose
Pectinic acid (polygalacturonoside, α → 1,4) (jelly-forming component of fruits)		Galacturonic acid
Polyethylene glycol terephthalate		
Polydimethylsiloxane		

or macromolecule is thus an average molecular weight, which may be determined by chemical analysis or by osmotic pressure or light-scattering measurements. When determined by chemical analysis or osmotic pressure measurement a *number-average molecular weight*, M_n, is found, which in a mixture containing n_1, n_2, n_3, ... moles of polymer with molecular weights M_1, M_2, M_3, ..., respectively, is defined by

$$M_n = \frac{n_1M_1 + n_2M_2 + n_3M_3 + \cdots}{n_1 + n_2 + n_3 + \cdots}$$
$$= \frac{\Sigma n_i M_i}{\Sigma n_i} \qquad (7.1)$$

The individual molecular weights M_1, M_2, ... cannot be determined separately – the equation merely explains the meaning of the value M_n.

In light-scattering techniques, larger molecules produce greater scattering; thus the weight (or, more strictly, the mass) rather than the number of the molecules is important, giving a *weight-average molecular weight*, M_w:

$$M_w = \frac{m_1M_1 + m_2M_2 + m_3M_3 + \cdots}{m_1 + m_2 + m_3 + \cdots}$$
$$= \frac{\Sigma n_i M_i^2}{\Sigma n_i M_i} \qquad (7.2)$$

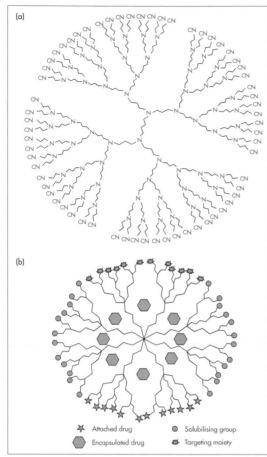

Figure 7.4 (a) A two-dimensional view of a dendrimer with 64 cyano functional groups. It is possible to trap small to medium-size molecules in dendrimers that have pores of appropriate dimensions between the branches of the structure. (b) A diagrammatic representation of possible sites for covalent attachment of drugs, solubilising groups and targeting moieties, and encapsulation of drugs.

(a) Reprinted by permission from Macmillan Publishers Ltd: *Nature*. Gibson HW. Architectural delights. *Nature* 1994;371:106, copyright 1994.

In equation (7.2) m_1, m_2, m_3, ... are the masses of each species, and m_i is obtained by multiplying the molecular weight of each species by the number of molecules of that weight; that is, $m_i = n_i M_i$. Thus the molecular weight appears as the square in the numerator of equation (7.2); the weight-average molecular weight is therefore biased towards larger molecules. Another consequence is that $M_w > M_n$; that is, the average molecular weight of a polymer measured by light scattering must be greater than that obtained by osmotic pressure measurements if the polymer is polydisperse (that is, contains a range of molecular weights). The ratio M_w/M_n expresses the degree of

Table 7.2 Number- and weight-average molecular weights for dextran fractions

Fraction	M_n	M_w	M_w/M_n
A	41 000	47 000	1.14
B	38 000	50 000	1.31
C	64 000	76 000	1.18
D	95 000	170 000	1.79
E	240 000	540 000	2.25

Reproduced from Wales M *et al*. Intrinsic viscosity-molecular weight relationships for dextran. *J Polymer Sci* 1953;10:229. Copyright Wiley-VCH Verlag GmbH & Co. KGaA. Reproduced with permission.

polydispersity. Table 7.2 shows actual values for the number-average and weight-average molecular weights for dextrans, microbial polysaccharides used therapeutically as plasma expanders.

7.1.3 Polymer mixtures or blends

Of course not all polymers are soluble or miscible with each other; some indeed de-mix when added together. The different phase behaviours that are realised with representative molecular architectures are shown in Fig. 7.5. Such mixtures produce solid polymeric structures such as films and membranes with distinctive morphologies and properties. When polymer blends are used as drug delivery matrices or as the basis of micro- and nanoparticles, it is important that polymer–polymer interactions are studied.

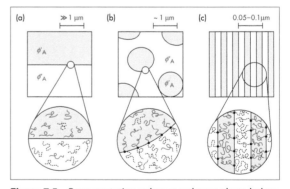

Figure 7.5 Representative polymer–polymer phase behaviour with different molecular architectures. Microphase separation (a) results when thermodynamically incompatible linear homopolymers are mixed. The covalent bond between blocks in a diblock copolymer leads to microphase segregation (c). A mixed architecture of linear homopolymers and the corresponding diblock copolymer produces a surfactant-like stabilised intermediate-scale phase separation (b).

7.1.4 Polymer solubility

The solubility of polymeric substances in water is determined by the same considerations that apply to smaller molecules. Those polymers that are sufficiently polar will be able to interact with the water to provide energy to remove individual polymer chains from the solid state.

Water-soluble polymers have an ability to increase the viscosity of solvents at low concentrations, to swell or change shape in solution, and to adsorb at surfaces. These are significant features of their behaviour, which we will deal with briefly.

Insoluble polymers or polymers with a low rate of solution are used more to form thin films, as film-coating materials, surgical dressings or membranes for dialysis or filtration, or to form matrices for envelop-

ing drugs to control their release properties, or simply as packaging materials.

Figure 7.6 illustrates the variety of morphologies that polymeric systems can adopt depending on the nature of the solvent, the polymer concentration and the nature of the polymer itself. Such diversity explains the wide range of uses in pharmacy and medicine.

Key points

- Polymers are substances of high molecular weight made up of repeating *monomer* units; they may be linear or branched, and separate linear or branched chains may be joined by crosslinks. Extensive crosslinking leads to a three-dimensional and often insoluble polymer network.

- Polymers in which all the monomeric units are identical are referred to as *homopolymers*; those formed from more than one monomer type are called *copolymers*. Homopolymers can be linear, star or branched; copolymers may be alternating copolymers, block copolymers or graft copolymers. *Dendrimers* are highly branched polymer constructs formed from a central spherical or quasi-spherical core.

- There is usually a range of sizes of the polymer chains in solution, i.e. the polymer solutions are *polydisperse*. As a consequence, the measured molecular weight varies depending on the experimental method used: techniques such as light scattering are more influenced by the larger molecules and give a *weight-average* molecular weight; others such as chemical analysis and osmometry give a *number-average* molecular weight.

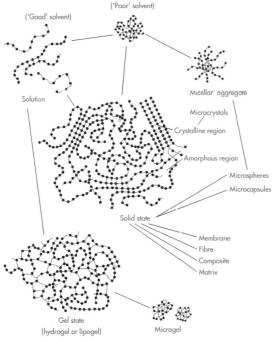

Figure 7.6. Representation of the variety of polymer morphologies in solution and in the gel (or microgel) or solid states. In solution the conformation of the polymer depends on the nature of polymer–solvent interactions and whether or not the polymer chains associate to form micellar aggregates. Crystals of polymer and microcrystals can be prepared, and gels can be formed from covalently crosslinked chains or polymer chains associated by hydrogen bonding or hydrophobic interactions. Listed are the forms in which most polymers can be fabricated: membranes, fibres, composites, matrices; microspheres and microcapsules can also feature, as discussed later in this chapter.

7.2 Water-soluble polymers

The rate of solution of a water-soluble polymer depends on its molecular weight: the larger the molecule, the stronger are the forces holding the chains together. More energy has to be expended to force the chains apart in the solvent. The greater the degree of crystallinity of the polymer, the lower the rate of solution.

The velocity of penetration (S) of a solvent into the bulk polymer obeys the relationship

$$S = kM^{-A} \tag{7.3}$$

where M is the polymer molecular weight, k and A being constants. The dissolution process, however, is more complicated than with ordinary crystalline materials. It is frequently observed that swollen layers and gel layers form next to the polymer (Fig. 7.7). If a drug is embedded in the polymer, the drug has to diffuse through these gel layers and finally through the diffusion layer.

It is the combination of slow solution rate and the formation of viscous surface layers that makes hydrophilic polymers useful in controlling the release rate of soluble drugs (see section 7.5). Choice of appropriate polymer molecular weight controls both the rate of dissolution and the viscosity of its resulting solution. A balance between rate of polymer solution and viscosity of the solution layer must be achieved in controlled-release systems. If the polymer solution rate is too slow, then soluble drug is leached out with little retardation.

The bulk viscosity of polymer solution is an important parameter also when polymers are being used as suspending agents to maintain solid particles in suspension by prevention of settling (see Chapter 6)

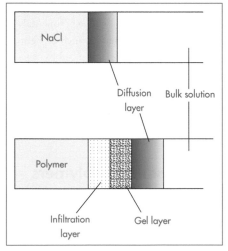

Figure 7.7 Penetration of solvent into (top) soluble crystalline material and (bottom) polymer compared.

and when they are used to modify the properties of liquid medicines for oral and topical use.

7.3 General properties of polymer solutions

7.3.1 Viscosity of polymer solutions

The rheology of colloidal solutions and suspensions has been discussed in Chapter 6. Here we consider the particular use of viscosity measurements to determine the average molecular weights and asymmetry of polymeric molecules.

The presence in solution of large macromolecular solutes has an appreciable effect on the viscosity of the solution. From a study of the viscosity as a function of polymer concentration it is possible to gain information on the shape or hydration of these polymers in solution and also their average molecular weight. The assumption is made in this section that the solution exhibits Newtonian flow characteristics.

As discussed in Chapter 6 (section 6.3), the viscosity of solutions of macromolecules is conveniently expressed by the *relative viscosity*, η_{rel}, defined as the ratio of the viscosity of the solution, η, to the viscosity of the pure solvent η_0; the *specific viscosity*, η_{sp}, defined as $\eta_{rel} - 1$; and the *reduced viscosity* η_{sp}/ϕ (where ϕ is the volume fraction, defined as the volume of the particles divided by the total volume of the solution). The ratio η_{sp}/ϕ for *ideal* solutions is independent of solution concentration. In *real* solutions the reduced viscosity varies with concentration owing to molecular interactions so it is usual to extrapolate plots of η_{sp}/ϕ versus ϕ to zero volume fraction. The extrapolated value is called the *intrinsic viscosity* $[\eta]$.

Einstein showed from hydrodynamic theory that for a dilute system of rigid, spherical particles

$$\eta_{rel} = 1 + 2.5\phi \tag{7.4}$$

i.e.

$$\lim_{\phi \to 0}(\eta_{sp}/\phi) = 2.5 \tag{7.5}$$

where ϕ is the volume fraction of the particles, defined as the volume of the particles divided by the total volume of the solution. In other words, the intrinsic viscosity $[\eta]$ of this ideal system is 2.5.

For polymers of high molecular weight, the value of η_{sp}/ϕ varies with solution concentration (which is directly related to ϕ). The concentration dependence is often expressed as

$$\eta_{sp}/c = [\eta] + k[\eta]^2 c \tag{7.6}$$

where k is a constant referred to as the Huggins' constant. At moderate concentrations a plot of η_{sp}/c against c is linear with a gradient equal to k. The value of this constant provides a useful indication of the extent of interaction between the polymer and the solvent; for flexible polymer molecules in a 'good' solvent (see below) k often has a value of approximately 0.35.

Departure of the limiting value of η_{sp}/ϕ from the theoretical value of 2.5 may result from either hydration of the particles, or from particle asymmetry, or from both.

A more general form of equation (7.4) allowing for *particle asymmetry* is

$$\eta_{rel} = 1 + \nu\phi \tag{7.7}$$

where the intrinsic viscosity $[\eta]$ is replaced by a shape factor ν related to the axial ratio of an ellipsoid. In the case of non-hydrated spheres ν reduces to 2.5.

The volume fraction is usually replaced by the weight concentration, c. For a macromolecule of hydrodynamic volume ν_h and molecular weight M, $\phi = c \, N_A \nu_h / M$ where N_A is the Avogadro constant.

Macromolecules are frequently hydrated, not only with chemically bound water but also with physically entrapped solvent. These two types of water have differing properties; the specific volume ν_0 (volume per gram) of the entrapped water may be considerably different from that of pure solvent, $\nu_1^{\ominus}$. The intrinsic viscosity of the *hydrated* macromolecule may be written as

$$[\eta] = \lim_{c \to 0}\left(\frac{\eta_{rel} - 1}{c}\right) = \nu(\bar{v}_2 + \partial_1 \nu_1^{\ominus}) \tag{7.8}$$

where ∂_1 is the number of grams of solvent per gram of dry macromolecular material and $\bar{v}_2$ is its partial specific volume.

If the particle can be assumed to be unhydrated, or if the degree of hydration can be estimated with certainty from other experimental techniques, equation (7.8) may be used to determine the asymmetry of the particle. Alternatively, if the macromolecule may be assumed to be symmetrical or its asymmetry is known from other techniques, then this equation may be used to estimate the extent of hydration of the macromolecule.

Shape and solvent effects

As the shape of molecules is to a large extent the determinant of flow properties, change in shape due to changes in polymer–solvent interactions and the binding of small molecules with the polymer may lead to significant changes in solution viscosity. The nature of the solvent is thus of prime importance in this regard. In so-called 'good' solvents, linear macromolecules will be expanded as the polar groups will be solvated. In a 'poor' solvent, the intramolecular attraction between the segments is greater than the segment–solvent affinity and the molecule will tend to coil up (Fig. 7.6). The viscosity of ionised macromolecules is complicated by charge interactions that vary with polymer concentration and additive concentration. Flexible charged macromolecules will vary in shape with the degree of ionisation. At maximum ionisation they are stretched out owing to mutual charge repulsion and the viscosity increases. On addition of small counterions, the effective charge is reduced and the molecules contract; the viscosity falls as a result. Some of the effects are illustrated later in this chapter in discussion of individual macromolecules.

The viscosity of solutions of globular proteins (which are more or less rigid) is only slightly affected by change in ionic strength. The intrinsic viscosity of serum albumin varies only between 3.6 and 4.1 cm^3 g^{-1} when the pH is varied between 4.3 and 10.5 and the ionic strength between zero and 0.50.

Viscosity in pharmacopoeial specifications

In cases where control of molecular weight is important, for example in the use of dextran fractions as plasma expanders,[3] a viscosity method is specified, for example, in the BP monograph. Staudinger proposed that the reduced viscosity of solutions of linear high polymers is proportional to the molecular weight of the polymer or its degree of polymerisation, p:

$$\frac{\eta_{sp}}{c} = K_m p \tag{7.9}$$

This empirical law has been modified to

$$\lim_{c \to 0} \frac{\eta_{sp}}{c} = [\eta] = KM^a \qquad (7.10)$$

where a is a constant in the range 0–2, which for most high polymers has a value between 0.6 and 0.8, $[\eta]$ is the intrinsic viscosity as defined previously, and M is the molecular weight of the polymer. Equation (7.10) is often referred to as the Mark–Houwink equation. For a given polymer–solvent system, K and a are constant. Values of these constants may be determined from measurements on a series of fractions of known molecular weight and hence the molecular weight of an unknown fraction can be determined by measurement of the intrinsic viscosity. The *viscosity-average molecular weight* is essentially a weight-average since the larger macromolecules influence viscosity more than the smaller ones. The intrinsic viscosity of Dextran 40 BP is stated to be not less than 16 cm³ g⁻¹ and not more than 20 cm³ g⁻¹ at 37°C, while that of Dextran 110 is not less than 27 cm³ g⁻¹ and not more than 32 cm³ g⁻¹.

 Key points

- Assuming that the polymer solution exhibits Newtonian flow properties, its viscosity can be expressed by:
  - the *relative viscosity*, η_{rel}, defined as the ratio of the viscosity of the solution, η, to the viscosity of the pure solvent η_0, i.e. $\eta_{rel} = \eta/\eta_0$
  - the *specific viscosity*, η_{sp}, of the solution defined by $\eta_{sp} = \eta_{rel} - 1$
  - the *intrinsic viscosity* $[\eta]$ obtained by extrapolation of plots of the ratio η_{sp} / c (called the *reduced viscosity*) against concentration c to zero concentration.
- If the polymer forms spherical particles in dilute solution then a plot of η_{sp}/ϕ against ϕ (the volume fraction) should have an intercept of 2.5; departure of the limiting value from this theoretical value may result from either hydration of the particles, or particle asymmetry, or both.

- A change in shape due to changes in polymer–solvent interactions and the binding of small molecules may lead to significant changes in solution viscosity. In 'good' solvents, linear macromolecules will be expanded as the polar groups will be solvated; in 'poor' solvents, the intramolecular attraction between the segments is greater than the segment–solvent affinity and the molecule will tend to coil up. Flexible charged macromolecules will vary in shape with the degree of ionisation.
- The intrinsic viscosity of solutions of linear high-molecular-weight polymers is proportional to the molecular weight M of the polymer as given by the *Mark–Houwink equation*, which may be used in the determination of the molecular weights of, for example, dextran fractions used as plasma expanders.

7.3.2 Gel formation

Concentrated polymer solutions frequently exhibit a very high viscosity because of the interaction of polymer chains in a three-dimensional fashion in the bulk solvent. These viscous crosslinked systems are termed *gels*. A gel is a polymer-solvent system containing a three-dimensional network of quite stable bonds that are almost unaffected by thermal motion. If such a polymer network is surrounded by the solvent (the system can be arrived at by swelling of solid polymer or by reduction in the solubility of the polymer in the solution) the system is a gel regardless of whether the network is formed by chemical or physical bonds. When gels are formed from solutions, each system is characterised by a critical concentration of gelation below which a gel is not formed. This concentration is determined by the hydrophile–lipophile balance of the polymer and the degree of regularity of the structure, by polymer–solvent interaction, by molecular weight and by the flexibility of the chain: the more flexible the molecule, the higher is the critical gelling concentration. The characteristic features of a gel include the considerable increase in viscosity above the gel point, the appearance of a rubber-like elasticity and, at higher polymer concentrations, a yield point stress. Under small stress the gel should retain its shape, but considerable deformation can occur at higher stress.

Type I and type II gels

Gels can be categorised into two groups, depending on the nature of the bonds between the chains of the network. Gels of type I are irreversible systems with a three-dimensional network formed by covalent bonds between the macromolecules. They include swollen networks, which have been formed by polymerisation of a monomer in the presence of a crosslinking agent.

Type II gels are heat-reversible, being held together by intermolecular bonds such as hydrogen bonds. Sometimes bridging by additive molecules can take place in these type II systems. Poly(vinyl alcohol) solutions gel on cooling below a temperature known as the gel point. The gel point can therefore be influenced by the presence of additives that can induce gel formation by acting as bridge molecules, as, for example, with borax and poly(vinyl alcohol). The gel point of polymers can also be increased or decreased by the addition of solvents that alter the polymer's affinity for the solvent (Table 7.3).

Table 7.3 Gel points of 10% poly(vinyl alcohol)

Solvent	Gel point (°C)
Water	14
Glycerol	64
Ethylene glycol	102

Reproduced from Pritchard JG. *Poly(vinyl alcohol): Basic Properties and Uses.* London: Macdonald; 1970.

Solutions of vinyl alcohol polymers in water are viscous mucilages that resemble those formed by methylcellulose; the viscosity of the mucilage is greatly increased by incorporating sodium perborate or silicate. Because of their gelling properties poly(vinyl alcohol) solutions are used as jellies for application of drugs to the skin. On application, the gel dries rapidly, leaving a plastic film with the drug in intimate contact with the skin. Plastic Film (Canadian Pharmacopoeia) is prepared from poly(vinyl alcohol) and other additives and is intended as a vehicle for acriflavine, benzocaine, ichthammol and other topical drugs.

Depending on the polymer, gelation can occur either with a fall or a rise in the temperature.

Crosslinked polymeric systems

If water-soluble polymer chains are covalently crosslinked, gels will be formed when the dry material interacts with water. The polymer swells in water but cannot dissolve as the crosslinks are stable. This expansion on contact with water has been put to many uses, such as in the fabrication of expanding implants from crosslinked hydrophilic polymers that imbibe body fluids and swell to a predetermined volume. These materials, such as the poly(hydroxyethyl methacrylate)s (poly(HEMA)s), are insoluble and chemically stable because of their three-dimensional structure (I and II) and do not dissolve. Implanted in the dehydrated state, these polymers swell to fill a body cavity or to give form to surrounding tissues. The gels may be used as vehicles for antibiotics, permitting protracted release of drug in the immediate environment of the implant. Antibiotic-loaded gels like this have been used in infections of the middle ear and other sites not readily reached by other methods of administration. Surgical suture material coated with antibiotic-containing hydrophilic gels acquires a chemotherapeutic role as the development of spread of infection along the suture fibre is prevented.

Structure I Poly(HEMA) crosslinked with ethylene glycol dimethacrylate (EGDMA)

Hydrophilic contact lenses (such as Soflens) are made from crosslinked poly(2-hydroxyethyl methacrylates). The emphasis in their development has been on their permeability to oxygen. They have also been used as reservoirs for drug delivery to the corneal surface. Conventional eye drop medication (see Chapter 9) has been modified over the years through the addition to formulations of a variety of viscosity-enhancing agents, polymers such as hydroxypropylmethylcellulose (HPMC), poly(vinyl alcohol) and silicones. These all prolong contact of drug with the cornea by increasing

$$
\begin{array}{ccc}
CH_3 & & CH_3 \\
| & & | \\
C-CH_2-CH-CH_2-C \\
| & | & | \\
C=O & C=O & C=O \\
| & | & | \\
O & NH & O \\
| & | & | \\
(CH_2)_2OH & CH_2 & (CH_2)_2OH \\
& | & \\
& NH & \\
CH_3 & | & CH_3 \\
| & C=O & | \\
CH_2-C-CH_2-CH-CH_2-C- \\
| & | \\
C=O & C=O \\
| & | \\
O & O \\
| & | \\
(CH_2)_2OH & (CH_2)_2OH
\end{array}
$$

Structure II Poly(HEMA) crosslinked with *N*, *N*′-methylene-bisacrylamide (BIS)

the viscosity of the medium and retarding the drainage of the tear fluid from the eye via the punctae.

Heterogels

As it is possible to produce macromolecular chains with segments that have different solubilities in a given solvent (copolymers), one would expect that concentrated solutions of such copolymers would behave in a manner different from that of a simple polymer. In block copolymers of the type AAABBBAAA, in which A is water-soluble and B is water-insoluble, the insoluble parts will tend to aggregate. If, for instance, a polystyrene–poly(oxyethylene) copolymer, comprising 41% polystyrene and 59% poly(oxyethylene), is dissolved at 80°C in butyl phthalate (a good solvent for polystyrene), a gel with a microscopic layer structure is formed at room temperature; in nitromethane the form

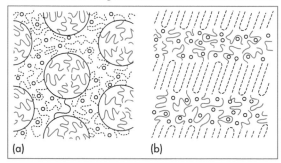

Figure 7.8 Structure of a copolymer of type A–B made from polystyrene and polyoxyethylene (a) in nitromethane (cylindrical structure) and (b) in butyl phthalate (layer structure). Nitromethane dissolves the poly(oxyethylene) part preferentially, but butyl phthalate dissolves the polystyrene part. (———) Polystyrene; (– – –), poly(oxyethylene); (○) solvent.

Reproduced with permission from Sadron F. *Angew Chem* 1963;2:248.

is somewhat different (Fig. 7.8a) as the nitromethane preferentially dissolves the poly(oxyethylene) chains.

Poly(oxyethylene)–poly(oxypropylene)–poly(oxyethylene) block copolymers, known commercially as Pluronic or poloxamer surfactants, are used as emulsifiers. Some form micellar aggregates in aqueous solutions above a critical micelle concentration, in which the hydrophobic central block associates with other like blocks, leaving the hydrophilic poly(oxyethylene) chains to the outside and protecting the inner core. Packing of these micelles in solution of high concentration leads to the reversible formation of gels, as shown in Fig. 7.9.

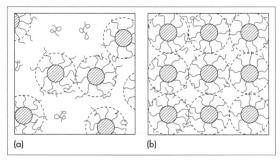

Figure 7.9 ABA-type copolymers: (a) micelles in dilute solution; (b) formation of a cubic-phase gel, by packing of micelles.

Syneresis

Syneresis is the term used for the separation of liquid from a swollen gel. Syneresis is thus a form of instability in aqueous and non-aqueous gels. Separation of a solvent phase is thought to occur because of the elastic contraction of the polymeric molecules; in the swelling process during gel formation, the macromolecules involved become stretched and the elastic forces increase as swelling proceeds. At equilibrium, the restoring force of the macromolecules is balanced by the swelling forces, determined by the osmotic pressure. If the osmotic pressure decreases, as on cooling, water may be squeezed out of the gel.

7.3.3 Polymer complexes

The varied structure and chemistry of polymers provide ample opportunity for complexes to form in solution. One example occurs when an aqueous solution of high-molecular-weight polyacids is mixed with polyglycols. The viscosity and pH of the solution of the equimolar mixture of polyacid and glycol remain the same with the increase in oligomer chain length up to a

Key points

- A gel is a polymer–solvent system containing a three-dimensional network that can be formed by swelling of solid polymer or by reduction in the solubility of the polymer in the solution.
- When gels are formed from solutions, each system is characterised by a critical concentration of gelation below which a gel is not formed.
- Gelation is characterised by a large increase in viscosity above the gel point, the appearance of a rubber-like elasticity and a yield point stress at higher polymer concentrations.
- Gels can be *irreversible* or *reversible* systems depending on the nature of the bonds between the chains of the network. Gels of *type I* are irreversible systems with a three-dimensional network formed by covalent bonds between the macromolecules (e.g. poly(HEMA) crosslinked with EGDMA); these polymers swell in water but cannot dissolve as the crosslinks are stable. *Type II* gels are heat-reversible, being held together by intermolecular bonds such as hydrogen bonds; gelation can be induced either by cooling (e.g. poly(vinyl alcohol)) or heating (e.g. water-soluble methylcelluloses) to the gel point. Solutions of some poly(oxyethylene)–poly(oxypropylene)–poly(oxyethylene) block copolymers form reversible gels by the close packing of their micelles when concentrated solutions are warmed.
- Swollen gels may exhibit *syneresis*, which is the separation of solvent phase from the gel.

critical point. The nature of the interaction is shown in (**III**); this occurs only when the polyethylene glycol molecules have reached a certain size.

Structure III Polycomplex formed by interaction of poly-acid and polyoxyethylene glycol

Such macromolecular reactions are highly selective and strongly dependent on molecular size and conformation. On mixing, some of the macromolecules might be involved in the complex while the rest will be free. The reason for compositional heterogeneity of the products could be the conformational transitions of macromolecules in the course of complex formation.

Interactions between macromolecules can occur in formulations, for example, when preparations are mixed. They can be put to good advantage in the synthesis of novel compounds. Polyethyleneimine and poly(acrylic acid) form a polyelectrolyte complex with salt-like bonds, as shown in (**IV**). If the complex is heated as a film, interchain amide bonds are formed

between the groups that formed electrostatic links. The non-ionised —COOH and —NH groups in the chain are the points of structural defects in the film.

Structure IV Complex formation between polyethyleneimine and poly(acrylic acid)

7.3.4 Binding of ions to macromolecules

Calcium is coordinated between certain uronic acid-containing polysaccharides (**V**), which can explain the tight binding of calcium and other multivalent ions in polysaccharide structures, and also how bivalent ions can induce gel formation in acidic polysaccharides such as alginic acid solutions.

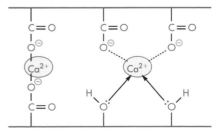

Structure V Calcium complexed in polysaccharides

It has been found that such interactions have dietary significance.

Clinical point

Dietary fibre from plants binds calcium in proportion to its uronic acid content. This binding by the non-cellulosic fraction of fibre reduces the availability of calcium for small-intestinal absorption, although colonic digestion of uronic acids liberates the calcium.[4] The pH dependence of the binding strongly suggests the involvement of carboxylic acid groups. Where daily fibre intakes vary between 50 and 150 g, with perhaps 30–110 mmol uronic acid, the binding capacity of fibre may exceed the total intake of calcium, which may be less than 20 mmol (800 mg) per day.

7.3.5 Interaction of polymers with solvents including water

As a consequence of their size, polymers interact with solvents in a more complex fashion than do smaller crystalline solutes. A given polymer may have no saturation solubility; it usually either dissolves completely or is only swollen by a given liquid. If the polymer is crosslinked, solution cannot occur and the polymer will only swell by imbibition of liquid to form a gel. Swelling decreases as the degree of crosslinking increases. Swelling is also a function of the solubility parameter of the liquid phase, and if the polymer is ionic, swelling will be dependent on the ionic strength of the solution, as shown in Fig. 7.10 for crosslinked hyaluronic acid (HA) gels. Increasing ionic strength decreases the repulsion between the chains and allows the polymer to shrink.

Highly polar polymers like poly(vinyl chloride) and some cellulose derivatives require polar liquids as solvents, in which dipole interactions or hydrogen bonding between polymer and solvent molecules occur. However, solvation does not necessarily lead to solution because the liquid, if it is to act as a solvent, must dissolve the solvated polymer. This process may be very slow because of the high viscosity of the partially solvated system.

Swelling of hydrogels and drug release

The relative mobility of a drug diffusing in the swelling hydrogel is given by the *swelling interface number*, Sw defined as

$$Sw = \frac{v \cdot \delta(t)}{D} \tag{7.11}$$

where v is the velocity of the moving front, $\delta(t)$ is the thickness of the rubbery layer (the infiltration and gel

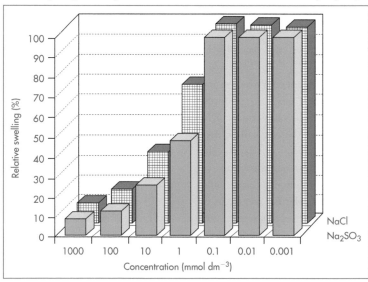

Figure 7.10 Relative swelling of hyaluronic acid hydrogels in different concentrations of NaCl and Na$_2$SO$_3$ solutions.

Reproduced from Tomer R *et al.* Electrically controlled release of macromolecules from cross-linked hyaluronic acid hydrogels. *J Control Release* 1995;33:405. Copyright Elsevier 1995.

layers represented in Fig. 7.7) at time t and D is the diffusion coefficient of the drug in the matrix.[5] When Sw $\gg$ 1, Fickian drug diffusion predominates, whereas when Sw $\ll$ 1, zero-order release kinetics are observed. The amount of drug released from a thin slab is expressed as an exponential:

$$\frac{M_t}{M_\infty} = kt^n \tag{7.12}$$

n varying from -0.5 to >1.0 where M_t/M_∞ is the fraction of drug and k is a constant.

It has been seen in Chapter 6 that the use of macromolecules as dispersion stabilisers depends in part on the osmotic forces arising from the interaction of solvated polymer chains as neighbouring particles approach (see Fig. 6.7). It is thus important to know how factors such as temperature and additives affect this interaction. Flory has given the free energy of dilution (the opposite process to the concentration effect discussed in section 6.2) as

$$\Delta G_1 = RT(k_1 - \psi_1)\phi_2 \tag{7.13}$$

where ϕ_2 is the volume fraction of polymer, and k_1 and ψ_1 are heat and entropy parameters, respectively.

It is sometimes convenient to define the temperature at which a polymer of infinite molecular weight just becomes insoluble in a given solvent; this temperature is the *Flory temperature* or *theta temperature*, θ, which may also be defined by

$$\theta = \frac{k_1 T}{\psi_1} \tag{7.14}$$

so that substituting in equation (7.13) we obtain the relationship between ΔG_1 and temperature:

$$\Delta G_1 = -RT\psi_1\left(1 - \frac{\theta}{T}\right)\phi_2 \tag{7.15}$$

ΔG_1 is therefore zero at the theta temperature when deviations from ideality vanish, that is, there are no polymer–polymer or polymer–solvent interactions. When $T = \theta$ there can thus be no stabilisation as molecules will interpenetrate without net interaction and will exert no forces on each other.

Not only do most linear polysaccharides tend to form spirals in solution, but in their tendency to associate they may form double helices, as does carrageenan, for instance. Under certain conditions of concentration and temperature the double helices may associate, forming gels. Possibilities exist for complex gel formation as with carrageenan, or of xanthan gum with locust bean gum. The locust bean gum molecule can associate over part of its length with the helix of xanthan, for example, while the other part of the molecule associates with another xanthan molecule, thereby acting as a bridging agent.

The firmness or strength of gels produced by such interactions will depend on the degree of interaction of the complex with water and the properties of the bridging units.

The ability to change the swelling characteristics of a polymer gel by heat, pH or application of electric current can be valuable in specialised delivery systems, as exemplified in Fig. 7.11, which shows the effect of temperature change on the swelling and de-swelling of a hydrogel, resulting in an on–off 'switching' mechanism.

The relationship between swelling and release in an electrically responsive hydrogel is shown in Fig. 7.12. The mechanism of the current-induced change in volume of the gel is shown in Fig. 7.12b.

Hydrophilic polymers as bulk laxatives

The ability of carbohydrates and other macromolecules to imbibe large quantities of water is put to use both medicinally and industrially; for example, in absorbent paper and sanitary towels, incontinence pads and surgical dressings. Medically, use is made of the swelling properties in the treatment of constipation and in appetite suppression. Three properties are of importance in the *in vitro* evaluation of bulk laxatives:

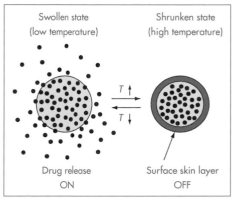

Figure 7.11 On–off switching mechanism for drug release.
Reproduced from Yoshida R *et al.* Pulsatile drug delivery systems using hydrogels. *Adv Drug Deliv Rev* 1993;11:85. Copyright Elsevier 1993.

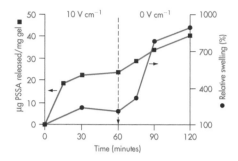

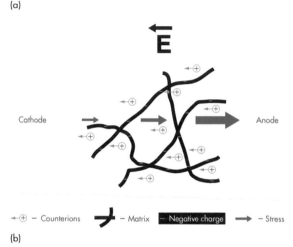

(a)

(b)

Figure 7.12 (a) Responsive swelling (●) and release (■) from poly(styrene sulfonic acid)-loaded hyaluronic acid hydrogels when an electric field of 10 V cm^{-1} was switched off. (b) The effect of an electric field on a polyelectrolyte network. The redistribution of ions causes shrinkage of the gel at the cathode and expansion at the anode.

(a) Reproduced from Tomer R *et al.* Electrically controlled release of macromolecules from cross-linked hyaluronic acid hydrogels. *J Control Release*, 1995; 33: 405. Copyright Elsevier 1995.

- the volume of water absorbed in the various media
- the viscosity and texture of the gel formed
- the ability of the gel to retain water.

The swelling properties of a sterculia-based preparation (Normacol) in various aqueous media and a comparison of Normacol with two other agents are shown in Fig. 7.13.

 Clinical point

It is desirable that colloidal bulk laxatives swell in the lower part of the small intestine and in the large intestine to cause reflex peristalsis, rather than in the stomach or duodenum; that is, they should swell in neutral rather than

acidic or alkaline conditions. In artificial intestinal juice, psyllium seed gum increased in volume 5–14 times, locust bean gum 5–10 times and methylcellulose 16–30 times in 24 hours. *In vivo* evaluation of methylcellulose and carboxymethylcellulose suggests that they have two advantages over the natural gums. Methylcellulose is more efficient as a bulk laxative because of its greater water-retentive capacity, whereas carboxymethylcellulose gives uniform distribution through the intestinal contents.

7.3.6 Adsorption of macromolecules

The ability of some macromolecules to adsorb at interfaces is made use of in suspension and emulsion stabilisation (see Chapter 6). Gelatin, acacia, poly (vinyl alcohol) and proteins adsorb at interfaces. Sometimes such adsorption is unwanted, as in the case of insulin adsorption on to glass infusion bottles and poly(vinyl chloride) infusion containers and tubing used in giving sets.

Clinical point

Adsorption of insulin to glass bottles and plastic intravenous (IV) tubing at slow rates of infusion is well documented. Adsorption ranges from 5% to 3.1% when 20 and 40 units respectively are added to 500 cm^3 of isotonic sodium chloride solution. Plastic IV tubing adsorbed 30% of 20 units and 26% of 40 units added to the same infusion bottles (Fig. 7.14). Adsorption occurs rapidly, within 15 seconds. Addition of albumin to prevent adsorption is now common practice. The albumin adsorbs at the glass or plastic surface and presents a more polar surface to the solution, thus reducing, but not always preventing, adsorption of the insulin (Fig. 7.15). The binding is considered to be a non-specific phenomenon that may occur on other inert materials such as polyethylene and glass.

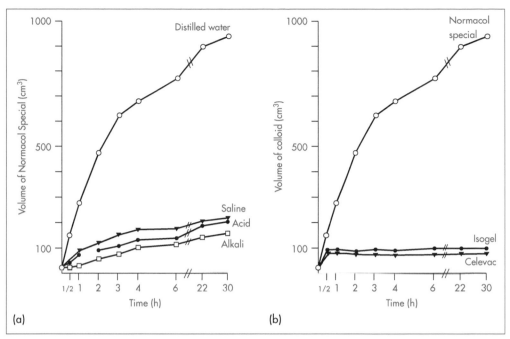

Figure 7.13 (a) The volume attained by 5 g of Normacol Special in various solutions over 30 hours. (b) The volumes attained by 5 g of Normacol Special, Isogel and Celevac in distilled water.

Reproduced from Ireson JD, Leslie GB. *Pharm J* 1970;205:540.

The adsorption of macromolecules at interfaces may be the reason why molecules such as those of HA can act as biological lubricants in joint fluids (see section

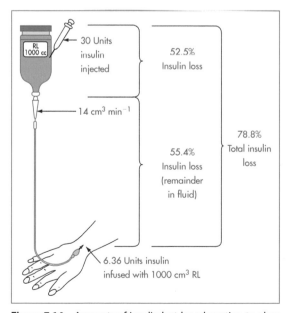

Figure 7.14 Amounts of insulin lost by adsorption to glass bottles and plastic intravenous tubing, following injection of 30 units of insulin. The patient receives only 6.36 units.

Reproduced from Petty C, Cunningham NL. *Anaesthesiology* 1974;40:400.

7.4.11). In healthy joints only 0.5 cm³ of synovial fluid is required to provide almost perfect lubrication; in diseased joints there are sometimes faults in this lubrication system and some research has been aimed at producing synthetic substitutes for synovial fluid. Polymer solutions provide one approach as their rheological characteristics more closely approach those of the natural fluid, which is non-Newtonian.

7.4 Water-soluble polymers used in pharmacy and medicine

In this section the properties of some specific polymers used in pharmacy and medicine will be discussed. This cannot be an exhaustive treatment of the subject, so choice of the macromolecular material for this section has been based partly on the degree of use but partly on the generally interesting features they display. The choice of a macromolecular material for a particular pharmaceutical use is often difficult because of the diversity of properties exhibited by the materials available. Figure 7.16 illustrates how the field can be narrowed to some extent by grouping the natural and synthetic materials of interest to the formulator. This

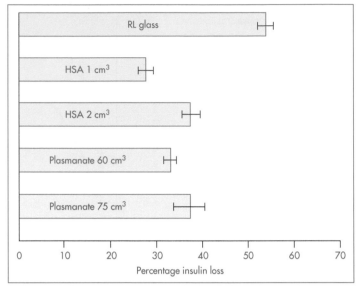

Figure 7.15 Prevention of insulin loss via adsorption by the addition of human serum albumin (HSA) or Plasmanate to 1000 cm³ of Ringer's lactate (RL) solution in a glass bottle. Insulin (30 units) was injected and measured at 5 minutes. Values represent means ± SEM. All HSA and Plasmanate values were significantly different from Ringer's lactate solution control ($p < 0.001$).

Reproduced from Petty C, Cunningham NL. *Anaesthesiology* 1974;40:400.

is, however, a very general guide, as the properties of individual macromolecules will, as discussed, often vary with pH, temperature, molecular weight and ionic strength. The most readily altered variable is, of course, the concentration of the macromolecule, whose effect on viscosity is illustrated for a range of compounds in Fig. 7.17. The most viscous material shown here is Carbopol 934.

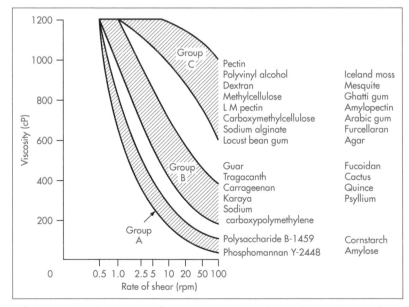

Figure 7.16 Effect of shear rate on the viscosity of gum solutions grouped according to their rheological behaviour.

Modified from Szezesniak AS, Farkas EH. Objective characterization of the mouthfeel of gum solutions. *J Food Sci* 1962;27:381. Copyright Wiley-VCH Verlag GmbH & Co. KGaA. Reproduced with permission.

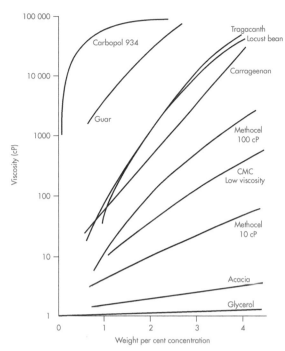

Figure 7.17 Viscosity of solutions of some pharmaceutical polymers and gums compared with glycerol plotted as a function of concentration.

Reproduced from Martin AN *et al.* Rheology. *Adv Pharm Sci* 1964;1:1.

7.4.1 Carboxypolymethylene (Carbomer, Carbopol)

Carboxypolymethylene is used as a suspending agent in pharmaceutical preparations and as a binding agent in tablets, and it is used in the formulation of prolonged-action tablets. It is a high-molecular-weight polymer of acrylic acid, containing a high proportion of carboxyl groups. Its aqueous solutions are acidic; when neutralised the solutions become very viscous, with a maximum viscosity occuring between pH 6 and 11. Electrolytes reduce the viscosity of the system and thus high concentrations of the polymer have to be employed in vehicles where ionisable drugs are present. A carbomer gel prolongs the contact time of drugs instilled into the eye.

7.4.2 Cellulose derivatives

Cellulose itself is virtually insoluble in water, but aqueous solubility can be conferred by partial methylation or carboxymethylation of cellulose.

Ethylcellulose is an ethyl ether of cellulose containing 44–51% of ethoxyl groups. It is insoluble in water but soluble in chloroform and in alcohol. It is possible to form water-soluble grades with a lower degree of substitution.

Methylcellulose samples are prepared by heterogeneous reaction that is usually controlled to allow substitution of, on average, about one-half of the hydroxyl groups. This leads to a product in which the methylated groups are not evenly distributed throughout the chains; rather, there are regions of high density of substitution (as in structure **VI**) that are hydrophobic in nature, and regions of low density of substitution that are hydrophilic in nature.

Structure VI Highly methylated region of the methylcellulose chain

Methylcellulose is thus a methyl ether of cellulose containing about 29% of methoxyl groups; it is slowly soluble in water. A 2% solution of methylcellulose 4500 has a gel point of about 50°C. High concentrations of electrolytes salt out the macromolecules and increase their viscosity; eventually precipitation may occur. Low-viscosity grades are used as emulsifiers for liquid paraffin and other mineral oils. High-viscosity grades are used as thickening agents for medicated jellies and as dispersing and thickening agents in suspensions.

Since methylcelluloses are poorly soluble in cold water, preliminary use of hot water ensures wetting of all portions of the particle prior to solution in cold water. The water-soluble methylcelluloses possess the property of thermal gelation; that is, they gel on heating while the natural gums gel on cooling. Methylcellulose exists in solution as long threadlike molecules hydrated by water molecules. On heating, the water of solvation tends to be lost; the 'lubricating' action of the hydration layer is also lost and the molecules lock together in a gel. Gelation is reversible on cooling. Variation in the alkyl or hydroxyalkyl substitution can be a means of controlling the gel points (Table 7.4). As the methoxyl content is lowered, the temperature of gelation increases and water solubility decreases. Unlike the ionic celluloses, the non-ionic alkylcelluloses possess surface activity. As the methoxyl content is reduced, the surface and

Table 7.4 Gel point and surface activity of cellulose derivatives

Derivative	Percentage —OCH$_3$	Percentage —OCH$_2$CH(OH)CH$_3$	Gel point[a] (°C)	Surface tension[b] (mN m^{-1})	Interfacial tension[c] (mN m^{-1})
Methocel MC	27.5–3.2	–	50–55	47–53	19–23
Methocel 60HG	28–30	7–12	55–60	44–50	18–19
Methocel 65HG	27–30	4–7.5	60–65	–	–
Methocel 70HG	24–27	4–8	66–72	–	–
Methocel 90HG	22–25	6–12	85	50–56	26–28

Reproduced from Windover FE. In: Davidson RL, Sittig M (eds) *Water Soluble Resins*. New York: Reinhold; 1962: 52ff.
[a]2% solution.
[b]Surface tension at 25°C.
[c]Interfacial tension versus paraffin oil at 25°C.

interfacial activities are also reduced, reflecting the importance of the hydrophobic moiety in determining surface activity.

Ethylhydroxyethylcellulose (EHMC) is an ether of cellulose with both ethyl and hydroxyethyl substituents attached via ether linkages to the anhydroglucose rings. It swells in water to form a clear, viscous colloidal solution. Preparation of solutions of cellulose derivatives requires hydration of the macromolecules, the rate of which is a function of both temperature and pH, as shown in the example in Fig. 7.18.

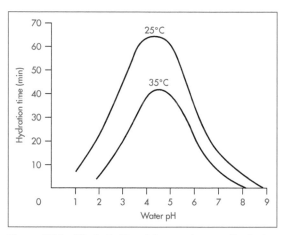

Figure 7.18 Effect of pH and temperature on the hydration time of fast-dissolving grades of hydroxyethylcellulose.
Reproduced with permission from Whistler RL (ed.) *Industrial Gums*, 2nd edn. New York: Academic Press; 1973.

Hydroxyethylcellulose (HEC) is soluble in hot and cold water but does not gel. It has been used in ophthalmic solutions. More widely used for the latter, however, is HPMC (hypromellose), which is a mixed ether of cellulose containing 27–30% of —OCH$_3$ groups and 4–7.5% of —OC$_3$H$_6$OH groups. It forms

a viscous colloidal solution. There are various pharmaceutical grades. For example, hypromellose 20 is a 2% solution that has a viscosity between 15 and 25 cSt (centistokes) at 20°C; the viscosity of a 2% hypromellose 15000 solution lies between 12 000 and 18 000 cSt. Hypromellose prolongs the action of medicated eye drops and is employed as an artificial tear fluid.

Sodium carboxymethylcellulose (NaCMC) is soluble in water at all temperatures. Because of the carboxylate group, its mucilages are more sensitive to change in pH than are those of methylcellulose. The viscosity of an NaCMC mucilage is decreased markedly below pH 5 or above pH 10.

7.4.3 Natural polymers: gums and mucilages

Gum arabic (acacia) has been used traditionally in pharmacy as an emulsifier. It is a polyelectrolyte whose solutions are highly viscous owing to the branched structure of the macromolecular chains; its adhesive properties are also believed to be due to, or in some way related to, this branched structure. Molecular weights between 200 000 and 250 000 Da (M_n) have been determined by osmotic pressure, values between 250 000 and 3 × 10^6 Da by sedimentation and diffusion, and values of 10^6 Da by light-scattering measurements which also point to the shape of the molecules as short stiff spirals with numerous side-chains. Arabic acid prepared from commercial gum arabic by precipitation is a moderately strong acid whose aqueous solutions have a pH of 2.2–2.7.

Whereas most gums are very viscous in aqueous solution, gum arabic is unusual in that, being extremely soluble, it can form solutions over a wide range of concentrations up to about 37% at 25°C. The marked variation in viscosity means that the gum arabic molecules must be flexible, with the ionic acid carboxyl groups distributed along the chain. At low pH the carboxyl groups are un-ionised. On increase of pH the carboxyl groups become progressively ionised and the folded chains expand owing to repulsion between the charged groups, causing an increase in viscosity. On addition of NaOH to the system the viscosity falls again as the concentration of counterion (Na^+) increases and effectively shields the acidic groups. The molecule then folds on itself. Similar falls in viscosity are exhibited on addition of sodium chloride. The effect of salt addition to the gum at fixed pH reflects the decrease in effective charge on the molecules of gum with resultant contraction and reduction in viscosity.

The gum arabic molecule is, in addition, surface-active: a 4% solution at 30°C has a surface tension of 63.2 mN m^{-1}. Addition of electrolytes makes the molecule more surface-active either by causing a change in conformation of the molecule at the interface, allowing closer packing, or by increasing the hydrophobicity of the molecule. It is an effective emulsifier, the stabilisation of the emulsion being dependent mainly on the coherence and elasticity of the interfacial film, which is by no means monomolecular.

Gum arabic is incompatible with several phenolic compounds; under suitable conditions it forms coacervates (see section 7.6.3) with gelatin and positively charged polyelectrolytes.

Gum tragacanth partially dissolves in water; the soluble portion is called tragacanthin and this can be purified by precipitation from water with acetone or alcohol. Tragacanthin is a highly viscous polyelectrolyte with a molecular weight of 800 000 Da (as determined by sedimentation measurements). It is one of the most widely used natural emulsifiers and thickeners. As its molecules have an elongated shape, its solutions have a high viscosity which, as with gum arabic, is dependent on pH. The maximum viscosity occurs at pH 8 initially, but because of ageing effects the maximum stable viscosity is near pH 5.

It is an effective suspending agent for pharmaceuticals and is used in conjunction with acacia as an emulsifier, the tragacanth imparting a high structural viscosity while the gum arabic adsorbs at the oil–water interface.

Clinical point

Tragacanth is also used in spermicidal jellies, acting both by immobilising spermatozoa and acting as a viscous barrier to spermatozoa. It is also used as an excipient in contraceptive preparations which contain chemical contraceptive molecules where its physical effect on spermatozoa reinforces the direct chemical action of the contraceptive agents.

Alginates. Although the solutions of alginate are very viscous and set on addition of acid or calcium salts, they are less readily gelled than pectin and are used chiefly as stabilisers and thickening agents. Propylene glycol alginate does not precipitate in acid and, as it is non-toxic, is widely used as a stabiliser for foodstuffs. The molecules are highly asymmetric, with molecular weights in the range 47 000–370 000 Da. Sodium alginate has the structure given in **VII**.

Structure VII Sodium alginate

Pectin is a purified carbohydrate product from extracts of the rind of citrus fruits and consists of partially methoxylated polygalacturonic acid (**VIII**). It has remarkable gelling qualities but is also used therapeutically, often with kaolin, in the treatment of diarrhoea. It has been established that the longer the pectin chains, the greater its capacity for gel formation. The presence of inorganic cations and the degree of esterification of the carboxyl groups are important factors; in the case of calcium pectate gel it can be assumed that the calcium or indeed other polyvalent cations can interlink the chains by binding through $COO^-\ldots Ca^{2+}\ldots{}^-OOC$ interactions. Thus a high degree of esterification will disfavour gelation in this case. In the absence of inorganic cations, however, a high degree of esterification aids gelation, suggesting that hydrophobic interactions cause the chains to associate.

Structure VIII Partially methylated chain of poly(galacturonic acid) of pectin

7.4.4 Chitosan

Chitosan is a polymer obtained by the deacetylation of chitin, one of the most abundant polysaccharides. Chitosan, or poly[α-(1,4)-2-amino-2-deoxy-D-glucopyranose], has the structure (**IX**). As might be expected, the degree of deacetylation has a significant effect on the solubility and rheological properties of the polymer. At low pH, the polymer is soluble, with the sol–gel transition occurring at approximately pH 7. Chitosan also has film-forming abilities and its gel- and matrix-forming abilities make it useful for solid-dosage forms, such as granules or microparticles.[6] The molecular weight, crystallinity and degree of deacetylation are all factors that can be varied to control the release rates from chitosan-based granules.

Structure IX The chemical structure of chitosan. The amine groups on the polymer have a pK_a in the range 5.5–6.5, depending on the source of the polymer

7.4.5 Dextran

Certain fractions of partially hydrolysed dextran are used as plasma substitutes or 'expanders'. Certain strains of *Leuconostoc meserentoides* are cultivated to synthesise dextran (**X**), which is a polymer of anhydroglucose, linked through α-1,6 glucosidic linkages. The chains are branched; on the average, one branch occurs for every 10–12 glucose residues. The intrinsic viscosity [η] is related to M by the relationship

$$[\eta] = 10^{-3}M^{1/2} \tag{7.16}$$

in the molecular weight range 20 000–200 000 Da. The dextrans produced by fermentation are hydrolysed and fractionated to give a range of products suitable for injection. Dextran, being a hydrophilic colloid, exerts an osmotic pressure comparable to that of plasma and

Structure X Dextran

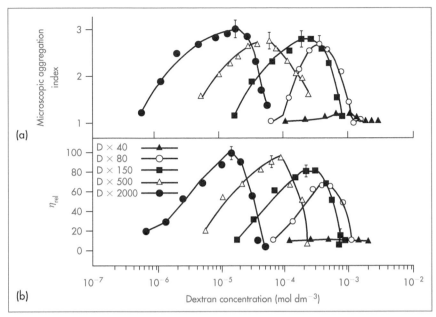

Figure 7.19 Variation of indices of red-cell aggregation with the concentration of five dextran fractions of different molecular weight: (a) microscopic aggregation index; (b) relative viscosity at a shear rate of 0.1 s^{-1}. Note that the maximum of each curve (that is, maximum aggregation of the red cells) corresponds to a well-defined concentration of a particular dextran fraction. Maxima in both indices of aggregation of red cells occur at about the same concentration of dextran fraction.

Reproduced with permission from Chien S. *Bib Anat Basel* 1973;11:244.

it is thus used to restore or maintain blood volume. Other substances that have been used in a similar way include hydroxyethyl starch, polyvinylpyrrolidone (PVP) and gelatin.

> ### ✚ Clinical point
>
> *Dextran injections* are sterile solutions of dextran with weight-average molecular weights of about 40 000–110 000 Da. Dextrans with a molecular weight of about 50 000 Da or less are excreted in the urine within 48 hours of injection. Dextran molecules with higher molecular weights disappear more slowly from the blood stream and are temporarily stored in the reticuloendothelial system.
>
> Dextran 70 (70 000 Da) and Dextran 110 (110 000 Da) are used to maintain blood volume, and Dextran 40 is used primarily to prevent intravascular aggregation of blood cells and for assisting capillary blood flow. This latter effect is the result of dextran adsorption and stabilisation of the erythrocyte

suspensions. If the higher-molecular-weight fractions exceed about 1% concentration in the blood, rouleaux (see photomicrograph) tend to form.

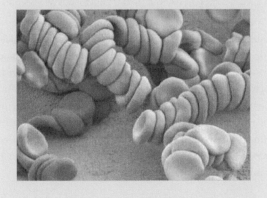

The sensitivity of blood to the concentration and molecular weight of dextran is clearly seen in Fig. 7.19, where aggregation and relative viscosity of red-cell suspensions are shown in the presence of varying amounts of five different dextrans. Molecular weight control is thus important and may be exercised by measurement of intrinsic viscosity, [η].

7.4.6 Iron–dextran complexes

Iron–dextran complexes are soluble, non-ionic and suitable for injection for the treatment of anaemia (Fig. 7.20); the complex is stable on storage in the pH range 4–11.

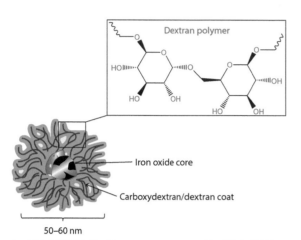

Figure 7.20 Conceptual drawing of an iron–dextran complex, showing the iron oxide core surrounded by a corona of dextran and carboxydextran molecules.

After Abdollah MRA et al. *Faraday Disc* 2014; 75:41–58; see also London E. *J Pharm Sci* 2004;93:1838–1846.

7.4.7 Polyvinylpyrrolidone

PVP is used as a suspending and dispersing agent, as a tablet-binding and granulating agent, and as a vehicle for drugs such as penicillin, cortisone, procaine and insulin to delay their absorption and prolong their action. It forms hard films that are utilised in film-coating processes. Chemically it is a homopolymer of *N*-vinylpyrrolidone (**XI**). It is available in a number of grades, designated by numbers ranging from K15 to K90. The K values represent a function of the mean molecular weight, and can be calculated from

$$\frac{\log \eta_{rel}}{c} = \frac{75K_0^2}{1 + 1.5K_0 c} + K_0 \qquad (7.17)$$

where c = concentration in grams per 100 cm^3 and η_{rel} is the viscosity relative to the solvent. $K = 1000K_0$. Viscosity is essentially independent of pH over the range 0–10 and aqueous solutions exhibit a high tolerance for many inorganic salts. Its wide solubility in organic solvents is unusual. The viscosity of a range of aqueous solutions of PVP is shown in Fig. 7.21.

Structure XI Polyvinylpyrrolidone

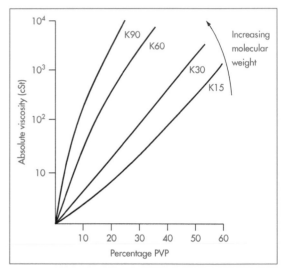

Figure 7.21 Viscosity of polyvinylpyrrolidone (PVP) solutions as a function of molecular weight (PVP K15 (mol wt 40 000 Da) to PVP K90 (mol wt 700 000 Da)) and concentration of the polymer in water.

Reproduced from Azorlosa JL, Martinelli AJ. In: Davidson RL, Sittig M (eds) *Water Soluble Resins*. New York: Reinhold; 1962.

PVP forms molecular adducts with many substances. Soluble complexes, called *iodophors*, are formed with iodine: the solubility of iodine is increased from 0.034% in water at 25°C to 0.58% by 1% PVP. The resulting iodophor retains the germicidal properties of iodine. It is thought that the iodine is held in a PVP helix in solution. The influence of two samples of PVP on the solubility of testosterone is shown in Fig. 7.22. The PVP correspondingly increases the rate of solution of the steroid from solid dispersions.

7.4.8 Polyoxyethylene glycols (macrogols)

Poloxyethyelene glycols are widely used in pharmaceutical formulations not only as solvents and bases for ointments and suppositories but also as molecules which can determine the lifetime of nanoparticles in the blood by adsorbing on to particle hydrophobic surfaces to prevent opsonin adsorption (see Chapter 14).

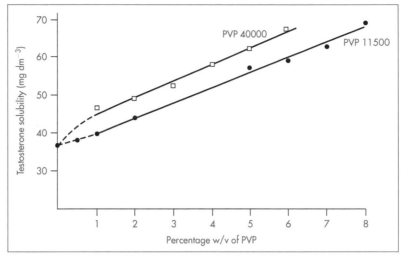

Figure 7.22 The influence of PVP 11500 and PVP 40000 on the aqueous solubility of testosterone at 37°C.
Reproduced from Hoelgaard A, Muller N. *Arch Pharm Chem* 1975;3:34.

Macrogols (polyoxyethylene glycols (PEGs), **XII**) are liquid over the molecular weight range 200–700 Da; the liquid members and semisolid members of the series are hygroscopic. Macrogol 200 has a hygroscopicity 70% of that of glycerol, but this decreases with molecular weight: the comparable value for Macrogol 1540 is only 30%. They are used as solvents for drugs such as hydrocortisone. The macrogols are incompatible with phenols and can reduce the antimicrobial activity of other preservatives. Higher-molecular-weight PEGs are more effective on a molecular basis as complexing agents. Up to four phenol molecules bind to each PEG molecule; the complex formed is of the donor–acceptor type. The semisolid and waxy members of the series may be used as suppository bases; in such cases their potential to interact with medicaments must be borne in mind.

$$HO(CH_2CH_2O)_n H$$

Structure XII Polyoxyethylene glycol

Use of PEGs, and other hydrophilic polymers, in high concentrations in formulations can influence the behaviour of drugs even when the drug is present as a physical mixture with the polymer. For example, combination of PEG 4000 with sulfathiazole increases the solution rate of sulfonamides (Fig. 7.23). Probable mechanisms include an increase in drug solubility or increased wetting of the drug surrounded by the hydrophilic polymer. Apart from these uses, the PEGs have turned out to be one of the most versatile water-

soluble polymers. They have been successful in modifying the behaviour of proteins, including monoclonal antibodies, in solution and in the circulation after being grafted to these molecules. The PEGs also prolong the circulation time of particulate delivery systems such as liposomes and nanoparticles through their adsorption or incorporation into the surface of these carriers, preventing the adsorption of opsonins and reducing uptake by the liver and spleen, as discussed in Chapter 12.

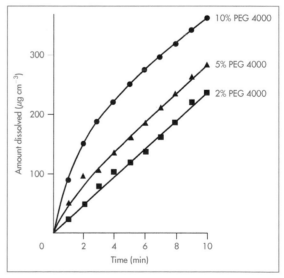

Figure 7.23 Dissolution rates of sulfathiazole (Form I)–polyethylene glycol 4000 physical mixtures.

Reproduced from Niazi S. Effect of polyethylene glycol 4000 on dissolution properties of sulfathiazole polymorphs. *J Pharm Sci* 1976;65:302. Copyright Wiley-VCH Verlag GmbH & Co. KGaA. Reproduced with permission.

7.4.9 Bioadhesivity of water-soluble polymers

Adhesion between a surface of a hydrophilic polymer, or a surface to which a hydrophilic polymer has been grafted or adsorbed, and a biological surface arises from interactions between the polymer chains and the macromolecules on the mucosal surface. From Fig. 7.24a it is clear that to achieve maximum adhesion there should be maximum interaction between the polymer chains of the bioadhesive (A) and the mucus (B). The charge on the molecules will be important, and for two anionic polymers maximum interaction will occur when they are not charged. Penetration and association must be balanced. Table 7.5 shows the adhesive performance of a range of polymers, many of which have been discussed in this chapter. Of these, two classes have been approved by the US Food and Drug Administration: anionic poly(acrylic acid) (carbophil) derivatives and the cationic chitosans. Poly-carbophil and carbomer (Carbopol 934P) have pK_a values of about 4.5 and display maximum muco-adhesivity at pH values where they are mostly un-dissociated[7] (Fig. 7.24b).

7.4.10 Viscous solutions and disorders of the eye

Anterior-chamber injections (intracameral injections)

Hypotony is defined as an intraocular pressure of 5 mmHg or less. Low intraocular pressure can adversely impact the eye in many ways, including causing accelerated cataract formation, maculopathy and discomfort.

Sodium hyaluronate, chondroitin sulfate and methylcellulose have been compared for maintaining the form of the anterior chamber of the eye in cases of hypotony. The rheological characteristics of the polymers used in the anterior chamber are key to success. Pseudoplastic fluids are ideal for maintaining the chamber form since they are more viscous at rest. Sodium hyaluronate and methylcellulose are pseudoplastic, while chondroitin sulfate displays Newtonian flow properties.

High viscosity is critical when the agent is applied in a thick layer to prevent mechanical damage to the corneal epithelium when an intraocular lens is drawn across the endothelium. Compression and shear are responsible for the damage[8]: thin layers of highly viscous HA convey the shear forces to the endothelium,

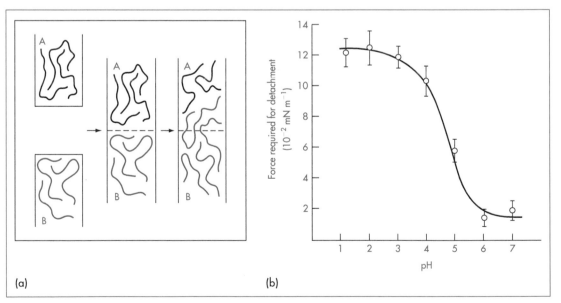

Figure 7.24 (a) Schematic representation of two phases, adhesive (A) and mucus (B), which adhere owing to chain adsorption and consecutive chain entanglement during mucoadhesion. (b) Effect of pH on *in vitro* bioadhesion of polycarbophil to rabbit gastric tissue.

(a) Reproduced from Peppas NA, Mikos AG. In: Gurney R, Junginger HE (eds) *Bioadhesion*. Stuttgart: Wiss. Verlagsgesellschaft; 1990. Copyright Elsevier 1990.

(b) From reference 7.

Table 7.5 Some representative mucoadhesives and their relative mucoadhesivities

Substance	Adhesive performance
Carboxymethylcellulose	Excellent
Carbopol	Excellent
Carbopol and hydroxypropylmethylcellulose	Good
Carbopol base with white petrolatum/ hydrophilic petrolatum	Fair
Carbopol 934 and EX 55	Good
Poly(methyl methacrylate)	Excellent
Polyacrylamide	Good
Poly(acrylic acid)	Excellent
Polycarbophil	Excellent
Homopolymers and copolymers of acrylic acid and butyl acrylate	Good
Gelatin	Fair
Sodium alginate	Excellent
Dextran	Good
Pectin	Poor
Acacia	Poor
Povidone	Poor
Poly(acrylic acid) crosslinked with sucrose	Fair

whereas thick layers provide a physical barrier to compression, as can be seen in Fig. 7.25. Clearly there are analogies to synovial fluid here.

Optiflex is one ophthalmic product containing sodium hyaluronate with a molecular weight of 4×10^6 Da in a sterile isotonic vehicle. When injected through a cannula it becomes less viscous, but it regains its viscosity in the anterior chamber of the eye. It is used for lubrication and protection of cells and tissue during surgical procedures.

Dry eye

In some patients, the supply of tear fluid (as discussed in Chapter 9), which comprises a largely aqueous solution containing protein, lipids and enzymes, is impaired. Tears spread over the surface of the cornea, which is hydrophobic. Tear films thin and break but the fluid is replenished by blinking. The film break-up time is variable but is more rapid in patients suffering from dry-eye syndrome. The tears contain phospholipids, which act as a surfactant, lowering the surface tension of the fluid and allowing spreading. The thin lipid layer on the surface of the tear film (like most lipid monolayers) also slows down evaporation of the aqueous medium beneath. Dry eye[9] (xerophthalmia[*]; Sjögren's syndrome) is caused when the tear film thins to such an extent that it ruptures, exposing the corneal surface to the air, as shown schematically in Figure 7.26. Drying out of patches on the corneal surface follows. This can be painful and must be avoided. Evaporation over 5–10 minutes can actually eliminate the tear film completely.[10]

Artificial tear fluids may replace the natural tear fluid with varying degrees of similitude. Most aim for formulations that have an appropriate viscosity, but these do not necessarily possess identical rheological

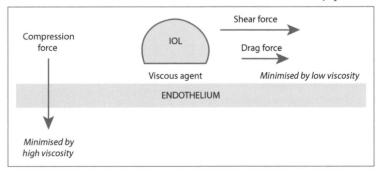

Figure 7.25 A diagram of the forces on an intraocular lens (IOL). The applied force on the lens is represented by two vectors: the compression force and the shear force. High viscosity transmits more of the shear force to the endothelial surface. The compression force is minimised by a high viscosity (note the similarity to synovial fluid) and the drag force is minimised by low viscosity.

[*] *Xeros*: Greek = dry.

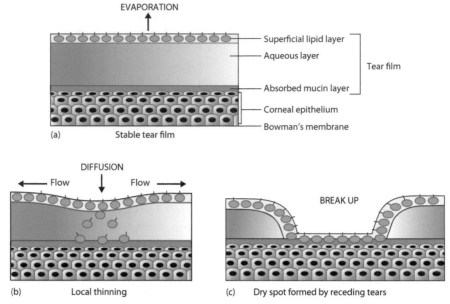

Figure 7.26 Schematic of (a) the effect of the lipid layer reducing evaporation of tear fluid; (b) the beginning of the thinning process; and (c) the eventual separation of the tear liquid, inducing the formation of dry spots on the cornea.

properties to those of natural tear fluids. HPMC is a component of many commercial replacement or 'artificial' tear products, as are the water-soluble macromolecules NaCMC (carmellose), poly(vinyl alcohol) and PVP.

Xerostomia

Another syndrome that requires replacement or supplementation of a natural fluid with an artificial substance is xerostomia ('dry mouth'). Normal saliva function and control are compromised in this condition. Saliva is a clear, usually alkaline and somewhat viscous secretion from the parotid, submaxillary, sublingual and smaller mucous glands of the mouth. In some cases xerostomia is caused by medication, especially by anticholinergics. Chemotherapeutic agents can also have a direct effect on salivary glands, reducing saliva output. Saliva consists primarily of water but contains enzymes and other proteins and electrolytes. It has a surface tension of around 58 mN m^{-1}. Saliva is essential for the normal 'feel' of the mouth and it assists lubrication, possesses antimicrobial activity and aids mucosal integrity. Saliva provides protection by constantly flushing non-adhered microbes, their toxins and nutrients from the mouth. It has also been suggested that the flow of saliva detaches adsorbed microbes from the teeth or prevents their adhesion, as shown in Fig. 7.27 Saliva contains a wide spectrum of

agents such as lactoferrin, lysozyme, histatins, cystatins, mucins, agglutinins, secretory leukocyte protei-

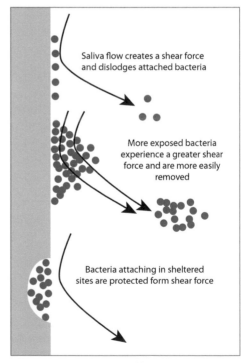

Saliva flow creates a shear force and dislodges attached bacteria

More exposed bacteria experience a greater shear force and are more easily removed

Bacteria attaching in sheltered sites are protected form shear force

Figure 7.27 Diagram of the effect of salivary flow in the normal mouth, dislodging bacteria adsorbed on teeth. Different situations are shown, with more exposed bacteria and bacteria in sheltered sites, such as crevices.

nase inhibitor, tissue inhibitors of proteinases, chitinase, peroxidases and calprotectin.

Dry mouth can be treated with artificial saliva, although these solutions, as can be imagined from the list of components of natural saliva, seldom truly mimic the properties of the natural lubricant and wetting material. Designed to behave as far as possible like natural saliva, commercially available artificial salivas mostly contain carboxymethylcellulose and hydroxyethylcellulose to increase viscosity. The rheological properties of saliva are, as one can imagine, quite complex, but these polymer additives do at least increase the residence time of the fluid. However, gel formulations that can prolong contact between the fluid and the oral mucosa are sometimes preferred.

7.4.11 Intra-articular hyaluronic acid

Synovial fluid is rheopexic – that is, stress increases with time in steady shear (see section 6.3). This is thought to be the result of protein aggregation with time and the influence of stress on the process. It is suggested[11] that there is a connection between the observed rheopexy and the remarkable lubrication properties of synovial fluid; one can envisage that the fluid that exists between two bony surfaces becomes more effective in 'cushioning' the contacts as its viscosity increases with the forces placed on it.

Products containing HA, such as Hyalgan, Artzal, Synvisc, Suplasyn, Hyalart and Orthovisc, have been developed for administration into the synovial space of joints to enhance the activity of the natural synovial fluid. The perception that higher-molecular-weight HA is superior to lower-molecular-weight species is based on the suggestion that high-molecular-weight HA normalises synovial fluid and results in effective joint lubrication. Higher-molecular-weight HAs are chemically crosslinked forms and are claimed to have a greater residence time in the joints.[12] *In vivo*, HA with a higher viscosity has been found to be more effective in lubricating joints.[13]

There is some controversy about modes of action. It has also been suggested that viscoelasticity does not in fact form the foundation of the beneficial properties of these injections.[14] This point is added because explanations of the behaviour of complex systems are fraught with confounding factors. One must, however, speculate from a reasoned base when necessary. It is

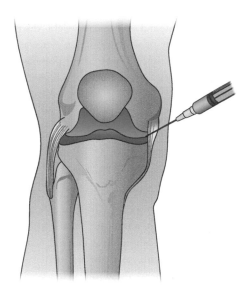

Figure 7.28 The site of administration of intra-articular injections of agents such as hyaluronic acid to lubricate the movement of the joints, as discussed in the text.

highly reasonable to conclude that one of the important properties of hyaluronan and hyaluronan solutions is their pseudoplastic behaviour. These then serve as lubricants when joint movements are slow and as shock absorbers when movements are fast[15] (Fig. 7.28).

7.4.12 Polymer crystallinity

Polymers form perfect crystals with difficulty, simply because of the low probability of arranging the chains in a regular fashion, especially at high molecular weights. Advantage can be taken of defects in crystals in the preparation of microcrystals. Microcrystalline cellulose (Avicel) is prepared by disruption of larger crystals. It is used as a tablet excipient and as a binder-disintegrant. Dispersed in water, it forms colloidal gels, and it can be used to form heat-stable oil-in-water (o/w) emulsions. Spheroids of microcrystalline cellulose with accurately controlled diameters can be prepared and drugs can be incorporated during preparation. The concept of crystallinity is potentially important when considering polymer membranes, as discussed below.

7.5 Water-insoluble polymers and polymer membranes

In defining the properties of polymers for drug formulation, certain characteristics are important. Obviously molecular weight and molecular weight distribution must be known, as these affect solvent penetration and crystallinity. The functionality of the polymer is best described by a series of parameters such as

- glass transition temperature, T_g
- tensile strength
- diffusion coefficient
- hardness (crystallinity)
- solubility.

Crystallinity defines several features of polymers: rigidity, fluidity, the resistance to diffusion of small molecules in the polymer, and degradation.

In hydrogels T_g can be measured and is a measure of polymer structure, crosslinking density, solvent content and polymer–solvent interactions, as can be seen from Table 7.6.

Table 7.6 Effect of hydrogel structure and characteristics on T_g

Feature	Effect on T_g
Presence of flexible groups in main chain	↓
Bulky, inflexible side-chains	↑
Flexible side-chains	↓
Increase in main-chain polarity	↑
Increase in crosslinking	↑
Plasticiser content	↓

7.5.1 Permeability of polymers

Hydrophobic polymers also play an important role in pharmacy. When these materials are used as membranes, containers or tubing material, their surfaces may come into contact with solutions. The surfaces of insoluble polymers are not as inert as might be thought. The interaction of drugs and preservatives with plastics depends on the structure of the polymer and on the affinity of the compound for the plastic. The latter is determined by the degree of crystallinity of the polymer, as permeability is a function of the degree of amorphous content of the polymer. The crystalline regions of the solid polymer present an impenetrable barrier to the movement of most molecules. Diffusing molecules thus have to circumnavigate the crystalline islands, which act as obstruc-

tions. The greater the volume fraction of crystalline material (ϕ_c), the slower the movement of molecules.

Diffusion

Diffusion in a non-porous solid polymer is of course a more difficult process than in a fluid because of the necessity for the movement of polymer chains to allow passage of the drug molecule, and it is therefore slower. The equation that governs the process is Fick's first law (see section 2.6, equation 2.63):

$$J = -D\frac{dc}{dx} \tag{7.18}$$

where J is the flux, D is the diffusion coefficient of the drug in the membrane and dc/dx is the concentration gradient across the membrane. If the membrane is of thickness l, and Δc represents the difference in solution concentration of drug at the two faces of membrane,

$$J = \frac{DK\Delta c}{l} \tag{7.19}$$

where K is the distribution coefficient of the permeant towards the polymer. Therefore, alteration of polymer/membrane thickness, coupled with appropriate choice of polymer, can give rise to the desired flux. Within a given polymer, permeability is a function of the degree of crystallinity, itself a function of polymer molecular weight. If P is the permeability of drug in a partially crystalline polymer (see Fig. 1.18, Chapter 1), the volume fraction of the crystalline regions being ϕ_c, and P_a is the permeability in an amorphous sample, then

$$\frac{P}{P_a} = (1 - \phi_c)^2 \tag{7.20}$$

Permeation of drug molecules through the solid polymer, which may be acting as a drug depot, is a function of the solubility of the drug in the polymer as

$$P = DK \tag{7.21}$$

Addition of inorganic fillers in which the drug is insoluble alters the overall solubility of the drug in the polymer and hence alters the permeation characteristics. The equation for overall solubility (S) is given by

$$S = S_f\phi_f + S_p\phi_p \tag{7.22}$$

where f refers to filler and p to polymer. Thus, when $S_f \rightarrow 0$, as happens when inorganic fillers such as zinc oxide are employed, an obstruction-type equation may be written:

$$\frac{S}{S_p} = 1 - \phi_f \qquad (7.23)$$

The natural permeabilities of polymers vary over a wide range and this widens the choice, provided one can select a polymer that is compatible with the tissues with which it comes into contact. Once a polymer has been chosen that gives a flux of drug sufficient to provide adequate circulating levels, use of fillers and plasticisers can give fine control of permeability (Table 7.7).

Table 7.7 Factors that influence diffusivity in polymers

Factor	Net effect on D
Increased polymer molecular weight	↓
Increased degree of crosslinking	↓
Diluents and plasticisers	↑
Fillers	↓
Increased crystallinity of polymers	↓
Increased drug molecular size	↓

The method of preparation also influences the properties of the film. Cast films of varying properties can be prepared by variation *inter alia* of the solvent power of the casting solution containing the polymer, although the complex processes involved in film formation are not yet fully understood. It is clear, however, that the conformation of the polymer chains in concentrated solution just prior to solvent evaporation will determine the density of the film, and the number and size of pores and voids. Drug flux through dense (nonporous) polymer membranes is by diffusion; flux through porous membranes will be by diffusion and by transport in solvent through pores in the film. With porous films, control can be exercised on porosity, and hence overall permeability, by the use of swelling agents. Dense membranes can be subjected to certain postformation treatments such as thermal annealing that modify their structural and performance characteristics.

The solubility of sterilising gases in polymers is important in determining the retention of residues that may, as in the case of ethylene oxide residues, be toxic. The quality control problems of polymers and plastics are considerable. Both the chemical and physical natures of the material have to be taken into account, as well as purity.

Permeability of polymers to gases

The permeability of polymers to the gaseous phase is of importance when the use of polymers as packaging materials is considered. Figure 7.29 shows oxygen penetration through a wide range of plastic materials, ranging from Teflon to dimethylsilicone rubber, which has the highest permeability. Ether, nitrous oxide, halothane and cyclopropane diffuse through silicone rubbers, and general anaesthesia in dogs has been achieved by passing the vapours of these substances through a coil of silicone rubber tubing, each end of which is placed in an artery or vein. Aspects of the permeability of polymeric films of interest pharmaceutically include the process of gas diffusion, water sorption and permeation and dialysis processes. With few exceptions, there is an inverse relationship between water-vapour transmission and oxygen permeability. Water-vapour permeability has been shown to be dependent on the polarity of the polymer. More polar films tend to be more ordered and less porous, hence less oxygen-permeable. The less polar films are more porous, permitting the permeation of oxygen but not necessarily of the larger water molecules. Being more lipophilic, the less polar films have less affinity for water. Because of the importance of water as a solvent and permeant species, much work has been directed towards the synthesis of polymeric membranes with controlled hydrophilic/hydrophobic balance. The hydrophilicity of the cellulose acetates is directly proportional to their —OH content and inversely proportional to the hydrophobic acetyl content (Table 7.8). Alternative approaches to alteration of characteristics of water permeability include the use of block copolymers where one can alter the ratio of hydrophilic polymer to increase transport rates of polar materials.

The affinity of drugs for plastics

Drugs may adsorb on to the surface of plastics or they may diffuse into the interior of the material. The affinity of drugs for plastics will vary with the structure

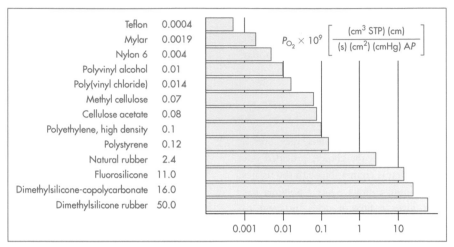

Figure 7.29 Permeation of oxygen through several polymer films. This illustrates the diversity of the properties of available polymers and shows the relatively high permeability of polydimethylsiloxane, a common component of prolonged-action drug devices.

Reproduced from Kesting R. *Synthetic Polymeric Membranes*. New York: McGraw-Hill; 1971.

of the drug: proteins, polypeptides and other hydrophilic or amphipathic molecules may adsorb, and smaller hydrophobic molecules *sorb*, that is enter the plastic. Chlorpromazine, for example, has a very high affinity for some materials used as tubing (Table 7.9). Silicone is actually very permeable to hydrophobic molecules and this can be put to good use in other areas, such as in controlled-release systems. The downside is that some drugs, e.g. steroids, are adsorbed from solutions passing through polyethylene tubing. In analytical chemistry such interactions can also be important in defining the accuracy of the method.

Glyceryl trinitrate, which has a high affinity for lipophilic plastics, migrates from tablets in contact with plastic liners in packages, causing a reduction of the active content of many tablets to zero. This peculiar migratory behaviour is due to the volatility of the drug; normally the drug molecules would only be able to be significantly affected by such transfer when in the solution state.

Table 7.8 Effect of hydroxyl and acetyl content on water permeability and sorption of moisture by cellulose acetates

Hydroxyl content (%)	Acetyl content (%)	Moisture sorption (%) at 95% relative humidity at 25°C	Water permeability D_1C_1 (10^{-7} g cm s^{-1})
7.2	34	19	12
5.9	36	17	7
4.6	38	14.7	4
3.3	40	12.6	2.5
2.0	42	10.5	1.5

Reproduced from Reid C, Breton E. Water and ion flow across cellulosic membranes. *J Appl Polymer Sci* 1959;1:133. Copyright Wiley-VCH Verlag GmbH & Co. KGaA. Reproduced with permission.

Table 7.9 Concentration of chlorpromazine in buffer solution after shaking with various polymers for 1 h at 22°C (original concentration 100 μmol dm^{-3})

Material	Chlorpromazine concentration (μmol dm^{-3})
Silicone tubing	1 ± 0.4
Latex tubing	16 ± 4.7
Poly(vinyl chloride) tubing	14 ± 1.0
Polyethylene tubing	60 ± 2.0
Polyethylene test tube	70 ± 3.8
Polyethylene stopper	77 ± 5.3
Plexiglas chippings	74 ± 4.3
Teflon chippings	81 ± 4.4
Polystyrene test tube	89 ± 1.2

Reproduced with permission from Krieglstein G *et al.* On the interaction of various drugs with synthetic materials used in pharmacological apparatus. *Arzneim Forsch* 1972;22:1538.

7.5.2 Ion-exchange resins

Synthetic organic polymers comprising a hydrocarbon crosslinked network to which ionisable groups are attached have the ability to exchange ions attracted to their ionised groups with ions of the same charge present in solution (Fig. 7.30). These substances, usually prepared in the form of beads, are ion-exchange resins and are insoluble in water, the aqueous phase diffusing into the porous resin beads. Because ions must diffuse into and out of the resin for exchange to occur, ions larger than a given size may be excluded from reaction by altering the nature of the crosslinks in the polymer. The resins may be either cation exchangers in which the resin ionisable group is acidic, for example, sulfonic, carboxylic (**XIII**) or phenolic groups, or anion exchangers in which the ionisable group is basic, either amine or quaternary ammonium groups.

The equations describing the equilibria involved are as follows:

Cation-exchange resin

$$POL - (SO_3^-)A^+ + B^+ \Longleftrightarrow POL - (SO_3^-)B^+ + A^+$$

Anion-exchange resin

$$POL - N(CH_3)_3^+X^- + Y^- \Longleftrightarrow POL - N(CH_3)_3^+Y^- + X^-$$

The equilibrium constant for the cation exchange resin is

$$K_{cation} = \frac{[POL - B^+][A^+]}{[POL - A^+][B^+]} \qquad (7.24)$$

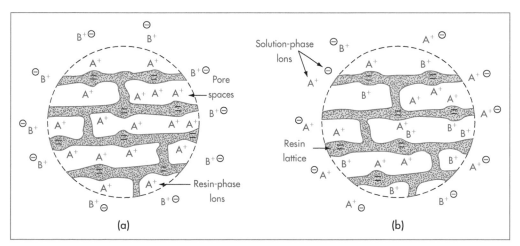

Structure XIII Sulfonic acid and carboxylic acid ion-exchange resins

Figure 7.30 Schematic diagram of a cation-exchange resin framework with fixed exchange sites prior to and following an exchange reaction: (a) initial state prior to exchange reaction with cation B$^+$; (b) equilibrium state after exchange reaction with cation B$^+$.

Modified from Weber WJ. *Physicochemical Processes for Water Quality Control*. New York: Wiley; 1972. Copyright Wiley-VCH Verlag GmbH & Co. KGaA. Reproduced with permission.

However, application of equation (7.24) is impossible because of the inaccessibility of the terms [POL-B$^+$] and [POL-A$^-$]. Some estimation of a resin's affinity for ions can be made using a standard ion such as lithium for cation-exchange resins. A selectivity coefficient, k, may be defined as

$$k = \frac{[B^+]_{resin}[A^+]_{solution}}{[A^+]_{resin}[B^+]_{solution}} \quad (7.25)$$

Even here there is a problem arising from the difficulty in the determination of the activity of the ions in the resin (because of the complexity of the environment) and the overall concentration of ion is generally used instead.

The ability of a resin to exchange one ion for another depends on its affinity for the ion and the concentration of ions in solution. Cation-exchange resins tend to have affinity in decreasing order for calcium, potassium, sodium, ammonium and hydrogen ions.

Pharmaceutical ion-exchangers

Anion-exchange resins such as polyamine methylene resin and polyaminostyrene have been used as antacids.

A polymeric ion-exchange resin, sevelamer (**XIV**), is used to reduce phosphate ion levels in patients with hyperphosphataemia following haemodialysis. It is a copolymer of 2-(chloromethyl)oxirane (epichlorohydrin) and prop-2-en-1-amine. The marketed form is a partial hydrochloride salt, being present as ≈40% amine·HCl and 60% sevelamer base. The amine groups of sevelamer become partially protonated in

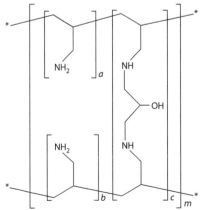

Structure XIV Sevelamer. The structure shows the exposed binding site for phosphates – the repeating and adjacent NH$_2$ groups

the intestine and interact with phosphorus molecules through ionic and hydrogen bonding.

Some other pharmaceutical ion exchangers are listed in Table 7.10.

Clinical point: **Compliance**

The dose both of calcium salts and of sevelamer is high, being 1.25 g for Calcichew tablets and 800 mg for sevelamer (Renegel; Renvela), and patients who are already on several medications have reported problems with compliance.[16] Sevelamer tablets are thus large and one patient reports: 'the tablets are so disgusting, their consistency is so disgusting – so disgusting that you don't want to take [them]'. The concept is good with the agents, but the compounds are insufficiently powerful adsorbents or ion-exchangers to allow dosage reduction. Tablets not taken are a negation of therapeutics. What is required are more powerful systems.

Clinical point

Administered orally, cation-exchange resins effect changes in the electrolyte balance of the plasma by exchanging cations with those in the gut lumen. In the ammonium form, cation-exchange resins are used in the treatment of retention oedema and for the control of sodium retention in pregnancy. Depletion of plasma potassium can be prevented by including a proportion of resin in the form of the potassium salt. These resins are also used (as calcium and sodium forms) to treat hyperkalaemia.

Ion-exchange resins are employed to form complexes with drug substances, especially basic drugs such as ephedrine, pholcodine (**XV**) and phenyltoloxamine (**XVI**) (an isomer of diphenhydramine) to prolong drug action. Pholtex is a sustained-action liquid

Table 7.10 Ion exchangers used in pharmacy

Name	Type	Comments	Trade name
Ammonium polystyrene sulfonate	Cation exchanger	Each gram exchanges 2.5 mEq Na^+	Katonium
Polycarbophil	Cation exchanger	Synthetic hydrophilic resin copolymer of acrylic acid, loosely crosslinked with divinyl glycol. Marked water-binding capacity	–
Calcium polystyrene sulfonate	Cation exchanger	Each gram exchanges about 1.3 mEq K^+	Calcium Resonium
Colestyramine	Anion exchanger	The chloride of a strongly basic anion-exchange resin containing quaternary ammonium groups attached to styrene-divinylbenzene copolymer	Questran
Polyamine–methylene resin	Anion exchanger	Effects a temporary binding of HCl + pepsin in the stomach, later released in the intestine	–
Sodium polystyrene sulfonate	Cation exchanger	Each gram exchanges 2.8–3.5 mEq K^+	Resonium A
Polyaminostyrene	Weak anion exchanger		–

utilising a sulfonic acid ion-exchange resin with pholcodine and phenyltoloxamine as resin complexes.

Structure XV Pholcodine

Structure XVI Phenyltoloxamine

The ion-exchange resin (Amberlite IRP-69 resin) has been used with betaxolol as an ophthalmic suspension. This formulation with 0.25% betaxolol gave levels of drug in the aqueous humour virtually identical to those with the 0.5% control.[17] The rate of release of basic drugs from cation-exchange resins depends on the diameter of the resin beads, on the degree of crosslinking within the resin, and on the pK_a of the ionisable resin group. The resin–drug complex may be tableted and administered orally; resin complexes have been used to mask the taste of bitter drugs and to reduce the nausea produced by some irritant drugs. Some types, such as polacrilin potassium (Amberlite IRP 88, sulfonated polystyrene resin) are used as tablet disintegrants because of the high degree of swelling the dry resins undergo on interaction with water.

Apart from these medical uses, ion-exchange resins are widely used in the removal of ionised impurities from water. Purified water may be obtained by passing through two columns containing a strong cation exchanger and a strong anion exchanger, respectively, or a column containing mixed resins. Anionic impurities in the water are replaced by OH^- from the anion exchanger and cations by H^+ from the cation-exchange resin. Dissolved salts are thus removed and replaced by H_2O molecules, but of course non-ionic impurities and colloidal material are not removed. Regeneration of the resins is accomplished using NaOH and HCl for the anion and cation exchangers, respectively.

7.5.3 Silicone oligomers and polymers

The silicones are examples of hydrophobic liquid polymers, although in high molecular weight they exist as waxes and resins. Silicones are polymers with a structure containing alternate atoms of silicon and oxygen; the dimethicones are fluid polymers with the general formula (**XVII**), in which each unit has two methyl groups and an oxygen atom attached to the silicon atom in the chain. The viscosity range extends from 0.65 cSt to 3×10^6 cSt. The dimethicones 20, 200, 350 and 1000 (the number representing the average viscosity in centistokes at 25°C) have rheological properties that allow them to be used in ophthalmology and in rheumatoid arthritis. Dimethicone 200 has been used as a lubricant for artificial eyes and to replace the degenerative vitreous fluid in cases of retinal detachment. It can also act as a simple lubricant in joints. More common uses are as barrier substances, silicone lotions and creams acting as water-repellent applications protecting the skin against water-soluble irritants. Methylphenylsilicone is used as a lubricant for hypodermic syringes. Glassware which has been treated with a thin film of silicone is rendered hydrophobic; solutions and aqueous suspensions thus drain completely from such vessels.

Structure XVII Dimethicone

Activated dimethicone (activated polymethylsiloxane) is a mixture of liquid dimethicones containing finely divided silica to enhance the defoaming properties of the silicone. The mechanism by which dispersion of colloidal silica antifoams improves their action is not well understood.

By varying the amounts of polymer in resin, a variety of products such as catheters, tubing materials for reconstructive surgery and membranes for drug reservoirs can be formed.

The release of lipophilic steroids from silicone elastomer matrices is dependent on the crosslinking density of the polymer and the content of filler, but also on the lipophilicity of the drug. A relationship between the solubility parameters of a number of drugs and their release rate is shown in Fig. 7.31.

An interesting application of the silicone fluids is their coformulation with adhesives to increase 'tack' and in elastomers to soften the product. Pressure-sensitive silicone adhesives are formed from the most highly crosslinked systems based on the structure **XVII**.

Other pressure-sensitive adhesives used in transdermal delivery device include those shown in Table 7.11.

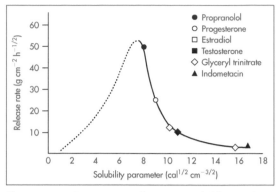

Figure 7.31 Comparative release rates of different drugs from a pressure-sensitive silicone matrix as a function of their solubility parameter.

Reproduced from Clauss LC. In: *Proceedings of the International Conference on Pharmaceutical, Ingredients and Intermediates (1990)*. Maarssen: Expoconsult; 1991: 116.

Table 7.11 Pressure-sensitive adhesives in transdermal patches

Adhesive class	Adhesive polymer
	Polyisoprene Polybutene Polyisobutylene
	Ethyl acrylate2-Ethylhexyl acrylate Isooctyl acrylate
	Polydimethylsiloxane Polysilicate resin Siloxane blends

Reproduced from Pfister WR *et al. Pharm Tech* 1992;16(1):42.

 Key points

- Water-soluble (hydrophilic) polymers are widely used in pharmacy, for example as suspending agents, emulsifiers, binding agents in tablets, thickeners of liquid dosage forms and in film coating of tablets. Important examples include: carboxypolymethylene (Carbomer, Carbopol), cellulose derivatives (methylcellulose, HPMC), natural gums and mucilages (acacia and tragacanth gums, alginates, pectin), chitosan, PVP and polyethylene glycols.

- Water-insoluble (hydrophobic) polymers are mainly used in packaging material and tubing, and in the fabrication of membranes and films. Important examples include ion-exchange resins and silicones (e.g. dimethicone).

- Important properties of hydrophobic polymers that affect their suitability for use in pharmacy are their permeability to drugs and gases and their tendency to adsorb drugs.

7.6 Some applications of polymeric systems in drug delivery

Control of the rate of release of a drug when administered by oral or parenteral routes is aided by the use of polymers that function as a barrier to drug movement.

7.6.1 Film coating

Aspects of film-coating technology have already been discussed in Chapter 1. Here we concentrate on the polymers used to achieve the desired release properties.

Polymer solutions allowed to evaporate produce polymeric films that can act as protective layers for tablets or granules containing sensitive drug substances or as a rate-controlling barrier to drug release. Film coats have been divided into two types: those that dissolve rapidly and those that dissolve very slowly and behave as dialysis membranes, allowing slow diffusion of solute or some delayed diffusion by acting as gel layers. Materials that have been used as film formers include shellac, zein, glyceryl stearates, paraffins and a range of anionic and cationic polymers such as the Eudragit polymers (**XVIII–XXI**). Newer materials used for the same purpose include cellulose acetate phthalate (CAP).

Different film coats applied to tablet surfaces can lead to quite different rates of solution. In Fig. 7.32, HPMC, an acrylic derivative, and zein are compared for their effect on sodium chloride dissolution from discs. Two plasticisers have been used: glycerin and diethyl phthalate. Times for 50% dissolution range from a few minutes to 450 minutes, indicating the

scope of the technique for retard formulations, and the possibility of unwittingly extending dissolution times by the injudicious choice of coating material.

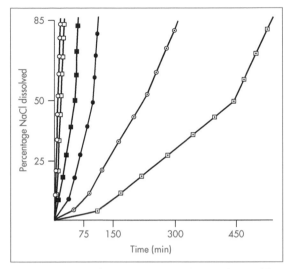

Figure 7.32 Dissolution of sodium chloride from tablets coated with hydroxypropylmethylcellulose (○), a vinyl polymer (●) and zein (◎) with glycerin as an additive, and the same polymers with diethyl phthalate as additive (□, ■, and ⊡, respectively).
Reproduced from Laguna O *et al. Ann Pharm Franc* 1975;33:235.

The process of film coating generally involves spraying the chosen polymer solution on to a bed of tablet cores. Several physical properties are important, for example, the viscosity and surface tension of the solutions will determine the droplet size and might also influence the spreading of the polymer on the tablet surfaces as well as its adhesion to the substrate. Additives are used to modify the native properties of the polymer solutions; in one example the addition of microcrystalline cellulose allowed a greater interaction with the tablet surface, probably through interaction with the same material in the tablet formulation. Polymer blends are used to tailor release rates of drugs from coated tablets. As with many pharmaceutical processes, matters are far from simple. Blended polymers may be incompatible, polymer dispersions may flocculate and plasticisers migrate. Ultimately the coated systems must be tested rigorously, with respect to their main functions, control of drug release rate, reduction of water permeability into the core and reduced oxygen permeability to minimise degradation.

MAA   MMA

Structure XVIII Poly(methacrylic acid, methyl methacrylate) 1 : 1 copolymer (Eudragit L12.5, L100)

MAA   EA

Structure XIX Poly(ethylacrylate, methacrylic acid) 1 : 1 (Eudragit L 30 D, L 100–55)

DMEMA   MMA/BMA

Structure XX Poly(butylmethacrylate, 2-dimethylaminoethyl methacrylate, methyl methacrylate) 1 : 2 : 1 (Eudragit E 100, E 12.5)

EA   MMA

Structure XXI Poly(ethylacrylate, methyl methacrylate) 2 : 1 (Eudragit E 30 D)

7.6.2 Matrices

The use of a barrier film coating is only one of several procedures that can be adopted to control release of drugs (Fig. 7.33). Various methods are shown schematically in Table 7.12. If hydrophobic water-insoluble polymers are used, the mechanism of release is the passage of drug through pores in the plastic, or by leaching or slow diffusion of drug through the polymer wall (Fig. 7.33b), as discussed earlier in this chapter. Release may also be effected by erosion of the polymer (Fig. 7.33c). When water-soluble polymers are employed, for example as hydrophilic matrices, the entry of water into the polymer is followed by swelling and gelation and the drug must diffuse through the viscous gel, a process obviously slower than diffusion through plain solvent.

Release of drugs from matrices

Equations describing the rate of drug release from hydrophobic and hydrophilic matrices are useful in determining which factors may be altered to change the measured release rate of drug. Higuchi[18] proposed the following equation for the amount of drug, Q, released per unit area of tablet surface in time t, from an insoluble matrix:

$$Q = \left[\frac{D\varepsilon}{\tau}(2A - \varepsilon C_s)C_s t \right]^{1/2} \quad (7.26)$$

D is the diffusion coefficient of the drug in the release medium, C_s is the solubility of drug in the medium, ε is the porosity of the matrix, τ is the tortuosity of the matrix and A is the total amount of drug in the matrix per unit volume.

If the same matrix is saturated with a solution of the drug (as in medicated soft contact lenses) the appropriate equation becomes, if C_0 is the concentration of drug solution:

$$Q = 2C_0\varepsilon \left(\frac{Dt}{\tau\pi} \right)^{1/2} \quad (7.27)$$

That is, for a given drug in a given matrix, $Q \propto t^{1/2}$. The more porous the matrix, the more rapid the release. The more tortuous the pores, the longer the path for diffusing molecules, the lower is Q. More soluble drugs diffuse more quickly from the matrix.

The extension of these equations to hydrophilic matrices is difficult because the conditions in a hydrophilic matrix change with time as water penetrates into it. If the polymer does not dissolve but simply swells and if the drug has not completely dissolved in the

Table 7.12 Depot forms employing polymeric films and matrices

Type	Materials[a]	Diagrammatic representation	Mechanisms
Barrier coating	Beeswax, glyceryl monostearate, ethylcellulose, nylon (Ultramid IC), acrylic resins (Eudragit retard)	drug / coating	Diffusion
Fat embedment	Glycerol palmitostearate (Precirol), beeswax, glycowax, castorwax, aluminium monostearate, carnauba wax, glyceryl monostearate, stearyl alcohol	drug / fat	Erosion, hydrolysis of fat, dissolution
Plastic matrix	Polyethylene Poly(vinyl acetate) Polymethacrylate Poly(vinyl chloride) Ethylcellulose	drug / polymer	Leaching, diffusion
Repeat action	Cellulose acetylphthalate	enteric coat	Dissolution of enteric coat
Ion exchange	Amberlite Dowex		Dissociation of drug–resin complex
Hydrophilic matrix	Carboxymethylcellulose Sodium carboxymethylcellulose Hydroxypropylmethylcellulose	hydrophilic polymer / drug	Gelation, diffusion
Epoxy resin beads	Epoxy resins	epoxy resin bead or microcapsule	Dissolution of resin or swelling, diffusion
Microcapsules	Polyamides, gelatin		
Soft gelatin depot capsules	Shellac–PEG Poly(vinyl acetate)–PEG		Diffusion

Modified from Ritschel WA. In: Ariens AJ (ed.) *Drug Design*, vol. IV. New York: Academic Press; 1974, with permission.
[a]Materials used are not all polymeric. The waxes are included for completeness; these depend on conferring a hydrophobic layer on the drug, tablet or granule to prevent access of solvent.

incoming solvent, diffusion of drug commences from a saturated solution through the gel layer, and

$$Q = \frac{D\varepsilon}{\tau}\left[\left(\left(\frac{2W_0}{V} - \varepsilon C_s\right)\right)tC_s\right]^{1/2} \qquad (7.28)$$

Equation (7.28) is similar to equation (7.26) except that the effective volume V of the hydrated matrix is used as this is not a fixed quantity. W_0 is the dose of the drug in the matrix. If the drug completely dissolves on hydration of the matrix, an analogue of equation (7.27) is used:

$$Q = \frac{2W_0}{V}\left(\frac{Dt}{\tau\pi}\right)^{1/2} \qquad (7.29)$$

In the initial stages of the process the rate of movement of water into the matrix may be important in determining release characteristics. When a homogeneous barrier wall is present diffusion through the walls has to take place and equations in section 7.5.1 apply.

7.6.3 Microcapsules and microspheres

Microencapsulation is a technique that, as its name suggests, involves the encapsulation of small particles of drug, or solution of drug, within a polymer film or coat. Microspheres, on the other hand, are solid but not necessarily homogeneous particles that can entrap drug. Although the terms tend to be used interchangeably, we retain the distinction here. Microspheres can be prepared also by a variety of techniques,

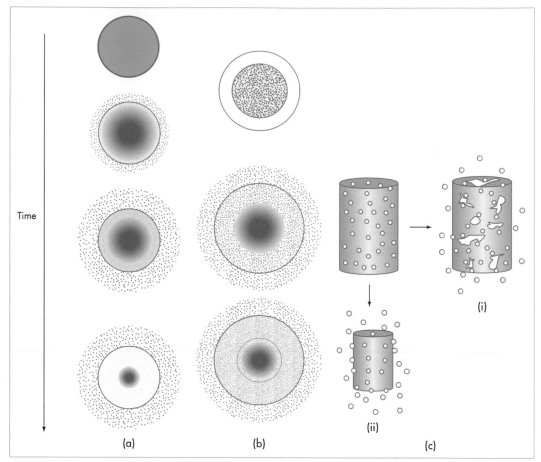

Figure 7.33 (a) Drug delivery from a matrix delivery device showing diagrammatically the depletion of drug from the system and the release of the drug. (b) Release from a typical reservoir system with a membrane controlling release from the internal store of drug. (c) Illustrating release from (i) a bulk-eroding system and (ii) a surface-eroding system.

After Brandon-Peppas L. Polymers in controlled drug delivery. *Med Plast Biomaterials* 1997;Nov.: 34, with permission.

discussed briefly below. Typical photomicrographs of poly(ε-caprolactone) microspheres are shown in Fig. 7.34. Three main processes can be considered:

1. *Coacervation* of macromolecules around the core material, this being induced by temperature change, solvent change or addition of a second macromolecule of appropriate physical properties.
2. *Interfacial* polymerisation of a monomer around the core material by polymerisation at the interface of a liquid dispersion.
3. *Spray coating and other methods* in which larger particles may be coated in suspension.

Any method that will cause a coherent barrier to deposit itself on the surface of a liquid droplet or a solid particle of drug may be applied to the formation

of microcapsules. Many so-called microencapsulation procedures result in the formation of macroscopic 'beads', which are simply coated granules.

Coacervation

Coacervation is the term used to describe the separation of macromolecular solutions into colloid-poor and colloid-rich (coacervate) phases when the macromolecules are desolvated. The liquid or solid to be encapsulated is dispersed in a solution of a macromolecule (such as gelatin, gum arabic, carboxymethylcellulose or poly(vinyl alcohol)) in which it is immiscible. A non-solvent, miscible with the continuous phase but a poor solvent for the polymer, under certain conditions will induce the polymer to form a coacervate (polymer-rich) layer around the disperse phase. This coating layer may then be treated to give

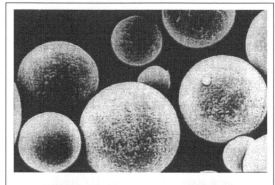

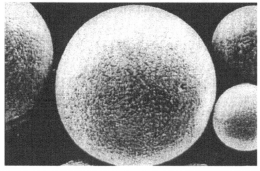

Figure 7.34 Scanning electron micrographs of bovine serum albumin-loaded microspheres prepared from a ternary blend of poly(ε-caprolactone). Protein entrapment efficiency and mean particle size were 28.6% and 2.9 μm, respectively.

Reproduced with permission from Huatan H *et al*. The microencapsulation of protein using a novel ternary blend based on poly (caprolactone). *J Microencapsul* 1995;12:557.

a rigid coat of capsule wall. This is the process of *simple coacervation*. Successful application of the technique relies on the determination of the appropriate conditions for coacervate deposition, which can be achieved not only by the addition of non-solvents such as ethanol and isopropanol and salts (sodium and ammonium sulfates) but also by the choice of macromolecules incompatible under selected conditions with the first species. The latter process is termed *complex coacervation*. In both simple and complex coacervation utilising hydrophilic macromolecules it is the decrease in solubility that results in deposition of the macromolecule layer at the particle–solution interface.

Desolvation of water-insoluble macromolecules in non-aqueous solvents leads to the deposition of a coacervate layer around aqueous or solid disperse droplets. Table 7.13 lists both water-soluble and water-soluble macromolecules that have been used in coacervation processes. Desolvation, and thus coacervation, can be induced thermally and this is the basis

of some preparative techniques. Conditions for phase separation are best obtained using phase diagrams.

Table 7.13 Materials used in coacervation microencapsulation

Water-soluble macromolecules	Water-insoluble macromolecules
Arabinogalactan	Cellulose acetate phthalate
Carboxymethylcellulose	Cellulose nitrate
Gelatin	Ethylcellulose
Gum arabic (acacia)	Poly(ethylene vinyl acetate)
Hydroxyethylcellulose	Poly(methyl methacrylate)
Poly(acrylic acid)	
Polyethyleneimine	
Poly(vinyl alcohol)	
Polyvinylpyrrolidone	
Methylcellulose	
Starch	

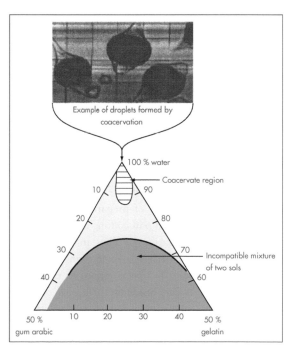

Figure 7.35 Ternary diagram showing complex coacervation region for mixtures of gum arabic and gelatin at pH 4.5; below the curved line the mixture separates into two sols (US Patent 2800457). Insert: Typical droplets formed by coacervation (Ronald T Dodge).

For example, in the region of pH 6, gelatin will be positively charged and gum arabic negatively charged. In admixture, complex coacervates will form under the conditions described in Fig. 7.35, which shows the partial phase diagram of the ternary system gum arabic–gelatin–water. The hatched area at the top of the phase diagram is the restricted region in which coacervation occurs. At higher concentrations of the macromolecules, macroscopic precipitates of the complex will occur.

Interfacial reaction

Reactions between oil-soluble monomers and water-soluble monomers at the oil–water interface of water-in-oil (w/o) or o/w dispersions can lead to *interfacial polymerisation,* resulting in the formation of polymeric microcapsules, the size of which is determined by the size of the emulsion droplets. Alternatively, reactive monomer can be dispersed in one of the phases and induced to polymerise at the interface, or to polymerise in the bulk disperse phase and to *precipitate* at the interface owing to its insolubility in the continuous phase. There are many variations on this theme. Probably the most widely studied reaction has been the interfacial condensation of water-soluble alkyl diamines with oil-soluble acid dichlorides to form polyamides. Representative examples of other wall materials are polyurethanes, polysulfonamides, polyphthalamides and poly(phenyl esters). The selection of polymer is restricted to those that can be formed from monomers with the requisite preferential solubilities in one phase so that polymerisation takes place only at the interface.

Physical methods of encapsulation

Various physical methods of preparing microcapsules such as spray drying and pan coating are available.

Pan-coating application of films to particles can only be used for particles greater than 600 µm in diameter. The process has been applied in the formation of sustained-release beads by application of waxes such as glyceryl monostearate in organic solution to granules of drug.

The *spray-drying* process involves dispersion of the core material in a solution of coating substance and spraying the mixture into an environment that causes the solvent to evaporate. In an analogous *spray-congealing* process the coating material is congealed thermally or by introducing the core coat mixture into a non-solvent mixture. Both processes can produce microcapsules in the size range 5000–6000 µm.

Spray polycondensation is a variant based on the polycondensation of surface-active monomers on a melamine–formaldehyde base on the surface of suspended particles during spray drying. A dispersion of the core material is prepared in a continuous phase containing aminoplast monomers or precondensates of relatively low molecular weight, in addition to other film-forming agents and catalyst. The reactive monomers derived from hexamethylol melamine derivatives are selectively adsorbed at the surface of the disperse phase. Spray drying at 150–200°C results in vaporisation of the water and causes simultaneous polycondensation of the monomers and precondensates by acid catalysis.

The preparation and properties of nanoparticles for drug delivery and targeting are discussed in Chapter 14.

General considerations

In all techniques discussed there are several factors which are of importance in relation to the use of the product as a drug delivery vehicle or carrier.

- the efficiency of encapsulation of the active ingredient
- the effect of the encapsulation process on the properties of the encapsulated agent
- the presence of potentially toxic residue (e.g. monomer, salts) in the final product
- the reproducibility of the process and ease of separation from the reaction mixture
- the biocompatibility of the encapsulating agent
- the biodegradability of the material (in some cases)
- the properties of the microcapsule in relation to use, size distribution, porosity and permeability of the wall.

Biodegradable polymers cannot always be induced to form microcapsules and a polymer found to be degradable in solid or film form may not be degradable when formed into microcapsules if the polymer chains are crosslinked. In their application in medicine, the permeability of the capsule wall is probably the most important feature of the product. The effects of the various parameters relating to wall material, capsule and environment on permeability are outlined in Table 7.14.

Protein microspheres

Aqueous solutions of proteins such as albumin can be emulsified in an oil and induced to form microspheres, either by crosslinking the protein molecules with glutaraldehyde or other agents or by coagulating the protein by heating. Incorporation of a drug within the initial protein solution results in drug-laden microspheres that are biodegradable. The particle size of the microspheres (generally 0.2–300 μm diameter) is determined by the size distribution of the initial emulsion.

Protein microspheres have been used for physical drug targeting, i.e. the entrapment of carrier and therefore drug in, for example, the capillaries of the lung. Microspheres greater than about 7 μm in diameter will be physically trapped in capillary beds. On intra-arterial injection of large microspheres, the blood supply to an organ is reduced; the process of chemoembolisation involves both blockage and delivery of drugs to the organ. External control over intravenously administered protein microspheres has been achieved

Table 7.14 General parameters affecting capsule wall permeability

Parameter	For lower permeability
Properties of wall polymer	
Density	Increase
Crystallinity	Increase
Crosslinking	Increase
Plasticiser content	Decrease
Fillers	Increase
Solvents used in film formation	Use good solvents versus poor
Properties of capsule	
Size	Increase
Wall thickness	Increase
Treatment	Utilise (e.g. crosslinking, sintering)
Multiple coatings	Utilise
Environmental properties	
Temperature	Decrease

Reproduced with permission from Vandegaer JE (ed.) *Microencapsulation, Processes and Applications.* New York: Plenum Press; 1974.

by incorporation of magnetite (Fe_3O_4) particles into the microspheres, which then respond to an externally applied magnetic field.

7.6.4 Rate-limiting membranes and devices

The use of rate-limiting membranes to control the movement of drugs from a reservoir has been referred to above. Implants of silicone rubber or other appropriate polymeric material in which drug is embedded can be designed by choice of polymer, membrane thickness and porosity, to release drug at preselected rates. The Progestasert device (Fig. 7.36c) was designed to be implanted into the uterine cavity and to release there 65 μg progesterone per day to provide contraceptive cover for 1 year. Progestasert was discontinued in 2001, but similar devices such as Mirena (Bayer) are available to deliver levonorgestrel. The Ocusert device and the Transiderm therapeutic system (also shown in Fig. 7.36) originated from the then Alza Corporation (USA) and rely on rate-limiting polymeric membranes to control drug release. The opportunities for prolonged release of drugs given by the oral route are fewer. The aim in oral dosage forms is for controlled rather than prolonged release, so that dosage frequency can be reduced or so that side-effects resulting from fast dissolution of drug can be minimised.

7.6.5 Eroding systems

Release of drug by erosion of the polymeric or macromolecular matrix in which a drug is dissolved or dispersed provides another mechanism for controlling drug absorption. Erosion, of course, demands some degree of solubility of the matrix to allow enzymes and other agents to penetrate. A typical bioerodible system would be that achieved by the molecular association of a CAP (a carboxylic acid polymer) with a poloxamer block copolymer such as Pluronic L101. This interaction is between the proton-donating CAP and the proton-accepting poloxamer. By varying the ratio of CAP to poloxamer, the erosion periods can be controlled from hours to days. Figure 7.37 shows the relationship between the percentage polymer eroded and the release of drugs from a 50 : 50 mixture of the polymers containing 10% of the drug metronidazole.

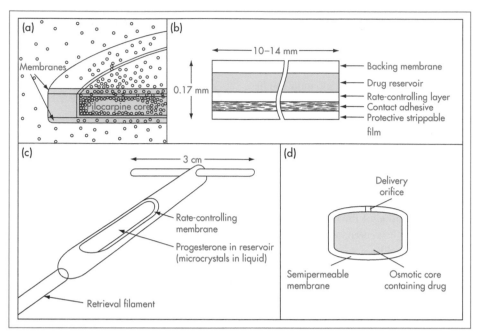

Figure 7.36 Examples of iconic drug delivery systems employing polymeric membranes. (a) Ocusert system for the eye with two rate-controlling membranes. (b) Transiderm system for transdermal medication with one rate-controlling layer. (c) The Progestasert device for intrauterine insertion in which the body of the device serves as the rate-controlling barrier. (d) The oral Oros device, in which the membrane is a semipermeable membrane that prevents drug transport, allowing water ingress only.

Computer simulation of eroding matrices (Fig. 7.38) can give an accurate representation of the process and can predict the position of the erosion front and the weight of the matrix.

More precise control of release than is possible with matrices has recently been achieved by the appli-

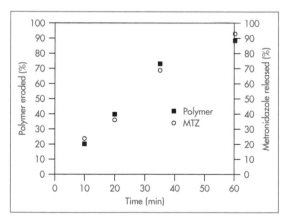

Figure 7.37 Characteristics of *in vivo* polymer erosion and metronidazole (MTZ) release from 50/50 CAP/Pluronic L101 films (with 10% metronidazole loading) in a dorsal rat model.

Reproduced from Gates KA *et al*. A new bioerodible polymer insert for the controlled release of metronidazole. *Pharm Res* 1994;11:1605, with kind permission from Springer Science and Business Media.

cation of several features of polymer physical chemistry, as discussed below.

7.6.6 Osmotic pumps

A variety of osmotic pumps have been described in the patent literature.[19,20] In the oral osmotic pump (Oros or Osmet) the drug is mixed with a water-soluble core material. This core is surrounded by a water-insoluble semipermeable polymer membrane in which is drilled a small orifice. Water molecules can diffuse into the core through the outer membrane to form a concentrated solution inside. An osmotic gradient is set up across the semipermeable membrane, with the result that drug is pushed out of the orifice (Fig. 7.39).

The core may be a water-soluble polymer, an inert salt or, as in the case of metoprolol fumarate,[21] the drug itself, whose saturated solution has an osmotic pressure of 32.5 atm. The osmotic tablet of nifedipine is described in detail in Fig. 7.40, which shows the semipermeable cellulose acetate coating, the swellable hydrogel layer of PEG and HPMC and the drug chamber containing nifedipine in HPMC and PEG.

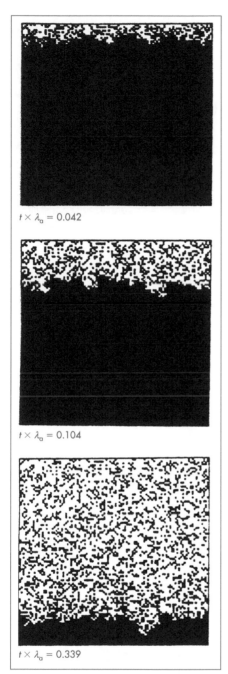

$t \times \lambda_a = 0.042$

$t \times \lambda_a = 0.104$

$t \times \lambda_a = 0.339$

Figure 7.38 Theoretical representation of a polymer matrix: changes during erosion (dark pixels = non-degraded areas, white pixels = degraded areas), where λ_a (a rate constant) = 2.7×10^{-7} s^{-1} for a sample containing 50% polyanhydride 1-3 bis(*p*carboxyphenoxypropane).

Reprinted with permission from Göpferich A *et al.* In: Cleland JL, Langer R (eds) *Formulation and Delivery of Proteins and Peptides.* ACS Symposium Series no. 567. Washington, DC: American Chemical Society; 1994. Copyright 1994 American Chemical Society.

For simple osmotic systems the initial zero-order delivery rate (dm/dt) is given by

$$\frac{dm}{dt} = \frac{A}{H} k (\pi_f - \pi_e) S_d \qquad (7.30)$$

where S_d is drug concentration in the system, π_f is the osmotic pressure of the formulation, π_e is the osmotic pressure of the environment (7.7 atm for isotonic saline at 37°C), k is the membrane permeability to water, H is the thickness of the membrane and A is its area. Calculated and experimental release rates are shown in Fig. 7.41.

One problem is that of controlling the transit of the device down the gastrointestinal tract, as individual subjects vary considerably in gastrointestinal transit times. If the system is designed to release drug over a period of 10 hours and total transit time in the gut is 5 hours, bioavailability will obviously be reduced.

7.6.7 Transdermal delivery systems

Several transdermal systems ostensibly dependent on rate-controlling membranes are available for the delivery of glyceryl trinitrate, hyoscine, estradiol, fentanyl and other drugs. The word 'ostensibly' is used as there is a debate about whether the barrier membrane in these devices is the rate-limiting step in absorption. The barrier properties of skin are so variable, however, that one advantage of rate-controlling systems is that they prevent too rapid dosing in patients with highly permeable skin. In those with less permeable skin, the systems probably act only as reservoirs. The wide range of agents listed in Table 7.15, has been supplemented by buprenorphine, testosterone, selegiline and 5-hydroxytryptophan among others.

Some of the devices and the bases of their design are shown in Fig. 7.42 (the Transiderm system is also shown in Fig. 7.36). There are two groups: membrane and matrix systems. Membrane systems generally consist of a reservoir, a rate-controlling membrane and an adhesive layer. Diffusion of the active principle through the controlling membrane governs release rate. The active principle is usually present in suspended form; liquids and gels are used as dispersion media. In matrix systems the active principle is dispersed in a matrix that consists either of a gel or of an adhesive film.

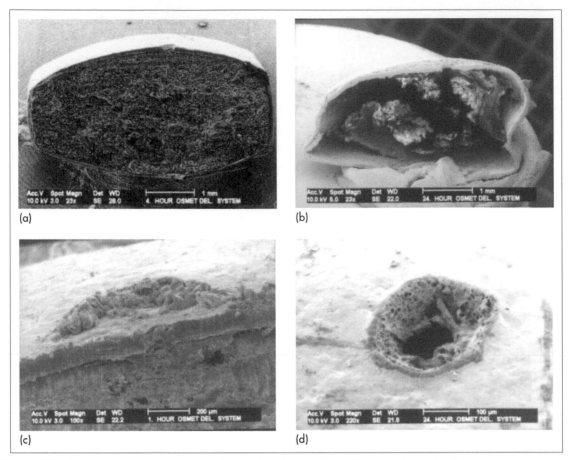

Figure 7.39 Low-power scanning electron micrographs of an oral osmotic pump (Osmet). (a) A section showing the semipermeable membrane, the osmotic core and the laser-drilled orifice. (b) The same, 8 hours after immersion in water. (c) The laser-drilled orifice. (d) Another view of the tablet via the orifice after 24 hours of immersion.

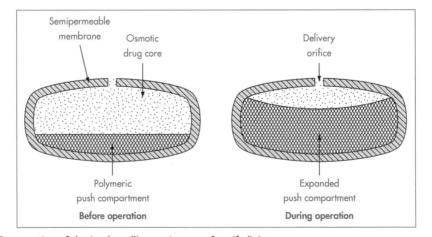

Figure 7.40 Cross-section of the 'push–pull' osmotic pump for nifedipine.

Table 7.15 Some transdermal drug delivery devices

Product	Drug	Adhesive	Adhesive use[a]	Marketing company
Antianginal				
Nitrodisc	GTN[b]	Acrylic	Rim	G. D. Searle
Nitro-Dur I	GTN	Acrylic	Rim	Schering-Plough
Nitro-Dur II	GTN	Acrylic	Matrix	Schering-Plough
Diafusor	GTN	Acrylic	Matrix	Lab Pierre Fabre Med
Minitran	GTN	Acrylic	Matrix	3M Riker
Transiderm-Nitro	GTN	Silicone	Face	Novartis
Nitroderm TTS	GTN	Silicone	Face	Novartis
Nitrol patch	GTN	Acrylic	Rim	Adria Lab.
NTS patch	GTN	Acrylic	Rim	Bolar, Major, Qualitest, Bio-Line, Goldline, Geneva, Rugby
Transdermal-NTG	GTN	Acrylic	Rim	Warner Chilcott Lab.
Nitrocine	GTN	Acrylic	Rim	Kremer Urban
Deponit	GTN	Polyisobutylene	Matrix	Schwarz/Wyeth
Frandol Tape	Isosorbide dinitrate	Acrylic	Matrix	Toaeiyo, Yamanouchi Pharm.
Motion sickness				
Trasiderm-Scop	Hyoscine	Polyisobutylene	Matrix	Novartis
Kimite-patch	Hyoscine	Polyisobutylene	Matrix	Myun Moon Pharm. Co.
Hypertension				
Catapress-TTS	Clonidine	Polyisobutylene	Matrix	Boehringer Ingelheim
Oestrogen therapy				
Estraderm	Estradiol	Polyisobutylene	Face	Novartis
Analgesia				
Duragesic	Fentanyl	Silicone	Face	Jansen Pharm.
Smoking cessation				
Nicotinell	Nicotine	Acrylic	Matrix	Novartis
Nikofrenon	Nicotine	Acrylic	Matrix	Novartis

Reproduced with permission from Foster WP *et al. Pharm Tech* 1992;16(1):42.
[a]Indicated as an adhesive laminated to an overlying backing substrate forming a rim around the matrix (rim): a drug-containing adhesive matrix laminated to a backing substrate (matrix); or an adhesive laminated to the face of a rate-controlling membrane (face).
[b]GTN = glyceryl trinitrate.

In Transiderm Nitro, the rate-controlling membrane is composed of a polyethylene–vinyl acetate copolymer having a thin adhesive layer (membrane type) (Table 7.15). The reservoir contains glyceryl trinitrate dispersed in the form of a lactose suspension in silicone oil. The Nitro-Dur system consists of a hydrogel matrix (composed of water, glycerin, poly (vinyl alcohol) and polyvinylpyrrolidone) in which a glyceryl trinitrate–lactose triturate is homogeneously dispersed.

In Nitro Disc, glyceryl trinitrate is distributed between microscopically small liquid compartments

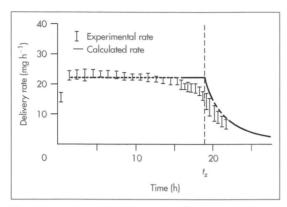

Figure 7.41 *In vitro* release rate of potassium chloride from elementary osmotic pumps in water at 37°C.

Reproduced from Theeuwes F. Elementary osmotic pump. *J Pharm Sci* 1975;64:1987. Copyright Wiley-VCH Verlag GmbH & Co. KGaA. Reproduced with permission.

and a crosslinked silicone matrix. In the approximately 10–200 μm sized micro compartments there is active ingredient also in the form of a lactose triturate, in an aqueous solution of PEG 400. The system is secured to the skin with the aid of a circular adhesive disc having a centrally located silicone matrix, not coated with adhesive. The system is termed a 'micro sealed drug delivery system'. The basis of the Deponit system[22] is shown in detail in Fig. 7.43.

7.6.8 Polymer fibres: electrospinning

We have discussed polymers as thin films, matrices, microspheres and nanospheres. In this section we treat briefly the concepts of the formation of polymer fibres

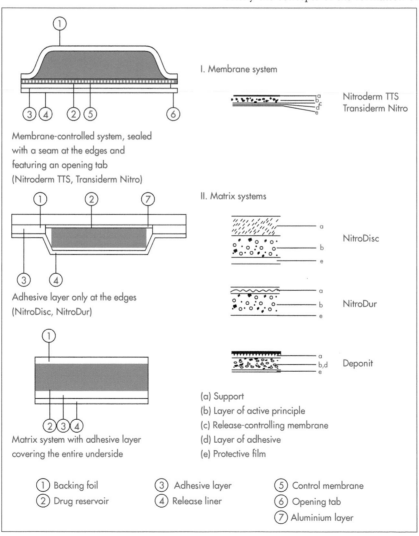

Figure 7.42 The structures of some commercial transdermal membrane-controlled and matrix systems (the structure of the Deponit TTS is shown in Fig. 7.43).

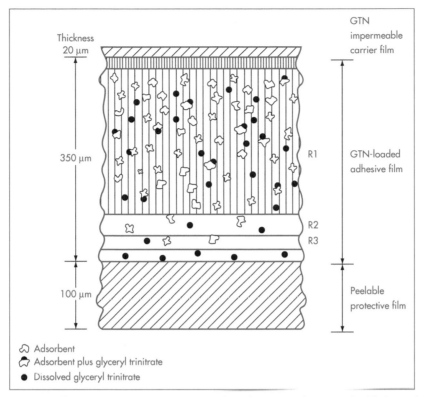

Figure 7.43 Cross-section of Deponit TTS. Deponit contains glyceryl trinitrate directly embedded in a lactose-containing adhesive film approximately 0.3 mm thick. In cross-section, the Deponit transdermal system, closely resembling a plaster, consists of three components in macroscopic proportions, the ratios of which are as given in the figure. The adhesive film is both a store of active ingredient and the release-controlling matrix.

Reproduced from Wolff M et al. In vitro and in vivo release of nitroglycerin from a new transdermal therapeutic system. *Pharm Res* 1985;2:23–29, with kind permission from Springer Science and Business Media.

which are being increasingly studied as delivery devices, or as materials for wound dressings, and transdermal delivery systems.

Electrospinning is an electrohydrodynamic process which uses electrostatic forces to drive fibres (or droplets) from a capillary via an electrically charged fluid jet. The topic of electrospinning has a long pedigree, dating from experiments in the 16th century when experiments were carried out on the effect of electric potential on beeswax and shellac in liquid form. As the name suggests, the phenomenon relates to the effect of electrostatic forces on a liquid droplet, a topic developed theoretically to understand the formation of Taylor cones (Fig. 7.44) and filaments which, if a polymer solution is in the capillary and the applied field is sufficiently strong, will be the basis of polymer fibres.

When an appropriately high voltage is applied to a liquid droplet, the liquid becomes charged, and elec-

trostatic repulsion counteracts the surface tension; the droplet is pulled out or stretched and at a critical point a stream (jet) of liquid erupts from the surface. This point is known as Taylor cone formation. As the jet travels towards the collector, tensile forces brought about by surface charge repulsion lead to a bending motion and the polymer chains in the jet orient to form microfibres or nanofibres depending on the polymer, its viscosity, surface tension and the capillary diameter; the polymer is then deposited on an earthed collector.

The current interest in the technique is that it allows the formation of fibres with a variety of internal structures and dimensions, these having potential for drug delivery and the application of drugs in novel ways. Some of these structures are shown in composite micrographs in Fig. 7.45.

A typical small-scale manufacturing device is shown in Fig. 7.46, which shows both monoaxial and

Key points

- Polymers may be used to control the rate of release of a drug when administered by oral or parenteral routes. Materials such as shellac, zein, CAP, glyceryl stearates, and a range of anionic and cationic polymers (Eudragits) form *film coats*, allowing slow diffusion of solute or delaying diffusion by acting as gel layers. *Matrices* may be formed by (1) hydrophobic water-insoluble polymers (e.g. poly(vinyl chloride), poly(vinyl alcohol), ethylcellulose) that release drug by slow diffusion through pores or through the polymer wall, or by erosion of the polymer and (2) water-soluble polymers (e.g. carboxymethylcellulose, HPMC) that swell in water to form viscous gels (hydrophilic matrices), from which drug is released by slow diffusion.
- Drug may also be slowly released from *microcapsules*, which encapsulate the drug as small particles or as a drug solution in a polymer film or coat, and *microspheres*, which are solid polymeric spheres that entrap drug. Microcapsules can be prepared by coacervation, by interfacial polymerisation or by spray coating.
- Rate-limiting membranes may be used to control the movement of drugs from a reservoir as in the Progestasert device designed to release progesterone into the uterine cavity, the Ocusert device for delivery to the eye and the Transiderm therapeutic system for transdermal medication.
- In oral *osmotic pumps* (Oros or Osmet) an osmotic gradient is set up across a semipermeable polymeric membrane that encloses a solution of drug in a water-soluble core material; the osmotic pressure developed as water diffuses into the core pushes the drug out of a small orifice drilled in the membrane.

coaxial processes, the former producing mainly monolithic fibres and the latter core-shell structures. Drug can be incorporated into the polymer (or indeed ceramic) materials to provide interesting geometries which can be manipulated for drug delivery.

What factors control the nature of the product? Those listed in Fig. 7.47 can be rationalised readily, *large-diameter fibres* being produced by increasing polymer concentration, increased molecular weight of the polymers, enhanced flow rate, increased needle diameter and increased viscosity of the solutions used. *Smaller-diameter fibres* form with increased field strength, increased conductivity of the solutions, enhanced solvent volatility, increased surface tension and the distance to the collector, as shown in Fig. 7.43. The physics is quite complex; however, it is important to know in more detail the outlines of the parameters concerned. The diameter of the fluid jet, *d,* is related to

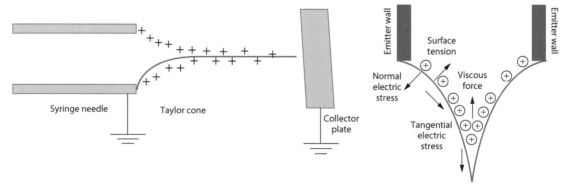

Figure 7.44 *Left:* The formation of a Taylor cone, showing the effect of the application of a high voltage to a needle tip, causing surface charges to accumulate on the liquid, leading to the deformation of the spherical drop into a cone. Increase in the voltage beyond this level causes the formation of a liquid jet. *Right:* The forces acting on the system which shape the nature of the jet include surface tension, viscous forces and normal and tangential electrical stresses.

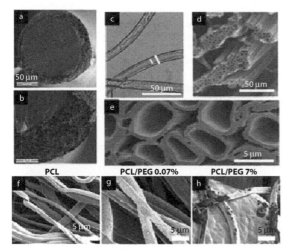

Figure 7.45 Photomicrographs of several fibrous structures prepared by electrospinning of polymers.

Reproduced from Chakraborty S *et al.* Electrohydrodynamics: a facile technique to fabricate drug delivery systems. *Adv Drug Deliv Rev* 2009;61:1043. Copyright Elsevier 2009.

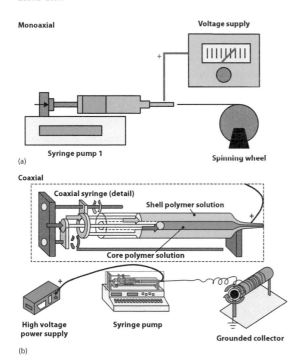

Figure 7.46 Two devices for electrospinning polymer solutions: (a) a monoaxial system in which a solution containing drug flows through a capillary to which a voltage is applied to form a monolithic fibre; and (b) the coaxial system in which the polymer can be made to surround a core system by the expedient of using a core drug polymer and a shell polymer solution. In both cases a collector which is grounded receives the fibres.

Reproduced from Chakraborty S *et al.* Electrohydrodynamics: a facile technique to fabricate drug delivery systems. *Adv Drug Deliv Rev* 2009;61:1043–1054. Copyright Elsevier 2009.

the flow rate, Q, of the fluid, the fluid density, ρ, and the applied field strength, E_∞, by the equation

$$d = (Q^3\rho/2\pi^2 E_\infty I)^{1/4} \cdot z^{-1/4} \qquad (7.31)$$

where z is an axial coordinate. The value of d determines the diameter of the fibre.

7.6.9 Polymers in wound dressings

The treatment of wounds is a complex topic, such are the variety of skin lesions and the types of wound dressings now available to aid the healing process. As many dressings involve synthetic or natural polymers and macromolecules and rely for some of their benefits on physical phenomena such as capillarity and wicking, it is appropriate to discuss these systems here. One of the purposes of a dressing is to keep the wound moist, to absorb exudate and to maintain gas exchange. The *British National Formulary* 68 states that 'advanced wound dressings' are designed to control the environment for wound healing, for example, to donate fluid (e.g. with hydrogels), maintain hydration (e.g. hydrocolloids) or to absorb wound exudate (e.g. alginates, foams).

Wound dressings can generally be classified[23] in groups depending on their nature and properties, e.g.:

- semipermeable films
- hydrocolloids
- alginates
- polymer foams
- hydrogels
- antimicrobial-releasing dressings.

There are naturally some overlaps in definitions and structures. We discuss a selection of structures here to illustrate their nature and variety.

Hydrocolloids

Hydrocolloids are composed of gel-forming substances such as gelatin or NaCMC. One product, Hydrofiber, is an NaCMC dressing with a high cohesive dry and wet tensile strength which absorbs up to 25 times its weight in fluid without losing its integrity. NaCMC is spun into fibres (see also alginates, below) and is produced in ribbon and sheet formats.

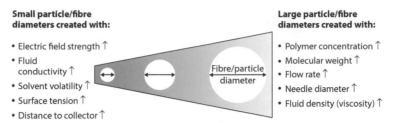

Figure 7.47 Factors affecting the diameter of the fibres produced by electrospinning.

Reproduced from Chakraborty S et al. Electrohydrodynamics: a facile technique to fabricate drug delivery systems. *Adv Drug Deliv Rev* 2009;61:1043–1054. Copyright Elsevier 2009.

Alginates

Alginates derived from seaweeds have been used pharmaceutically for many years. The alginates which are polyelectrolytes – composed of two sugars, L-glucuronic acid and D-mannuronic acid – form highly absorbent strong gels, which *inter alia* minimise bacterial contamination. Sodium alginates are soluble, but binding to calcium results in hydrated poorly soluble systems in the form of gels, beads, films and fibres. Calcium alginate fibres are made by extruding sodium alginate solutions through spinnerets into calcium-containing solutions where the fibres precipitate. This approach can be used to prepare zinc alginate and silver alginate fibres.

Foam dressings

Polyurethane is most commonly used to prepare foam dressings. Synthaderm is a 'synthetic skin' of a modified polyurethane foam, hydrophilic on one side and hydrophobic on the other (Fig. 7.48). The hydrophilic side is placed in contact with the wound. The system[24]: (a) maintains a high humidity at the dressing interface; (b) removes excess exudate; (c) allows gaseous

exchange; and (d) provides insulation; moreover, it is impermeable to bacteria, the outer surface remaining dry, unlike some saturable dressings.

Lyofoam is a similar product[25] – a soft, hydrophobic, polyurethane foam sheet 8 mm thick. The side of the dressing that is to be placed in contact with the skin or wound has been heat-treated to collapse the cells of the foam, and thus enable it to absorb liquid by capillarity. The dressing is freely permeable to gases and water vapour but resists the penetration of aqueous solutions and wound exudate. In use, the dressing absorbs blood or other tissue fluids, and the aqueous component is lost by evaporation through the back of the dressing.

Hydrogels

Hydrogel dressings are most commonly able to conform to the shape of a wound. A secondary, non-absorbent dressing is needed. These dressings are generally used to donate liquid to dry sloughy wounds and facilitate debridement of necrotic tissue; some also have the ability to absorb very small amounts of exudate. Hydrogel sheets have a fixed structure and limited fluid-handling capacity.

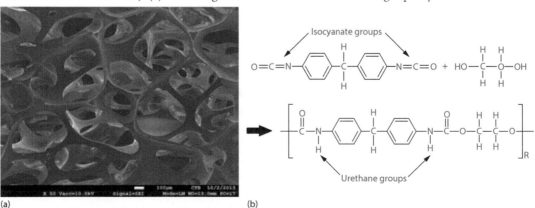

(a)   (b)

Figure 7.48 (a) Polyurethane foam and (b) the molecular structure of polyurethane.

(a) Reproduced from www.centexbel.be, with permission.

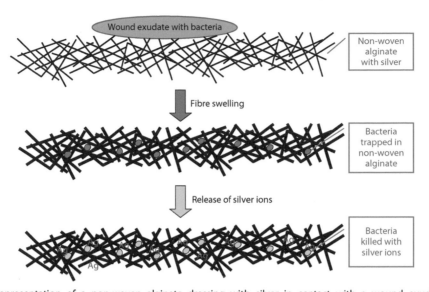

Figure 7.49 Representation of a non-woven alginate dressing with silver in contact with a wound exudate containing bacteria, which are trapped in the swollen alginate as the fibres expand where the released silver then acts.

Reproduced from Qin Y. Silver-containing alginate fibres and dressings. *Int Wound J* 2005;2:172–176. Copyright Wiley-VCH Verlag GmbH & Co. KGaA. Reproduced with permission.

Crosslinked dextran gels are insoluble hydrophilic gels that can be partially depolymerised to the required molecular weight. The gel is produced in a bead shape; the degree of crosslinking determines the water uptake and pore size. Dextranomer (Debrisan) is a crosslinked dextran with pores large enough to allow substances with a molecular weight of less than 1000 Da to enter the beads. Each gram of beads abstracts approximately 4 cm^3 of fluid. Applied to the surface of secreting wounds, dextranomer removes by suction various exudates that tend to impede tissue repair, while leaving behind high-molecular-weight materials such as plasma proteins and fibrinogen.

Antimicrobial-releasing dressings

Dressings containing antimicrobials such as polihexanide (polyhexamethylene biguanide) or dialkylcarbamoyl chloride are available for use on infected wounds (see *British National Formulary*). Cadexomer is a dextrin derivative which forms a complex with iodine, cadexomer–iodine, which, like povidone–iodine, releases free iodine when it is exposed to wound exudate. The free iodine acts as an antiseptic on the wound surface; the cadexomer particles embedded in the dressing structure also absorb wound exudate and encourage de-sloughing.

Silver bonded to alginates can form antimicrobial dressings and work as shown in Figure 7.49.

Wicking

Wicking describes the cumulative action of capillarity in drawing liquid into matrices. In this section we refer to wicking as the process whereby moisture is moved by capillary action from the inside (wound-facing) to the external surface of a dressing. Figure 7.50 reminds us pictorially and graphically of the effect of the diameter of channels on the extent of capillary rise and the fact that channels, especially in fibres and composites, may be asymmetric.

To be absorbed in this way the fibres or other structures of the dressing must be wetted by the liquid. The last diagram of Fig. 7.50 shows an uneven channel that will occur in real systems. The Lucas–Washburn equation describes capillary flow in a bundle of parallel cylindrical tubes as one would find in several dressing structures. It provides the relationship between the time, t, it takes a liquid with surface tension, γ, and viscosity, η, to travel the distance L in a capillary whose diameter is D

$$L^2 = \frac{\gamma D t}{A\eta} \tag{7.32}$$

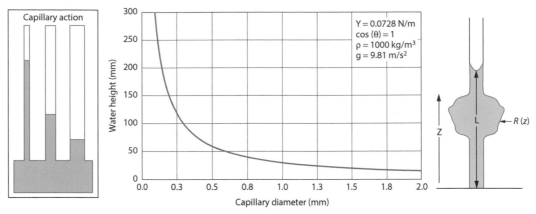

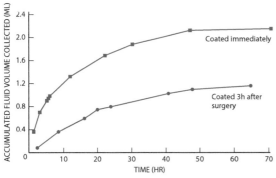

Figure 7.50 From left to right: the effect of capillary action on the liquid rise via capillaries with channels of different diameters; a graph showing calculated water heights for one system as a function of capillary diameter; and a more complex liquid pathway.

Not surprisingly, various substrates, e.g. packed beds, fibre mats or foams, may show different wicking behaviours due to the shape and dimensions of their flow paths.

When a dry porous medium is brought into contact with a liquid, it will start to absorb the liquid at a rate which decreases over time (Fig. 7.51). For a bar of material with cross-sectional area, A, that is wetted on one end, the cumulative volume, V, of absorbed liquid after a time, t, is

$$V = AS\sqrt{t} \tag{7.33}$$

where S is the sorptivity of the medium (in $m\,s^{-1/2}$ or $mm\,min^{-1/2}$).

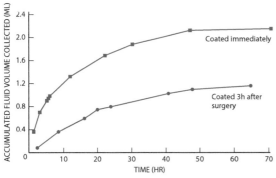

Figure 7.51 Fluid uptake as a function of time in two experiments with crosslinked dextran gels , the upper plot showing the uptake data as a function of time when the system is covered by an impermeable strip, whereas the lower shows the results when the layer is applied 3 h after surgery. Amongst other things the results demonstrate the importance of the mode of application and the use of backing films.

After Wang PY. *Clin Mater* 1987;2:91–102.

The quantity $i = V/A$ (which has the dimension of length) is called the *cumulative liquid intake*. The wetted length, x, of the bar, that is, the distance between the wetted end of the bar and the so-called *wet front*, is dependent on the fraction, f, of the volume occupied by liquid. This number f is the porosity of the medium; the wetted length is then

$$x = \frac{i}{f} = \frac{S}{f}\sqrt{t} \tag{7.34}$$

Some authors use the quantity S/f as the sorptivity. The above description is for the case where gravity and evaporation do not play a role.

Capillary-action dressings act by a wicking process. These dressings consist of an absorbent core of hydrophilic fibres sandwiched between two low-adherent wound-contact layers to ensure no fibres are shed on to the wound surface. Wound exudate is taken up by the dressing and retained within the highly absorbent central layer. Some examples of wound dressing structures are described below.

Wound-dressing structures: Vacutex, Cerdak and Mextra

The technologies now involved have increased the efficacy of wound products. Figure 7.52 demonstrates some of these developments in describing several commercial products, Vacutex, Cerdak and Mextra. The process of capillary transport of the liquid exudate (including bacteria) is described in the previous section.

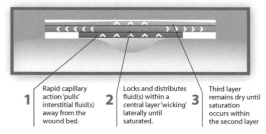

1. Rapid capillary action 'pulls' interstitial fluid(s) away from the wound bed.
2. Locks and distributes fluid(s) within a central layer 'wicking' laterally until saturated.
3. Third layer remains dry until saturation occurs within the second layer

(a) Vacutex

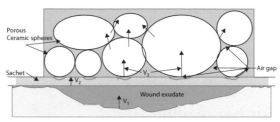

Porous Ceramic spheres

Sachet

V_2

V_3

Air gap

Wound exudate

V_1

(b) Cerdak

FOUR LAYER CONSTRUCTION

1. Fluid repellent backing layer
2. Absorbent layer
3. Distribution layer
4. Wound contact layer

Four phase absorption and retention

(c) Mextra, a 'superabsorbent' dressing

Figure 7.52 (a) Liquid removal by capillary action of fluid from the wound, first by vertical wicking and then by lateral (horizontal) wicking action; (b) to act as a reservoir for the liquid porous ceramic spheres are incorporated into one layer to aid also the extraction process; (c) a four-layer design, showing the wound contact layer, the liquid distribution layer, the absorbent layer and a fluid-repellent backing layer.

Bacterial uptake into dressings along with fluid ingress will depend on the characteristics of the dressing and the nature of the bacteria concerned. Not surprisingly, the transport of bacteria in porous media varies with the size and shape of the organism as well as the nature of the dressing.

Summary

Although there is no strict boundary line, we have divided polymers into water-soluble polymers and water-insoluble systems, typified respectively by materials used to prepare viscous solutions and those that function as barrier membranes or containers. In the first case we have considered the factors controlling their properties: the influence of molecular weight (distribution), branching, charge, flexibility, ionic strength and pH on solution properties. In the case of water-soluble polymers, the main concern has been with solute transport through the polymer bulk. Equations dealing with viscosity and with diffusion have been cited. The variety of pharmaceutical uses of polymers has been described, and the variety of morphologies that polymers can adopt has been emphasised: solutions, gels, microcrystals, crystals, fibres and dendrimers.

When a polymer is being characterised for pharmaceutical use, therefore, much more than its molecular weight distribution should be determined. Its end use will, of course, determine the tests to be applied. The sheer versatility of polymers and the variety of chemical structures and physical forms they can adopt open up fascinating possibilities for the development of novel delivery systems, from nanoparticles (discussed in Chapter 14) to macroscopic and microscopic systems with biodegradable, biocompatible, erodible, leachable, hydrophobic, hydrophilic and all the other characteristics we have discussed in this chapter, which lead one to conclude that their utility is limited only by our ingenuity.

References

1. Svenson S, Tomalia DA. Dendrimers in biomedical applications – reflecting on the field. *Adv Drug Deliv Rev* 2005;57:2106–2129.
2. Menoge AR *et al*. Dendrimer based drug and imaging conjugates: design considerations for nanomedical applications. *Drug Discov Today* 2010;15:171–185.
3. McCahon R, Hardman J. Pharmacology of plasma expanders. *Anesth Intensive Care Med* 2007;879–881.
4. James WP *et al*. Calcium binding by dietary fiber. *Lancet* 1978;1:638–639.
5. Peppas NA, Khare AR. Preparation, structure and diffusional behavior of hydrogels in controlled release. *Adv Drug Deliv Rev* 1993;1:11–35.

6. Chaubal M. Using chitosan as an excipient for oral drug delivery. *Drug Deliv Technol* 2003;3:32–34, 36.

7. Lueßen HL *et al*. Bioadhesive polymers for the peroral delivery of peptide drugs. *J Control Release* 1994;29:329–338.

8. Hammer ME, Burch TG. Viscous corneal protection by sodium hyaluronate, chondroitin sulfate and methylcellulose. *Invest Ophthalmol Vis Sci* 1984;25:1329–1332.

9. Tabbara KF, Sharara N. Dry eye syndrome. *Drugs Today* 1998;34:447.

10. Holly FJ. Formation and rupture of the tear film. *Exp Eye Res* 1973;15:515–525.

11. Oates KMN *et al*. Rheopexy of synovial fluid and protein aggregation. *Interface* 2006;3:164–174.

12. Aviad AD, Houpt JD. The molecular weight of therapeutic hyaluronan (sodium hyaluronate): how significant is it? *J Rheumatol* 1994;21:297–301.

13. Mori S *et al*. Highly viscous sodium hyaluronate and joint lubrication. *Int Orthop* 2004;26:116–121.

14. Allard S, O'Regan M. The role of elastoviscosity in the efficacy of viscosupplementation for osteoarthritis of the knee: a comparison of Hylan G-F 20 and a lower molecular weight hyaluronan. *Clin Ther* 2000;22:792–795.

15. Biomet Inc. Technical literature: Fermathron™. fr.biomet.be/befr-medical/befr-biomaterials/befr-fermathron (accessed 17 September 2009).

16. Lindberg M, Lindberg P. Overcoming obstacles for adherence to phosphate binding medication in dialysis patients: a qualitative study. *Pharm World Sci* 2008;30:571–576.

17. Jani R *et al*. Ion exchange resins for ophthalmic delivery. *J Ocul Pharmacol* 1994;10:57–67.

18. Higuchi T. Mechanism of sustained-action medication. Theoretical analysis of rate of release of solid drugs dispersed in solid matrices. *J Pharm Sci* 1963;52:1145–1149.

19. Santus G, Baker RW. Osmotic drug delivery: a review of the patent literature. *J Control Release* 1995;35:1–21.

20. Gupta BP *et al*. Osmotically controlled drug delivery systems with associated drugs. *J Pharm Pharm Sci* 2010;13:571–588.

21. Theeuwes F *et al*. Osmotic delivery systems for the alpha-adrenoceptor antagonists metoprolol and oxyprenolol: design and evaluation of systems for once-daily administration. *Br J Clin Pharmacol* 1985;19(Suppl):69S–76S.

22. Wolff M *et al*. *In vitro* and *in vivo* release of nitroglycerin from a new transdermal therapeutic system. *Pharm Res* 1985;2:23–29.

23. Abdelrahman T, Wilson H. Wound dressings: principles and practice. *Surgery* 2011;29:491–495.

24. Turner TD. Synthaderm – an 'environmental' dressing. *Pharm J* 1982;228:206–208.

25. Myers JA. Lyofoam – a versatile polyurethane foam surgical dressing. *Pharm J* 1985;235:270.

Further reading

Chakraborty S *et al*. Electrohydrodynamics: a facile technique to fabricate drug delivery systems. *Adv Drug Del Rev* 2009;61:1043–1105.

Liechty WB *et al*. Polymers for drug delivery. *Annu Rev Chem Biomol Eng* 2010;1:149–173.

Mogoşanu GD, Grumezescu AM. Natural and synthetic polymers for wounds and burns dressings. *Int J Pharm* 2014;463:127–136.

Siepmann F *et al*. Polymer blends for controlled release coatings. *J Control Rel* 2008;125:1–15.

Tong L *et al*. Choice of artificial tear formulations for patients with dry eye. *Cornea* 2012;31(Suppl. 1): S32–S36.

Zaman M *et al*. Advances in drug delivery via electrospun and electrosprayed materials. *Int J Nanomed* 2013;8:2997–3017.

8

Drug absorption basics and the oral route

This chapter provides basic information on the physicochemical mechanisms of drug absorption and how the processes of absorption are affected by the physicochemical properties of the drug and its formulation, and importantly, by the interaction of the drug with both the aqueous phase and absorbing membranes. The nature of the barrier membranes varies, however, and while they share the same basic structures, differences in detail can determine the extent of absorption at different sites in the gastrointestinal (GI) tract. The oral route, as the most frequently used and most acceptable route of drug administration, is discussed here in some detail. The influence of the following intertwined parameters in determining bioavailability should become clear:

- the rate and extent of dissolution of the drug, an essential prelude to absorption
- the rate of gastric emptying and its importance in the dynamics of the absorption process
- the site of absorption, especially in relation to the influence of pH.

The pH of the contents of the GI tract and the effect of pH on the ionisation of the drug (discussed also in Chapter 4) are crucial. The application of the so-called pH-partition hypothesis – and its limitations – should be understood, so that the effects of the nature of the drug and the medium on absorption can be assessed. In the case of the oral route, the effect of concomitant medication (e.g. H_2 antagonists, antacids), which might alter the pH of the gut contents, can be approximated by calculating the change in the drug ionisation. The word 'approximated' is used deliberately because the multiple factors involved in absorption from the GI tract mean that the theoretical equations can only explain each process in part.

Absorption, whether it is from the GI tract, the buccal mucosa or the rectal cavity, generally requires the passage of the drug in a molecular form across one or more barrier membranes and tissues. Most drugs are presented to the body as solid or semisolid dosage forms and obviously these must first release the drug contained within them. Tablets or capsules will disintegrate, and the drug will then dissolve either completely or partially and at a greater or lesser rate. Many tablets contain granules or drug particles that deaggregate to facilitate the solution process. If the drug has the appropriate physicochemical properties, it will pass by passive diffusion from a region of high concentration to a region of low concentration across the membrane separating the site of absorption from tissues containing the blood supply. Soluble drugs can, of course, also be administered as solutions, but it should be remembered that drugs can precipitate from solution formulations as they interact with biological fluids.

The special features of other routes of administration are dealt with in Chapter 9. A brief summary of the general properties of biological membranes and drug transport, knowledge of which is important in understanding all absorption processes, is given here. Where attempts have been made to quantify absorption, equations are presented, but the derivations of most equations have been omitted.

8.1 Biological membranes and drug transport

Biological membranes confine the aqueous contents of cells and separate them from an aqueous exterior phase. To achieve this, membranes are lipoidal in nature. To allow nutrients to pass into the cell and waste products to move out, biological membranes are selectively permeable. Membranes have specialised transport systems to assist the passage of water-soluble materials and ions through their lipid interior. Lipid-soluble substances can pass by passive diffusion through the membrane from a region of high concentration to one of low concentration. Biological membranes differ from polymer membranes in that they are composed of small amphipathic molecules, phospholipids (Fig. 8.1) with two hydrophobic chains and cholesterol or other related structures, which associate into lipoidal bilayers in aqueous media. Embodied in the matrix of lipid molecules are proteins, which are generally hydrophobic in nature, embedded in the matrix of lipid molecules. Glycoproteins provide a hydrophilic element to the external membrane; cells have a net negative surface charge.

Cholesterol is a major component of most mammalian biological membranes. Cholesterol forms complexes with phospholipids and its presence reduces the permeability of phospholipid membranes to water, cations, glycerol and glucose. The shape of the cholesterol molecule allows it to fit closely in bilayers with the hydrocarbon chains of unsaturated fatty acids (Fig. 8.1).

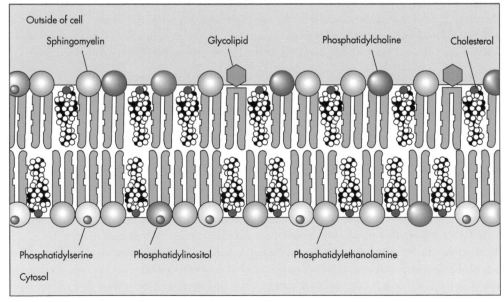

Figure 8.1 Model of a biological membrane showing the different compositions of the interior and exterior sides. Glycolipids are seen on the outside, while phosphatidylserine and phosphatidylinositol predominate on the cytosolic side. See Fig. 8.2 for an impression of the membrane surface appearance.

Cholesterol condenses and rigidifies membranes without solidifying them. Its removal causes the membrane to lose its structural integrity and to become highly permeable. The flexibility of biological membranes is one of their important features, giving them their ability to re-form and to adapt to changed environments, a vital part of their function. The dynamic characteristics of biological membranes are due to their unique construction from small amphipathic molecules. On stretching (as with a soap film), the molecules at the surfaces become less concentrated in the bilayer but then are rapidly replenished from the bulk phase to maintain the original tension. That is, they are dynamic structures. Figure 8.2 shows a diagram of the 'fluid mosaic' model of a biological membrane.

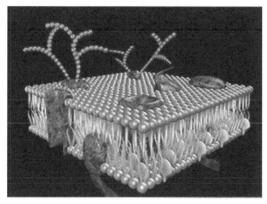

Figure 8.2 Representation of the 'fluid mosaic' model of a biological membrane, showing embedded protein and protruding glycoproteins.
From Funhouse Films, with permission.

Although most of the data on permeation of non-electrolytes across biological membranes can be explained on the basis of the membrane behaving as a continuous hydrophobic phase, a fraction of the membrane may be composed of aqueous channels. These are effectively pores that offer a pathway parallel to the diffusion pathway through the lipid. In the absence of flow of water in one direction or the other, these pores play a minor part in the transfer of most drugs, although in the case of ions and charged drugs such as the quaternary ammonium compounds the pore pathway must be important. The fluid mosaic model of membranes allows the protein–lipid complexes to form either hydrophilic or hydrophobic 'gates' to allow transport of materials with different characteristics.

Overall, membrane permeability is controlled by the nature of the membrane, its degree of internal bonding and rigidity, its surface charge and the nature of the drug (solute) being transported. There are some similarities between solute transport in biological membranes and in synthetic membranes. As we have discussed in Chapter 7, the permeation of drugs and other molecules through hydrophobic membranes made of polydimethylsiloxane, for example, depends primarily on the solubility of the drug in the membrane. Drugs with little affinity for the membrane are unlikely to permeate, although in porous membranes, such as those of cellophane or collagen, even drugs with little affinity for the polymer may be transported through the pores.

Most biological membranes bear a surface negative charge, so one would imagine that this might influence permeation. Membranes with un-ionised surfaces (such as cellophane) or positively charged surfaces such as collagen have different permeability characteristics for ionic drugs. Crucially, anionic solutes permeate faster than cationic solutes. With amphoteric drugs such as sulfisomidine and sulfamethizole, a similar order of permeation may be observed depending on the pH of the medium, namely: un-ionised > anionic > cationic form. In acidic media the membrane is positively charged and cationic drugs will therefore be repelled from the surface.

In biological membranes, one might expect some preference for cationic drugs, other things being equal, but we have to remember that biological membranes are more complex and more dynamic than synthetic membranes and there are many confounding factors. One of these, which is outside the scope of this book, is the existence of efflux mechanisms centred on P-glycoprotein 'pumps'. Some drugs are ejected from cells by the efflux pump, so that these drugs have a lower apparent absorption than predicted on physicochemical grounds. Some excipients (e.g. surfactants such as polysorbate 80) interact with these proteins, so both drug and excipients must be studied for their effect on the efflux pump activity.

In Chapter 4 we examined some relationships between the lipophilicity of drugs and their activity, controlled by their ability to pass across lipid barriers. Although of the same basic construction, biological membranes in different sites in the body serve different functions and thus one might expect them to have different compositions and physicochemical properties, as indeed they do. Tissues derived from the ectoderm (the epidermis, the epithelium of nose and mouth and the anus, and the tissues of the nervous system) have protective and sensory functions. Tissues evolved from the endoderm, such as the epithelium of the GI tract, have evolved mainly to allow absorption.

8.1.1 Lipophilicity and absorption

If one measures the absorption of a sufficiently wide range of substances in a series, one generally finds that there is an optimal point in the series for absorption. In other words, a plot of percentage absorption versus $\log P$ would be parabolic, with the optimum value designated as $\log P_o$ (Fig. 8.3). By noting the values of optimal partition coefficient for different absorbing membranes and surfaces, one can deduce something about their nature. Some values are given in Table 8.1.

Table 8.1 Ideal lipophilic character of drugs (log P_o) in different regions of the body

System	Solute or drug	Log P_o (octanol/water) for maximal transport
Buccal cavity (human)	Bases	5.52 (undissociated)
		3.52 (dissociated)
	Acids	4.19 (undissociated)
Epidermis (human)	Steroids	3.34
Whole skin (rabbit)	Non-electrolytes	2.55
Small intestine (rat)	Sulfonamides	2.56–3.33
Stomach (rat)	Barbiturates	2.01
	Acids	1.97
Cornea (rabbit)	Steroids	2.8
Biliary excretion	Sulfathiazoles	0.60
Milk/plasma	Sulfonamides	0.53
Prostatic/plasma ratio	Sulfonamides	0.23

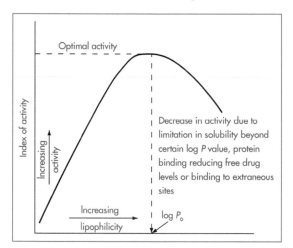

Figure 8.3 Parabolic nature of a typical activity–log P plot: the decrease in biological activity beyond the optimal log P_o is probably due to the factors listed.

The parabolic nature of activity–log P plots is due to a combination of factors: with drugs with high log P values, protein binding, low solubility and binding to extraneous sites cause a lower measured activity than if it were possible to take the drug and place it at the receptor without it having to traverse the various lipid and aqueous hurdles that it has to overcome on its way to the site of action.

Molecular weight and drug absorption

The larger drug molecules are, the poorer will be their ability to traverse biological membranes. The change of permeability with increasing molecular size is shown in Fig. 8.4.

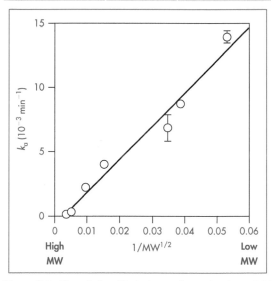

Figure 8.4 The relationship between the molecular weight of compounds and absorption rate constant. The membrane studied is the rat kidney surface, but similar plots hold for other sites.

Reproduced from Nishida K *et al.* Absorption characteristics of compounds with different molecular weights after application to the unilateral kidney surface in rats. *Eur J Pharm Biopharm* 2004;58:705–711. Copyright Elsevier 2004.

In a survey of over 2000 drugs, only 11% had molecular weights above 500 Da, and only 8% had molecular weights above 600 Da. Lipinski *et al.*[1] devised the so-called 'rule of 5', which refers to the drug-like properties of molecules. It states that *poor* oral absorption is more likely when the drug molecule:

- has more than five hydrogen-bond donors (—OH groups or —NH groups)
- has a molecular weight > 500 Da
- has a log $P > 5$
- has more than 10 H-bond acceptors.

Note that all the numbers are factors of 5, hence the name of the rule. Compounds that are substrates for transporters are exceptions to the rule.

8.1.2 Permeability and the pH-partition hypothesis

If, in the first instance, the plasma membrane is considered to be a strip of lipoidal material, homogeneous in nature and with a defined thickness, one must assume that only lipid-soluble agents will pass across this barrier. As most drugs are weak electrolytes it is to be expected that the un-ionised form (U) of either acids or bases, the lipid-soluble species, will diffuse across the membrane, while the ionised forms (I) will be rejected. This is the basis of the *pH-partition hypothesis,* in which the pH dependence of drug absorption and solute transport across membranes is considered. The equations of Chapters 2 and 4 are relevant here.

For weakly acidic drugs such as acetylsalicylic acid (aspirin) and indometacin, the ratio of ionised to un-ionised species is given by the equation

$$pH - pK_a = \log\frac{[\text{ionised form}]}{[\text{un-ionised form}]}$$

$$= \log\frac{[I]}{[U]} \tag{8.1}$$

For weak bases the equation takes the form

$$pK_a - pH = \log\frac{[\text{ionised form}]}{[\text{un-ionised form}]}$$

$$= \log\frac{[I]}{[U]} \tag{8.2}$$

One can calculate from these equations (and equations 2.45 and 2.47) the relative amounts of absorbable and non-absorbable forms of a drug substance ([U] and [I], respectively), given the prevailing pH conditions in the lumen of the gut or the site of absorption. The profiles for un-ionised drug (%) versus pH for several drugs are given in Fig. 8.5. In very broad terms, one would expect acids to be absorbed from the stomach and bases from the intestine.

A comparison of the intestinal absorption of several acids and bases at various pH values (Table 8.2) indicates the expected trend. Surprisingly, however, it will be seen that salicylic acid is absorbed from the rat intestine at pH 8, although with a pK_a of 3.0 it is virtually completely ionised at this pH. There are two explanations: one is that absorption and ionisation are both dynamic processes and that the small amount of un-ionised drug absorbed is replenished; the second is that the bulk pH is not the actual pH at the membrane. Nevertheless, instilling solutions of different pH directly into the lumen of the rat stomach indicates the correct qualitative trends of absorption (62% absorption at pH 1 for salicylic acid and 13% at pH 8). Similarly, Box 8.1 shows that the absorption of

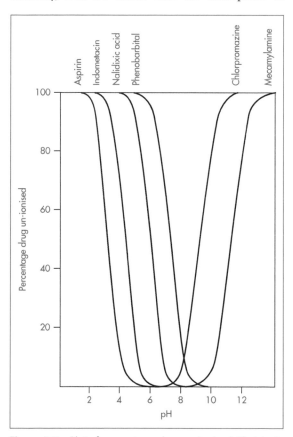

Figure 8.5 Plot of percentage drug un-ionised (that is, in its lipid-soluble form) as a function of solution pH, for the acidic drugs aspirin, indometacin, nalidixic acid and phenobarbital, and for the basic drugs chlorpromazine and mecamylamine.

acetylsalicylic acid is much greater than one would expect from a calculation of the pH dependency of its ionisation.

Table 8.2 Intestinal absorption of acids and bases in the rat at several pH values

Acid/base	pK_a	Percentage absorption			
		pH 4	pH 5	pH 7	pH 8
Acids					
Salicylic acid	3.0	64	35	30	10
Acetylsalicylic acid (aspirin)	3.5	41	27	–	–
Benzoic acid	4.2	62	36	35	5
Bases					
Amidopyrine	5.0	21	35	48	52
Quinine	8.4	9	11	41	54

Box 8.1 Calculation of percentage ionisation

Absorption values for acetylsalicylic acid at pH 4, 5, 7 and 8 are quoted in Table 8.2. The amount of drug in the un-ionised form at these pH values is obtained from equation (8.1). For example, at pH 4,

$$4 - 3.5 = \log \frac{[I]}{[U]}$$

$$\therefore \frac{[I]}{[U]} = 3.162$$

Percentage un-ionised

$$= \frac{[U] \times 100}{[U] + [I]} = \frac{100}{1 + \frac{[I]}{[U]}}$$

$$= \frac{100}{1 + 3.162} = \frac{100}{4.162} = 24.03\%$$

In the same way, we find 3.07% un-ionised at pH 5; 0.032% at pH 7; and less than 0.009% un-ionised at pH 9. Absorption is much greater than one would expect, being 41% at pH 4 and 27% at pH 5, although the trend is as predicted.

In attempts to explain away discrepancies between theoretical prediction and observed results we have already hinted that a local pH exists at the membrane surface that differs from the bulk pH (see below). This local pH is due to the attraction of hydrogen ions by the negative groups of membrane components so that, in the intestine, while the bulk pH is around 7 the surface pH is nearer 6. A 'virtual' surface pH can be calculated, which will allow results such as those in Table 8.2 to be explained. If we take as another example salicylic acid, again calculating the percentage of un-ionised species by equation (8.1), we obtain the following figures (taken from Table 8.2):

pH	4	5	7	8
Percentage un-ionised	9.09	0.99	0.0099	0.001
Percentage absorbed	64	35	30	10

To have 30% of this compound in its un-ionised form when the bulk pH is 7 would require a surface pH of about 3.4, which is lower than anticipated. Again, however, we must remember that absorption and ionisation processes are dynamic processes. As the un-ionised species are absorbed, so the level of [U] in the bulk falls and, because of a shift in equilibrium, more of the un-ionised species appears in the bulk. In fact, if a pH of 5.3 is taken as the pH of the absorbing surface, the results in Table 8.2 become more explicable, as we discuss in the next section.

8.1.3 Problems with the quantitative application of the pH-partition hypothesis

There are several reasons why the pH-partition hypothesis cannot be applied quantitatively in practical situations. Some are discussed here.

Variability in pH conditions

The variation in the stomach pH in human subjects is remarkable, bearing in mind that each pH unit represents a 10-fold difference in hydrogen ion concentration. While the normally quoted range of stomach pH is 1–3, studies using pH-sensitive radiotelemetric capsules have shown a greater spread of values, ranging up to pH 7, as seen in Fig. 11.2 in Chapter 11. This means that the dissolution rate of many drugs will vary markedly in individuals – this is indeed one of the reasons for individual-to-individual variation in drug availability.

The scope for variation in the small intestine is less, although in some pathological states the pH of the duodenum may be quite low, owing to hypersecretion of acid in the stomach. Table 8.3 lists the normal pH of the blood and of different regions of the GI tract.

Table 8.3 pH of blood and contents of the human alimentary tract	
Sample	pH
Blood	7.35–7.45
Buccal cavity	6.2–7.2
Stomach	1.0–3.0
Duodenum	4.8–8.2
Jejunum and ileum	7.5–8.0
Colon	7.0–7.5

pH at membrane surfaces

Data on the relationship between absorption and pH of the intestinal contents on the one hand, and the percentage of drug in the un-ionised state on the other, can generally be rationalised if the apparent pH is reduced below the pH of the intestine. As described above, this pH 'shift' is due to the existence of a pH at the membrane surface lower than that of the bulk pH. One might expect that the hydrogen ion concentration at the surface would be greater (and hence pH lower) at the membrane surface as hydrogen ions would accumulate near anionic groups, leading to an effect that can be quantified by the equation

$$[H^+]_{surface} = [H^+]_{bulk} \exp\frac{-F\zeta}{RT} \qquad (8.3)$$

where F is the Faraday constant, R is the gas constant, T is absolute temperature and ζ is the zeta potential of the surface (see Chapter 6). Thus, in terms of pH,

$$pH_{surfce} = pH_{bulk} + \frac{\zeta}{60} \qquad (8.4)$$

where ζ is expressed in millivolts.

The secretion of acidic and basic substances in many parts of the gut wall is also a complicating factor, as the local pH in the region of the microvilli of the small intestine will undoubtedly influence the absorption of weak electrolytes. A drug molecule in the bulk will diffuse towards the membrane surface and so meet different pH conditions from those in the bulk phase. Whether or not this influences the extent of absorption will depend on the pH changes and the pK_a of the drug in question. The negative charge on the membrane will attract small cations towards the surface and small anions will be repelled; one might thus expect some selectivity in the absorption process. The existence of this 'microclimate' has been questioned, but experimental evidence for its existence has been obtained from the use of microelectrodes, which revealed the existence of a layer on the (rat) jejunum with a pH of 5.5 when the pH of the bathing buffer was 7.2. The existence of this more acid layer has also been demonstrated on the surface of the human intestine.

Other complications include convective water flow and unstirred layers, discussed below.

Convective water flow

The movement of water molecules into and out of the GI tract will affect the rate of passage of small molecules across the membrane. The reasons for water flow are the differences in osmotic pressure between blood and the contents of the lumen, and differences in hydrostatic pressure between lumen and perivascular tissue, resulting, for example, from muscular contractions. It can be appreciated that the absorption of water-soluble drugs will be increased if water flows from the lumen across the mucosa to the blood side, provided that drug and water are using the same route. Water movement is greatest within the jejunum.

Unstirred water layers

A layer of relatively unstirred water lies adjacent to all biological membranes. The boundary between the bulk water and this unstirred layer is indistinct but, nevertheless, it has a real thickness. During absorption, drug molecules must diffuse across this layer and then on through the lipid layer. The overall rate of transfer is the result of the resistance in both water layer and lipid layer. The flux, J, for a substance across the unstirred layer is given by the expression

$$J = (C_1 - C_2)\frac{D}{\delta} \qquad (8.5)$$

where C_1 and C_2 are the concentrations of the substance in the bulk water phase and in the unstirred water layer, respectively, D is the diffusion coefficient and δ is the effective thickness of the unstirred layer. The flux of molecules that pass by passive diffusion through the lipid membrane can be written as

$$J = C_2 P_c \tag{8.6}$$

where P_c is the permeability coefficient. The rate of absorption must equal the rate of transport across the unstirred layer; that is,

$$J = (C_1 - C_2)\frac{D}{\delta} = C_2 P_c \tag{8.7}$$

The rate of movement across the unstirred layer, as can be seen from the equations, is proportional to D/δ; the rate of absorption is proportional to P_c. Compounds with a large permeability coefficient may be able to penetrate across cell membranes much faster than they can be transported through the unstirred layer. Under these circumstances diffusion through the water layer becomes the rate-limiting step in the absorption process. Neglect of the unstirred layer causes errors in the interpretation of experimental flux data.

Effect of the properties of the drug

Drugs must be in their molecular form before diffusional absorption processes take place. We would expect bases to be more soluble than acids in the stomach, but it is impossible to generalise in this way. Although the basic form of a drug as its hydrochloride salt should be soluble to some extent in this medium, this is not always so. Indeed, the free bases of, for example, chlortetracycline, dimethylchlortetracycline and methacycline are more soluble than their corresponding hydrochlorides in the pH range of the stomach (see Chapter 4). It has been shown that mean plasma levels following administration of the free base and the hydrochloride of these tetracyclines reflect the differences in solubility, the bases giving higher levels. The reason is most likely that discussed in section 4.7.2, namely the influence of high ionic strength on the solubility of the drug substance (the common ion effect). As absorption of the tetracyclines takes place mainly from the duodenum, it is vital that they reach the intestine in a dissolved or readily soluble form, as their solubility is low at the pH conditions prevailing in the duodenum (pH 4–5).

The presence of buffer components in the formulation also creates a pH microenvironment around dissolving particles that may aid drug dissolution. If dissolution is the rate-limiting step in the absorption process, this will be significant in determining absorption. Bulk pH will then give little help in calculating the solution rate on the basis of a knowledge of saturation solubilities in bulk conditions.

Other complicating factors

The very high area of the surface of the small intestine also upsets the calculation of absorption based on considerations of theoretical absorption across identical areas of absorbing surface. The sheer complexity of the situation precludes mathematical precision, yet the pH-partition hypothesis is useful, especially in predicting what follows from a change in bulk pH – for example, on ingestion of antacids or drugs such as histamine receptor antagonists (H_2 blockers) that reduce gastric acid secretion. The extent of the change in pH after administration of one of the first in the class, cimetidine, can be seen from Fig. 8.6, which shows a rise in resting pH from below 2 to near neutrality. The effect in turn depends on the formulation used. The fact that aspirin, an acid with a pK_a of 3.5, is absorbed from the small intestine is due partly to the massive surface area available for absorption which allows significant absorption to occur, even

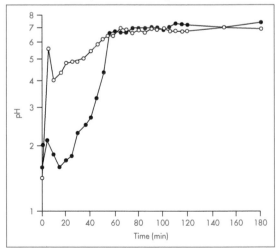

Figure 8.6 Intragastric pH after administration of (○) effervescent cimetidine and (●) standard cimetidine, plotted as median values from 13 patients with gastro-oesophageal reflux given 800 mg orally of the preparations.
Reproduced from Ström M *et al*. Intragastric pH rise with effervescent citrate-cimetidine. *Lancet* 1991;337:433.

Key points

- Biological membranes are composed primarily of phospholipids and cholesterol, forming a lipoidal bilayer in which proteins are embedded; as a consequence they have a hydrophilic negatively charged exterior and a hydrophobic interior. They are selectively permeable, allowing nutrients to pass into the cell and waste products to move out.

- Lipid-soluble agents can cross the membrane by passive diffusion; in addition there are pores that offer an alternative diffusion pathway that is particularly important for the transference of ions and charged drugs, such as the quaternary ammonium compounds. Overall, the permeability is controlled by the nature of the membrane, its degree of internal bonding and rigidity, its surface charge and the nature of the solute being transported.

- A plot of percentage absorption versus log P for drugs within a series is generally parabolic; optimum absorption occurs at log P_o. A relationship between the properties of a drug and its extent of absorption was devised by Lipinski *et al.* – the 'rule of 5'. *Poor* absorption is likely when the drug has a molecular weight > 500 Da, more than 5 H-bond donors, a log $P > 5$ and more than 10 H-bond acceptors.

- The pH-partition hypothesis assumes that only lipid-soluble agents will cross the membrane, which for simplicity is considered to be a strip of lipoidal material. It is therefore expected that un-ionised forms of either acidic or basic drugs will diffuse across the membrane, while the ionised forms will be rejected.

- Absorption is sometimes much greater than predicted from the pH-partition hypothesis. There are several possible reasons for this:
  - The pH of the stomach may be higher than the normally quoted range of 1–3.
  - The pH at the membrane surface is lower than the bulk pH; there may also be secretion of acidic and basic substances in parts of the gut wall.
  - The movement of water molecules, due to differences in osmotic pressure between blood and the contents of the lumen and differences in hydrostatic pressure between the lumen and the perivascular tissue, affects the rate of absorption of small molecules.
  - A layer of unstirred water lies adjacent to the membrane, which is an additional barrier across which molecules must diffuse during their absorption.
  - Although we would expect that bases would be more soluble than acids in the stomach, this may not always be the case because, for example, of the common ion effect.
  - A variety of other factors may complicate the absorption process, including the complex nature and very high area of the surface of the small intestine and the properties of the drug, for example, its stability in the GI tract, its binding to mucin or complexation with bile salts and the formation of ion pairs.

though the percentage of absorbable species is very low, and partly to the dynamics of the process referred to earlier.

A warning, however, about other complications: drugs that (1) are unstable in the GI tract (for example, erythromycin); (2) are metabolised on their passage through the gut wall; (3) are hydrolysed in the stomach to active forms (namely prodrugs); and (4) bind to mucin or form complexes with bile salts may not always be absorbed in the manner expected.

Ion pairing

The interaction of drugs in the charged form with other ions to form absorbable species with a high lipid solubility is a possible explanation for the ability of molecules such as quaternary ammonium compounds, ionised under all pH conditions, to be usefully absorbed. The origin of the ions that pair with drug ions is not clear, but there is evidence that ion-pair formation will aid absorption.

One could assume that small organic ions are absorbed through water-filled pores or channels in the membrane, but the effective diameter of such pores means that large drug ions would be excluded from this route. Although membranes are impermeable to large organic ions, nevertheless ion-pairing between a drug ion and an organic ion of opposite charge forming an absorbable neutral species is possible.

Two ionic species A^+ and B^- may exist in solution in several states:

$$A : B \quad \rightleftharpoons \quad A^+, B^- \quad \rightleftharpoons \quad A^+ B^- \quad \rightleftharpoons \quad A^+ + B^-$$

| undissociated species | 'tight' ion pair | 'loose' ion pair | free ions |

The formation of tight or loose ion pairs will depend on solvent–ion interactions: hydrophobic ions might be encouraged to form ion pairs by the mechanism of *water-structure-enforced ion pairing*, in which the water attempts to minimise the disturbance on its structuring, and achieves this end by reducing the polarity of the species in solution by ion-pair formation. Ion pairing in highly structured solvents, then, is due not to an electrostatic interaction but to a solvent-mediated effect. The significance of the phenomenon is that ion pairs have the property of being almost neutral species, so that the ion pair can partition into an oily phase when its parent ionic species cannot, a property that is important in drug absorption and

drug extraction procedures, and that is put to use in chromatography.

The two reactions below are examples of (i) a quaternary amine pairing with a weak acid, and (ii) an alkyl sulfate with a weak base, both under pH conditions in which the solute is charged:

(i) $RCOO^- + N^+(C_4H_9)_4 \rightleftharpoons RCOON(C_4H_9)_4$

(ii) $RNH_3^+ + {}^-O_3SO(CH_2)_{11}CH_3 \rightleftharpoons$
$$RNH_3O_3SO(CH_2)_{11}CH_3$$

| hydrophilic | ion-pair agent |
| solute | hydrophobic pair |

Figure 8.7 shows clearly the effect of chloride ion and other anions such as methane sulfonate on the apparent partition coefficient of chlorpromazine. The nature of the anion significantly affects the partitioning of the drug. Ion pairing in the GI tract obviously could influence absorption.

8.2 The oral route and oral absorption

8.2.1 Drug absorption from the gastrointestinal tract

The oral route is the most widely used and convenient route of drug administration for those drugs that can survive the acid of the stomach, that are resistant to enzymatic attack and that are absorbed across GI membranes. The primary function of the GI tract is the digestion and absorption of foods and other nutrients and it is not easy to separate these from that of drug delivery. Indeed, the natural processes in the gut frequently influence the absorption of drugs. This is not surprising when it is considered that, on average, approximately 500 g of solid and up to 2.5 litres of fluid are ingested each day. As well as this oral intake, litres of endogenous fluid are excreted each day into the intestine.

The pH of the gut contents and the presence of enzymes, foodstuffs, bile salts, fat and the microbial flora will all influence drug absorption. The complexity of the absorbing surfaces means that a simple physicochemical approach to drug absorption remains an approach to the problem and not the complete picture, as described above. Whatever the limitations

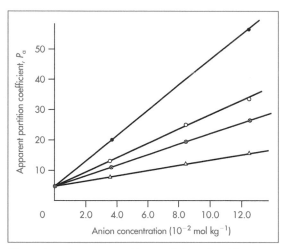

Figure 8.7 Apparent partition coefficients for chlorpromazine between *n*-octanol and aqueous buffers at pH 3.9, in the presence of various anions at 30°C: ○, chloride; ●, propanesulfonate; ⊗, ethanesulfonate; △, methanesulfonate.

Reproduced from Murthy LS, Zografi G. Oil-water partitioning of chlorpromazine and other phenothiazine derivatives using dodecane and n-octanol. *J Pharm Sci* 1970;59:1281. Copyright Wiley-VCH Verlag GmbH & Co. KGaA. Reproduced with permission.

of theory – and one should not expect simple theories to hold in the complex and dynamic circumstances that are involved in drug absorption – theory provides a starting point in rationalising the behaviour of drugs in the GI tract. While most drugs are absorbed by passive diffusion across the lipid membranes separating the gut contents from the rest of the body, certain molecules that resemble naturally occurring substances are actively transported by special mechanisms.

We first consider the physiological situation that might impinge on passive drug absorption. The delivery of macromolecules, including peptides and proteins, is treated in Chapter 13.

Particulate absorption from the gut

While the general rule is that only drugs in solution are absorbed from the GI tract, colloidal particles, some viruses, bacteria and prion proteins can gain entry in low amounts to the lymphatic system through absorption by the specialised cells (M cells) in the gut-associated lymphoid tissue (GALT) and also by enterocytes under certain conditions. In studies in rats, for example, model polystyrene particles above 300 nm in diameter were absorbed in minute amounts, with maximal absorption with particles around 50 nm. Comparisons of uptake between carboxylated microspheres and non-ionic systems, showed lower uptake of the former through the lymphoid tissue of the GI tract. Size is a key parameter: uptake increases with decreasing particle diameter. Adsorption of hydrophilic block copolymers on to polystyrene markedly reduces the uptake by intestinal GALT. Modification of the surface with specific ligands, such as by covalent attachment of tomato lectin molecules has indicated enhanced uptake following their binding to, and internalisation by, enterocytes. The ability to decrease and increase uptake is clear evidence of a phenomenon which has the potential for further control to allow it to be exploited fully for drug or vaccine delivery. The evidence to date with nanoparticles as carrier systems for labile drugs such as proteins by the oral route remains to be substantiated.

A lengthy discussion of this route of uptake is outside the scope of this book, but it is a route that is likely to be increasingly explored as a means of delivering proteins and perhaps genes in carrier nanoparticles, and for oral vaccination. It has yet to fulfil its promise.[2] If the level of incorporation of the active ingredient is low and uptake is relatively low (a maximum perhaps of 5%) and if drug is released before uptake, this limits the absorption of the gut-labile active considerably. However, we should be aware that excipients such as titanium dioxide (rutile) have been found to be absorbed by the GALT, and we should be aware of the *potential* at least for other materials also to be taken up.

8.2.2 Structure of the gastrointestinal tract

We first consider the physiological situations and the structure and function of the GI tract that might impinge on passive drug absorption.

Figure 8.8 diagrammatically represents the GI tract and some of the factors involved in the process of drug absorption from this complex milieu. The stomach is not an organ that has evolved for absorption; the main site of absorption is the small intestine.

The *stomach* may be divided into its two main parts: (1) the body of the stomach, which is in effect a receptacle or hopper, which includes pepsin- and HCl-secreting areas; and (2) the pyloris (a churning chamber), the mucus-secreting area of the gastric mucosa. The stomach varies its luminal volume with the content of food and this is one reason why food intake can be so important in relation to drug absorption; the stomach of adults may contain a few millilitres or a litre or more of fluid. Hydrochloric acid is liberated from the parietal cells at a concentration of 0.58%, or 160 mmol dm^{-3}. The gastric glands produce some 1000–1500 cm^3 of gastric juice per day. It is in this somewhat chaotic environment that pharmaceutical dosage forms find themselves. Some of the events that result are shown in Fig. 8.8b.

The *small intestine* is divided anatomically into three sections: duodenum, jejunum and ileum. Histologically there is no clearly marked transition between these parts. All three are involved in the digestion and absorption of foodstuffs, absorbed material being removed by the blood and the lymph. The absorbing area is enlarged by surface folds in the intestinal lining that are macroscopically apparent: the surfaces of these folds possess villi and microvilli (Fig. 8.9). It has been calculated that, with a maximum of 3000 microvilli per cell in the epithelial brush border (so called because of its physical appearance), the number

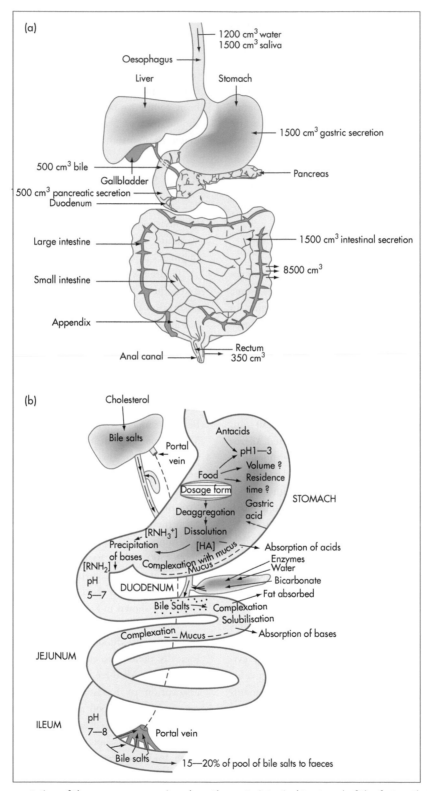

Figure 8.8 Representation of the processes occurring along the gastrointestinal tract, and of the factors that must be taken into account in considering drug absorption.

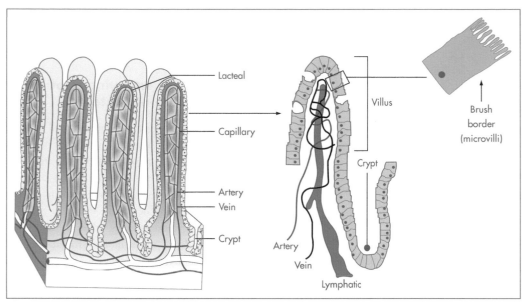

Figure 8.9 Representation of the epithelium of the small intestine at different levels of magnification. From left to right: the intestinal villi and microvilli that comprise the brush border.

of microvilli in the small-intestine mucosa, even of the rat, is 2×10^8 per mm^2. Although one would expect organic acids to be absorbed only from the stomach, where they will exist in the un-ionised lipid-soluble and membrane-diffusible form, the enormous surface area in the intestine allows significant absorption of acidic drugs from the intestine even though (as noted earlier) the fraction of un-ionised molecules is very small.

Over the entire length of the large and small intestines and the stomach, the brush border has a uniform coating (3 nm thick) of mucopolysaccharides that consist of multibranched polymeric chains. This coating layer appears to act as a mechanical barrier to bacteria, cells or food particles, or as a filter. Whatever its function, the weakly acidic, sulfated mucopolysaccharides influence the charge on the cell membrane and complicate the explanations of absorption.

The goblet cells of the epithelium form mucus; secretions are stored in granule form in the apical cell region and are liquefied on contact with water to form mucus, which is composed of protein and carbohydrate and acts as a protective mechanism for the gut surface. Its role in the absorption of drugs is unclear.

The *large intestine* is concerned primarily with the absorption of water and the secretion of mucus to aid the intestinal contents to slide down the intestinal 'tube'. Villi are therefore completely absent from the large intestine, but there are deep crypts distributed over its surface.

Differences in the absorptive areas and volumes of gut contents in experimental animals are important when comparing experimental results on drug absorption in various species and in humans.[3] The all-important extrapolation to the human animal is complex. The human small intestine has a calculated active surface area of approximately 100 m^2. No analogous calculations are available for the most commonly used laboratory animals, although the surface area of the small intestine of the rat is estimated to be 700 cm^2.

Passive transport, carrier-mediated transport and specialised transport

In discussing the pH-partition hypothesis, it has been considered that drugs are absorbed by passive diffusion through epithelial cells – the enterocytes of the GI tract, for example. In fact, there is the possibility of some passage of drugs by way of the tight junctions (the paracellular route) and there are transcellular carrier-mediated uptake mechanisms as well as endocytosis. Figure 8.10 summarises these.

8.2.3 Bile salts and fat absorption pathways

Fat is absorbed by special mechanisms in the gut. The bile salts that are secreted into the jejunum are efficient

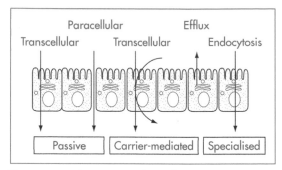

Figure 8.10 Gastrointestinal membrane transport. Transport through the enterocyte barrier can be divided into active, passive and specialised transport; and into the paracellular and transcellular routes. Efflux mechanisms can reduce absorption by these routes.

emulsifiers and disperse fat globules, allowing the action of lipase at the much-increased globule surface. Medium-chain triglycerides are thought to be directly absorbed. Long-chain triglycerides are hydrolysed, and the monoglycerides and fatty acids produced form mixed micelles with the bile salts and are absorbed either directly in the micelle or, more probably, brought to the microvillus surface by the micelle and transferred directly to the mucosal cells, the bile salts remaining in the lumen. The bile salts are reabsorbed in the ileum and transported via the portal vein back into the bile salt pool.

There have been suggestions that lipid-soluble drugs may be absorbed by fat absorption pathways. Certainly, administration of drugs in an oily vehicle can significantly affect their absorption, increasing it in the case of griseofulvin and ciclosporin, but decreasing it in the case of vitamin D.

8.2.4 Gastric emptying, motility and volume of contents

The volume of the gastric contents will determine the concentration of a drug that finds itself in the stomach. The time the drug or dosage form resides in the stomach will determine many aspects of absorption. If the drug is absorbed lower down the gut, the residence time will determine the delay before absorption begins; if the drug is labile in acid conditions, longer residence times in the stomach will lead to greater stability; if the dosage form is non-disintegrating then retention in the stomach can influence the pattern of absorption. Gastro-retentive dosage forms are designed to achieve that control (see section 8.3.2).

The stomach empties liquids faster than solids. The rate of transfer of gastric contents to the small intestine is retarded by the activity of receptors sensitive to acid, fat, osmotic pressure and amino acids in the duodenum and the small intestine, and stimulated by material that has arrived from the stomach. Gastric emptying is a simple exponential or square-root function of the volume of a test meal – a pattern that holds for meals of variable viscosity. To explain the effect of a large range of substances on emptying, an osmoreceptor has been postulated that shrinks in hypertonic solutions and swells in hypotonic solutions.

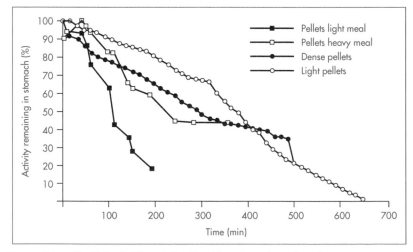

Figure 8.11 Gastric emptying of pellets of different density with various sizes of meal.

Reproduced with permission from Wilson CG, Washington N. *Physiological Pharmaceutics*. Chichester: Ellis Horwood; 1989.

Acids in test meals have been found to slow gastric emptying; acids with higher molecular weights (for example, citric acid) are less effective than those, such as HCl, with very low molecular weights. Natural triglycerides inhibit gastric motility, linseed and olive oils being effective. The formulation of a drug may thus influence drug absorption through an indirect physiological effect. The nature of the dose form – whether solid or liquid, whether acid or alkaline, whether aqueous or oily – may thus influence gastric emptying. The question of gastric emptying and transit down the GI tract has assumed further importance in relation to the design and performance of sustained-release preparations. The transit of pellets of different densities,[4,5] for example, is shown in Fig. 8.11 and illustrates the influence of both density and food intake.

Food, then, affects not only transit but also pH. The effect of a meal on the hydrogen ion concentration of the stomach contents is shown in Fig. 8.12; the effect of two antacids on gastric volume and pH is shown in Table 8.4. When considering the effect of an antacid, therefore, the effect of volume change and pH change and the effect on gastric emptying must all be considered. In designing delivery systems all these factors have ideally to be taken into account.

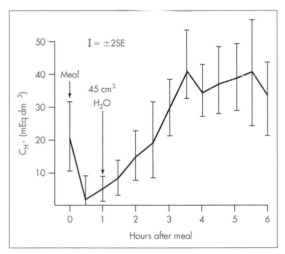

Figure 8.12 Hydrogen ion concentrations (C_{H^+}) at intervals after a test meal (mean results are shown ±2 SEM); the zero samples were taken just before the meal was begun, and the 1-hour sample just before 45 cm³ of water.

Modified with permission from Fordtran J. Antacid pharmacology in duodenal ulcer. Effect of antacids on postcibal gastric acidity and peptic activity. *N Engl J Med* 1966;274:921.

Table 8.4 Effects of antacids on gastric volume and pH in the rat[a]

	Water	Maalox	Amphojel
Volume (cm³)	0.29 ± 0.03	1.8 ± 0.3	4.0 ± 0.2
pH	2.2 ± 0.2	7.4 ± 0.1	4.7 ± 0.2

[a]Ten rats per group. Measurements on gastric contents made 20 minutes after the third hourly dose of 1 cm³ water or antacid by gastric intubation.

Reproduced from Hava M, Hurwitz A. The relaxing effect of aluminum and lanthanum on rat and human gastric smooth muscle *in vitro. Eur J Pharmacol* 1973;22:156. Copyright Elsevier 1973.

 Key points

- The oral route is the most convenient route of drug administration for those drugs that can survive the acid of the stomach, that are resistant to enzymatic attack, and that are absorbed across GI membranes. Prediction of absorption rates is complicated, however, by the complexity of the absorbing surfaces and the presence of enzymes, foodstuffs, bile salts, fat and microbial flora.
- Absorption is influenced by the volume of the gastric contents, the rate of gastric emptying and the effect of food on the pH of the stomach contents.
- Although most drugs are absorbed by passive diffusion through epithelial cells, there is also the possibility of absorption by passage through tight junctions (paracellular absorption), by transcellular carrier-mediated uptake mechanisms and by endocytosis.
- Special mechanisms operate for the absorption of fat that involve mixed micelle formation with bile salts.

8.3 Oral dosage forms

A variety of modified-release oral dosage forms are discussed in other chapters of this book. Here we briefly touch on the conventional delivery systems used in the great majority of cases, namely tablets, capsules, suspensions and liquids, whose production and properties have also been discussed in earlier chapters. In the main, conventional – that is to say, fast-release – products are used as a means of administering large and small doses of drugs in convenient forms, to provide stable systems and reliable dosing. For very low-dose drugs (such as oral contraceptives) there is the problem even today of ensuring that the drug is dispersed evenly in the bulk powder or granules used for tableting, because of the phenomenon of particle segregation. On the other hand, it is possible by appropriate design of the dosage form to alter the pharmacokinetics that the drug would otherwise exhibit. Modified-, sustained-, delayed- or controlled-release forms (these descriptors are used interchangeably) can be used by the oral route to prolong the release and thus the action of drugs, so reducing the frequency of dosing with drugs having a short intrinsic half-life. One of the oldest forms of delayed-release product is the enteric-coated tablet or capsule. These have a polymer coat whose solubility is pH-dependent, this becoming porous or soluble in the lower intestine or colon. Other film coats and non-disintegrating matrix forms are dealt with in Chapter 7.

The preparation and formulation of tablets and capsules can be either straightforward or complex depending on the nature of the drug and the excipients. Particular problems arise with labile drugs that might be affected by moisture, low-dose drugs and dose forms containing more than one active ingredient, with the potential for the interaction between the drugs themselves or with the excipient materials, as discussed in Chapter 1. A cartoon of a typical coated tablet is shown in Fig. 8.13, which in a simple way illustrates the potential for problems, not least the uneven distribution of drug, the potential for drug–excipient interactions, drug–drug interactions even in the solid state, when more than one agent is incorporated into the dose form, and issues of overall stability, mostly discussed in earlier chapters.

 Clinical point

Controlled-release formulations can moderate toxicity, prolong the activity of a drug and often have great benefits, as has been shown in clinical trials of prednisone in controlled release, reducing morning stiffness in the joints of patients with rheumatoid arthritis, when compared to conventional release forms, as shown in Fig. 8.14.

8.3.1 The Biopharmaceutical Classification System (BCS)[6]

With the plethora of drugs now available and being tested, there was a need to assist drug developers to make decisions about the manner in which to deliver drugs by the oral route. Through the work of Gordon Amidon and colleagues, a valuable classification system was developed to relate drug intestinal absorption to the physical properties of drugs. Drugs were characterised into four types or classes, as shown in Table 8.5. The ideal drugs fall within class I. Different strategies must be adopted to formulate drugs in other classes to achieve efficient oral absorption.

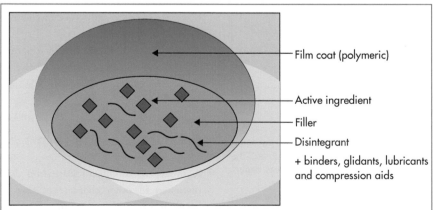

Figure 8.13 A cartoon of a conventional film-coated tablet, showing just some of the ingredients commonly found and the range of possibilities for interactions, such as drug–excipient, excipient–excipient, and changes in the polymer film coat.

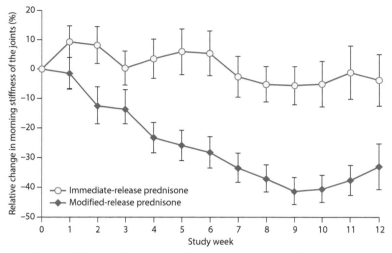

Figure 8.14 Index of stiffness relief in a 10-week clinical trial comparing immediate-release and modified-release oral prednisone tablets. The differences were found to be clinically relevant.

Reproduced from Buttgereit F *et al*. Efficacy of modified-release versus standard prednisone to reduce duration of morning stiffness of the joints in rheumatoid arthritis (CAPRA-1): a double-blind, randomised controlled trial. *Lancet* 2008;371:205–214.

Table 8.5 The four BCS drug classes	
Class I: High solubility, high permeability	Class II: Low solubility, high permeability
Class III: High solubility, low permeability	Class IV: Low solubility, low permeability

There are, of course, drugs that are at the boundaries of these classifications: it is clear too that properties will vary widely within classes. The commonly seen grid is as shown in Fig. 8.15, where GI permeability is plotted not against drug solubility itself but against the *dose/solubility ratio*. Very poorly soluble drugs may be

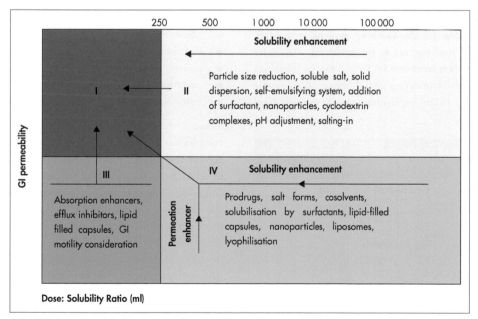

Figure 8.15 A BCS-type plot of the four classes of drug with suggested techniques to enhance absorption. Class II compounds benefit from particle size reduction, soluble salt formation and solubilisation by surfactants; class III drugs require absorption enhancers and efflux inhibitors, *inter alia*; class IV drugs require a range of techniques to attempt to enhance absorption, as shown.

Table 8.6 BCS classification of some well-known drugs

Class I	Class II	Class III	Class IV
Chloroquine	Carbamazepine	Aciclovir	Coenzyme Q_{10}
Diltiazem	Danazol	Atenolol	Ciclosporin A
Metoprolol	Glibenclamide	Captopril	Ellagic acid
Paracetamol	Ketoconazole	Cimetidine	Furosemide
Propranolol	Nifedipine	Metformin	Ritonavir
Theophylline	Phenytoin	Neomycin B	Saquinavir
Verapamil	Troglitazone	Ranitidine	Taxol

therapeutically effective orally if their dose is very low. High-dose drugs with a low solubility present the greatest pharmaceutical challenge. The figure also shows some of the stratagems to be adopted to achieve better absorption.

Table 8.6 lists some well-known drugs and their classification.

Of course, absorption is determined in part by the nature of the formulation used to deliver the drug. Formulation, as indicted in the legend to Fig. 8.15, can be used to enhance bioavailability, but there are also differences in the propensity of dose forms to display problems of bioavailability, especially with drugs which are themselves difficult to be absorbed. Table 8.7 shows those systems with high, medium and low potentials for problems, the order being self-evident from our understanding of the issues already discussed in terms of GI transit, pH, gastric emptying and other important factors, such as food intake.

Table 8.7 Relative potential of oral medicines to display bioavailability problems

High	Intermediate	Low
Enteric-coated tablets	Suspensions	Solutions
Sustained-release tablets	Chewable tablets	
Complex formulations	Capsules	
Slowly disintegrating tablets		

8.3.2 Variability in responses to oral medications

In this chapter so far we have discussed the difficulty in the strict application of physicochemical equations in spite of the fact that the physical chemistry is vitally important in understanding the processes occurring in drug absorption. One of the issues is the dynamic nature of absorption of drug and movement of dose forms down the GI tract. Smith and Rawlins' 1973 book, *Variability in Human Drug Response*,[7] succinctly explained the many reasons for the variation between individuals following the administration of identical medicines, which result from differences in:

- absorption
- distribution
- metabolism
- excretion
- tissue sensitivity.

These are in addition to problems with patient or carer compliance with medication regimes. Physiological, genetic and physicochemical variations can be crucial in determining the successful outcome of treatment. In cases where the effective dose and toxic doses are close then it is important that we understand better the processes involved. Here we are concerned mainly with absorption and how appropriate formulations can modulate differences. Figure 8.16 emphasises, in this case with ciclosporin, the importance of the product, which is a particular issue with drugs with a narrow therapeutic window. Chapter 16 returns to this topic when dealing with generic medicines and biosimilars.

Ciclosporin is an immunosuppressant cyclic peptide that has an oral bioavailability of around 15% in

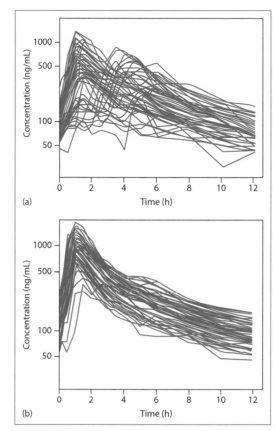

Figure 8.16 Plasma concentration of ciclosporin following oral administration of (a) Sandimmun and (b) Neoral, showing the improvement with the newer formulation, but the still large variation between individual liver transplant patients.

Reproduced from Trull AK *et al.* Absorption of cyclosporin from conventional and new microemulsion oral formulations in liver transplant recipients with external biliary diversion. *Br J Clin Pharmacol* 1995;39:627–631. Copyright Wiley-VCH Verlag GmbH & Co. KGaA. Reproduced with permission.

its amorphous and unformulated form. This is in contrast to the majority of (non-cyclic) peptides, which have little or no oral availability. Ciclosporin, being poorly water-soluble, is difficult to formulate as an oral product. It has been available in several innovative forms: an emulsion-forming (Sandimmun) and a microemulsion-forming product (Neoral), as discussed in Chapter 6 (section 6.4.6). Neoral oral solution contains, in addition to ciclosporin, DL-α-tocopherol, ethanol, polyoxyethylated 40, hydrogenated castor oil, maize oil (corn oil mono-, di-, triglycerides) and propylene glycol. The oral concentrate forms a microemulsion. Neoral soft gelatin capsules also contain the above excipients and these also form microemulsions *in vivo*.

Clinical point

Figure 8.16 shows the variability of absorption after oral administration of Sandimmun and also with the improved microemulsion system, Neoral. The latter is less variable, that is, it improves the quality of effect but there is still variability. Reproducibility of effect is extremely important in transplantation patients to avoid underdosing and transplant rejection. In transplantation patients, initial treatment is by way of intravenous dosing and later maintenance through the oral route.

It is logical to assume that the absorption of the drug would be improved by its formulation in a microemulsion form, where the lipid droplets are in the nanometre rather than micrometre size range. A simple surface area effect would operate – the smaller droplets, having a larger surface area per unit weight, present a greater surface from which the ciclosporin can diffuse directly into intestinal absorbing tissue. It has been suggested that, with the microemulsion, inhibition of metabolism in the gut wall leads to higher availability.

Clinical point

Several formulations of ciclosporin are available. The *British National Formulary* 68 (p. 619)[8] warns:

Patients should be stabilised on a particular brand of oral ciclosporin because switching between formulations without close monitoring may lead to clinically important changes in blood-ciclosporin concentration. Prescribing and dispensing of ciclosporin should be by brand name to avoid inadvertent switching. If it is necessary to switch a patient to a different brand of ciclosporin, the patient should be monitored closely for changes in blood-ciclosporin concentration, serum creatinine, blood pressure, and transplant function.

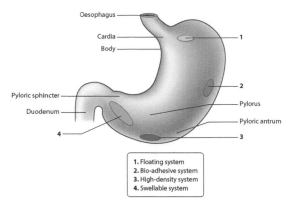

Figure 8.17 Representation of the four main types of gastro-retentive dose forms: floating systems, bioadhesive systems, high-density systems and swellable gel-like systems.

Sandimmun is listed primarily as an intravenous injection but Sandimmun capsules and oral solution are available direct from Novartis for patients who cannot be transferred to a different oral preparation, of which there are Capimune and Deximune, as well as Neoral. It is not always straightforward to determine the ingredients of such formulations, which makes it difficult for pharmacists and physicians. The warning for the intravenous preparation – 'observe patients for signs of anaphylaxis for at least 30 minutes after starting infusion and at frequent intervals thereafter' – is due, as discussed in Chapter 12, to the presence of Cremophor EL, which can induce anaphylaxis in a minority of individuals.

As one of the sources of variation in absorption from the gut is the behaviour of the dosage form in the GI tract, the gastric emptying time, the time for transit in the intestine, the effect of food and concomitant therapies, not to mention gender and age all contribute to the inability to predict outcomes. Logarithmic plots of blood levels have to be read with caution.

Gastro-retentive products can go some way to make gastric emptying times less crucial. Drug is presented to the stomach and intestine as a solution. Four main categories of retentive system are shown in Fig. 8.17:

1. floating systems
2. bioadhesive systems
3. high-density systems
4. swellable systems.

These attempt to overcome the normal patterns of GI transit, particularly that of gastric emptying.

8.3.3 Targeting to sites in the gastrointestinal tract

Enteric-coated systems were the first to achieve targeting of delivery by preventing the dissolution of the dosage form in the stomach, until these units experience the higher pH of the intestine. Targeting to the colon is desirable for the treatment of ulcerative colitis and other pathologies of the gut. Some of the

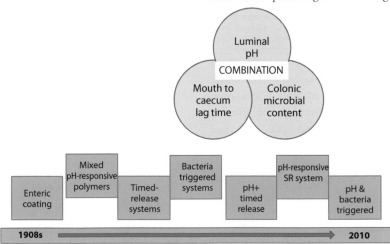

Figure 8.18 The evolution of the development of delivery strategies to target drugs to the colon using the differences in the pH of the gastrointestinal lumen in different regions, the transit times in the gut and the possibility of using the colonic microbiota to initiate release of drug or active drugs released in the vicinity of the colon. SR = sustained-release.

Adapted from Basit AW, McConnell EL. Drug delivery to the colon, Chapter 18. In Wilson CG, Crowley PJ (eds) *Controlled Release in Oral Drug Delivery*. New York: Springer-CRS; 2011, with kind permission from Springer Science and Business Media. See also: Florence AT. A short history of controlled release, pp. 1–26, in the same book.

approaches adopted over the last few decades are represented in Fig. 8.18.

Sulfasalazine represents one drug used in the management of inflammatory bowel diseases. Its activity is generally considered to lie in its metabolic breakdown product, 5-aminosalicylic acid, released in the colon (Fig. 8.19).

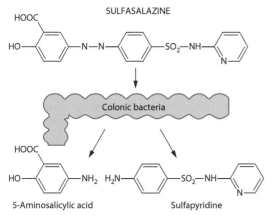

SULFASALAZINE

Colonic bacteria

5-Aminosalicylic acid   Sulfapyridine

Figure 8.19 Sulfasalazine and the formation of its active metabolite as a result of the action of colonic bacteria.

Key points

- Conventional oral delivery systems such as tablets, capsules, suspensions and liquids are fast-release formulations. The release

of drug can be prolonged in order to reduce the frequency of dosing by enteric coating or the use of non-disintegrating matrix forms.

- Particular problems arise in the formulation of oral dosage forms containing labile drugs that might be affected by moisture, low-dose drugs and dose forms containing more than one active ingredient, with the potential for the interaction between the drugs themselves or with the excipient materials.

- The BCS[6] is a valuable aid in choosing a strategy for the formulation of oral dosage forms. Drugs are classified as high solubility, high permeability (class I); low solubility, high permeability (class II); high solubility, low permeability (class III); and low solubility, low permeability (Class IV).

8.4 Buccal and sublingual absorption

Mouthwashes, toothpastes and other preparations are introduced into the oral cavity for local prophylactic and therapeutic reasons. It is not known to what extent components of these formulations are absorbed and give rise to systemic effects. The absorption of drugs through the oral mucosa, however, provides a route for

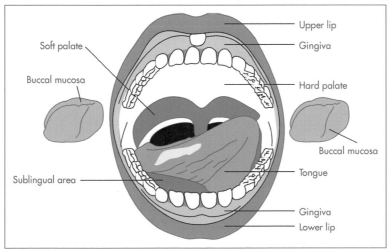

Figure 8.20 The anatomy of the oral cavity, including the buccal, sublingual and gingival cavities.

Reproduced from Kunth K *et al.* Hydrogel delivery systems for vaginal and oral applications. Formulations and biological considerations. *Adv Drug Deliv Rev* 1993;11:137. Copyright Elsevier 1993.

systemic administration that avoids exposure to the GI system. Drugs absorbed in this way bypass the liver and have direct access to the systemic circulation. The sublingual, buccal and gingival tissues are shown diagrammatically in Fig. 8.20. The oral mucosa functions primarily as a barrier, however, and it is not a highly permeable tissue, resembling skin more closely than the gut in this respect (Fig. 8.21) Table 8.8 lists some commercially available sublingual and buccal delivery systems. Mucosal adhesive systems have been studied for administration of buprenorphine through the gingiva.

8.4.1 Mechanisms of oral mucosal absorption

The oral mucosa comprises:

- a mucus layer over the epithelium
- a keratinised layer in certain regions of the oral cavity
- an epithelial layer
- a basement membrane
- connective tissue
- a submucosal region.

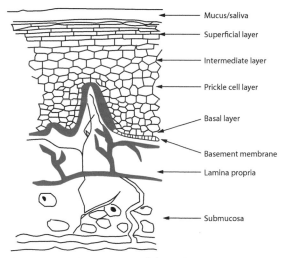

Figure 8.21 The structures of the oral mucosa.*

While cells of the oral epithelium and epidermis are capable of absorbing material by endocytosis, it does not seem likely that drugs or other solutes would be transported by this mechanism across the entire stratified epithelium. It is also unlikely that active transport processes are operative in the oral mucosa. There is considerable evidence that most substances are absorbed by simple diffusion. The linear relationship between percentage absorption through the buccal epithelium and log P of a homologous series is seen in Fig. 8.22. For example, the buccal absorption of some basic drugs increases (Fig. 8.23), and that of acidic drugs decreases, with increasing pH of their solutions.

Table 8.8 Commercially available drug-delivery systems for systemic delivery by the oral mucosal route			
Mucosal site	**Drug**	**Proprietary name**	**Dosage form**
Sublingual	Glyceryl trinitrate	Nitrostat	Tablets
		Lenitral spray	Spray
		Susadrin	Bioadhesive tablets
	Isosorbide dinitrate	Risordan	Tablets
		Sorbitrate	Chewable tablets
		Isocard spray	Spray
	Erythritol trinitrate	Cardiwell	Tablets
	Nifedipine	Adalat	Tablets
	Buprenorphine	Temgesic; Subutex	Tablets
	Apomorphine HCl	Apomorphine	Tablets
Buccal	Prochlorperazine	Buccastem	Bioadhesive tablets
		Tementil	Solution
	Phloroglucinol	Spasfon-Lyoc	Lyocs
	Oxazepam	Seresta Expidet	Lyophilised tablets
	Lorazepam	Temesta Expidet	Lyophilised tablets
	Methyltestosterone	Metandren	Tablets
	Nicotine	Nicorette	Chewing-gum

Modified from Ponchel G. Formulation of oral mucosal drug delivery systems for the systemic delivery of bioactive materials. *Adv Drug Deliv Rev* 1994;13:75. Copyright Elsevier 1994.

---

* When reading papers on the possible buccal delivery of drugs − typical of which might be insulin − which may be promising in animal models, note that rats are not appropriate models as they have a keratinised buccal mucosa.

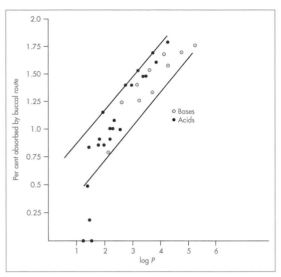

Figure 8.22 Relationship between the log *P* of solute and the percentage absorption through the buccal mucosa of human subjects for bases (○) and acids (●).

Plotted from data from Lien E *et al.* Buccal and percutaneous absorption. *Drug Intell Clin Pharm* 1971;5:38, with permission.

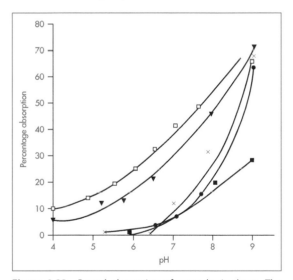

Figure 8.23 Buccal absorption of some basic drugs. The drugs were dissolved in buffered solutions of different pH and placed in the mouth of human subjects; absorption rates were determined from the decrease of drug concentration in expelled solutions: □, chlorphenamine (pK_a = 8.99); ▼, methadone (pK_a = 8.25); ×, amfetamine (pK_a = 9.94); ●, pethidine (pK_a = 8.72); ■, nicotine (pK_a = 8.02).

Reproduced with permission from Beckett AH, Triggs EJ. Buccal absorption of basic drugs and its application as an *in vivo* model of passive drug transfer through lipid membranes. *J Pharm Pharmacol* 1976;19:31S.

Experiments with some analgesics showed that the highly lipid-soluble etorphine was absorbed several times more rapidly from the buccal cavity than the less lipid-soluble morphine.[9] Impressive absorption has been obtained with glyceryl trinitrate (which exerts its pharmacological action 1–2 minutes after sublingual administration), methacholine chloride, isoprenaline, some steroids such as desoxycortisone acetate[10] and 17β-estradiol (at one-quarter of its normal oral dose), morphine, captopril and nifedipine.

It has been claimed that an oil/water partition coefficient in the range 40–2000 (log *P* of 1.6–3.3) is optimal for drugs to be used by the sublingual route. Drugs with a log *P* greater than 3.3 are so oil-soluble that it is difficult for sufficiently high levels of drug to be soluble in the aqueous salivary fluids. Drugs less lipophilic than those with a log *P* of 1 would not be absorbed to any great extent and would thus require large doses by this route. A comparison of the sublingual/subcutaneous dose ratio serves as an index of the usefulness of the route.[11] For example, cocaine with a *P* of 28 requires a sublingual/subcutaneous dosage ratio of 2 to obtain equal effects; atropine with a *P* of 7 requires 8 times the subcutaneous dose; and for codeine (*P* ≈ 2) over 15 times the subcutaneous dose must be given sublingually.

An oromucosal spray: Sativex

Structures of tetrahydrocannabinol (THC) **(I)** and cannabidiol **(II)**, active components of Sativex oromucosal spray

The only cannabis product for medicinal use licensed in the UK and increasingly in other countries is Sativex, containing tetrahydrocannabinol (THC, **I**) and cannabidiol (**II**), mainly for the relief of pain in multiple sclerosis. The spray is a solution of the cannabis extracts in a vehicle consisting of propylene glycol and ethanol flavoured with peppermint oil. Table 8.9 shows the C_{max} and t_{max} of the THC compared to inhaled extract and the very different results from smoking cannabis (note that the doses are different!).

Orodispersible films

Orodispersible films show promise because of their versatility for personalised medication. They can be

Table 8.9 Pharmacokinetic parameters for Sativex, vaporised tetrahydrocannabinol (THC) extract and smoked cannabis

	C_{max} THC (ng mL^{-1})	t_{max} THC (min)	AUC (0-t) THC ng/mL/min
Sativex (providing 21.6 mg THC)	5.40	60	1362
Inhaled vaporised THC extract (providing 8 mg THC)	118.6	17.0	5987.9
Smoked cannabis[a] (providing 33.8 mg THC)	162.2	9.0	No data

[a]Huestis *et al. J Analyt Toxicol* 1992;16:276–282.

fabricated on a small scale. Casting solutions containing hypromellose, carbomer and glycerol are used for example. Poorly soluble drugs such as diazepam can be prepared in film form using ethanol as cosolvent. The water-soluble active pharmaceutical ingredients as well as ethanol influence the viscosity of the casting solution, the mechanical properties and disintegration times of the orodispersible films. Chapter 15 discusses an *in vitro* testing procedure for the determining the mechanical strength of such films.

Nicotine gum

Nicotine in a gum vehicle, when chewed, is absorbed through the buccal mucosa; nicotine levels obtained are lower than those obtained by smoking cigarettes and the high peak levels are not seen. Buccal glyceryl trinitrate has been found to be an effective drug. The buccal route has the advantages of the sublingual route – the buccal mucosa is similar to sublingual mucosal tissue – but a sustained-release tablet can be held in the cheek pouch for several hours if necessary. Mucosal adhesive formulations can have obvious advantages.

Orally disintegrating tablets

Tablets which are designed to disintegrate rapidly in the mouth frequently do so within 30 seconds of placing the dose on the tongue. Some are made by lyophilisation procedures from solutions or suspensions of the active ingredient. This mode of administration again avoids the passage of solid-dose forms down the GI tract and hence can minimise some of the variables we have discussed.

 Key points

- Absorption of drugs through the oral mucosa provides a route for systemic administration that avoids exposure of the drug to the GI tract, and also metabolism in the liver.
- The oral mucosa functions primarily as a barrier and is not highly permeable. Most drugs are absorbed by simple diffusion.
- There is a linear relationship between percentage absorption through the buccal epithelium and log *P* for a homologous series of drugs. Buccal absorption of basic drugs increases and that of acidic drugs decreases with increasing pH of their solutions.
- The optimum log *P* for drugs to be administered by the sublingual route is between 1.6 and 3.3.

Summary

We have considered the basic mechanisms of absorption that apply to all routes of administration, dealing with the factors that depend on the drug itself, its chemical and physicochemical characteristics, the nature of the medium and the subtle differences in biological barriers that drugs experience *in vivo*. While the equations that relate to many of the processes are given, it is emphasised that the dynamic processes of drug absorption – dynamic in two senses, in that the drug is moving down the GI tract at the same time as it is being absorbed – deny us a physicochemical 'theory of everything'. Nonetheless, estimates are valuable in understanding what is going on.

The emphasis on the oral route of delivery and sublingual and buccal delivery provided details of the underlying processes. The following chapter considers parenteral (non-oral) routes of drug administration. In all of these, the actual processes of absorption of drug once it reaches the absorbing surface are the same as those discussed in the present chapter. Sometimes the route to that surface, such as after inhalation, is very tortuous, as we discuss in the next chapter, and sometimes, as with topical preparations, there is a more direct contact between the formulation and the barrier to be overcome. In all, there are at least four important factors: the drug, the route and the formulation (both its physical form and the excipients it contains). These four factors feature as strongly in the discussions in the next chapter.

References

1. Lipinski CA *et al*. Experimental and computational approaches to estimate solubility and permeability in drug discovery and development settings. *Adv Drug Deliv Rev* 2001;4:63–26.
2. Florence AT. Nanoparticle uptake by the oral route: fulfilling its potential? *Drug Discov Today: Technology* 2005;2:75–81.
3. Kararli TT. Comparison of the gastrointestinal anatomy, physiology, and biochemistry of humans and commonly used laboratory animals. *Biopharm Drug Dispos* 1995;16:351–380.
4. Davis SS *et al*. Transit of pharmaceutical dosage forms through the small intestine. *Gut* 1986;27:886–892.
5. Davis SS *et al*. The effect of food on the gastrointestinal transit of pellets and an osmotic device (Osmet). *Int J Pharm* 1984;21:331–340.
6. Amidon GL *et al*. A theoretical basis for a biopharmaceutical classification system: the correlation of *in vitro* drug product dissolution and *in vivo* bioavailability. *Pharm Res* 1995;12:413–420.
7. Smith SE, Rawlins MD. *Variability in Human Drug Response*. London: Butterworths, 1973.
8. *British National Formulary 68*. London: British Medical Association and the Royal Pharmaceutical Society, September 2014–March 2015.
9. Dobbs EH *et al*. Uptake of etorphine and dihydromorphine after sublingual and intramuscular administration. *Eur J Pharmacol* 1969;7:328.
10. Gibaldi M, Kanig JL. Absorption of drugs through the oral mucosa. *J Oral Ther Pharmacol* 1965;31:440–450.
11. Speirs CF. Oral absorption and secretion of drugs. *Br J Clin Pharm* 1977;4:97–100

Further reading

Freire AC *et al*. Does sex matter? The influence of gender on gastrointestinal physiology and drug delivery. *Int J Pharm* 2011;415:15–28.

Pinto JF. Site-specific drug delivery systems within the gastrointestinal tract: from the mouth to the colon. *Int J Pharm* 2010;395:44–52.

Sattar M *et al*. Oral transmucosal drug delivery: current status and future prospects, *Int J Pharm* 2014;471:498–506.

Varum FJO *et al*. Oral modified release formulations in motion. The relationship between gastro-intestinal transit and drug absorption. *Int J Pharm* 2010;395:26–36.

Wilson CG, Crowley PJ (eds) *Controlled Release in Oral Drug Delivery*. New York: Springer-CRS, 2011.

9

In Chapter 8 we discussed the basic mechanisms of drug absorption across biological membrane barriers. Whatever route of delivery and absorption, the basic principles are the same in terms of the determinants of drug transport across membranes. These are dependent on the physical chemistry and nature of the drug, the environment in which the drug finds itself and the nature of the membrane. In this chapter we look at a range of other routes used to administer formulations for both systemic and local use. We deal here with the particular issues with the following routes:

- intravenous (IV) and intra-arterial (IA)
- subcutaneous (SC) and intramuscular (IM)
- topical
- ocular
- aural
- vaginal
- rectal
- respiratory
- nasal
- intrathecal.

Factors affecting drug absorption after delivery of the drug by these routes, often in special formulations, are important, particularly with regard to the comparative advantages and disadvantages of the different routes. More recent specialist devices for specific interventions, such as drug-eluting stents, are considered here as they apply to many of the concepts discussed in earlier chapters.

9.1 Intravenous and intra-arterial administration

The venous route is used for several reasons: it is the most direct route into the blood and thus in emergencies rapid administration of life-saving drugs such as streptokinase is by IV injection. It is of course used in all clinical studies where possible, as the baseline for bioavailability studies. Bioavailability is measured against the values obtained by the IV route. Antibiotics may be given by this route, often over a period of time. It is also the mode of administration of drugs that cannot be given orally, such as many cytotoxic drugs that are toxic to the gut epithelium and proteins that are not absorbed by the oral route. The main physicochemical issues of the route revolve around: (a) the physical and chemical stability of drugs given by infusion in admixture with common fluids such as dextrose; (b) the stability of admixtures when drugs are combined in the same giving set; and (c) tonicity and haemolytic activity. Aqueous solutions, suspensions and emulsions may be employed intravenously. There is a limiting size for any particulate system, which is below 1 μm. The issue of stability is frequently one of physical stability, such as arises with a pH dependency of solubility (discussed in Chapter 4) and with drug–drug interactions (Chapter 11).

 Clinical point

IA injection of BCNU (carmustine; *bis*-chloronitrosourea) in the treatment of malignant glioma results in levels of drug that are four times greater than those following IV infusion, but arguments persist about the relative clinical risks and benefits of IA administration of this drug. The rationale in liver cancer treatment for IA administration is that liver tumours derive their blood supply from the hepatic artery, unlike normal tissue. Two commonly used drugs are fluorouracil and floxuridine.

Microspheres loaded with drugs such as doxorubicin have been used experimentally to optimise delivery by this route.

IA drug administration can be used when venous access cannot be established, as in paediatric patients. It also has a use in cancer chemotherapy, and is sometimes employed in conjunction with IV therapy. Injection into an artery leading directly to an organ such as the liver provides the rationale for its use in cancer chemotherapy.

9.1.1 Implantable infusion pumps

Such devices are implanted under the skin in the lower abdomen and designed to deliver infusate containing the appropriate drug at a constant rate (usually 1 cm^3 per day) into an artery or vein. The Infusaid implantable pump was originally devised for the long-term administration of heparin but has since found application for a wide variety of drugs.[1] The device consists of a relatively small (9 × 2.5 cm) titanium disc that is

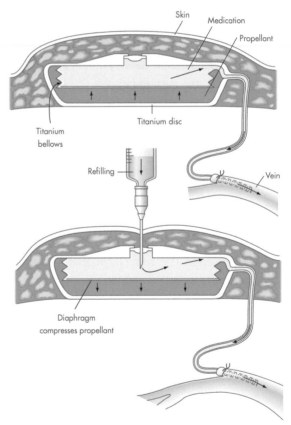

Figure 9.1 Diagrammatic representation of the Infusaid implantable infusion pump during operation (top) and during refilling (bottom).

Reproduced with permission from Blackshear PJ, Rhode TH. In: Burk SD (ed.) *Controlled Drug Delivery*, vol. 2, *Clinical Applications*. Boca Raton, FL: CRC Press; 1983: 11.

Key points

- The venous route is the most direct route into the blood and is used in emergencies for rapid administration of life-saving drugs; it is also the baseline for bioavailability studies and the mode of administration of drugs that cannot be given orally, e.g. many cytotoxic drugs that are toxic to the gut epithelium, and proteins.
- Aqueous solutions, suspensions and emulsions may be employed intravenously, but there is a limiting size for any particulate system, which is below 1 μm.
- IA drug administration can be used when venous access cannot be established, as in paediatric patients. It also has use in cancer chemotherapy.

Table 9.1 Widely used drugs that may be incompletely absorbed after intramuscular injection

Ampicillin	Digoxin[a]
Cefaloridine	Insulin[a]
Cefradine	Phenylbutazone
Chlordiazepoxide	Phenytoin[a]
Diazepam	Quinidine
Dicloxacillin	

[a] Clinically important problems have been demonstrated with these.

divided into two chambers by cylindrical titanium bellows that form a flexible but impermeable barrier between the compartments (Fig. 9.1). The outer compartment contains Freon (chlorofluorocarbon propellants); the inner compartment contains the infusate and connects via a catheter to a vein or artery through a series of filters and flow-regulating resistance elements. The vapour pressure above the liquid propellant remains constant because of the relatively constant temperature of the body, and hence a constant pressure is exerted on the bellows, ensuring a constant rate of delivery of infusate into the blood stream. The propellant is replenished as required by a simple percutaneous injection through the skin.

9.2 Intramuscular and subcutaneous injection

The IM and SC routes of administration have long been regarded as efficient because they bypass the problems encountered in the stomach and intestine. Early views that SC and IM administration of drugs resulted in only local action at the site were dispelled by Benjamin Bell, who wrote in 1858 in the *Edinburgh Medical Journal* that 'absorption from the enfeebled stomach may not be counted on; we possess in sub-

cutaneous injections a more direct, rapid and trustworthy mode of conveying our remedy in the desired quantity to the circulatory blood'. We now know that not all drugs are efficiently or uniformly released from IM or SC sites. Some of the drugs that are not fully absorbed from their IM sites are listed in Table 9.1.

Where differences in bioavailability between IM, SC, oral or IV delivery occur, the clinical importance is most significant when the route of administration is changed from one to another. Such changes are most important in drugs with a low therapeutic index, such as digoxin and phenytoin.

The various regions into which injections are given are shown in Fig. 9.2. The SC region has a good supply of capillaries, although it is generally agreed that there are few, if any, lymph vessels in muscle proper. Drugs with the optimal physicochemical characteristics can diffuse through the tissue and pass across capillary walls and thus enter the circulation by way of the capillary supply.

If it is reasonably assumed that drug absorption proceeds by passive diffusion of the drug, it can be considered to be a first-order process. Thus the rate of absorption is proportional to the concentration, C, of drug remaining at the injection site:

$$\frac{dC}{dt} = -k_a C \tag{9.1}$$

where k_a is the first-order rate constant. The half-life of the absorption process is

$$t_{0.5} = \frac{0.693}{k_a} \tag{9.2}$$

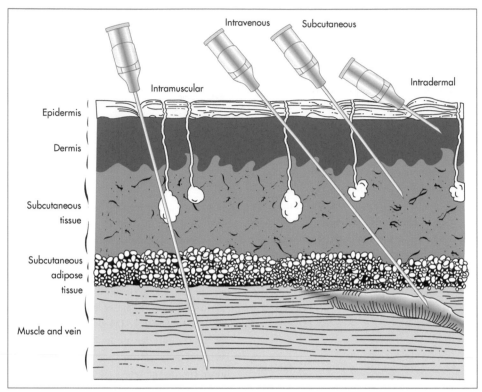

Figure 9.2 Routes of parenteral medication, showing the tissues penetrated by intramuscular, intravenous, subcutaneous and intradermal injections; the needles, with bevel up, penetrate the epidermis (cuticle), consisting of stratified epithelium with an outer horny layer, the corium (dermis or true skin) consisting of tough connective tissue, elastic fibres, lymphatic and blood vessels, and nerves, the subcutaneous tissue (tela subcutanea) consisting of loose connective tissue containing blood and lymphatic vessels, nerves and fat-forming cells, the fascia (a thin sheet of fibrous connective tissue) and the veins, arteries and muscle.

Modified with permission after Quackenbush DS. In: Martin EW (ed.) *Techniques of Medication*. Philadelphia: Lippincott; 1969.

Drug absorption is 90% complete when a time equivalent to three times the half-life has elapsed.

Both dissolution and diffusion are important parameters in defining bioavailability of species by the IM or SC routes. Soluble neutral compounds disperse from IM sites according to size: Table 9.2 shows that mannitol, a small molecule, rapidly diffuses from the site of injection; inulin disperses less rapidly; and

Table 9.2 Influence of molecular size on clearance from intramuscular sites

Substance	Molecular weight	Fraction cleared (5 min)
Mannitol	182	0.70
Inulin	3 500	0.20
Dextran	70 000	0.07

dextran (molecular weight 70 000 Da), as might be expected, disperses more slowly.

With smaller molecules, those with molecular weights in the range 100–1000 Da, molecular size is a factor, but a minor one, in controlling release of drugs, but it assumes greater importance with proteins and other macromolecules, as discussed in Chapter 13. To achieve slow release of low-molecular-weight drugs they may be attached to a macro-molecular backbone. Hydrophilic molecules such as those listed in Table 9.2 will be transported to the blood after diffusing through muscle fibres and then through the pores in the capillary walls, being incapable of absorption through the lipid walls. The transport through the capillary wall is the rate-limiting step in most cases; the larger the molecule, the more slowly it diffuses (as seen from equation 2.64) and the greater difficulty it has in traversing the aqueous pore in the capillary walls or the cell junction. The pores account for only 1% of the available surface of the capillary wall.

Absorption of weak electrolytes across the capillary walls follows the expected patterns, uptake of more lipid-soluble agents being relatively fast. Hydrophobic drugs may bind to muscle protein, leading to a reduction in free drug and perhaps to prolongation of action. Dicloxacillin is 95% bound to protein, while ampicillin is bound to the extent of 20%; as a consequence, dicloxacillin is absorbed more slowly from muscle than is ampicillin.

The significance of the diffusion phase through muscle tissue was demonstrated by Duran Reynolds who, in 1928, observed that dye solutions injected together with hyaluronidase spread out more rapidly and over a greater distance in the tissue than in the absence of the enzyme. The enzyme achieves its effect by breaking down the hyaluronic acid in intercellular spaces, thus leading to a decrease in viscosity and so easing the passage of small molecules in the matrix.

9.2.1 The importance of site of injection

The region into which the injection is administered is complex, being composed of both aqueous and lipid components. Muscle tissue is more acidic than normal physiological fluids. Measurement of percutaneous muscle surface pH (pH_m) using microelectrodes indicates a mean value of 7.38; patients with peripheral vascular disease demonstrated a mean pH_m of 7.16. pH_m reflects the IM ion concentrations but is stated to be higher than the actual IM pH, which may be as low as 6.4. The pH of the region will determine whether drugs will dissolve in the tissue fluids or precipitate from formulations. In some cases precipitation will occur and may be the cause of the pain experienced on injection (see Chapter 12). The rate of solution here, as in many other routes, therefore determines how quickly the drug begins to act or, in some cases, over which period of time it acts. The deliberate reduction of the solubility of a drug achieves prolonged action by both routes.

9.2.2 Vehicles

Many drugs for IM administration are formulated in water-miscible solvents such as polyethylene glycol (PEG) 300 or 400, propylene glycol or ethanol mixtures. Dilution by the tissue fluids may cause the drug to precipitate. Drugs formulated as aqueous solutions by adjustment of pH will only transiently alter the pH at the injection site. Three main types of formulation are used for IM and SC injections: aqueous solutions, aqueous suspensions and oily solutions. Rapid removal of aqueous vehicles is to be expected, the drug being left perhaps as a precipitate. If the vehicle is non-aqueous and is an oil such as sesame oil, or another vegetable or a mineral oil, the oil phase disperses as droplets in the muscle and surrounding tissue, and is eventually metabolised.

The rate-determining step in the absorption of drug esters such as fluphenazine decanoate (which has an aqueous solubility of about 1 part per million) is the hydrolysis of the drug at the surface of the oil droplet. Hydrolysis of the fluphenazine decanoate to its soluble alcohol therefore depends on the state of dispersion and surface area of the droplets.

A recent addition to long-acting injections for schizophrenia, paliperidone palmitate (**I**) takes a different approach using nanocrystals of the insoluble drug which will be deposited in the muscle tissue and hydrolysed by esterases.

 Clinical point

Dispersing the droplets of sustained-release oil-based injections by rubbing the site of injection or by vigorous exercise can result in excessive dosage, with toxic effects. Exercise also causes increased blood flow and, as absorption is a dynamic process requiring the sweeping away of the drug from the localised absorption site, this increased flow increases the rate of drug dispersal.

Structure I Paliperidone palmitate

9.2.3 Blood flow in muscles

Different rates of blood flow in different muscles mean that the site of IM injection can be crucial. Resting blood flow in the deltoid region is significantly greater than in the gluteus maximus muscle; flow in the vastus lateralis is intermediate. The difference between blood flow in the deltoid and gluteus is of the order of 20% and is likely to be the reason why deltoid injection of lidocaine has been found to give higher blood levels than injection into the lateral thigh. Therapeutic plasma levels for the prevention of arrhythmia with a dose of 4.5 mg kg^{-1} of a 10% solution of lidocaine were achieved only following deltoid injection.

> ### Clinical point
>
> The age of the patient should influence the behaviour of the injection, as ageing affects vascular blood flow and fatty deposits, but age has not been specifically isolated as a factor in studies to date. In some disease states it is possible to predict that the outcome of an IM injection might be different from that in other patients. For example, in patients with circulatory shock, hypotension, congestive heart failure and myxoedema, where blood flow to skeletal muscle is decreased, one might anticipate lower bioavailability.

9.2.4 Formulation effects

Crystalline suspensions of fluspirilene, some steroids and procaine benzylpenicillin can be prepared in different size ranges to produce different pharmacokinetic profiles following IM or SC injection, as discussed above. Variability in response to a drug, or differences in response to a formulation from different manufac-

turers, can be the result of the nature of the formulation. Some years ago, in one trial diazepam as Valium (Roche) produced plasma levels ranging from about zero to 160 ng cm^{-3} 90 minutes after injection into muscle (Fig. 9.3). The formulation contained diazepam dissolved in an ethyl alcohol–propylene glycol mixture. Upon injection, this solvent is absorbed and the drug precipitates (see Chapter 11). Injection of the formulation into the fatty tissue of the buttock can result in poor dispersal of drug, as the drug would have little opportunity for dissolution in that environment. Accordingly, the depth of the injection is significant. If, in addition, the blood supply to the region is limited, there will be an additional restriction to rapid removal. An alternative formulation of diazepam (Stesolid) containing a surface-active agent as a solubiliser has a greater bioavailability than a non-aqueous solution form of the drug (Diapam).

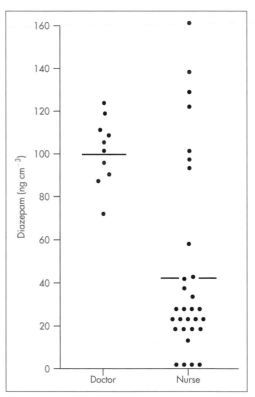

Figure 9.3 Plasma diazepam levels 90 minutes after intramuscular injection by one doctor and several nurses, showing the importance of technique and site of injection, which was variable in the latter group (individual values; horizontal lines denote average levels).

Redrawn with permission from Dundee JW *et al.* Plasma diazepam levels following intramuscular injection by nurses and doctors. *Lancet* 1974;2:1461.

Clinical point

Additives can influence dispersion, the solubiliser undoubtedly in the case of Stesolid reducing precipitation of the drug at the site of injection and thus increasing the rate of solution. Reports of marked difference in side-effects and adverse reactions to diazepam formulations are due to the additives present, either indirectly or directly.

Controlled delivery from SC or IM sites may be achieved by dissolving a lipophilic drug in an oil phase, as discussed above, or encapsulating the drug in liposomes, niosomes or biodegradable microspheres. These techniques are discussed in Chapters 6 and 7.

9.2.5 The case of insulin

Insulin is a classic example of what can be achieved by manipulation of the properties of a drug and its formulation. Modification of the crystallinity of insulin allows control over its solubility and duration of action. An acid-soluble formulation of insulin was introduced for clinical use in 1923. It had a short duration of action and attempts were then made to prolong the action. In 1936, Hagedorn and his colleagues found that insulin complexed with zinc and protamine from the trout (*Salmo irideus*) formed an amorphous precipitate at neutral pH. When injected subcutaneously, the insulin was slowly released from the complex into the blood and was active for about 36 hours. The prolonged-acting insulins introduced since the advent of protamine-zinc insulin (PZI) have been designed to have intermediate durations of action (Table 9.3).

The long-acting insulins in use today are mainly protamine insulin and zinc insulins. Protamine insulins are the salt-like compounds formed between the acid polypeptide (insulin) and the polypeptide protamine, which consists primarily of arginine. They are used in the form of neutral suspensions of protamine insulin crystals (isophane insulin).

Isophane insulin is produced by titration of an acidic solution of insulin with a buffered solution of protamine at neutral pH until so-called isophane precipitation occurs; that is, no insulin or protamine is present in the supernatant. Under these conditions the precipitate consists of rod-shaped crystals. Crystalline forms of insulin free from foreign protein were developed in 1951. Under conditions of high zinc ion

Table 9.3 Pharmaceutical injections of insulin BP					
Preparation	**pH**	**Buffer**	**Description**	**Onset (h)**	**Duration of effect (h)**
Insulin injection	3.0–3.5	–	Solution	~0.5–1	6–8
Neutral injection	6.6–7.7	Acetate	Solution	~0.5–1	6–9
Protamine zinc	6.9–7.4	Phosphate	Amorphous particles; rod-shaped crystals	~5–7	36
Globin zinc	3.0–3.5	–	Solution	~2	18–24
Isophane	7.1–7.4	Phosphate	Rod-shaped crystals (about 20 µm long)	~2	28
Zinc suspension (amorphous) 'Semilente'	7.0–7.5	Acetate	Amorphous particles (2 µm diameter)	~1	12–16
Zinc suspension 'Lente'	7.0–7.5	Acetate	Amorphous particles (30%) Rhombohedral crystals (70%)	~2	24
Zinc suspension (crystalline) 'Ultralente'	7.0–7.5	Acetate	Rhombohedral crystals (about 20 µm across)	~5–7	36
Biphasic	6.6–7.2	Acetate	Insulin in solution (25%) Rhombohedral crystals (75%)	~1	18–22

Modified from Stewart GA. Historical review of the analytical control of insulin. *Analyst* 1974;99:913, with permission of the Royal Society of Chemistry.

Clinical point

1   Variable insulin activity may result from the mixing of PZI and soluble insulin in a syringe prior to administration. It has been suggested that this variability is due to the combination of the soluble insulin with excess protamine. As a general rule, insulin formulations of different pH should not be mixed.

2   Absorption of insulin is faster from injections administered subcutaneously in the arms than into the thighs. Insulin absorption in some patients may be poor because the SC tissue can act as a mechanical barrier to diffusion and as an active site of degradation.

concentration (10 times that normally used to crystallise insulin) and in the absence of citrate and phosphate ions, rhombohedral crystals of insulin are formed in acetate buffer (IZS crystalline). By adjustment of the pH during the crystallisation stage, the insulin is produced as an amorphous precipitate (IZS amorphous) that has a duration of action of up to 16 hours. Various mixtures can be used providing modified durations of actions, as in biphasic insulin. Insulin zinc suspensions are incompatible with PZI and isophane insulin, both of which act as a buffer that destroys the zinc complex.

Figure 9.4 is a diagrammatic representation of the events following SC administration of a soluble human insulin existing initially as a hexameric zinc–insulin complex.

The use of insulins in solution obviates the potential source of error that arises when drawing a suspension into a syringe, but soluble insulins have the drawback that they must be stored at acid pH. Figure 9.5 shows the solubility–pH profiles for soluble insulin and a trilysyl derivative. Injected subcutaneously, the insulin precipitates as amorphous particles. The pH of insulin preparations influences their stability, solubility and immunogenicity.

9.2.6 Long-acting contraceptives

There is a series of progestogen-only contraceptives which display a variety of techniques of formulation and delivery, namely:

- Depo-Provera, an aqueous medroxyprogesterone acetate suspension delivered by deep IM injection,

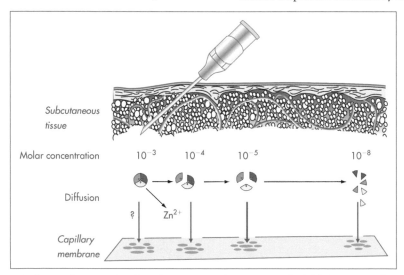

Figure 9.4 Suggested scheme of events after the subcutaneous administration of soluble human insulin: the concentration of hexameric zinc-insulin, which is the predominant form of insulin in soluble insulin (40 or 100 units – i.e. 0.6 mmol dm^{-3}), decreases as diffusion of insulin occurs and as a result the hexamer dissociates into smaller units; to achieve monomeric insulin requires a 1000-fold dilution. The importance of the association state is that the larger species have more difficulty dispersing and passing through the capillary membrane.

Reproduced with permission from Brange J et al., Monomeric insulins and their experimental and clinical implications. Diabetes Care, 1990; 13: 923.

Clinical points

1 After IM administration, short-acting insulin is absorbed about twice as rapidly as after SC injection, and therefore the IM route is used in the management of ketoacidosis in those cases where continuous IV infusion cannot be established. After SC injection, absorption of short-acting insulin varies considerably depending in particular on the site of injection. Patient-to-patient variability is as great with these preparations as the variations in the absorption rate of intermediate-acting insulins. This can lead to difficulty in control.

2 Flocculation of Humulin N insulin and of NPH insulin leads to changes in the appearance of vials (a frosting) and signals a problem, that of loss of potency and thus control. In affected samples it was found that the insulin concentration ranged from 6 to 64 U mL^{-1}, where in normal samples within narrow margins the concentration was 110 U mL^{-1}.

Key points

- The IM and SC routes avoid problems encountered in the stomach and intestine; however, not all drugs are efficiently or uniformly released from IM or SC sites.
- Drugs with the optimal physicochemical characteristics can diffuse through the SC tissue and enter the circulation by way of the extensive capillary supply in this region.
- Drug absorption proceeds by passive diffusion and can be considered to be a first-order process; the rate of absorption is proportional to the concentration of drug remaining at the injection site.
- The bioavailability of species by the IM or SC routes is influenced by dissolution and diffusion. The rate of dispersion of soluble neutral molecules from the injection site and their transport through the capillary wall (the rate-limiting step in most cases) is determined by molecular size: the larger the molecule, the more slowly it diffuses.
- Hydrophilic molecules are incapable of absorption through the lipid walls and enter the blood stream through the pores in the capillary walls. Hydrophobic drugs may bind to muscle protein, leading to a reduction in free drug and perhaps to prolongation of action.
- The pH at the injection site will determine whether drugs will dissolve in the tissue fluids or precipitate from formulations; precipitation may be the cause of the pain experienced on injection.
- The main types of formulation used for IM and SC injections are aqueous solutions, aqueous suspensions and oily solutions, from which drugs can diffuse slowly for long action. Many drugs for IM administration are formulated in water-miscible solvents such as PEG 300 or 400, propylene glycol or ethanol mixtures; dilution by the tissue fluids may cause the drug to precipitate.
- The site of IM injection can be crucial because of different rates of blood flow in different muscles.
- The nature of the formulation can cause variability in response to a drug, or differences in response to a formulation from different manufacturers.

which is repeated every 12 weeks for long-term contraception

- Noristerat, an oily injection of norethisterone acetate injection given by deep IM injection, repeated once every 8 weeks

- Sayan Press, a suspension of medroxyprogesterone acetate injected SC into the anterior thigh or abdomen, which is repeated every 13 weeks.

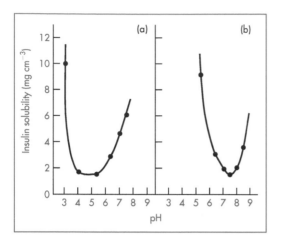

Figure 9.5 The solubility dependence of (a) insulin and (b) trilysyl insulin, a chemically modified insulin with an iso-electric point of 7.4 compared with the isoelectric point of unmodified insulin of 5.3.

Reproduced with permission from Fischel-Ghodsian F, Newton JM. Simulation and optimisation of a self-regulating insulin delivery system. *J Drug Targeting* 1993;1:67.

These show the potential for very slow release, the duration being a factor of drug, dose and formulation, which must include the control of particle size distribution for the two suspensions and drug solubility, as we have discussed elsewhere.

Nexplanon subdermal implant

To achieve even longer-term action there are implants such as Nexplanon, which allows contraceptive cover over 36 months, delivering subdermally etonogestrel from a soft, flexible sterile ethylene vinyl acetate (EVA)

copolymer core, surrounded by an EVA skin. It also contains barium sulfate as a radiopaque material for location during its lifetime (Fig. 9.6).

In Chapter 8 we referred briefly to human variability in responses to drugs and medication, particularly by the oral route with the vagaries of the behaviour of the gastrointestinal tract. Apart from genetic and racial factors, and factors related to age and concomitant pathologies, one additional factor that is evident with the lipophilic steroids used in contraception is illustrated clearly in Fig. 9.7 – the effect of obesity. Plasma levels of etonogesterel from implants were much reduced in obese women.

9.3 Transdermal delivery

A comprehensive account of the pharmaceutics and biopharmaceutics of topical preparations is not possible here. This section is restricted in scope to the physicochemical principles involved both in the process of treating the skin and in systemic medication by the *transdermal* or *percutaneous* route.

Formulation of topical vehicles for the potent drugs applied to the skin is now a more exact art. It is readily demonstrated that the vehicle in which the drug is applied influences the rate and extent of absorption. However, topical formulations can change rather rapidly once they have been spread on the skin, and absorption of some excipients and evaporative loss of water cause the breakdown of original structures.

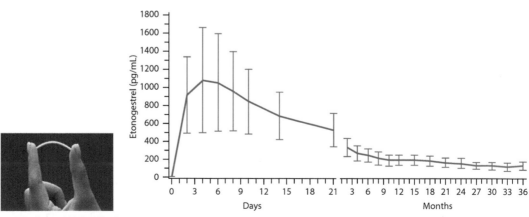

Figure 9.6 Mean (± SD) Serum concentration–time profile of etonogestrel after insertion of Nexplanon (a photograph of a subdermal implant is shown) during 36 months of use.

From data on Nexplanon, MSD.

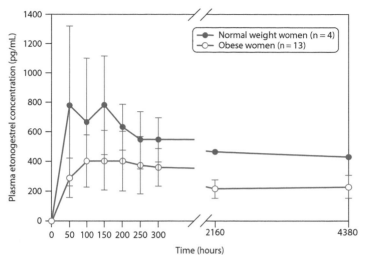

Figure 9.7 Human variability: the pharmacokinetics of etonogestrel in women of normal weight versus women categorised as obese.
Reproduced from S. Mornar et al. *Am. J Obstet Gynecol* 2012;207:110e1–110e6.

Before any drug applied topically can act either locally or systemically it must penetrate the barrier layer of the skin, the stratum corneum (Fig. 9.8). This behaves like a passive diffusion barrier with no evidence of metabolic transport processes; drugs are absorbed by transcellular or intercellular pathways.

Penetration of water and low-molecular-weight non-electrolyte solutes through the epidermis is proportional to their concentration, and to the partition coefficient of the solute between tissue and vehicle.

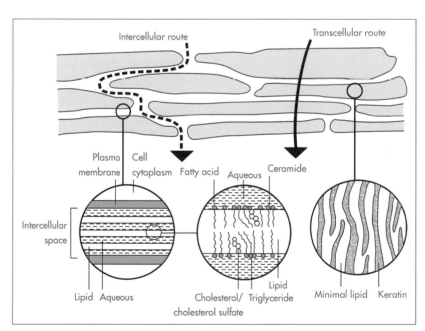

Figure 9.8 'Bricks and mortar' model of the stratum corneum, illustrating possible pathways of drug permeation through intact stratum corneum (transcellular and tortuous intercellular pathways) and the lamellar structure of intercellular lipids.
Reproduced from Moghimi HR *et al*. A lamellar matrix model for stratum corneum intercellular lipids II. Effect of geometry of the stratum corneum on permeation of model drugs 5-fluorouracil and oestradiol. *Int J Pharm* 1996;131:117. Copyright Elsevier 1996.

A form of Fick's law describes steady-state transport through the skin:

$$J = \frac{DP}{\delta}\Delta C_V \qquad (9.3)$$

where J is the solute flux, D is the solute diffusion coefficient in the stratum corneum (values range from 1×10^{-12} to 1×10^{-17} m^2 s^{-1} for human stratum corneum), P is the solute partition coefficient between skin and vehicle and δ is the thickness of the stratum corneum. ΔC_v is the difference in solute concentration between vehicle and tissue? This relation is obtained as shown in Derivation Box 9A.

Before steady-state penetration is achieved, the rate builds up over a period of time and a lag phase will be apparent (Fig. 9.9). The lag time, τ, does not indicate the point at which steady state is achieved, which, as shown in Fig. 9.9, is obtained by extrapolation. The linear portion of the graph can be described by an equation relating the total amount absorbed at time t, Q_t, to $\Delta C, P, \delta, t$ and D. From equation (9.3), as $Q_t = Jt$,

$$Q_t = \frac{DP\Delta C_V}{\delta} t \qquad (9.4)$$

But from Fig. 9.9 it is obvious that the time to be substituted is the time over which steady-state flux has been maintained; namely, $t - \tau$. Thus we write

$$Q_t = \frac{DP\Delta C_V}{\delta}(t - \tau) \qquad (9.5)$$

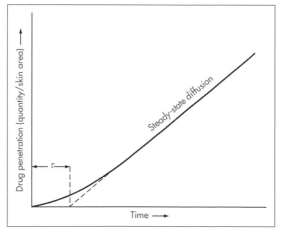

Figure 9.9 Drug penetration–time profile for an idealised drug diffusing through human skin; once steady-state diffusion occurs Q_t can be obtained using equation (9.4), where t = (time elapsed − τ).

As the lag time, τ, has been shown to be equal to $\delta^2/6D$, the drug's diffusion coefficient D is readily obtained from data such as those shown in Fig. 9.7. Values of τ range from a few minutes to several days, so lag times are of obvious clinical relevance.

9.3.1 Routes of skin penetration

Drug molecules may penetrate the skin not only through the stratum corneum but also by way of the hair follicles or through the sweat ducts, but these offer only a comparatively minor route because they represent such a small fraction of the surface area. Only in the case of molecules that move very slowly through the stratum corneum may absorption by these other routes predominate. Passage through damaged skin is increased over normal skin. Skin with a disrupted epidermal layer will allow up to 80% of hydrocortisone to pass into the dermis, whereas only 1% is absorbed through intact skin.

The physicochemical factors that control drug penetration include the hydration of the stratum corneum, temperature, pH, drug concentration and the molecular characteristics of the penetrant and the vehicle. The stratum corneum is a heterogeneous structure containing about 40% protein (keratin, a disulfide-crosslinked linear polypeptide), about 40% water and 18–20% lipids (principally triglycerides and free fatty acids, cholesterol and phospholipids). Hydration of the stratum corneum is one determinant of the extent of absorption: increased hydration decreases the resistance of the layer, presumably by causing a swelling of the compact structures in the horny layer.

 Clinical point

Occlusive dressings increase the hydration of the stratum corneum by preventing water loss by perspiration; certain ointment bases are designed to be self-occluding. The use of occlusive films can increase the penetration of corticosteroids by a factor of 100 and of lower-molecular-weight drugs up to fivefold.

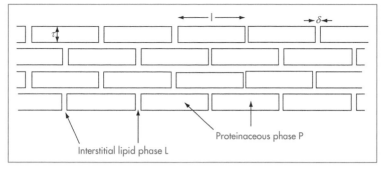

Figure 9.10 Idealised model of the stratum corneum. Lipid (L) and proteinaceous (P) parts of the stratum corneum are represented; this model is used to derive model equations for drug transport across this layer (see text).

Reproduced from Michaels AS *et al.* Drug permeation through human skin, theory and *in vitro* experimental measurement. *A I Chem J* 1975;21:985. Copyright Wiley-VCH Verlag GmbH & Co. KGaA. Reproduced with permission.

In the idealised model of the stratum corneum shown in Fig. 9.10, L represents the lipid-rich interstitial phase and P the proteinaceous phase. If $\rho = P_L/P_P$ (the ratio of the partition coefficients of the drug between vehicle and the L and P phases) and D_L and D_P are the diffusion coefficients of the drug in these phases, the flux through stratum corneum of average thickness (40 µm) is found to reduce to

$$J = 0.98\rho \frac{D_L}{D_P} \ (\mu g\, cm^{-2}\, h^{-1}) \qquad (9.6)$$

when $\rho(D_L/D_P)$ is very small. When $\rho(D_L/D_P)$ is very large, the flux becomes

$$J = (2.3 \times 10^{-4} \rho \frac{D_L}{D_P} \ (\mu g\, cm^{-2}\, h^{-1}) \qquad (9.7)$$

which emphasises the importance of both the partition coefficient and diffusion coefficient of the drug in the absorption process.

9.3.2 Influence of the drug

The diffusion coefficient of the drug in the skin will be determined by factors such as molecular size, shape and charge; the partition coefficient will be determined not only by the properties of the drug but also by the vehicle as this represents the donor phase, the skin being the receptor phase. The quantity ρ can be approximated by experimentally determined oil/water partition coefficients. Substances that have a very low oil solubility will have lower rates of penetration.

The major pathway of transport for water-soluble molecules is transcellular, involving passage through cells and cell walls. The pathway for lipid-soluble molecules is presumably the endogenous lipid within the stratum corneum, the bulk of this being intercellular. Increase in the polar character of the molecule decreases permeability, as seen from the data on steroids in Table 9.4, in which progesterone and hydroxyprogesterone and deoxycortone and cortexolone should be compared. Each pair differs only by a hydroxyl group. The lipid/water partition coefficients of the drugs in Table 9.4 decrease as the number of hydroxyl groups increases, but a simple lipid/water partition coefficient is not an ideal guide, as the stratum corneum is a complex system, as described above. If a substance is more soluble in the stratum corneum than in the vehicle in which it is presented, however, the concentration in the first layer of the skin may be higher than that in the vehicle. If depletion of the contact layers of the vehicle occurs, then the nature of the formulation will dictate how readily these are replenished by diffusion and, therefore, will dictate the rate of absorption.

The penetration rates of four steroids through intact abdominal autopsy skin were, in the order of their physiological activity, betamethasone 17-valerate (**II**) > desonide > triamcinolone acetonide (**III**) > hydrocortisone (**IV**).

Structure II Betamethasone 17-valerate

Table 9.4 Permeability constants of steroids

Steroid	Structure	Permeability constant, κ_P (10^{-6} cm^{-2} h^{-1})
Progesterone		1500
Hydroxyprogesterone		600
Deoxycortone		450
Cortexolone		75

Reproduced by permission from Macmillan Publishers Ltd from Scheuplein R. Permeability of the skin: a review of major concepts and some new developments. *J Invest Dermatol* 1976;67:672.

Structure III Triamcinolone acetonide

Structure IV Hydrocortisone

Of 23 esters of betamethasone (**V**), the 17-valerate ester possesses the highest topical activity. The vasoconstrictor potency of betamethasone 17-valerate is 360 (fluocinolone acetonide = 100), that of betamethasone 0.8, of its 17-acetate 114, of the 17-propionate 190, and of the 17-octanoate 10. The peak activity coincides with an optimal partition coefficient, one that favours neither lipid nor aqueous phase.

Structure V Betamethasone

Note that the order of systemic and transdermal biological activities can be quite different. And of course the esters of certain steroids can result in startling differences in activity.

1 Triamcinolone is five times more active systemically than hydrocortisone, but has only one-tenth of its topical activity.
2 Betamethasone is 30 times as active as hydrocortisone systemically but has only four times the topical potency.
3 Triamcinolone acetonide has a topical activity 1000 times that of the parent steroid because of its favourable lipid solubility.

9.3.3 Influence of the vehicle

Consideration of equation (9.3) shows immediately that the vehicle has an influence on the absorption of the drug: if the vehicle is changed so that the drug becomes less soluble in it, P increases and so permeability increases. The vehicle is more dominant in topical therapy than in most routes of administration because the vehicle remains at the site, although not always in an unchanged form. Evaporation of water from a water-in-oil base would leave

drug molecules immersed in the oily phase. Oil-in-water emulsion systems may invert to water-in-oil systems, in such a way that the drug would have to diffuse through an oily layer to reach the skin. Volatile components are driven off, probably altering the state of saturation of the drug and hence its activity. Drug may precipitate owing to lack of remaining solvent. This all means that theoretical approaches very much represent the simplest or, in thermodynamic terms, 'ideal' cases.

Formulations

Many modern dermatological formulations are washable oil-in-water systems. Simple aqueous lotions are also used as they have a cooling effect on the skin. Ointments are used for the application of insoluble or oil-soluble medicaments and leave a greasy film on the skin, inhibiting loss of moisture and encouraging the hydration of the keratin layer. Aqueous creams combine the characteristics of the lotions and ointments. A classification of semisolid bases is given in Fig. 9.11.

The descriptions 'ointment' and 'cream' have no universally accepted meaning and generally refer to the completed formulation. Ointments are generally composed of single-phase hydrophobic bases, such as pharmaceutical grades of soft paraffin or microcrystalline paraffin wax.

'Absorption' bases have an alleged capacity to facilitate absorption by the skin, but the term also

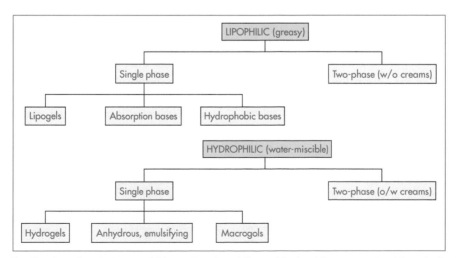

Figure 9.11 Classification of topical semisolid bases into lipophilic and hydrophilic systems in either single-phase or two-phase forms.

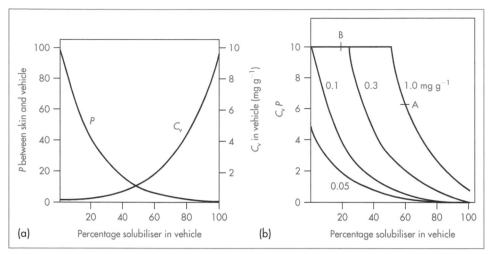

Figure 9.12 (a) Drug partition coefficient and solubility dependence on vehicle composition for the 'ideal' case. (b) Predicted relative steady-state penetration (C_vP) as a function of vehicle composition for the 'ideal' case. Point A represents a formulation containing 1.0 mg g^{-1} and 60% solubiliser. On threefold dilution with a base containing no solubiliser, point B is arrived at, where C_vP is higher.

Reproduced with permission from Poulsen BJ. In: Ariens EJ (ed.) *Drug Design*, vol. 4. New York: Academic Press; 1973.

alludes to their ability to take up considerable amounts of water to form water-in-oil emulsions. Lipogels are gels prepared by dispersion of long-chain fatty-acid soaps such as aluminium mono-stearate in a hydrocarbon base. Hydrogels prepared from Carbopols or cellulose derivatives are discussed in Chapter 7.

Thermodynamic activity in topical products

The complexity of many of the topical bases means that a simple physicochemical explanation of their influence on the release of medicament is not always possible. It is not difficult, however, to ascertain the effect of the base and to highlight the problem. The interactions between the physical properties of the base and the drug are exemplified by the effect of propylene glycol in simple bases, shown in Fig. 9.12, where the percentage of the glycol acting as a solvent for the drug significantly affects permeation.

The thermodynamic activity of the drug is the ultimate determinant of its biological activity. If the solubility of the drug in the base is increased by addition of propylene glycol, then its partition coefficient, P, towards the skin is reduced. On the other hand, increasing the amount that can be incorporated in the base is an advantage and the concentration (C_v) gradient is increased. It is apparent that there will be an optimum amount of solubiliser. The optimum

occurs at the level of additive that just solubilises the medicament. Addition of excess results in desaturation of the system, and a decrease in thermodynamic activity. As the total amount of drug in the vehicle is increased from 0.5 to 1.0 mg g^{-1} (Fig. 9.12b), more propylene glycol has to be added to cause a decrease in C_vP. From Fig. 9.12b one could postulate that threefold dilution of a formulation containing 1.0 mg g^{-1} and 60% solubiliser with a base with no solubiliser would cause the thermodynamic activity to increase. The vehicle affects penetration only when the release of drug is rate-limiting.

In situations where all of the activity gradient is in the applied phase, skin properties play no part. In these cases drug concentration in the vehicle, the diffusion coefficient of the drug in the system and the solubility of the drug are the significant factors. Where these factors are not important, the only significant factor involving the vehicle is the thermodynamic activity of the drug contained in it. Using the simplest model, for a solution of concentration C applied to an area A of the skin, the steady-state rate of penetration, dQ/dt, is given by

$$\frac{dQ}{dt} = \frac{PCDA}{\delta} \tag{9.8}$$

δ being the thickness of the barrier phase. An equivalent form of this equation expresses release in terms of the thermodynamic activity, a, of the agent in the vehicle:

$$\frac{dQ}{dt} = \frac{a}{\gamma} \frac{DA}{\delta} \qquad (9.9)$$

where γ is the activity coefficient of the agent in the skin barrier phase. Ointments containing finely ground particles of drug where the thermodynamic activity is equal to that of solid drug will have the same rate of penetration, provided that the passage of the drug in the barrier phase is rate-limiting.

Drug release from complex vehicles

In more complex vehicles the activity a is impossible to determine and other approaches must be adopted. For example, in emulsions the relative affinity of drug for the external and internal phases of the emulsion is an important factor. A drug dissolved in an internal aqueous phase of a water-in-oil emulsion must be able to diffuse through the oily layer to reach the skin. Three cases can be considered: solution, suspension and emulsion systems.

1. Release from *solutions* is most readily understood and quantified by equations of the form

$$\frac{dQ}{dt} = C_0 \left(\frac{D}{\pi t} \right)^{1/2} \qquad (9.10)$$

and

$$Q = 2C_0 \left(\frac{Dt}{\pi} \right)^{1/2} \qquad (9.11)$$

where C_0 is the initial medicament concentration in solution, D is the diffusion coefficient and t is the time after application of the vehicle. As D is inversely proportional to the viscosity of the vehicle, one would expect that drug release would be slower from a viscous vehicle.

2. If a drug in *suspension* is to have any action it must have a degree of solubility in the base used. An aged suspension of a drug will therefore have a saturated solution of the drug present in the continuous phase. Release of medicament in these conditions is given by

$$\frac{dQ}{dt} = \kappa_{sp} \left(\frac{C_0 C_s D}{2t} \right)^{1/2} \qquad (9.12)$$

where C_s is the total solubility of the drug in the vehicle and C_0 is the concentration in the vehicle. This equation applies only when $C_s \ll C_0$. Only material in solution penetrates the stratum corneum and the depleted layer in the vehicle is replenished only by solution of particles and diffusion of the drug molecules to the depleted layer.

3. The equations for *emulsion-type* vehicles are discussed in Chapter 6.

9.3.4 Dilution of topical steroid preparations

 Clinical point

Inappropriate dilution of carefully formulated creams and ointments may result in changes in stability and effectiveness. An example would be clobetasol propionate formulated in a base containing the optimum amount of propylene glycol. The solubilities of the steroid as a function of propylene glycol concentration are shown in Fig. 9.13. A 1 in 2 dilution of a 0.05% cream, with a vehicle containing water and no propylene glycol, will precipitate a large proportion of the steroid. The same principles apply to steroids presented in a fatty-acid propylene glycol base.

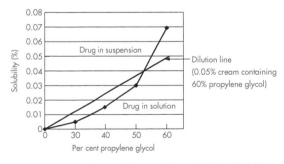

Figure 9.13 A diagram showing the solubility of clobetasol propionate as a function of propylene glycol concentration. The dilution line shows that, if a 0.05% cream containing 60% propylene glycol is diluted with a base not containing the glycol, the drug will be precipitated.
Data from Busse M. *Pharm J* 1978;220:25.

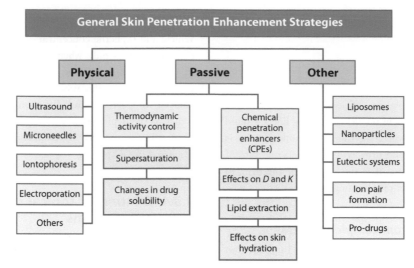

Figure 9.14 Physical, passive and other means of improving the absorption of drugs or their penetration, e.g. via microneedles, iontophoresis, electroporation or by penetration enhancers or formulation techniques.
Reproduced from Hadgraft J, Lane M. Skin: the ultimate interface. *Phys Chem Chem Phys* 2011;13:5215–5222.

Enhancing skin penetration

The many techniques for enhancing the penetration of drugs through the skin are summarised in Fig. 9.14 and can be used as an *aide mémoire* for the whole topic of transdermal drug delivery.

9.3.5 Transdermal medication: patches and devices

The ease with which some drugs can pass through the skin barrier into the circulating blood means that the transdermal route of medication is a possible alternative to the oral route. Theoretically there are several advantages:

- For drugs that are normally taken orally, administration through the skin can eliminate the vagaries that influence gastrointestinal absorption, such as pH changes and variations in food intake and intestinal transit time.
- A drug may be introduced into the systemic circulation without initially entering the portal circulation and passing through the liver.
- Constant and continuous administration of drugs may be achieved by a simple application to the skin surface.
- Continuous administration of drugs percutaneously at a controlled rate should permit elimination of pulse entry into the systemic circulation, an effect that is often associated with side-effects.

- Absorption of medication can be rapidly terminated whenever therapy must be interrupted.

Not all drugs are suitable for transdermal delivery. The limitations of the route are indicated in Table 9.5, which compares the percutaneous absorption of a range of drugs, from aspirin (only 22% of which is absorbed, even after 120 hours) to chloramphenicol, of which only 2% is absorbed. The transdermal route is now routinely used for a range of drugs, including oestrogens, clonidine and nicotine. The four basic forms of patch systems are shown in Fig. 9.15.

Maximum flux from a saturated aqueous system of several drugs was estimated to be 300 µg cm^{-2} h^{-1} and from a mineral-oil system 250 µg cm^{-2} h^{-1}. Using

Table 9.5 Percutaneous absorption of a range of drugs in humans

Drug	Percentage dose absorbed (120 h)
Aspirin	22
Chloramphenicol	2
Hexachlorophene	3
Salicylic acid	23
Urea	6
Caffeine	48

Reproduced with permission from Beckett AH *et al.* Comparison of oral and percutaneous routes in man for the systemic administration of ephedrine. *J Pharm Pharmacol* 1972;24:65P.

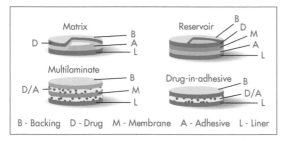

Figure 9.15 The four main types of transdermal patch: matrix, reservoir, multilaminate and drug-in-adhesive designs. The matrix and reservoir systems are cut away to show the drug.

Illustration courtesy of 3M.

a 'patch' with a rate-limiting polymeric membrane, delivery is controlled to 40–50 µg cm^{-2} h^{-1}; that is, it is presented to the skin at that rate. A 10 cm^2 device will therefore deliver 0.4–0.5 mg h^{-1}. Control of release can be exercised by altering the membrane's properties and by changing the pH of the reservoir solution for a drug such as hyoscine (Fig. 9.16).

Iontophoresis

Iontophoresis is the process by which the migration of ionic drugs into tissues such as skin is enhanced by the use of an electric current, a technique that has found application favour in facilitating the delivery of peptides and proteins. A typical iontophoretic device is shown in Fig. 9.17.

Current can be applied in a continuous manner using either direct current (e.g. 0.1 mA cm^{-2}) or pulsed (0.1 mA cm^{-2}; 2000 Hz) to either solutions or

gels of a drug. Enhancement of migration results from several possible sources, of which two are:

1. convective flow (electro-osmosis)
2. current-induced increases in skin permeability.

The flux of drug can be increased by increasing current density. With drug molecules (up to a molecular weight 1000 Da), the fraction of total current flowing that is carried by the drugs is small because of competition from smaller ions. Electro-osmosis probably plays a greater role here. Figure 9.18 shows the effect of pH, osmolality and current density on the transport of the nonapeptide buserelin through stratum corneum.

9.3.6 Ultrasound and transdermal penetration

Therapeutic ultrasound has been found[2] first to expand and then collapse air bubbles in the stratum corneum (the process of cavitation) (Fig. 9.19). Cavitation tends to liquefy the solid fats and allows molecules such as insulin to pass through the skin at levels that in diabetic rats cause blood sugar lowering. The permeability of the skin was found to increase as the frequency of ultrasound decreased and no long-term damage was caused.

9.3.7 Jet injectors

Invented in 1947 as a needle-free method of delivering drugs to the skin,[3] jet injection techniques have received renewed attention recently. They perhaps

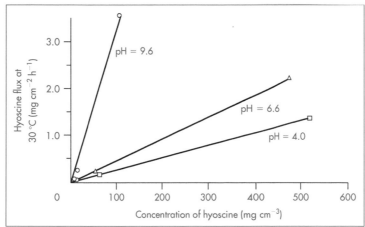

Figure 9.16 The effect of hyoscine concentration and pH on the flux of hyoscine across a membrane; increasing the pH increases the flux as ionisation is decreased.

Reproduced from Michaels AS *et al.* Drug permeation through human skin, theory and in vitro experimental measurement. *A I Chem J* 1975;21:985. Copyright Wiley-VCH Verlag GmbH & Co. KGaA. Reproduced with permission.

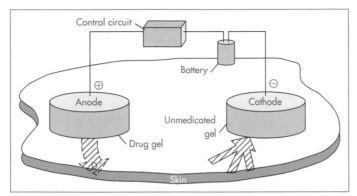

Figure 9.17 The major components of an iontophoretic drug delivery system. To optimise iontophoretic transdermal drug delivery, the drug should be charged. It should be applied under an electrode of the same polarity, and a counterelectrode opposite in charge to the drug must be placed at an indifferent site on the body. Electric current must be allowed to flow for an appropriate duration at a level minimising skin irritation. Iontophoresis can deliver neutral drugs by inducing solvent flow (electro-osmosis) that results from the migration of ionic species in the applied field. Drug candidates for iontophoretic transdermal delivery must usually be in a salt form with adequate aqueous solubility, be stable in an aqueous environment, and be sufficiently potent to allow therapeutic doses to be delivered at an acceptable current density.

Reproduced from Lattin GA *et al.* Electronic control of iontophoretic drug delivery. *Ann N Y Acad Sci* 1991;618:450. Copyright Wiley-VCH Verlag GmbH & Co. KGaA. Reproduced with permission.

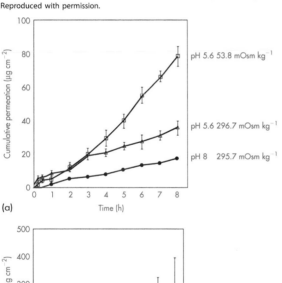

(a)

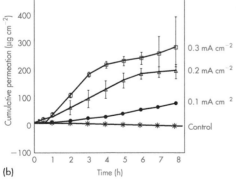

(b)

Figure 9.18 (a) The influence of donor pH and ionic strength of the donor medium on buserelin (a nonapeptide) permeation. (b) Continuous iontophoresis and release of buserelin through the stratum corneum, showing the effect of increasing the current.

Reproduced from Knoblauch P, Moll F. In vitro pulsatile and continuous transdermal delivery of buserelin by iontophoresis. *J Control Release* 1993;26:203. Copyright Elsevier 1993.

have not lived up to recent promise, because of a certain unreliability of drug penetration, drug collection or pooling on the skin[4] and rebound of particles from the skin surface. The systems are based on the high-velocity ejection of particles from the injector, through an orifice. Drug delivery is then due to either or both of skin 'failure' and flow through the skin.[4] The theoretical maximum velocity (v) of the jet is related to the pressure (P) in the nozzle and the density (ρ) of the liquid by

$$v = \left(\frac{2P}{\rho}\right)^{1/2} \tag{9.13}$$

but the velocity is affected by diameter of the orifice and is reduced by turbulence and friction.

Microneedles

When drug molecules have no natural tendency to penetrate the skin (hydrophilic molecules, proteins and oligopeptides and antigens), it is possible to take advantage of the development of microneedles fabricated, for example, from silicon, metal or polymers in solid or hydrogel form. There are five main categories of microneedle, as shown in Fig. 9.20:

1. solid
2. coated
3. dissolving

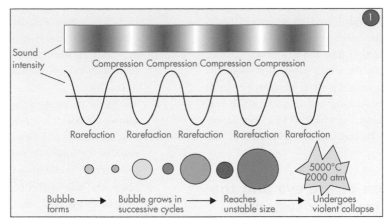

Figure 9.19 The process of cavitation leading to bubble collapse and change in fat structures and expulsion of drug.

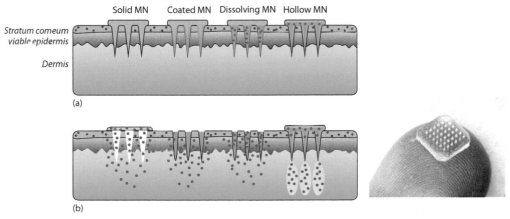

Figure 9.20 Diagram of the four types of microneedle (MN) showing (a) their structure: solid, coated. dissolving and hollow; and (b) their mode of behaviour once inserted into the skin. There are other configurations undergoing development. Right: photograph of a typical microneedle patch.

4. hollow
5. hydrogel-based systems.

These penetrate the stratum corneum, the viable epidermis and the dermis (Fig. 9.20). In the case of solid forms, their use is to make passages in these layers to allow a topical preparation to penetrate physically without invoking the processes discussed above. Other forms are coated with a drug so that the drug dissolves when inserted; dissolving systems contain the drug in the fabric of the needle and hollow needles allow drug from a reservoir to become available.[*]

9.4 Topical treatment of the nails: transungual therapy

Treatment of fungal infections of the nail requires special topical approaches. It is a subject that has been the subject of several reviews. The same basic parameters hold for ensuring delivery via the nail as through the skin, but Murdan in her review[5] concludes: 'The permeability of the compact, highly keratinised nail plate to topically applied drugs is poor and drug uptake into the nail apparatus is extremely low. Topical therapy is worth pursuing, however, as local action is required in many nail disorders.' Research aimed at enhancing ungual drug uptake following topical

[*] For further information, see Kim Y-C *et al*. Microneedles for drug and vaccine delivery. *Adv Drug Del Rev* 2012;64:1547–1568; Tuan-Mazlelaa T-M *et al*. Microneedles for intradermal and transdermal drug delivery. *Eur J Pharm Sci* 2013;50:623–637.

application may be divided into three approaches[6]: (1) understanding the physicochemical factors that influence drug permeation into the nail plate; (2) the use of chemical enhancers which cause alterations in the nail plate, thus assisting drug permeation; and (3) the use of drug-containing nail lacquers which are brushed on to nail plates and which act as a drug depot from which drug can be continuously released into the nail.

9.5 Medication of the eye and the eye as a route for systemic delivery

The eye is not, of course, a conduit for the administration of drugs to the body, although it has been explored for the systemic delivery of peptides and proteins such as insulin. It is considered here because absorption of drugs does occur from medication applied to the eye, producing sometimes toxic systemic effects, although often the desired local effect is on the eye or its component parts. We will consider the factors affecting drug absorption from the eye, and those properties of formulations that affect drug performance. A wide range of drug types are placed in the eye, including antimicrobials, antihistamines, decongestants, mydriatics, miotics and cycloplegic agents.

Drugs are usually applied to the eye in the form of drops or ointments for local action. The absorbing surface is the cornea. Drug absorbed by the conjunctiva enters the systemic circulation. It is useful to consider some of the properties of the absorbing surfaces and their environment.

Key points

- The barrier layer of the skin is the stratum corneum, which behaves like a passive diffusion barrier. The physicochemical factors that control drug penetration include the hydration of the stratum corneum, temperature, pH, drug concentration and the molecular characteristics of the penetrant and the vehicle.
- Penetration of water and low-molecular-weight non-electrolyte solutes through the epidermis is proportional to their concentration, and to the partition coefficient of the solute between tissue and vehicle; solute flux can be calculated using a form of Fick's law.
- The major pathway of transport for water-soluble molecules is *transcellular*, involving passage through cells and cell walls. The pathway for lipid-soluble molecules is the endogenous lipid within the stratum corneum, the bulk of this being *intercellular*. Increase in the polar character of the molecule decreases permeability by this route. Drug molecules may penetrate the skin not only through the stratum corneum but also by way of the hair follicles or through the sweat ducts, but these offer only a comparatively minor route.
- The vehicle in which the drug is applied influences the rate and extent of absorption; formulations can change rapidly once they have been spread on the skin, with absorption of some excipients and evaporative loss of water.
- Many dermatological formulations are washable oil-in-water systems. Simple aqueous lotions are also used as they have a cooling effect on the skin. Ointments are used for the application of insoluble or oil-soluble medicaments; aqueous creams combine the characteristics of the lotions and ointments. Other vehicles, such as suspensions and emulsions, may be used and equations predicting drug release from these have been given.
- In addition, transdermal medication may be achieved using patches (matrix, reservoir, multilaminate or drug-in-adhesive) and jet injectors, and may be enhanced by iontophoresis or by ultrasound.

9.5.1 The eye

The eye (Fig. 9.21) has two barrier systems: a blood–aqueous barrier and a blood–vitreous barrier. The former is composed of the ciliary epithelium, the epithelium of the posterior surface of the iris and blood vessels within the iris. Solutes and drugs enter

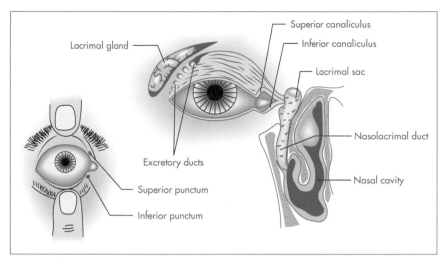

Figure 9.21 Diagrams of parts of the eye of importance in medication: the superior and inferior punctae are the drainage ports for solutions and tear fluids, and medicaments can drain via the canaliculi into the nasolacrimal duct and then to the nasal cavity, from whose surfaces absorption can occur.

Modified with permission from Robinson JR (ed.) *Ophthalmic Drug Delivery Systems*. Washington, DC: American Pharmaceutical Association; 1980.

the aqueous humour at the ciliary epithelium and at blood vessels. Many substances are transported out of the vitreous humour at the retinal surface. Solutes also leave the vitreous humour by diffusing to the aqueous humour of the posterior chamber.

Figure 9.21 is a diagrammatic representation of those parts of the eye involved in drug absorption. The cornea and the conjunctiva are covered with a thin fluid film, the tear film, which protects the cornea from dehydration and infection. Cleansed corneal epithelium is hydrophobic, physiological saline forming a contact angle of about 50° with it, and it has, in this clean condition, a critical surface tension of 28 mN m^{-1}. The aqueous phase of tear fluid is spread by blinking.

Tears

Tears comprise inorganic electrolytes – sodium, potassium and some calcium ions, chloride and hydrogen carbonate counterions – as well as glucose. The macromolecular components include some albumin, globulins and lysozyme. Lipids that form a monolayer over the tear fluid surface derive from the Meibomian glands, which open on to the edges of the upper and lower lids. This secretion consists mainly of cholesteryl esters with low melting points (35°C) due to the predominance of double bonds and branched-chain structures.

Tear fluid

Tears are released from the Meibomian glands in the eye. Tears are important for lubrication of the eye.

When we blink the tear film is replenished and re-spread, thus compensating for evaporation of the aqueous film and preventing the drying that would otherwise occur. In some patients, the supply of tear fluid, comprising a largely aqueous solution containing protein, lipids and enzymes, is impaired. Tears spread over the surface of the cornea, which is hydrophobic. The tears contain phospholipids, which act as a surfactant, lowering the surface tension of the fluid and allowing spreading. The thin lipid layer on the surface of the tear film (like most lipid monolayers) also prevents or slows down evaporation of the aqueous medium beneath. Dry eye[7] (xerophthalmia; Sjögren's syndrome) is caused when the tear film thins to such an extent that it ruptures, exposing the corneal surface to the air. Drying out of patches on the corneal surface follows. This can be painful and must be avoided. Evaporation over 5–10 min can actually eliminate the tear film completely.[8]

Artificial tear fluids

Artificial tear fluids may replace the natural tear fluid with varying degrees of similitude. Most aim for formulations that have an appropriate viscosity, but not necessarily identical rheological properties. Hydroxypropylmethylcellulose (HPMC) is a component of many commercial replacement or 'artificial' tear products, as are the water-soluble macromolecules carboxymethylcellulose, polyvinyl alcohol (PVA) and polyvinylpyrrolidone (PVP). Trehalose[9] has also been studied as an agent for amelioration of the symptoms of dry eye. Trehalose is one of those molecules which, because of its hydrophilicity, increases the surface tension of water, but at 0.8 mol L^{-1} it has a viscosity of only ≈ 2 cP at 30°C. The aim is usually to reproduce the wetting and rheological properties of tear fluids, but in this case wetting is not enhanced. Increased concentrations, however, will have higher viscosities.

 Clinical point

Tear fluid lies on the surface of the cornea and its importance lies in the possibility that components of formulations or drugs themselves can so alter the properties of the corneal surface, or interact with components of the tear fluid, that tear coverage of the eye is disrupted. When this occurs the so-called dry-eye syndrome (xerophthalmia) may arise, characterised by the premature break-up of the tear layer, resulting in dry spots on the corneal surface.

9.5.2 Absorption of drugs applied to the eye

The cornea, which is the main barrier to absorption, consists of three parts: the epithelium, the stroma and the endothelium. Both the endothelium and the epithelium have a high lipid content and, as with most membranes, they are penetrated by drugs in their un-ionised lipid-soluble forms. The stroma lying between these two structures has a high water content, however, and thus drugs that have to negotiate the corneal barrier successfully must be both lipid-soluble and water-soluble to some extent (Fig. 9.22).

Tears have some buffering capacity so, as we noted before, the pH-partition hypothesis has to be applied with some circumspection. The acid-neutralising power of the tears when 0.1 cm^3 of a 1% solution of a drug is instilled into the eye is approximately equivalent to 10 μL of a 0.01 mol dm^{-3} strong base. The pH for either maximum solubility (see Chapter 4) or maximum stability (see Chapter 3) of a drug may well be below the optimum in relation to acceptability and activity. Under these conditions it is possible to use a buffer with a low buffering capacity to maintain a low pH adequate to prevent change in pH due to alkalinity of glass or carbon dioxide ingress from the

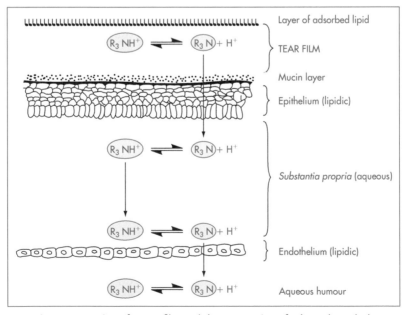

Figure 9.22 Diagrammatic representation of a tear film and the penetration of a base through the cornea; in this example R_3N represents a drug such as homatropine.

Modified with permission from Moses RA. *Adler's Physiology of the Eye*, 5th edn. St Louis: Mosby; 1970.

air. When such drops are instilled into the eye, the tears will participate in a fairly rapid return to normal pH.

Clinical point

In agreement with the pH-partition hypothesis, raising the pH from 5 to 8 results in a two- to threefold increase in the amount of pilocarpine reaching the anterior chamber. It is also found, however, that glycerol penetration increases to the same extent. The clue to why this should be so lies in the effect of the buffer solutions on lacrimation. Increased tear flow reduces the concentration of drug in the bathing fluid; loss of drug solution through the punctae and nasolacrimal ducts does not affect concentration, as the whole fluid drains away.

Solution concentration is reduced only by diffusion of drug across the cornea or conjunctiva or by tear inflow. The pH 5 solution induced more tear flow than the pH 8 solution; thus the concentration gradient is reduced and transport of both ionised and non-ionic drugs is less at pH 5. At pH 11, absorption of pilocarpine is reduced because of the irritant effects of this solution on the eye.[10] Mechanical irritation can produce the same effects and this can override the influence of other formulation factors.

Aqueous humour

As the examples above have shown, both water-soluble and lipid-soluble drugs can enter the aqueous humour. The pH-partition hypothesis thus accounts only imperfectly for different rates of entry into the aqueous humour. Sucrose and raffinose pass through the leaky ciliary epithelium and reach steady-state aqueous/plasma concentration ratios of 0.2 and 0.3, respectively. Lipid-soluble drugs, including chloramphenicol and some tetracyclines, can achieve higher concentrations as they can enter by both pathways. Penicillins, however, reach only low aqueous/plasma concentration ratios because they are removed from aqueous humour by absorption through the ciliary epithelium. Proteins are excluded, so that protein binding of ophthalmic drugs limits their absorption.

9.5.3 Influence of formulation

Pilocarpine activity has been compared in various formulations. Figure 9.23 shows some of the results on formulations, including results on ointments designed to prolong the contact of the drug with the cornea. One of the most difficult problems is to design vehicles that will retard drainage and prolong contact. Viscous polymer vehicles help to some extent but are not the complete answer. The rate of drainage of drops deceases as their viscosity increases and these factors contribute to an increased concentration of the drug in the precorneal film and aqueous humour.[11] The magnitude of the concentration increase was small considering the 100-fold change in the viscosity, and it was concluded that the viscosity of the solution is not as important a factor in bioavailability as was previously thought.

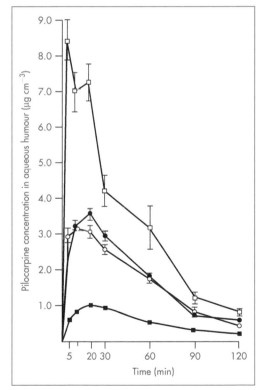

Figure 9.23 Aqueous humour levels of pilocarpine after dosing with 10^{-2} mol dm^{-3} ointment and solution in intact and abraded eyes. ●, 25 mg of ointment, intact eyes; ○, 25 mg of ointment, abraded eyes; ■, 25 mm^3 of solution, intact eyes; □, 25 mm^3 of solution, abraded eyes; all points represent an average of 8–16 eyes.

Reproduced from Sieg JW, Robinson JR. Vehicle effects on ocular drug bioavailability II: Evaluation of pilocarpine. *J Pharm Sci* 1977;66:1222–1228. Copyright Wiley-VCH Verlag GmbH & Co. KGaA. Reproduced with permission.

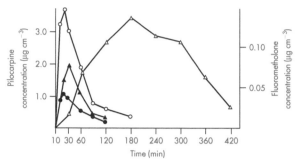

Figure 9.24 Aqueous humour levels after dosing with pilocarpine and fluorometholone in ointment and aqueous solution. ●, 10^{-2} mol dm^{-3} pilocarpine solution; ○, 10^{-2} mol dm^{-3} pilocarpine ointment; ▲, saturated fluorometh-olone solution; △, 0.1% fluorometholone ointment.

Reproduced from Sieg JW, Robinson JR. Vehicle effects on ocular drug bioavailability II: Evaluation of pilocarpine. *J Pharm Sci* 1977;66:1222–1228. Copyright Wiley-VCH Verlag GmbH & Co. KGaA. Reproduced with permission.

The results of incorporating pilocarpine (**VI**) (a relatively water-soluble drug) and fluorometholone (a lipophilic drug) into a water-in-oil ointment base can be compared in Fig. 9.24. Pilocarpine is thought to be released only when in contact with aqueous tear fluid, whereas the steroid, being soluble in the base, can diffuse through the base to replenish the surface concentrations and thus produce a sustained effect.

Structure VI Pilocarpine (pK_a = 7.05)

Polymeric vehicles

Hydrophilic polymeric vehicles, such as PVA and HPMC, are used in ophthalmic formulations.[12] PVA increases the effectiveness of the drug substance, most likely by slowing the drainage rate of the eye drops. The viscosity of Newtonian fluids should be greater than 4.4 cP to influence drainage times, with a maximum effect at 100 cP. HPMC has been found to enhance the activity and reduce the effective dose of neomycin sulfate required to prevent infection of corneas of experimental animals (Table 9.6).

The influence of log *P* of beta-blockers (Table 9.7) on their permeation coefficients into conjunctiva and cornea is shown in Fig. 9.25. In humans, the conjunctiva has 17 times the surface area of the cornea and therefore it absorbs significant amounts of drug. Work has centred on increasing corneal permeability or

Table 9.6 Calculated effective dose (ED$_{50}$) of neomycin sulfate required to prevent infection in 50% of rabbit corneas when incorporated into various vehicles

Vehicle	Derived values (mg base per cm³)	
	ED$_{50}$	95% confidence limits
HPMC, 0.5%	0.50	0.403–0.620
PVA, 1.4%	1.00	0.750–1.330
PVP, 1.4%	1.10	0.89–1.35
Distilled water	1.03	0.84–1.27

Reproduced from Bach FC *et al.* The influence of vehicles on neomycin sulfate prevention of experimental ocular infection in rabbits. *Am J Ophthalmol* 1970;69:659. Copyright Elsevier 1970.

✚ Clinical point

Eye drops are often formulated to be isotonic with tear fluid, but deviations from tonicity do not cause major problems, although hypertonicity may cause stinging of the eye and hypotonicity may increase the permeability of the cornea. Some ingredients may increase the permeability of the cornea. Surfactants are known to interact with membranes to increase the permeability: benzalkonium chloride has surfactant properties and may well have some effect on corneal permeability, although its primary purpose is as a bacteriostat and bactericide. Chlorhexidine acetate and cetrimide, both of which are surface-active, are also used.

retention of the drug (or product) in the conjunctiva sac. Appropriate doses of drug can achieve a degree of corneal or conjunctival selectivity, represented in Fig. 9.25c by the ratio *C/J*. Increasing lipophilicity increases the *C/J* ratio.

The prodrug approach

Attempts have been made to improve the performance of drugs used in the eye. One approach has been to modify the drug substance to increase its ability to penetrate the corneal barrier. In Fig. 9.26, the results of application of 0.5% epinephrine (adrenaline) (**VII**) and

Table 9.7 Log *P* values of beta-blockers (in increasing order of lipophilicity)

Compound		Log *P*
Sotalol		−0.62
Atenolol		0.16
Nadolol		0.93
Pindolol		1.75
Acebutolol		1.77
Metoprolol		1.88
Timolol		1.91
Oxprenolol		2.07
Levobunolol		2.40
Labetalol		2.55
Alprenolol		2.61
Propranolol		3.21
Betaxolol		3.44

0.16% of the dipivoyl derivative of epinephrine (dipivefrine) (**VIII**) are shown. The more hydrophobic derivative is absorbed to a greater extent and is then hydrolysed to the active parent molecule in the aqueous humour.

Structure VII   Epinephrine (adrenaline)

Derivatives of pilocarpine such as the hexadecanoyl-oxymethylene chloride (**IX**) similarly show the advantages of the epinephrine prodrug.

Structure VIII   Dipivoyl epinephrine (dipivefrine; compare with Structure VII)

Reservoir systems

Eye drops and eye ointments have their limitations, thus other means of delivering drugs to the eye have been developed. These include reservoirs such as contact lenses and the Ocusert device. Figure 9.27 traces

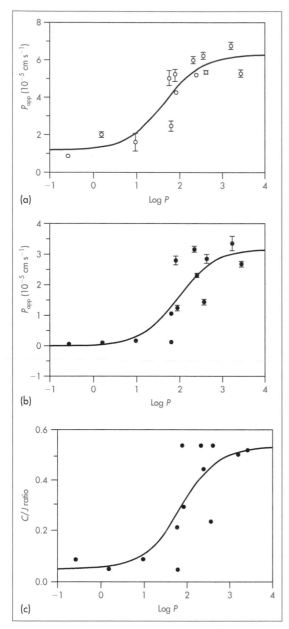

Structure IX Pilocarpine derivatives

Soft contact lenses

Since the advent of soft contact lenses, attempts have been made to use these as drug reservoirs[13]; a drug such as pilocarpine is imbibed from solutions into the polymer matrix and when this is placed in the eye the drug leaches out, generally over a period of up to 24 hours. Levels of prednisolone applied in a copolymer of 2-hydroxyethyl methacrylate and N-vinyl-2-pyrrolidone were compared with levels in aqueous humour, cornea and iris after applications of prednisolone in solution. When the drug was incorporated into the lens, aqueous and corneal levels of the drug were two- to threefold higher 4 hours after insertion. Figure 9.28 shows data for the delivery of the prostaglandin latanoprost, illustrating the levels achieved over 30 days from a contact lens. Issues discussed in Chapter 7 should be refreshed to appreciate the mechanism of drug release from polymeric systems and the means of rationalising their physicochemical behaviour. The results in the figure show prolonged action but marked differences in concentration of the drug over the 30-day duration.

Ocusert

The Ocusert device (Fig. 9.29) releases controlled amounts of pilocarpine over a period of 7 days and is designed for the treatment of glaucoma. It comprises a drug reservoir in which pilocarpine is embedded in an alginic acid matrix, and this is bounded by two rate-controlling membranes of polymer (vinyl acetate–ethylene copolymer). It is inserted into the lower conjunctival sac of the eye. The rate-controlling membranes are subject to strict quality control during manufacture and their thicknesses adjusted to give the appropriate flux of drug, either 20 or 40 µg h^{-1}. The difference between the two available systems is effected by altering the amount of di-(2-ethylhexyl)phthalate in the polymer; increasing the concentration of this plasticiser increases the permeability to pilocarpine.

Figure 9.25 Influence of drug lipophilicity (log P) on the permeability coefficients (P_{app}) of beta blockers across (a) the conjunctiva and (b) the cornea of the pigmented rabbit. Plot (c) shows the influence of log P on the ratio of the corneal (C) and conjunctival (J) permeability coefficients.

Reproduced with permission from Wong W *et al.* Lipophilicity influence on conjunctival drug penetration in the pigmented rabbit: a comparison with corneal penetration. *Curr Eye Res* 1991;6:571.

the fate of drugs delivered in systems to the eye and some of the issues that must be take into account in their use.

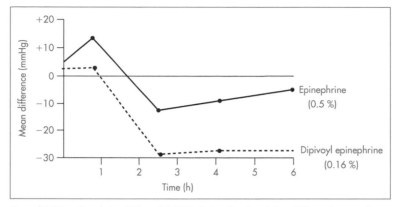

Figure 9.26 The action of 0.5% epinephrine (**VI**) and 0.16% dipivoyl epinephrine (**VII**) on intraocular pressure.

Reproduced with permission from McClure DA. In: Higuchi T, Stella V (eds) *Prodrugs as Novel Drug Delivery Systems*. Washington, DC: American Chemical Society; 1975. Copyright 1975 American Chemical Society.

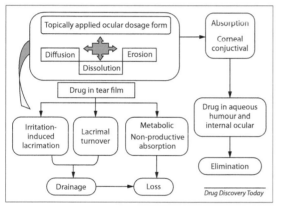

Figure 9.27 Illustration of the systems that release a drug by diffusion, erosion or dissolution, entering the tear film and being absorbed by the conjunctival tissue, and showing the means of loss of drug by drainage and elimination. One other relevant factor is that devices can induce lacrimation, thus increasing tear flow and diluting released drug.

Reproduced from Gupta H, Aqil M. Contact lenses in ocular therapeutics. *Drug Discov Today* 2012;17:522–527. Copyright Elsevier 2012.

Figure 9.28 The effect of changes in lens pretreatment to produce different levels of latanoprost for the treatment of glaucoma over a 1-month period. Data from rabbit eyes. For comparison, the average concentration over 24 hours was about 12 mg mL^{-1} using topical drops.

Reproduced from Ciolino JB *et al.* In vivo performance of a drug-eluting contact lens to treat glaucoma for a month. *Biomaterials* 2014;35:432–439. Copyright Elsevier 2014.

9.5.4 Systemic effects from eye drops

Most of the dose applied to the eye in the form of drops reaches the systemic circulation and typically less than 5% acts on ocular tissues.

 Clinical point

Atropine toxicity resulting from the use of eye drops to dilate the pupil has been reported,[14] as has a rise in blood pressure in premature infants following the use of 10% phenylephrine eye drops in preparation for ophthalmoscopy.[15] The mucosa in the eye, nose and mouth of infants is much thinner and more permeable to a drug than is, say, the skin. Drugs placed in the eye, nose or mouth, moreover, may bypass the metabolic transformations which may inactivate the drug given orally. Reduction in exercise tachycardia in normal volunteers is induced following administration of 0.5% timolol eye drops, showing the significant effects of beta-blockers.

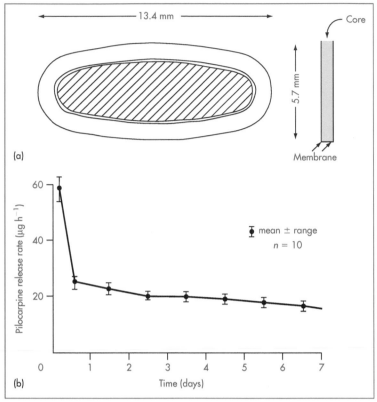

Figure 9.29 (a) Dimensions and structure of the Ocusert device. (b) A release rate profile over 1 week.
Reproduced from Snell JW, Baker RW. Diffusional systems for controlled release of drugs to the eye. *Ann Ophthalmol* 1974;6:1037.

Key points

- Drugs (including antimicrobials, anti-histamines, decongestants, mydriatics, miotics and cycloplegic agents) are usually applied to the eye in the form of drops or ointments for local action.

- The eye has two barrier systems: a blood–aqueous barrier and a blood–vitreous barrier.

- The absorbing surface is the cornea, which comprises an epithelium, a stroma and an endothelium; the epithelium and endothelium have high lipid contents and are penetrated by drugs in their un-ionised form; the stroma lying between the two other structures has a high water content. Thus drugs that have to negotiate the corneal barrier successfully must be both lipid-soluble and water-soluble to some

extent. Tears have some buffering capacity, so the pH-partition hypothesis has to be applied with some circumspection.

- Some ingredients of ophthalmic formulations, e.g. surfactants, may increase the permeability of the cornea.

- Reservoir systems, including soft contact lenses and the Ocusert device, may be used for sustained delivery to the eye.

9.6 The ear (the aural route)

Medications are administered to the ear only for local treatment. Drops and other vehicles administered to the ear will occupy the external auditory meatus, which is separated from the middle ear by the tympanic membrane (Fig. 9.30).

Various factors affect drug absorption from the ear or action in it. The sebaceous and apocrine glands of the mucosa secrete an oily fluid that, when mixed with

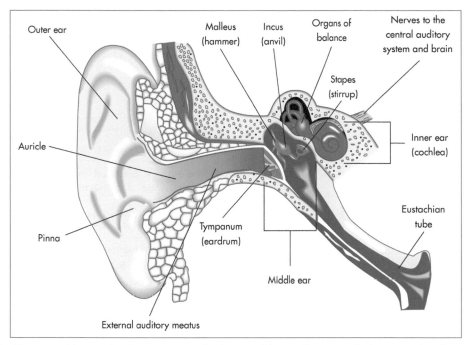

Figure 9.30 The ear and its associated structures; medications would normally enter only the external auditory meatus.

exfoliated cells of the stratum corneum, forms the cerumen or wax composed of, *inter alia*, fats, fatty acids, protein, pigment, glycoprotein and water. The acidic environment of the ear skin surface (around pH 6), sometimes referred to as the acid mantle of the ear, is thought to be a defence against invading micro-organisms.

Various ceruminolytic agents achieve their action by partially dissolving the wax. Several commercial ear drops contain surfactants such as poloxamers or sodium dioctyl sulfosuccinate (docusate sodium) to assist in the process. In otitis media, infection of the Eustachian tube is involved; antibiotic treatment is indicated along with oral analgesics. There is little evidence that topical analgesics give faster relief, suggesting poor absorption. However, cefmetazole sodium, a cephamycin antibiotic, passes through the membrane into the inner ear of the guinea pig. The concentration of the drug in the inner ear fluid indicated that a larger amount of the drug reached the inner ear by this means than when it was administered intraperitoneally.

9.7 Absorption from the vagina

The vagina cannot be considered to be a route for the systemic administration of drugs, although oestrogens for systemic delivery have been applied intravaginally. Certain medicaments are, however, absorbed when applied to the vaginal epithelium as it is permeable to a wide range of substances, including steroids, prostaglandins, iodine and some antibiotics.[16] Econazole and miconazole are both also appreciably absorbed.

The epithelial layer of the vagina (Fig. 9.31a) comprises the lamina propria and a surface epithelium of non-cornified, stratified squamous cells (Fig 9.31b). The thickness of the epithelium increases after puberty and then again after menopause. The surface area is increased by folds in the epithelium and by microridges. The pH in the vagina decreases after puberty, varying between pH 4 and 5 depending on the point in the menstrual cycle and also on the location within the vagina, the pH being higher near the cervix. There is little fluid in the vagina. The absorbing surface is under constant change, therefore absorption will be variable. While the presence of mucus is likely to retard absorption, there is unlikely to be other material in the vagina which will inhibit absorption. The uterine and pudendal arteries are the main sources of blood to the vagina; the venous plexus that surrounds the vagina empties into the internal iliac veins. Lymph vessels drain the vagina, and vaginal capillaries are found in close proximity to the basal epithelial layer.

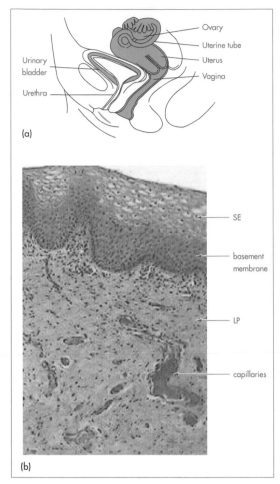

(a)

(b)

Figure 9.31 (a) Anatomy of the urethra and vagina; drug delivery systems for both are available. (b) For other than local vaginal treatment, transport through the absorbing membrane structure (squamous epithelium (SE) lamina propria (LP) and muscularis (not shown)) is important in securing systemic levels of drug; inadvertent absorption after local therapy is, of course, possible.

9.7.1 Vaginal delivery systems

Conventional vaginal delivery systems include vaginal tablets, foams, gels, suspensions and pessaries. Vaginal rings (Fig. 9.32) have been developed to deliver contraceptive steroids. These commonly comprise an inert silicone elastomer ring that is covered with an elastomer layer containing the drug. In some systems a refinement has been to add a third, rate-modifying layer to the external surface of the ring, as shown. Some systems contain both an oestrogen and progestogen.

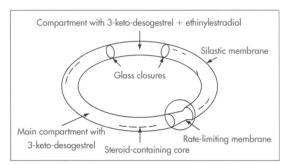

Figure 9.32 A combined contraceptive vaginal ring for the slow release of 3-keto-desogestrel (etonogestrel) and ethinylestradiol.
Reproduced from Sam AP. Controlled release contraceptive devices: a status report. *J Control Release* 1992;22:35. Copyright Elsevier 1992.

Hydrogel-based vaginal pessaries to deliver prostaglandin E_2 (to assist in ripening of the cervix prior to labour), progesterone and bleomycin have been developed.

Tablets for vaginal use have included hydroxypropylcellulose or sodium carboxymethylcellulose and poly(acrylic acid) (such as Carbopol 934) as excipients. Micropatches in the size range 10–100 μm diameter prepared from albumin, collagen or dextrose will gel on contact with vaginal mucosal surfaces and adhere, prolonging contact between the delivery system and the absorbing surface.[17]

9.8 Inhalation therapy

The respiratory system provides a route of entry into the body for a variety of airborne substances but is also a route of medication. The large contact area of its surfaces extends to more than 30 m^2. The surfaces have been described[18] as 'gossamer-thin membranes' that separate the lung air from the blood, which courses through some 2000 km of capillaries in the lungs. There is consequently an 'exquisite degree of intimacy between the lung tissue and blood and the atmospheric environment'. The route is thus used for rapid relief of asthmatic conditions, where both local and systemic effects are required, for chronic therapy, and for the administration of peptides and proteins.

Orally administered corticosteroids are effective in the treatment of chronic bronchial asthma. The inhalation route has been widely used in attempts to avoid systemic side-effects, such as adrenal suppression, but evidence suggests that inhaled steroids are absorbed systemically to a significant extent. The respiratory tract epithelium has permeability characteristics similar to those of the classical biological membrane, so lipid-soluble compounds are absorbed more rapidly than lipid-insoluble molecules. Cortisone, hydrocortisone and dexamethasone are absorbed rapidly by a non-saturable diffusion process from the lung; the half-time of absorption is of the order of 1–1.7 minutes. Quaternary ammonium compounds, hippurates and mannitol have absorption half-times, in contrast, of between 45 and 70 minutes.

Relative to the gastrointestinal mucosa the pulmonary epithelium possesses a high permeability to water-soluble molecules, which is an advantage with drugs such as sodium cromoglicate (**X**), a bischromone with two carboxylic acid groups and a pK_a of approximately 1.9. The drug is well absorbed from the lungs with a clearance rate of about 1 hour, even though the molecule is completely ionised at physiological pH. The free acid is very insoluble in both polar and non-polar solvents and has virtually no lipid solubility. Because of this, and the insolubility of the un-ionised form, very little of an oral dose of sodium cromoglicate is absorbed. Powder swallowed after inhalation therefore contributes little to the systemic dose and is subsequently excreted in the urine and bile.

NaOOC O O COONa
OH
O OCH₂CHCH₂O O

Structure X Sodium cromoglicate (DSCG; sodium cromoglycate; cromolyn sodium)

Drugs administered by inhalation are mostly intended to have a direct effect on the lungs. However, the efficiency of inhalation therapy is often not high because of the difficulty in targeting particles to the sites of maximal absorption. Only about 8% of the inhaled dose of sodium cromoglicate administered from a Spinhaler device reaches the alveoli.

Crude inhalers have been used for medicinal purposes for at least two centuries. Solutions of volatile aromatic substances with a mild irritant action, inhaled as vapour rising from hot aqueous solutions, have been used for many years. Particles from the older nebulisers would settle without reaching the patient's face (a 100 μm particle of unit density settles in still air

at a velocity of 8 cm s⁻¹). The duration of existence of a suspension of particles of size around 10 μm is so brief that the upper limit of aerosols of therapeutic interest is well below this size. Special devices are required to generate these.

9.8.1 Physical factors affecting deposition of aerosols

Figure 9.33 shows the order of maximum size of particles that can penetrate to various parts of the respiratory tract, from trachea to alveoli. The major processes that influence deposition of drug particles in the respiratory tract are, as illustrated in Fig. 9.34,

- the *interception* of particles
- their *impaction* on epithelial surfaces
- their *gravitational settling*
- electrostatic attraction
- Brownian diffusion.

The passage of an aerosol particle from the alveolar sac into the blood stream is illustrated diagrammatically in Fig. 9.35.

When a particle contacts the walls of the airways it is removed from the airstream; this process can occur during inspiration or expiration of a single breath, or

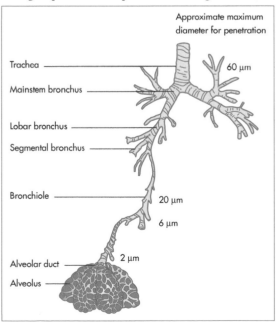

Figure 9.33 Deposition of particles in various anatomical regions of the respiratory tract from bronchus to alveoli according to particle size.

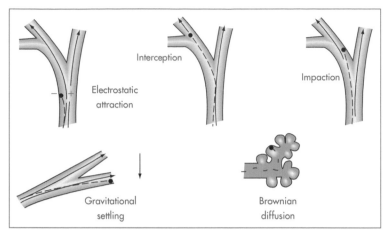

Figure 9.34 Representation of the major processes of particle deposition in the respiratory tract, as discussed in the text.

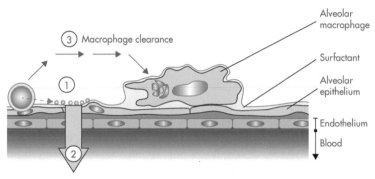

Figure 9.35 Diagram of the fate of an aerosol particle in a surfactant-coated alveolar sac. The particle dissolves after landing (1) and is taken up into the alveolar epithelial cell layer (2), transported by transcytotic vesicles into the pulmonary lymph and then into the blood via the capillary endothelium. Alveolar macrophages remove residues.
Reproduced from Ruge CA, Kirch J, Lehr CM. *Lancet Resp Med* 2013;1:402–413.

later if the particle has been transferred to unexhaled lung air. Deposition increases with duration of breath holding and depth of breathing, hence the instruction to patients to breathe deeply when using their inhalers.

As flowing air moves in and out, inertial forces within the nasopharyngeal chamber and at the points of branching of the airways, or wherever the direction of flow changes, result in the collision of particles with surfaces. Along the narrower airways, particles are removed by gravity. Very fine particles may be exhaled.

The next sections present a more detailed account of deposition in the airways. There is no unified theory that predicts exactly what is occurring, but each subset of events is governed by an equation that demonstrates the key parameters of the aerosol. This section is included for completeness to illustrate the physico-chemical basis of therapy of the lung.

Physical diameter and aerodynamic diameter

The aerodynamic diameter of a particle, d_a, is related to the particle diameter (d) and density (ρ) by the equation

$$d_a = \rho^{0.5} d \tag{9.14}$$

To overcome problems of powder flow and agglomeration, porous particles (i.e. particles with a low density) have been developed. Equation (9.14) shows that a particle of 10 μm diameter with a density of 0.1 g cm^{-3} has an aerodynamic diameter of around 3 μm.

Gravitational settling

Fine particles falling through the air under the force of gravity do so at a constant velocity such that the resistance of the air balances the mass of the particle.

Table 9.8 Terminal velocity (μ_t) of spherical particles of unit density in air

Diameter (µm)	μ_t (cm s^{-1})
20	1.2
10	2.9×10^{-1}
4	5×10^{-2}
1	3.5×10^{-3}
0.6	1.4×10^{-3}
0.1	8.6×10^{-5}

Reproduced from Hatch TF, Gross P. *Pulmonary Deposition and Retention of Inhaled Aerosols*. New York: Academic Press; 1964.

The following equation relates particle diameter, d, and density, ρ, to terminal velocity, μ_t:

$$\mu_t = \frac{\rho g d^2}{18\eta} \tag{9.15}$$

where g is the gravitational constant and η is the viscosity of the air. For air, $\eta = 1.9 \times 10^{-7}$ N m^{-2} s and therefore

$$\mu_t - 2.9 \times 10^6 \rho d^2 \quad (\text{m s}^{-1}) \tag{9.16}$$

Table 9.8 shows the terminal velocities for particles of a range of diameters from 20 to 0.1 µm, reinforcing the importance of small size in preventing removal of particles before entry into the lower reaches of the respiratory tract. In still air, a cloud of powder particles of about 20 µm diameter takes a few seconds to settle, whereas powder of around 1 µm diameter takes approximately 60 seconds.

Sedimentation

As the particles of drug move with the air in laminar flow in the airways, they fall under the force of gravity a distance equal to $\mu_t t$, where t is the time of travel. If the tube (or part of the bronchial tree) in which they move is of radius R and is inclined at an angle ψ to the horizontal, the maximum distance of fall will no longer be $2R$ but $2R/\cos \psi$. The ratio, r, of the distance of fall to the maximum distance for deposition to be achieved is thus

$$r = \frac{\mu_t t \cos \psi}{2R} \tag{9.17}$$

The probability of deposition by sedimentation is proportional to this ratio; the closer μ_t is to

$2R/\cos \psi$, the greater the likelihood of deposition by this mechanism. If the particles are evenly distributed over the cross-section of an airstream, it is theoretically possible to calculate the probability of deposition in tubular airways and in a spherical alveolus. Individual tubes are of course randomly positioned with reference to the horizontal and therefore an average value of ψ is used. Airflow is also not always laminar, and orderly deposition will not always occur, but in spite of these problems the following calculations of percentage sedimentation (S) may usefully be quoted. If $S = 55\%$ when $d = 2$ µm and the deposition diameter is 1.0 µm, then for 1 µm particles $S = 29\%$, and for 0.5 µm particles $S = 10\%$. Sedimentation, of course, reduces in importance as the drug particle size decreases.

Diffusion

The effectiveness of deposition by diffusion increases as particle size is reduced, which contrasts with the above. There must therefore be a particle diameter for which both processes have a combined minimum value; this occurs with particles approximately 0.5 µm in diameter. Particles of this size have the minimum probability of deposition in the upper respiratory tract.

Inertial impaction

When, during breathing, the airflow suddenly changes direction, a drug particle will continue in its original direction of flow owing to its inertia. In this way the particle may impact on the channel wall. In curved tubes the particle in an airstream that experiences a sudden bend suffers a similar fate, and the effective stopping distance at right angles to the direction of travel, h_s, is given by

$$h_s = \frac{\mu_t \mu \sin \theta}{g} \tag{9.18}$$

where μ is the velocity of the airstream with particles approaching a bend of angle θ. The term $\mu \sin \theta$ is therefore a component of initial particle velocity at right angles to the direction of airflow. The probability of inertial deposition, I, is proportional to the ratio of stopping distance, h_s, to the radius, R, of the airway; that is

$$I \propto \frac{h_s}{R} \propto \frac{\mu_t \mu \sin \theta}{gR} \tag{9.19}$$

from a calculation similar to that discussed above for sedimentation. Calculated inertial deposition shows a dependence on particle size as follows: 10 μm particles 50%, 7 μm particles 33%, leading to 20% for 5 μm particles, and 1% for 1 μm particles.

9.8.2 Experimental observations

Although the complexity of the respiratory system prevents a precise mathematical approach to the problem, many clinical studies clearly demonstrate the importance of particle size, as one would anticipate from the preceding sections.

Particles of hygroscopic materials are removed more effectively than are non-hygroscopic particles, because of the growth of these particles by uptake of water from the moist air in the respiratory system. Apart from its importance in determining the efficiency of an aerosol in reaching the alveoli, particle size may be critical in determining response because of the influence of particle size on rate of solution.

The effect of particle size on the fate of particles inhaled from an aerosol is shown in Fig. 9.36.

When used by patients, the Spinhaler delivers about 25% by weight of sodium cromoglicate, which is normally dispersed as particles below 6 μm in diameter, about 5% being less than 2 μm diameter. The mass medium diameter (and geometric standard deviation) of the sodium cromoglicate particle batches used were, respectively, 2 ± 1.2 and 11.7 ± 1.1 μm.

Clinical point

There is no doubt that the biological effect of small particle material is dramatically greater than that of coarser material, hence the importance of storage conditions of drug cartridge capsules to prevent aggregation of the drug particles. Although the Spinhaler is designed to break up aggregates, its efficiency will be reduced if moisture uptake is increased by storage in humid conditions. If aerosols of drug with large particles (11 μm diameter) are administered, up to 66% of the dose will end up in the mouth.

An alternative dry-powder aerosol device is illustrated in Fig. 9.37 and the mechanism of dispersion of powdered drug in a Ventodisk or Becodisk system is shown in Fig. 9.38.

Types of pressurised aerosol

In two-phase systems the propellant forms a separate liquid phase, whereas in the single-phase form the liquid propellant is the liquid phase containing the drug in solution or in suspension in the liquefied propellant gas. The vapour pressure of metered-dose inhalers determines the aerosol droplet size, which, as discussed above, has an important influence on the efficiency of deposition in the lungs. The requirement of the Montreal Protocol in 1989 for the replacement of chlorofluorocarbon (CFC) propellants in pressurised metered-dose inhalers with hydrofluoroalkanes (HFAs) because of the ozone-depleting properties of CFCs led to a substantial review of the formulation of these devices as a consequence of major differences in physical and chemical properties of these propellants.[19] The properties of the two most widely used HFAs, HFA 227 and HFA 134a, are summarised in Table 9.9.

The vapour pressure above an aerosol system in which there is an equilibrium between the liquefied propellant and its vapour can be calculated using Raoult's law,

$$p = p_i^{\ominus} x_i$$

where p_i is the partial vapour pressure of a component i in the vapour phase, x_i is the mole fraction of that component in solution and $p_i^{\ominus}$ is the vapour pressure of the pure component. Its application to this type of aerosol system is illustrated in Example 9.1.

Binary mixtures of hydrofluoroalkanes show behaviour that approaches ideality.[20] Figure 9.39a shows the vapour pressure–composition plots for a mixture of the propellants HFA 134a (tetrafluoroethane) and HFA 227 (heptafluoropropane); the linearity of the plots indicates that Raoult's law is obeyed over the temperature range examined. It is frequently necessary to include a cosolvent such as alcohol in the aerosol formulation to enhance the solvent power of the propellant blend.[21] Figure 9.39b shows large positive deviations from Raoult's law due to interactions between the components of the formulation. In practical terms such behaviour is beneficial as it enables

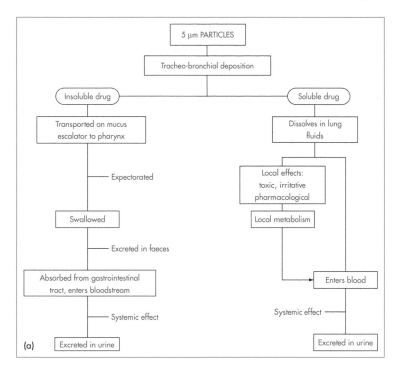

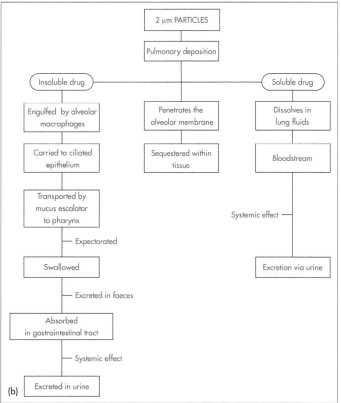

Figure 9.36 The fate of particles of (a) 5 μm and (b) 2 μm in diameter deposited in alveoli.
Reproduced from Clark DG. *Proc Eur Soc Study Drug Toxic* 1974;15:252.

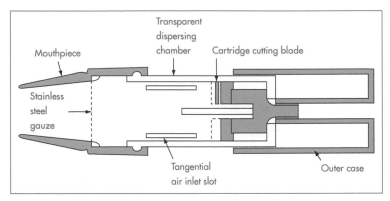

Figure 9.37 Longitudinal view of the Rotahaler.

Reproduced from Hallworth GW. An improved design of powder inhaler. *Br J Clin Pharmacol* 1977;4:689. Copyright Wiley-VCH Verlag GmbH & Co. KGaA. Reproduced with permission.

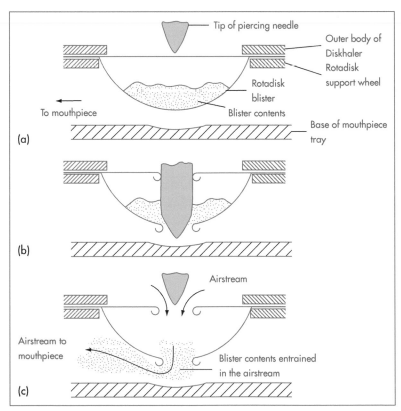

Figure 9.38 Dispersion of Ventodisk or Becodisk contents by breath actuation: a cross-section of a Diskhaler is shown with a disc located on the support wheel. (a) A disc is located beneath an aperture in the body of the Diskhaler through which a piercing needle enters. (b) The needle penetrates the upper and lower surfaces of the blister. (c) The patient inhales through the device and pierced blister, entraining the blister contents into the airstream.

Reproduced with permission from Farr SJ *et al.* In: Florence AT, Salole EG (eds) *Routes of Drug Administration*. London: Wright; 1990.

Table 9.9 Physicochemical properties of hydrofluoroalkanes

Propellant	Molecular formula	Molecular weight	Boiling point (°C) at 1.013 bar (1 atm)	Gauge vapour pressure (psig) at 20°C
HFA 134a	$C_2H_2F_4$	102.0	−26.5	68.4
HFA 227	C_3HF_7	170.0	−17.3	56.0

Data from reference 19.

 Example 9.1 Calculation of the vapour pressure of a mixture of hydrofluoroalkanes

Assuming ideal behaviour, calculate the vapour pressure at 20°C above an aerosol mixture consisting of 30% w/w of HFA 134a (tetrafluoroethane, molecular weight 102 Da) with a vapour pressure of 68.4 psig and 70% w/w of HFA 227 (heptafluoropropane, molecular weight 170 Da) with a vapour pressure of 56.0 psig. Convert the pressure into pascals using the relationship between the various units of pressure shown in Box 9.1.

Answer

For the two propellants HFA 134a and HFA 227 with respective vapour pressures $p_{134}^{\ominus}$ and $p_{227}^{\ominus}$ we have

$$p_{134} = p_{134}^{\ominus} x_{134}$$

$$p_{227} = p_{227}^{\ominus} x_{227}$$

where p_{134} and p_{227} are the partial pressures of components HFA 134a and HFA 227 respectively, and x_{134} and x_{227} are the mole fractions of these components in the liquid phase.

Amount of HFA 134a in mixture = 30/102 = 0.2941 mole

Amount of HFA 227 in mixture = 70/170 = 0.4118 mole

$x_{134} = 0.2941/0.7059 = 0.4166$

$x_{227} = 0.4118/0.7059 = 0.5834$

From Dalton's law of partial pressures, the total vapour pressure P is the sum of the partial pressures of the component gases, assuming ideal behaviour. Thus,

$$p = p_{134}^{\ominus} x_{134} + p_{227}^{\ominus} x_{227}$$

and hence

$$P = (68.4 \times 0.4166) + (56.0 \times 0.5834) = 61.17 \, \text{psig}$$

Converting pressures into pascals (Pa) using

$$\text{psia} = \text{psig} + 14.7 \quad \text{and} \quad 1 \, \text{psia} = 6894.76 \, \text{Pa}$$

we obtain

$$P = 5.23 \times 10^5 \, \text{Pa}$$

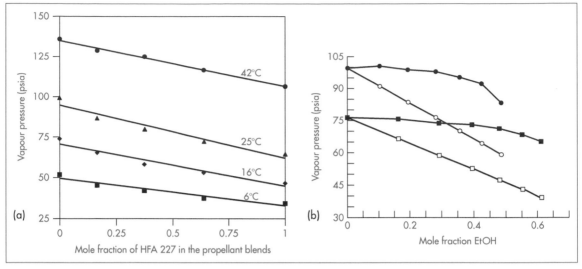

Figure 9.39 (a) Plots of vapour pressure versus mole fraction of HFA 227 for propellant systems composed of HFA 134a and HFA 227 at 6, 16, 25 and 42°C showing ideality of mixing (Raoult's law obeyed). (b) Plots of vapour pressure of HFA 134a (circles) and HFA 227 (squares) versus mole fraction of ethanol at 21.5°C. Solid symbols represent experimental data; open symbols represent theoretical values calculated assuming ideal (Raoult's law) behaviour.

(a) From Williams RO, Lie I. *Int J Pharm* 1998; 166:99–103.

(b) From Vervaet C, Byron PR. *Int J Pharm* 1999; 186:13–30.

Box 9.1 Pressure units

In practice, pressure is expressed in terms of a wide range of units. The SI unit is the pascal (Pa), where $1\ Pa = 1\ N\ m^{-2}$. Pressure should usually be converted to this unit before substitution into equations. The relationship of other commonly used pressure units to the pascal is as follows:

$1\ bar = 10^5\ Pa$

$1\ mmHg = 1\ torr = 133.32\ Pa$

$1\ atmos = 1.013 \times 10^5\ Pa$

$1\ psi^* = 6894.76\ Pa$

Standard atmospheric pressure is 760 mmHg $= 760\ torr = 1.013\ bar = 1.013 \times 10^5\ Pa$.

*It is common to report vapour pressure of propellants as pounds per square inch gauge, psig. Gauge pressure uses the actual atmospheric pressure as the zero point for measurement and hence atmospheric pressure (14.7 psi at sea level) must be added to measurements quoted in psig to obtain the absolute pressure in pounds per square inch, psia, i.e.
psia = psig + 14.7

---

substantial addition of ethanol without reduction in vapour pressure and aerosol performance.

Optimisation of vapour pressure, drug stability, solubility and spray patterns takes place during the design stage. Other ingredients of the formulation can include surfactants to act as solubilisers, stabilisers or lubricants to ease the passage of the particles when emitted from the valve.

The Autohaler has been devised as a breath-activated pressurised inhaler system because of the difficulty experienced by some patients in coordinating manual operation of an aerosol with inhalation. The Autohaler is activated by the negative pressure created during the inhalation phase of respiration and is specifically designed to respond to shallow inhalation in those with restricted pulmonary capacity.

Nebulisers[22]

Modern nebulisers for domestic and hospital use generate aerosols continuously for chronic therapy of respiratory disorders. A Venturi-type system is shown in Fig. 9.40 and an ultrasonic device in Fig. 9.40b. The particle size distribution and hence efficiency of such systems vary with the design and sometimes with the mode of use. Hence adequate monitoring of particle size is important. *In vitro* analysis of the particle size distribution of aerosols and nebulisers is discussed in Chapter 15.

Other mechanisms of generating solid or liquid aerosols are available, such as vibrating mesh devices

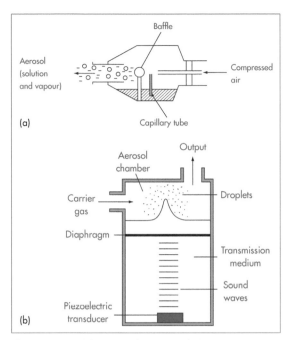

(a)

(b)

Figure 9.40 Schematic diagrams of (a) a Venturi-type nebuliser and (b) an ultrasonic nebuliser.

Modified with permission from Egan DF. *Fundamentals of Respiratory Therapy*, 3rd edn. New York: Mosby; 1977.

where the material to be inhaled is directed via the mesh, as shown simply in Fig. 9.41.

 Key points

- The respiratory tract epithelium has permeability characteristics similar to those of the classical biological membrane, so lipid-soluble compounds are absorbed more rapidly than lipid-insoluble molecules.
- Compared with the gastrointestinal mucosa, the pulmonary epithelium possesses a relatively high permeability to water-soluble molecules.
- The efficiency of inhalation therapy is often low because of the difficulty in targeting particles to the sites of maximal absorption.
- The major processes that influence deposition of drug particles in the respiratory tract are interception, impaction, gravitational settling, electrostatic attractions and Brownian diffusion.

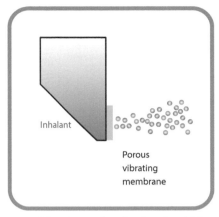

Inhalant

Porous vibrating membrane

Figure 9.41 Vibrating mesh technology in which a mesh/membrane with 1000–7000 laser-drilled holes vibrates at the exit of a liquid reservoir, forcing a mist of very fine droplets through the holes. For further discussion, see www.ers-education.org (Vicellio L. *Breathe* 2006; 2:253–260).

- Deposition of particles in the various regions of the respiratory tract is dependent on particle size and size distribution; this will be affected by the nature of the aerosol-producing device and the formulation. Particles of hygroscopic materials are removed from the airstream more effectively than are non-hygroscopic particles because of their growth through uptake of water from the moist air in the respiratory tract.
- Delivery devices include pressurised aerosols and nebulisers.

9.9 The nasal route

Two main classes of medicinal agents are applied by the nasal route:

1. drugs for the alleviation of nasal symptoms
2. drugs that are inactivated in the gastrointestinal tract following oral administration and where the route is an alternative to injection, such as for peptides and proteins.

Intranasal beclometasone dipropionate in a dose as low as 200 µg daily is a useful addition to the therapy of perennial rhinitis. Considerable attention is being paid to the delivery by the nasal route of peptides and proteins such as insulin, luteinising hormone-releasing hormone (LHRH) analogues such as nafarelin, as

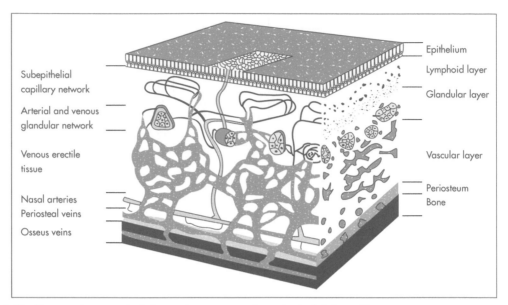

Figure 9.42 The vascular network of the nasal mucous membrane in the inferior turbinate.

well as vasopressin, thyrotropin-releasing hormone analogues and adrenocorticotrophic hormone.

Figure 9.42 shows the structures involved in delivery by the nasal route. Formulations have to be efficiently delivered to the epithelial surfaces: what physical factors affect the utility of this route? Factors such as droplet or particle size that affect deposition in the respiratory tract are involved if administration is by aerosol, but formulations may also be applied directly to the nasal mucosa. The physiological condi-

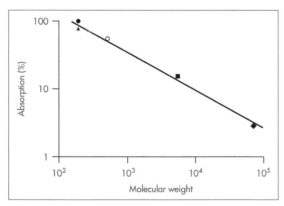

Figure 9.43 Correlation between the percentage dose absorbed after nasal administration and molecular weight: ●, 4-oxo-4H-1-benzopyran-2-carboxylic acid (chromocarb); ▲, p- aminohippuric acid; ○, sodium cromoglicate; ■, inulin; ♦, dextran; $r = -0.996$.

Reproduced from Fisher AN *et al*. The effect of molecular size on the nasal absorption of water-soluble compounds in the albino rat. *J Pharm Pharmacol* 1987;39:357. Copyright Wiley-VCH Verlag GmbH & Co. KGaA. Reproduced with permission.

tion of the nose, its vascularity and mucus flow rate are therefore of importance. So too is the formulation used – the volume, concentration, viscosity, pH and tonicity of the applied medicament can affect activity.[23] As the condition of the nasal passages changes with changes in the environment, temperature and humidity, it is clearly not an ideal route for absorption of drugs or vaccines, but may be the only feasible route for some agents. As with all routes, however, absorption decreases with the increasing molecular weight of the active, as seen in Fig. 9.43 for a series of model molecules.

The air passages through the nasal cavity begin at the nares (nostrils) and terminate at the choanae (posterior nares). Immediately above the nares are the vestibules, lined by skin that bears relatively coarse hairs and sebaceous glands in its lower portion. The hairs curve radially downward, providing an effective barrier to the entry of relatively large particles. The division of the nasal cavity exposes the air to maximal surface area. As in the other parts of the respiratory tree, sudden changes in the direction of airflow cause impingement of large particles through inertial forces. The respiratory portion of the nasal passage is covered by a mucous membrane that has a mucous blanket secreted in part by the goblet cells. The ciliary streaming here is directed posteriorly so that the nasal mucus is transported towards the pharynx. Figure 9.44 shows the fractional deposition of inhaled particles in the

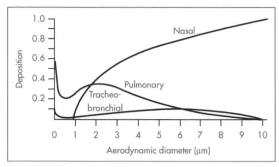

Figure 9.44 Regional deposition of inhaled particulate matter as a function of particle size; nose breathing at 15 respirations per minute and 730 cm³ tidal volume (the 'pulmonary compartment' refers to deposition beyond the terminal bronchiole).

Reproduced with permission from Muir CDF. *Clinical Aspects of Inhaled Particles.* London: Heinemann; 1972.

nasal chamber as a function of their particle size. A diameter of not less than 10 μm minimises the loss of drug to the lung. In the external nares, removal of particles occurs on nasal hairs; further up inertial deposition takes place; and in the more tortuous upper passages deposition is assumed to be by inertia and sedimentation.

Comparison of the nasal route with other routes has been made in some instances. Desmopressin (1-desamino-8-D-arginine vasopressin), administered as 20 μg dose, elicits a response equivalent to approximately 2 μg administered by IV injection. A greater dose of virus is required to obtain an equivalent response to a nasal vaccine than when administered by other routes. The role of the intranasal route for the delivery of peptides and proteins has been widely researched (see Chapter 13); as can be inferred from above, the bioavailability of desmopressin acetate ranges from 9% to 20% in humans, buserelin 6% and salmon calcitonin 3% when compared with the IM route. Penetration enhancers can lead to increases in uptake, but insulin's bioavailability in human subjects ranges from only 3% to 13% depending on the study involved.

In the treatment of nasal symptoms the patient adjusts the dose so that, perhaps, the theoretical bases of droplet and particle retention are less vital. Although formulation of the nasal drops, or sprays from plastic squeeze-bottles must obviously influence the efficiency of medication, little work has in the past been carried out relating formulation to the effect of intranasal medicines. Microsphere delivery systems have received

some attention, however, with special interest being directed to bioadhesive microsphere carriers.

9.10 Rectal absorption of drugs

Drugs administered by the rectal route in suppositories are placed in intimate contact with the rectal mucosa, which behaves as a normal lipoidal barrier. The pH in the rectal cavity lies between 7.2 and 7.4, but the rectal fluids have little buffering capacity. As with topical medication, the formulation of the suppository can have marked effects on the activity of the drug. Factors such as retention of the suppository for a sufficient duration of time in the rectal cavity also influence the outcome of therapy; the size and shape of the suppository and its melting point may also determine bioavailability.

The once traditional suppository base cocoa butter (theobroma oil) is a variable natural product that undergoes a polymorphic transition on heating. It is primarily a triglyceride. Four polymorphic forms exist: γ, m.p. 18.9°C; α, m.p. 23°C; β′, m.p. 28°C; and the stable β form, m.p. 34.5°C. Heating above 38°C converts the fat to a metastable mixture solidifying at 15–17°C instead of 25°C, and this subsequently melts at 24°C instead of at 31–35°C. Reconversion to the stable β-form takes 1–4 days depending on storage conditions.

Modern bases include polyoxyethylene glycols of molecular weight 1000–6000 Da and semisynthetic vegetable fats. The appropriate bases must be selected carefully for each substance. The important features of excipient materials are melting point, speed of crystallisation and emulsifying capacity. If the medicament dissolves in the base, it is likely that the melting point of the base will be lowered, so that a base with a melting point higher than 36–37°C has to be chosen. If the drug substance has a high density, it is preferable that the base crystallises rapidly during production of the suppositories to prevent settling of the drug. Preservatives, hardening agents, emulsifiers, colouring agents and materials which modify the viscosity of the base after melting are common formulation additives.

9.10.1 The rectal cavity

The rectum is the terminal 15–19 cm of the large intestine. The mucous membrane of the rectal ampulla, with which suppositories and other rectal

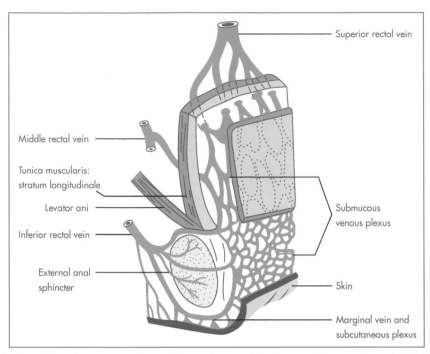

Figure 9.45 Blood supply to the rectum and anus. The significance of the location of the superior and the inferior rectal veins is discussed in the text.

Reproduced with permission from Tondury G. *Topographical Anatomy*. Stuttgart: Thieme; 1959.

medications come into contact, is made up of a layer of cylindrical epithelial cells, without villi.

Figure 9.45 shows the blood supply to the rectal area. The main artery to the rectum is the superior rectal (haemorrhoidal) artery. Veins of the inferior part of the submucous plexus become the rectal veins, which drain to the internal pudendal veins. Drug absorption takes place through this venous network. Superior haemorrhoidal veins connect with the portal vein and thus transport drugs absorbed in the upper part of the rectal cavity to the liver; the inferior veins enter into the inferior vena cava and thus bypass the liver. The particular venous route the drug takes is affected by the extent to which the suppository migrates in its original or molten form further up the gastrointestinal tract, and this may be variable. The rectal route therefore does not necessarily, or even reproducibly, avoid the liver.

A schematic representation (Fig. 9.46) shows the processes occurring following insertion of a suppository into the rectum. Cocoa butter suppositories usually liquefy within a few minutes, but the drug is not necessarily released from solution or suspension, as the fat in this case is not emulsified or absorbed.

Surfactants may be required to aid dispersal of the fat and thus when this base is used the physicochemical properties of the drug are important. The rate-limiting step in drug absorption for suppositories made from a fatty base is the partitioning of the dissolved drug from the molten base, not the rate of solution of the drug in the body fluids.

The influence of the aqueous solubility on *in vitro* release from fat-based suppositories is shown in Fig. 9.47, the results being collated from the study of 35 drugs grouped into classes I–V in decreasing order of water solubility. The results may be explained as follows. The water-soluble active substances will be insoluble in the fatty base, while the less water-soluble material will tend to be soluble in the base, and will thus diffuse from the base more slowly. Water-soluble drugs are better absorbed from a fatty excipient than from a water-soluble one, and ethyl nicotinate, for example, which is lipid-soluble, is absorbed faster from a water-soluble excipient.

In a study of the various physical properties of suppositories, the most important parameter for the bioavailability of paracetamol was found to be rheological properties at 37°C. The relationship between the

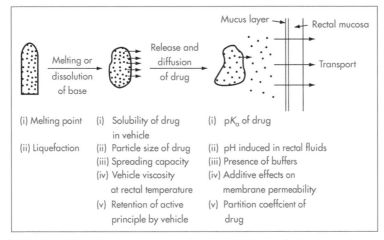

Figure 9.46 Schematic representation of rectal absorption of an active principle from a suppository, and the factors at each stage likely to affect the bioavailability of the drug.

Modified from Jaminet F. In: Guillot BR, Lombard AP (eds) *The Suppository*. Paris: Maloine; 1973.

excretion of paracetamol (APAP; N-acetyl-*p*-aminophenol) and the rheology of the excipient drug suspension is shown in Fig. 9.48. The greater the limiting shear stress, τ, of the system, the lower the bioavailability of the drug.

Apparatus for studying the many variables in suppository formulation has been designed to measure rates of release *in vitro*. Both a circulating dissolution apparatus and a dialysis device utilising an aqueous and a non-aqueous phase have been described, and are discussed in Chapter 15. As the suppository base is heated before moulding, certain effects can be noted

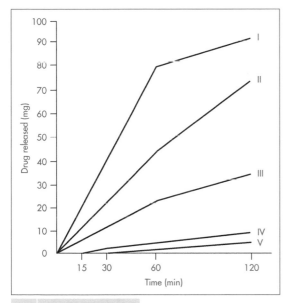

Type	Solubility in water
I	1 in 1
II	1 in 10
III	1 in 10 to 1 in 100
IV	1 in 100 to 1 in 1000
V	1 in 1000 to 1 in 10 000

Figure 9.47 Release of drugs of varying solubilities from fat-based suppositories of equal active agent content.

Modified from Voigt R, Falk G. *Pharmazie* 1968;23:709.

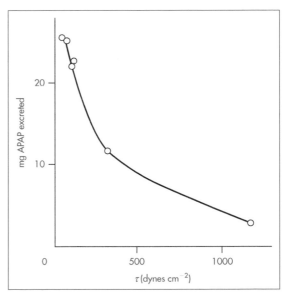

Figure 9.48 Variation of the excretion of APAP (paracetamol) in the urine 2 hours after rectal administration of a formulation as a function of the limiting shear stress, τ, of the excipient–drug mixture at 37°C.

Modified with permission from Moës A. *J Pharm Belg* 1974;29:319.

that are unique to this type of medication. Testosterone dissolves when hot in the semisynthetic excipient Witepsol H, to give, on cooling, crystals of about 2–3 μm in diameter. After dissolution in theobroma oil, the drug does not crystallise on cooling but remains dissolved as a solid solution. In the former case, high absorption rates are obtained, while in the latter poor absorption is achieved.

Absorption from the rectum depends on the concentration of drug in absorbable form in the rectal cavity and, if the base is not emulsified, on the contact area between molten excipient and rectal mucosa. Addition of surfactants may increase the ability of the molten mass to spread and tends to increase the extent of absorption. Significant increases in absorption can be obtained with polyoxyethylene sorbitan monostearate (polysorbate 60), sodium lauryl sulfate and cetyltriethylammonium (cetrimonium) bromide. Surfactants increase wetting and spreading and may increase the permeability of the rectal mucosal membrane.

A study of the effect of polyoxyethylene glycols on the rectal absorption of un-ionised sulfafurazole demonstrated the importance of the affinity of the drug substance for base and for rectal mucosa. As the amount of Macrogol 4000 (polyoxyethylene glycol 4000) was increased, the partition coefficient (lipid/vehicle) fell and absorption decreased correspondingly, because the affinity of the drug for the suppository base increased and its tendency to partition to the rectal lipids decreased. In a similar way, incorporation of water-soluble drug into a water-in-oil emulsified suppository base tends to decrease bioavailability as the drug is transferred in dispersed aqueous droplets in the molten base.

Deliberate incorporation of water into a formulation gives rise to the possibility that, on storage, water will be lost by evaporation and drug may crystallise as a result. Reactions between components of the formulation are more likely to occur in the presence of moisture than in its absence.

9.10.2 Incompatibility between base and drug

Various incompatibilities have been noted with polyoxyethylene glycol bases. Phenolic substances complex with glycol, probably by hydrogen bonding between the phenolic hydroxyl group and the glycol ether oxygens. Polyoxyethylene glycol bases are incompatible with tannic acid, ichthammol, aspirin, benzocaine, clioquinol and sulfonamides. High concentrations of salicylic acid alter the consistency of the bases to a more fluid state.

Glycerogelatin bases are prepared by heating together glycerin, gelatin and water. Although primarily used *per se* as an intestinal evacuant, the glycerogelatin base may be used to deliver drugs to the body. For this purpose the United States Pharmacopeia XVIII specified two types of gelatin to avoid incompatibilities. Type A is acidic and cationic, with an isoelectric point between pH 7 and 9; type B is less acidic and anionic, with an isoelectric point between pH 4.7 and 5. Use of untreated gelatin renders the base incompatible with acidic and basic drugs.

9.11 Drug administration to brain, spinal cord and tissues

Administration of drugs in solution by intrathecal catheter provides an opportunity to deliver drugs to the brain and spinal cord. Relatively hydrophilic drugs such as methotrexate ($\log P = -0.5$) that do not cross the blood–brain barrier in significant amounts have been infused intrathecally to treat meningeal leukaemia, and baclofen ($\log P = -1.0$) to treat spinal cord spasticity. High lumbar cerebrospinal fluid concentrations are achieved as a result. Figure 9.49 shows

Clinical point

The hygroscopicity of some hydrophilic bases such as the polyoxyethylene glycols (each oxygen can interact with up to 4 water molecules under certain circumstances) results in the abstraction of water from the rectal mucosa. This causes a stinging sensation and discomfort and probably affects the passage of drugs across the rectal mucosa. The hygroscopicity of the glycols decreases as the molecular weight increases. The problem may be overcome by the incorporation of water into the base, although the presence of water may affect drug stability. Glycerogelatin bases are also hygroscopic.

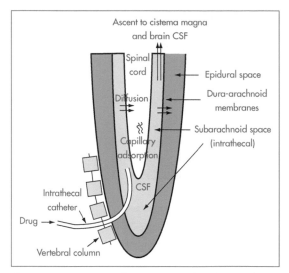

Figure 9.49 Anatomical structures and pathways of drug movement important in intrathecal drug administration; the lower part (sacral, lumbar) of the spinal cord is shown in this diagram.

Reproduced from Kroin JS. Intrathecal drug administration. Present use and future trends. *Clin Pharmacokinet* 1992;22:319, with kind permission from Springer Science and Business Media.

the anatomy of the epidural space and routes of drug transport. The spinal cerebrospinal fluid has a small volume (70 cm^3) and a relatively slow clearance (20–40 cm^3 h^{-1}) of hydrophilic drugs.

The intrathecal route is more invasive than IV, IM or SC routes. Both percutaneously implanted catheters and subcutaneously implantable pumps have been used to reduce the risk of infection on repeated puncture.

Diffusion of the drug following administration intrathecally is critical in determining activity. The cerebrospinal fluid pharmacokinetics of three drugs (morphine, log $P = 0.15$; clonidine, log $P = 0.85$; and baclofen, log $P = -1.0$) were found to be similar, leading to the suggestion that bulk flow mechanisms may be the dominant factor in determining distribution.

9.11.1 Brain implants

The brain offers many challenges in terms of treatment systemically because of the power of the blood–brain barrier to resist entry of certain drugs. It might be assumed that direct implantation of delivery systems into the brain, e.g. to treat brain tumours, might

always be effective. However, the physical and chemical phenomena that control the transport of drugs in the brain tissue are complex and not fully understood.[**] The physicochemical issue is not necessarily the release of drug from any reservoir (e.g. polymer wafers) but the subsequent diffusion and spread of the drug into the surrounding tumour or other tissues.

A large variety of processes can be involved in the transport of the drug once it is released from the dosage form to its target site(s), including:

- diffusion within the extracellular space
- reversible and irreversible binding to the extracellular matrix (which comprises long-chain macromolecules)
- degradation of the dose form (implant or wafer) (e.g. by enzymes or hydrolysis)
- passive or active uptake into central nervous system cells (by diffusion or receptor-mediated internalisation)
- release from endolysosomes into the cytosol
- diffusion and convection within the cytosol of the cells
- uptake into the cell nuclei (where appropriate)
- bulk flow within the extracellular space
- direction-dependent drug transport (anisotropy), because the brain is not one homogeneous mass

and, of course, elimination into the blood stream.

Figure 9.50 shows the arrangement of Gliadel implants in brain tissue and the pathways of diffusion and interaction of a drug released from an implant in the brain.

The poor diffusion characteristics of one agent, human nerve growth factor, in the brain obviates the use of implants, as shown clearly in Fig. 9.51. This would require more direct intervention and application of the drug used as a prospective drug for the treatment of Alzheimer's disease.

9.11.2 Cardiovascular drug-eluting stents

A *stent* is a mesh 'tube' inserted into any natural passage such as a ureter or an artery to prevent or counteract a flow constriction. Cardiovascular stents are wire mesh tubular devices that are employed to

[**] An excellent overview on the importance of diffusion and related processes has been given by Tao and Nicholson (Tao L, Nicholson C. *J Theor Biol* 2004;229:59–68).

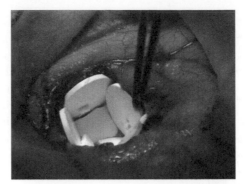

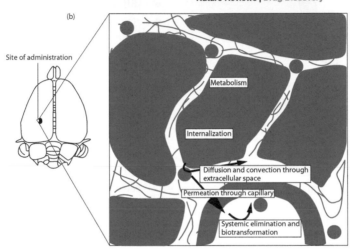

Figure 9.50 (a, top) Implants of the polyanhydride-based Gliadel wafers containing carmustine (BCNU); drug release is controlled both by diffusion of the drug and erosion of the polymer matrix. (b, bottom) The pathways of diffusion and interaction of a drug released from implants. The results of the complex pathways in the brain tissues are shown by the data in Fig. 9.51.

(a) Reproduced with permission from Lesniak MS, Brem H. Targeted therapy for brain tumours. *Nature Rev Drug Discov* 2004;3:499–508.

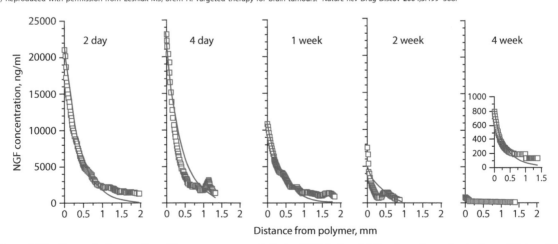

Figure 9.51 Concentration profiles of human nerve growth factor (NGF) in the vicinity of a polymer implant over 28 days. The solid lines represent the calculation of diffusion/elimination from days 2 and 4 and steady-state conditions thereafter. Note the small distance where levels are significant, some 1–2 mm from the implant surface.

Reproduced from Krewson CE, Saltzman WM. Transport and elimination of recombinant human NGF during long-term delivery to the brain. *Brain Res* 1996;727:169–181. Copyright Elsevier 1996.

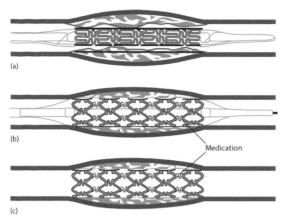

(a)

(b)

Medication

(c)

Figure 9.52 (a) A stent is mounted on a balloon catheter and advanced to the narrowed portion of the heart artery. (b) The balloon is inflated and the stent is expanded, opening the narrowed section of the artery. (c) The balloon is deflated and removed; the stent is embedded into the wall of the artery and stays in position.

Reproduced with permission from Maisel WH, Laskey WK. Cardiology patient page. Drug-eluting stents. *Circulation* 2007;115:e426–e427.

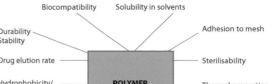

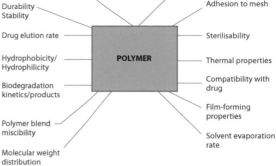

Factors in the development of new polymers for extended release in drug eluting stents

Biocompatibility   Solubility in solvents

Durability
Stability   Adhesion to mesh

Drug elution rate   Sterilisability

Hydrophobicity/
Hydrophilicity   **POLYMER**   Thermal properties

Biodegradation
kinetics/products   Compatibility with drug

Film-forming
properties

Polymer blend
miscibility   Solvent evaporation
rate

Molecular weight
distribution

Figure 9.54 The range of properties of importance in the design of new polymers for slow release of drugs on stents.
Redrawn from Udipi K *et al. J Biomed Mater Res A* 2007; 85A:1064–1071.

enlarge diseased arteries. Early versions of cardiovascular stents caused problems of provoking clot formation and restenosis, a renewed narrowing of the vessel. A relatively new form of drug delivery has appeared in the form of 'coated stents' in which polymer coatings on the mesh are used to deliver drugs such as sirolimus (a drug that can prevent restenosis) directly to tissues (Fig. 9.52).

Some designs of stent use several polymers in several layers to control drug release, as in Fig. 9.53.

Some of the factors of importance in the design of new polymers for slow release of drugs on stents are shown in Fig. 9.54.

Summary

The routes discussed in this chapter are sometimes simpler, and perhaps sometimes more complex than the oral route. In several of those we have covered there is a more intimate contact between the formulation and the absorbing surface – as in the topical and rectal routes – so the formulation and the thermodynamic activity of the drug in the vehicle become more directly important. In essence:

- Each route has its own special characteristics. Administration of the same dose of drug by different routes usually produces significantly different pharmacokinetics.

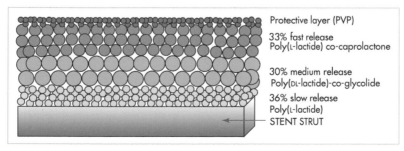

Protective layer (PVP)
33% fast release
Poly(L-lactide) co-caprolactone

30% medium release
Poly(DL-lactide)-co-glycolide

36% slow release
Poly(L-lactide)
STENT STRUT

Figure 9.53 A diagrammatic representation of a polymer-coated stent (the Infinitum stent). The stent structure is coated with three different layers of polymers that have different functions from the outermost coat, which contains no drug but protects the underlying structures.

- The optimal lipophilicity of a drug to traverse the barrier membrane depends on the nature of the membrane.

- Some barriers as in the eye are complex, having the characteristics of typical lipid barriers, interspersed with more aqueous hurdles.

- In some cases, as with IM injections, the nature of the tissue into which the drug is injected, whether fatty or aqueous, is key to the process of transferring drug into the blood.

- No one equation can yet predict the pharmacokinetic profile of a drug delivered by a particular route in a particular formulation, but the equations presented in this chapter help to show the effect of key parameters.

- The overriding importance of lipophilicity is clear when drug is absorbed in molecular form.

- When drug is delivered as a suspension (as in an aerosol), the paramount importance of particle size in first getting the drug to the site of action is clear; once it has reached that site, its rate of solution and its lipophilicity are again important.

- There is no escaping the fact that the diffusion coefficient and flux of the active entity in the tissues concerned in each route of drug delivery have a paramount effect on the success or otherwise of a route. The body's many biological and physical barriers present what we sometimes refer to as the complex realities of drug delivery and targeting, a topic to which we return in later chapters.

References

1. Balch CM *et al*. Continuous regional chemotherapy for metastatic colorectal cancer using a totally implantable infusion pump. A feasibility study in 50 patients. *Am J Surg* 1983;145:285–290.
2. Mitragotri S *et al*. Ultrasound-mediated transdermal protein delivery. *Science* 1995;269:850–853.
3. Figge FHJ, Barnett DJ. Anatomic evaluation of a jet injection instrument designed to minimise pain and inconvenience of parenteral therapy. *Am Pract* 1948;3:197–206.
4. Shramm J, Mitragotri S. Transdermal drug delivery by jet injectors: energetics of jet formation and penetration. *Pharm Res* 2002;19:1673–1679.
5. Murdan S. Drug delivery to the nail following topical application. *Int J Pharm* 2002;236:1–26.
6. Elkeeb R *et al*. Transungual drug delivery: current status. *Int J Pharm* 2010;384:1–8.
7. Tabbara KF, Sharara N. Dry eye syndrome. *Drugs Today* 1998;34:447.
8. Holly FJ. Formation and rupture of the tear film. *Exp Eye Res* 1973;15515–525.
9. Matsuo T *et al*. Trehalose eye drops in the treatment of dry eye syndrome. *Ophthalmology* 2002;109:2024–2029.
10. Sieg JW, Robinson JR. Vehicle effects on ocular drug bioavailability II: Evaluation of pilocarpine. *J Pharm Sci* 1977;66:1222–1228.
11. Chrai SS, Robinson JR. Binding of sulfisoxazole to protein fractions of tears. *J Pharm Sci* 1976;65:437–439.
12. Snell JW.. Ophthalmic drug delivery systems. *Drug Deliv Res* 1985;6:245–261.
13. Hull DS *et al*. Ocular penetration of prednisolone and the hydrophilic contact lens. *Arch Ophthalmol* 1974;92:413–416.
14. German E, Siddiqui N. Atropine toxicity from eyedrops. *N Engl J Med* 1970;282:689.
15. Borromeo-McGrail V *et al*. Systemic hypertension following ocular administration of 10% phenylephrine in the neonate. *Paediatrics* 1973;51:1032–1036.
16. Benziger DP, Edelson J. Absorption from the vagina. *Drug Metab Ther* 1983;141:37–68.
17. Kunth K *et al*. Hydrogel delivery systems for vaginal and oral applications. Formulations and biological considerations. *Adv Drug Deliv Rev* 1993;11:137–167.
18. Cox JSG *et al*. Disodium cromoglycate (Intal). *Adv Drug Res* 1970;5:115–196.
19. McDonald KJ, Martin GP. Transition to CFC-free metered dose inhalers-into the new millennium. *Int J Pharm* 2000;201:89–107.
20. Williams RO, Lie L. Influence of formulation additives on the vapor pressure of hydrofluoroalkane propellants. *Int J Pharm* 1998;166:99–103.
21. Vervaet C, Byron P. Drug–surfactant–propellant interactions in HFA-formulations. *Int J Pharm* 1999;186:13–30.
22. O'Callaghan C, Barry PW. The science of nebulised drug delivery. *Thorax* 1997;52(Suppl. 2):S31–S44.
23. Constantino HR *et al*. Intranasal delivery: physicochemical and therapeutics aspects. *Int J Pharm* 2007;337:1–14.

10

Paediatric and geriatric formulations

Human variability in responses to drugs is well known, as we have discussed, so that the average patient becomes a myth. There is a pressing need for the greater personalisation of medicine and medicines. There has been much emphasis on genetic routes to reveal differences in patients' sensitivities to certain drugs or idiosyncratic abreactions to medication. However, in order to make use of the information when it becomes freely available and intelligible there is a need for a greater variety and flexibility of dosage forms to deliver more tailored doses and predictable bioavailability, as well as to provide dosage forms for the age-related and disease-related differences in absorption and kinetics. This chapter covers some aspects of formulation in paediatric and geriatric practice, and discusses attempts to personalise medication, but it is not a guide to the whole subject of paediatric or geriatric therapy. We deal with the need for special formulations for individual cases and some of the more general needs of the population at the different ends of the age spectrum. This has been termed 'age-specific' medicine. Here we naturally emphasise the pharmaceutics and explore the systems devised to facilitate safe dosing in these contrasting age groups.

10.1 Introduction

If there was ever a case of continued emphasis on pharmaceutics it is the need to design patient-specific medicines, not least in relation to dose and dosage form. Very low doses of potent drugs pose a problem of their accurate measurement. The possibility of errors in medication increases with the number of manipulations and calculations required, so even simple technologies that provide dosing systems to avoid the large dilutions that are frequently necessary in paediatric care would be of benefit. There is now a wide range of excipients and active agents available and also a much broader range of methods of formu-

lation and modes of delivery of drugs. We can now also characterise and manipulate materials in more exact ways, as we hope earlier chapters have proved. The emphasis on early and late life here does not preclude the need for all patients to be assessed more closely and medication (drug and dose form) to be person-specific. The advances in pharmaceutical sciences aid this goal.

Childhood covers more than a decade of life and there are large changes in metabolism, weight, height, gastric pH, gastric emptying, sensitivity to drugs and excipients, and many other parameters. Old age can span decades. Unfortunately, many formulations for children have had perforce to be prepared from products designed for adults; the same applies for the elderly, who may have difficulties in swallowing or have problems that demand modified approaches to medication. We do not deal here in any detail with the differences in the pharmacokinetic, pharmacodynamic or metabolic aspects of drugs in these different categories of patients but these often necessitate the use of controlled-release formulations or individualised therapies, covered in detail in other texts. The drivers of formulation choice are outlined in Fig. 10.1.

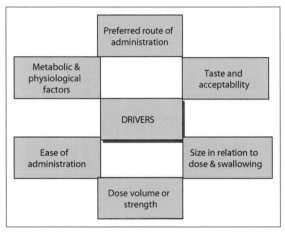

Figure 10.1 The matrix of drivers for special formulations.

10.2 Paediatric medication

Children are far from being a homogeneous group. They range from:

- preterm newborn infants (premature: average weight <3.4 kg)
- full-term infants (neonates: 0–27 days)
- infants and toddlers (28 days to 23 months: 3.4–12.4 kg)
- children from 2 to 11 years (12.4–39 kg)
- adolescents from 12 to 16/18 years (on average 39–72 kg for males and 60 kg for females).

Formulations are not designed or selected in isolation from the biological realities. There are age-related developmental changes in the pharmacokinetics[1,2] and pharmacodynamics of drugs. Changes occur in gastric acidity, drug clearance and receptor expression. Many of these changes are relevant to drug absorption.

Neonatal stomachs are achlorhydric soon after birth, so the absorption of acid-labile drugs may be increased. The rate of gastric emptying falls as infants get older, being faster in the neonate than in adults, but slower in infants and children than in adults. This has consequences with some formulations. Because the liver takes up a relatively large percentage of body volume in infants, clearance rates often exceed those in adults. It is clear then that extrapolation of results from adult data sets in terms of absorption or the behaviour of both drugs and dose forms is hazardous. Many of these issues are discussed in more detail in a review on the topic of developing paediatric medicines.[3]

A study over 60 years ago illustrated differences in the absorption of penicillin in neonates and children (Fig. 10.2). One of the key causes is the achlorhydria in neonates so that the acid-labile penicillin survives the passage through the stomach and can explain the results of elevated levels in neonates compared to infants and children up to 13 years old.

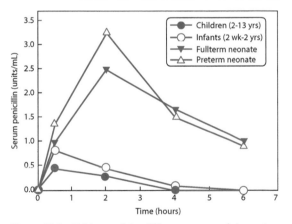

Figure 10.2 Evidence of the different extents of absorption of a weight-related dose of penicillin (a single 22 000 U kg^{-1}) administered to preterm or full term neonates infants and children, the result of the achlorhydria in the neonates.

Reproduced from Huang NN, High RH. Comparison of serum levels following the administration of oral and parenteral preparations of penicillin to infants and children of various age groups. *J Pediatr* 1953;42:657–669. Copyright Elsevier 1953.

Figure 10.3 illustrates the variety of approaches to paediatric dosing using solutions, powder, granules (accumulation) or dividing solid-dose forms ('partition'). The scheme makes clear the options available to achieve precise incremental dosing, for example, by using mini-tablets whose quantity for delivery in a capsule can be adjusted appropriately.

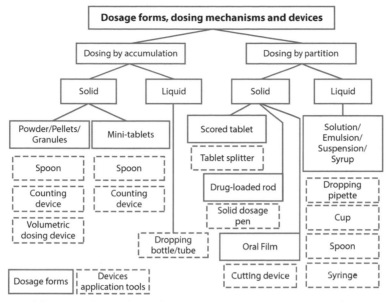

Figure 10.3 A diagram of the approaches to dosing for individual patients using an 'accumulation' or 'partition' approach.

Reproduced from Wening K, Breitkreuz J. Oral drug delivery in personalized medicine: unmet needs and novel approaches. *Int J Pharm* 2011;404:1–9. Copyright Elsevier 2011.

10.2.1 Acceptability of paediatric medication

Acceptability is driven by the characteristics of the patient (age, ability, disease type and state) and by the characteristics of a medicinal product, such as:

- palatability
- ease of swallowing (size and shape, integrity of dosage form, e.g. film coating)
- appearance (e.g. colour, shape, embossing)
- complexity of modification prior to administration (if required)
- required dose (e.g. the dosing volume, number of tablets, break marks)
- required dosing frequency and duration of treatment
- selected administration device (if any)
- primary and secondary container closure system
- actual mode of administration.

This list would apply to medicines designed for the elderly also.

10.2.2 Extemporaneous formulations

Extemporaneous formulations are frequently prepared from tablets, capsules and injections to produce medicines suitable for an individual child or for groups of children. In spite of pharmacists' expertise in formulation and production, preparations made extemporaneously (except in emergencies) without the fullest quality control should be considered unacceptable in the 21st century. Cutting tablets for any age too is not always the optimal way forward. Nonetheless, it is the pharmacist's role to provide appropriate medicine for individuals and the possibilities to prepare novel dose forms in hospitals and other environments is increasing. Three-dimensional printing of films and tablets will increasingly be a powerful tool.

Figure 10.4 illustrates some of the basic approaches used when converting existing formulations of tablets, capsules and injections into alternative forms. It may be that the contents of an injection can be incorporated directly into a suitable vehicle. The same may be true of soft gelatin capsules, whose contents may be amenable to emulsification depending on their nature. In a survey of extemporaneously prepared dosage forms it was found that 66% were aqueous suspensions, 22% solutions, 4% powders, 1.2% oils and 0.2% capsules,[4] most for paediatric patients. These included:

- midazolam
- vancomycin
- clonidine hydrochloride
- diazoxide

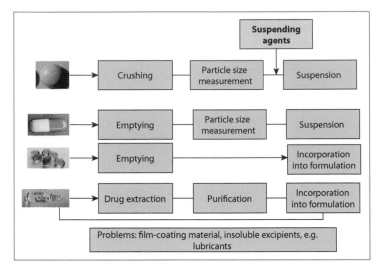

Figure 10.4 Stratagems applied when there is a need to convert existing dosage forms into medicines for children or the elderly: crushing of tablets, emptying hard and soft gelatin capsules or in a few cases extracting the active substance from products when the active is unavailable in pure chemical form. In all cases key parameters should be determined: stability, particle size distribution of granules and powders, purity of drug substance.

● clobazam

● warfarin.

Many had neither chemical nor microbiological supporting data.

Developing paediatric medicines: liquid or solid oral forms?

Liquid formulations are often favoured because of the ease of administration and acceptability to the child. Taste masking is more of an issue with liquid formulations, but solid-dose forms can be difficult to swallow and may lodge in the young oesophagus. Liquid formulations suffer somewhat from variability of measurement of dose, although oral injectors can reduce this frequent domestic error. The teaspoon is far from a standard measure, delivering in use between 2.5 and 9 mL. If tablets are crushed to provide drug for extemporaneous formulations, the process must be standardised as far as possible and the particle size distribution must be evaluated as minimal quality procedures. Often the issue is to reduce doses, but also to provide a dosage form that aids swallowing in both the young and the elderly.

The importance of solvent choice

Figure 10.5 shows clearly the possible effect of solvents in extemporaneous preparations, in this case of oxandrolone (**I**) which degrades hydrolytically. Earlier chapters discuss the question of stability – the chemical

stability of drug substances and excipients and the physical stability of formulations. The example here is simply to illustrate the marked effect in practice of the choice of suboptimal solvents, even the simple solvents discussed in this case.

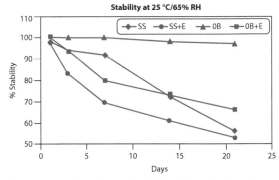

Figure 10.5 The chemical stability of oxandrolone (structure **I**) prepared with four different solvents: SS, Simple Syrup; SS + E, Simple Syrup with 8% ethanol; OB, Orablend (Paddock Laboratories, USA); OB + E, Orablend with 8% ethanol. Orablend itself comprises purified water, sucrose, glycerin, sorbitol, flavouring, microcrystalline cellulose, carboxymethylcellulose sodium, xanthan gum, carrageenan, calcium sulfate, trisodium phosphate, citric acid and sodium phosphate as buffers, dimethicone antifoam emulsion. Preserved with methylparaben and potassium sorbate.

Reproduced from Garg A et al. Development of an extemporaneous oral liquid formulation of oxandrolone and its stability evaluation. *Burns* 2012;37:1150–1153. Copyright Elsevier 2012.

Structure I Oxandrolone

Clearly, given the complexity of some of the vehicles used, this is not a textbook example which explains the data, but in practical terms it highlights the importance of appropriate assays and stability assessments in extemporaneous preparations.

>
> **Clinical point The case of oral captopril solutions**
>
> Oral liquid captopril formulations for paediatric patients used in UK hospitals have been found to have variable stability, partly as a result of *variability of the purity of the captopril* used.[5] Even with a single source of drug, stability after 1 month at room temperature ranged from 71.5% to 100%, although with storage at 5 ± 3°C the range was narrowed (82–99.7%). At the latter storage temperatures, the formulation is stable for 2 years. Captopril oxidation is catalysed by metal ions, hence the value of ethylenediaminetetraacetic acid and avoidance of contact with metal ions.
>
> Apparently, a variety of unlicensed captopril products have been used in 13 tertiary paediatric cardiac centres in the UK and 13 large hospitals referring patients to these centres: four hospitals dispensed captopril tablets by crushing and dissolving in water before administration, and the other 22 used nine different liquid formulations. As the authors conclude,[6] this degree of inconsistency raises 'issues about optimal captopril dosing and potential toxicity, such that its use may influence paediatric cardiac surgical and interventional outcomes'.

Excipients

There are some restrictions in the range of excipients that can be used in paediatric formulations.[7] As neonates do not metabolise alcohol efficiently, ethanol should be used with caution. There have been reports of injury to the gastrointestinal tract of neonates; thus, hypertonic solutions should not be used.

>
> **Clinical point Ethanol in paediatric medicines**
>
> The American Academy of Pediatrics Committee on Drugs recommendation[8] is that the quantity of ethanol contained in a single dose of a drug preparation should not produce a blood concentration greater than 25 mg 100 mL^{-1}. A suitable alternative is a less toxic solvent such as glycerin. Preservatives are not contraindicated in formulations for children generally, but should be used only when necessary. However the product may require refrigeration and proper storage conditions must be followed and the hazards associated with administering a preparation that has passed its beyond-use date known.

Dose in paediatric medication

Low doses can cause many difficulties, not least in the reliable measurement of small volumes per dose. In the case of insulin, the lowest dose that could be reproducibly delivered has been studied.[9,10] The smaller the dose, the less accurate it is; it has been suggested that, for the lowest dose, insulin should be given diluted for greater accuracy of dose measurement. Insulin pens accurately delivery 5 U doses but showed no advantage in terms of accuracy over syringes. For other proteins there are questions of solution viscosity that might dictate choice of dosing method (see Chapter 13).

Case study Isoniazid absorption in young children

The abstract of a paper by Notterman *et al.* reads (verbatim):

In an 8-month-old infant with tuberculosis meningitis treatment with isoniazid was unsuccessful and was associated with lower than expected plasma concentrations of isoniazid (measured concentration 0.1 microgram/mL). The infant had received isoniazid as a crushed tablet admixed with apple sauce. Oral administration of the parenteral solution of isoniazid (Nydrazid, Squibb) mixed in apple juice produced a higher isoniazid concentration (2.9 micrograms/mL) and the child improved clinically. Pharmacokinetic studies in two subjects were performed after oral administration of three formulations:

(1) an isoniazid tablet crushed and mixed with apple sauce,

(2) parenteral isoniazid solution mixed with apple juice, and

(3) a commercially available syrup containing isoniazid and pyridoxine (P-I-N Forte, Lannett).

Of the three oral preparations, the syrup produced the highest peak concentrations (8.3 and 6.9 micrograms/mL). The crushed tablet in apple sauce produced the lowest peak concentrations (1.4 and 2.4 micrograms/mL). Administration of crushed isoniazid tablets with food may be associated with impaired gastrointestinal absorption, lower than expected isoniazid concentrations, and treatment failure. There are issues of the particle size or granule size in the case of the crushed tablets and of the effect of the apple sauce, as suggested, on gastrointestinal (GI) absorption. One of the key issues when using crushed tablets or the contents of capsules is the determination of particle size distributions so that different batches at least consist of the same size as far as possible.

Source: Notterman DA *et al.* Effect of dose formulation on isoniazid absorption in two young children. *Pediatrics* 1986;77:850–852.

Case study Fatality from administration of labetalol and crushed Extended-Release Nifedipine

This case involved not an infant but a 38-year-old female, but it illustrates dramatically the potential dangers in both children and adults of misusing special formulations.

Case summary

A 38-year-old woman with multiple medical problems presented to the hospital in acute respiratory distress and was diagnosed with acute pulmonary edema and pneumonia. After initial stabilization, her medications were changed to oral hydralazine, labetalol, and nifedipine XL. These medications were crushed and administered through a nasogastric tube. The patient developed worsening bradycardia with hypotension and experienced asystolic cardiac arrest. She was resuscitated; however, the following morning, another dose of labetalol and nifedipine XL was crushed and administered through the nasogastric tube. She again developed worsening bradycardia with hypotension and ultimately died.

Source: Schier J. *Ann Pharmacother* 2002;37:1420–1423.

As the author concludes, there may be synergistic effects following simultaneous administration of a beta-blocker and a calcium-channel blocker. The release characteristics of the nifedipine controlled-release product were destroyed on crushing, resulting in the rapid release of the total drug amount.

Tablets designed for division

The use of mini-tablets, 3 mm in diameter, to aid swallowing has been investigated in children aged 2–6 years.[11] Such products also avoid, as we have discussed, the need for subdivision of adult dose forms. Recent developments have also led to new tablets designed for division, as shown in Fig. 10.6.

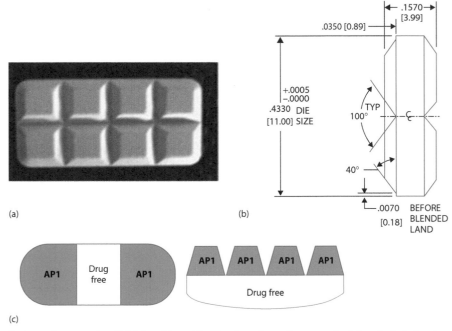

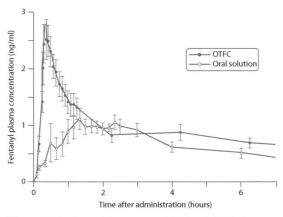

(a)

(b)

(c)

Figure 10.6 Design of rectangular divisible tablets: (a) side view along shortest axis; (b) technical drawing providing the design to make splitting accurate and another prototype system; and (c) systems which provide drug-free regions to aid the accurate breaking of the tablet. API = active pharmaceutical ingredient.

a) and b) from Kayitake E *et al Int J Pharm* 2009;370:41-47 with permission from Elsevier; c: modified from Solomon L and Kaplan AS, US Patent 2010; 0713547B2

10.2.3 Other routes of administration

Oral mucosal delivery

Delivery to the oral mucosa has been discussed in Chapter 8. Its use in infants has some advantages. Oral transmucosal fentanyl citrate is used as an anaesthetic premedication in children undergoing surgery and painful diagnostic or therapeutic procedures within a monitored care setting. Rapid drug absorption is achieved through the oral mucosa (Fig. 10.7).

Sublingual

The advantages of sublingual and buccal administration have also been discussed in Chapter 8. There can be occasions when this route is appropriate, such as for comatose babies who cannot swallow.

Figure 10.7 An oral transmucosal fentanyl citrate lozenge (OTFC) administered and compared with an oral solution.

Reproduced with permission from: Streisand JB *et al.* Absorption and bioavailability of oral transmucosal fentanyl citrate. *Anesthesiology* 1991; 75:223–229.

 Clinical point

Sublingual sugar has been found to be a useful alternative to intravenous dextrose and superior to orally administered sugar to correct hypoglycaemia in children in the tropics. Bioavailabilities were 84% for sublingual compared to 38% from oral sugar[12]; one explanation is that the sublingual route is rich in transport systems for sugar. These transporters are saturable and prevent overdose. A 40% dextrose gel has more recently been trialled in hypoglycaemic neonates,[13] administered by rubbing the gel on to the buccal surface. It is suggested that dextrose (the D-isomer of glucose) might be more rapidly absorbed sublingually than the disaccharide sucrose (structures below).

Glucose

Fructose

Sucrose

Subcutaneous injection

The skin of children is thinner and their subcutaneous tissue thickness is lower compared to adults, hence shorter syringe needles (e.g. 4 mm) are employed to avoid unwanted results of injection into intramuscular tissue. Insulin injections should be given into the subcutaneous tissue and optimally avoid deposition into other sites (see Chapter 9). Measurements that have been made of combined skin and subcutaneous tissue show large variations with respect to body mass index at all sites (arm, thigh, abdomen and buttock),[14] hence making personalised medicine more difficult. We have discussed above the use of insulin pens and the advantages that these may bring to young diabetic patients.

Intramuscular injection

There is little information on the difference between intramuscular administration of many drugs in different age groups. However, the time to reach peak drug levels after intramuscular injection of ampicillin, cefalexin, cefaloridine and benzylpenicllin is equivalent in neonates, children and adults. It is known that neonates have less muscular mass and subcutaneous fat and higher water content, which should affect solubility and diffusion of drugs deposited in depots.

Transdermal delivery

Patches

Transdermal administration can provide a non-invasive method for paediatric drug delivery. Delgado-Charroe and Guy[15] state that 'the competent skin barrier function in term infants and older children limits both water loss and the percutaneous entry of chemicals including drugs; but the smaller doses required by children eases the attainment of therapeutic concentrations'. Fentanyl, buprenorphine, clonidine, scopolamine, methylphenidate, oestrogens, nicotine and tulobuterol have been formulated as patches for paediatric use. The 'immature and rapidly evolving skin barrier function in premature neonates represents a significant formulation challenge' and this group suffers from a lack of approved transdermal formulations.

Microneedles

Microneedles, which have been discussed in Chapter 9, have several advantages over conventional systems. Microneedles fabricated by one of a variety of techniques are now being used in practice to provide a means of administering drugs or vaccines which may be poorly absorbed across the stratum corneum. For the young or old with needle phobia the small size of the microneedle patch and their painless application demonstrate advantages over conventional systems.

Intranasal delivery

Intranasal fentanyl has been used for pain relief in the treatment of burns and procedures during treatment, such as the removal of dressings in paediatric patients as an alternative to oral morphine. The ideal paediatric analgesic should be potent and have a quick onset, a short duration of action and minimal side-effects.

Ophthalmic route

The eye of the newborn is about two-thirds of its adult size; it reaches adult size at ages 3–4 years. There is a ready risk of systemic side-effects with ocular delivery of drops, as drugs after absorption enter a smaller circulating blood volume; it has been found with timolol that in young children blood levels range from 3.5 to 34 ng mL^{-1}, much higher than average levels of 2.45 ng mL^{-1} in adults. It is thus important that concentrations of active in eye drops are appropriate for the age of the child and that drop size variations (often dictated by the surface tension and viscosity of the drops as well as the nature of the dropper) are minimised.[16]

Inhalation

Drugs can be delivered via the respiratory tract by the methods discussed in Chapter 9. However, the dispar-

Dosage form	Preterm newborn infants	Term newborn infants (0d-28d)	Infants and Toddlers (1m-2y)	Children (pre school) (2-5y)	Children (school) (6-11y)	Adolescents (12-16/18y)
Liquids for nebulisation	Applicable with problems	Probably applicable, not preferred	Good applicability	Best and preferred applicability	Good applicability	Probably applicable, not preferred
pMDI with spacer / holding chamber	Not applicable	Probably applicable, not preferred	Good applicability	Best and preferred applicability	Good applicability	Good applicability
DPI	Not applicable	Not applicable	Probably applicable, not preferred	Good applicability	Best and preferred applicability	Best and preferred applicability

Figure 10.8 The appropriateness of forms of inhalation for various age groups, a figure modified from the EMA Committee for Medicinal Products for Human Use 2006. pMDI, pressurised metered-dose inhaler; DPI, dry powder inhaler.

Reproduced from Leiner S. A respiratory product for children – development and submission experiences. *Int J Pharm* 2014;469:263–264. Copyright Elsevier 2014.

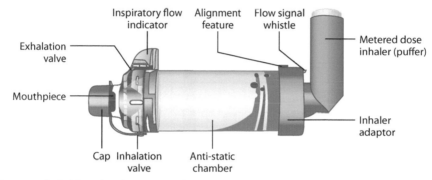

Figure 10.9 Diagram of a holding chamber or spacer for use with a pressurised metered-dose inhaler, showing the inhalation valve mentioned in the text and the adapters for the inhaler.

ity in the sizes of children and their tolerance to aerosols formed by nebulisers or pressurised devices varies. Recent consensus about the applicability of the various approaches in the range from preterm neonates to adolescent children is summarised in Fig. 10.8.

Spacers (or holding chambers), as shown in Fig. 10.9, are used in inhalation therapy for both adults and children. These chambers reduce the velocity of the aerosol particles and also allow more complete evaporation of solvent so that the particle size is smaller than when used without such as device. Most chambers have one-way valves that open during inspiration, closing during expiration. Spacers are easier to use by children than pressurised metered-dose inhalers.[*]

The reference in the figure legend to the antistatic chamber reveals the issue with some chambers, in which electrostatic charges attract aerosol particles to the surface of the chambers – often plastic – a problem that can be obviated by treating the interior surface of the chamber with detergent or other agents. Figure 10.10 demonstrates the influence of spacers on the lung deposition of the aerosol. The advantages in this case are clear, but with over 100 inhaler/drug combinations available for inhalation therapy it is not easy to provide hard and fast, quantitative rules! However, the facts in some studies are quite stark with lung deposition of salbutamol[17]: even with chambers reaching maximally around 10%, there is significant variability, in older children reaching around 15% but fluctuating from child to child. The inhaler matters, as does the spacer, as shown in Figs 10.11 and 10.12.

[*] For a more detailed account, see Pedersen P *et al*. The ADMIT series – issues in inhalation therapy 5: inhaler selection in children with asthma. *Primary Care Resp J* 2010;19:209–216.

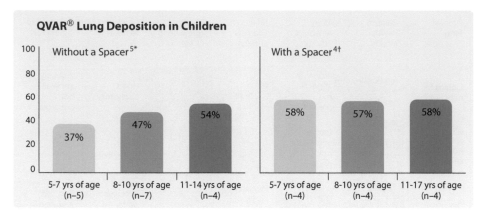

Figure 10.10 The influence of spacers on lung deposition from an aerosol of beclometasone dipropionate.

Reproduced from www.qvar.com, using data from [5*]Devadason SG *et al. Eur Respir J* 2003;21:1007–1011 and [4†]Roller CM *et al. Eur Respir J* 2007;29:299–306.

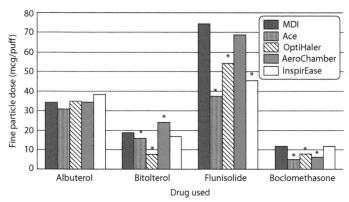

Figure 10.11 The dose of fine particles in a study of four drugs delivered via a range of spacers compared with a metered-dose inhaler (MDI).

Reproduced from Ahrens R *et al.* Choosing the metered-dose inhaler spacer or holding chamber that matches the patient's need: evidence that the specific drug being delivered is an important consideration. *J Allergy Clin Immunol* 1995;96:288–294. Copyright Elsevier 1995.

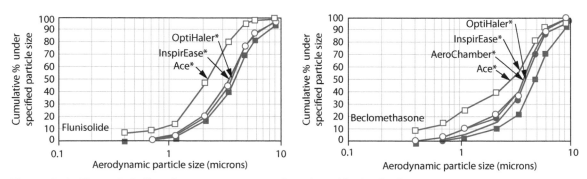

Figure 10.12 The marked effect of some spacers on aerodynamic particle size distribution.

Reproduced from Ahrens R *et al.* Choosing the metered-dose inhaler spacer or holding chamber that matches the patient's need: evidence that the specific drug being delivered is an important consideration. *J Allergy Clin Immunol* 1995;96:288–294. Copyright Elsevier 1995.

10.3 The elderly and their medication

The term 'elderly' covers an even longer span of life than does the category 'paediatric', and it has been suggested by Wooten[18] that there are two subdivisions, the young elderly (from 70 to 85 years) and the old elderly (from 85 years onward).

10.3.1 Changes with age that affect medication

There are many reasons why specialised or tailored medicines are required for the elderly patient. There are physiological and other changes which occur with ageing that often complicate pharmaceutical care, including the following which impact on absorption of drugs, as can be deduced from earlier chapters:

- changes to the oral cavity (e.g. xerostomia: reduction in saliva)
- changes to the oesophagus (e.g. delayed passage of dosage forms)
- decrease in gastric acid production (hence increase in gastric pH)
- reduced gastric emptying time
- intestinal changes (e.g. reduced surface area).

Figure 10.13 lists these and other changes on ageing which impinge on medication. These effects are in addition to the problems of comorbidity and consequent polypharmacy[19] (hence drug–drug interactions and compliance) and alterations in physical and biological factors which also affect absorption, distribution, excretion and metabolism and thus pharmacokinetics.

Complicating factors

Xerostomia

Xerostomia and delayed oesophageal emptying may have relevance for the use of certain oral medications, such as fast-dissolving dosage forms or buccal and sublingual forms. Here paucity of fluid intake may slow the release of drug in the oral cavity.

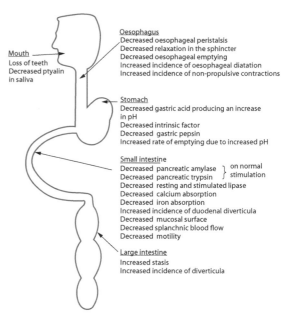

Figure 10.13 The principal changes in gastrointestinal function with age.
Reproduced with permission from Macdonald ET, Macdonald JB. *Drug Treatment in the Elderly*. Chichester: John Wiley; 1982.

Oesophageal transit

The elderly are more susceptible to the lodging of tablets and capsules in the oesophagus than are younger patients. This is not necessarily the fault of the dose form, but can be the result of taking the tablet with no or too little water. The variability of water intake in 108 female subjects in a trial of a film-coated placebo tablets when they were free to use whatever volume they wished is shown in Fig. 10.14.[20] However, as discussed in Chapter 12, some dosage forms can themselves have adhesive properties and adverse effects may be exacerbated in the elderly patient.

Difficulties in swallowing are a problem not only in the young but also in the elderly[21] with dysphagia** and those in particular with dementia. Patients may simply refuse to take their oral solid medications. Fast-dissolving formulations administered sublingually can be one solution to the problem (Fig. 10.15); such formulations are frequently bioequivalent to the conventional oral forms. The problems of xerostomia may, however, compromise outcomes. There remains the need for a range of different drug formulations, for initial titration and subsequent treatment.[22]

** Swallowing dysfunction is discussed in a review by Stegemann S *et al*. Swallowing dysfunction and dysphagia is an unrecognized challenge of oral drug therapy. *Int J Pharm* 2012;430:187–206.

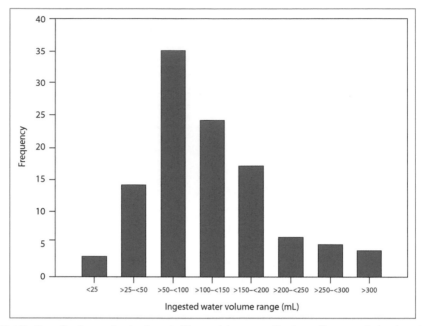

Figure 10.14 Distribution of volume of water ingested by participants swallowing a film-coated placebo tablet in a study of oesophageal transit.

Reproduced from Perkins AC *et al*. The use of scintigraphy to demonstrate the rapid esophageal transit of the oval film-coated placebo risedronate tablet compared to a round uncoated placebo tablet when administered with minimal volumes of water. *Int J Pharm* 2001;222:295–239 with permission. Copyright Elsevier 2001.

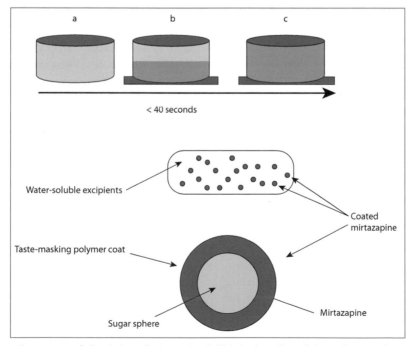

Figure 10.15 Top: the process of dissolution of mirtazapine SolTab in the saliva of the oral cavity: the penetration of water (stages a, b c) takes less than 40 seconds. Bottom: the structure of these fast-dissolving systems.

Reproduced from Frijlink HW. Benefits of different drug formulations in psychopharmacology. *Eur Neuropsychopharmacol* 2003;13:S77–S84 with permission. Copyright Elsevier 2003.

Alternative routes of administration may be employed. The transdermal route has been promoted for use in the older population. There are apparently few differences in the permeability of the skin: the need to adapt doses for use in the elderly relates more to changes in cardiovascular, renal and hepatic change.[23]

Achlorhydria

The incidence of achlorhydria is found in up to 20% of elderly patients and hypochlorhydria in 20% of patients over 70 years of age. Around 11% of the elderly have a median fasting gastric pH of above 5.[24] Intestinal transit may be slowed in the elderly. The effects of these many changes may be self-cancelling or may be significant. Much will depend on the drug. It is difficult to predict effects, largely because individual patient data are not available, hence the 'myth of the average'.

10.3.2 Enteral feeding

While the main use of enteral feeding is to enhance nutrition in patients unable to take food normally, enteral feeding tubes also allow the administration of drugs to such patients.[25] This poses many pharmaceutical problems, however. Different feeding tubes have different destinations (Fig. 10.16) and hence it is important to choose the correct site for the administration of the drug, depending on the characteristics of the medication. Even though drugs may be absorbed maximally in the intestine, bypassing the stomach may result in poor absorption as the drug will not have the opportunity to dissolve in the acidic environment of the stomach.

Liquid formulations and solid-dosage forms can be administered this way, and with caution several medications can be given at the same time. Nevertheless, drug–nutrient interactions can take place, there can be problems with the osmolality of the liquids administered, and there can be blockage of the tubes (Table 10.1).

Osmolality of enteral feeding formulae

The osmolality of enteral feeding formulae is important because of its influence on the gastrointestinal tract. Osmolality is expressed in mOsm kg^{-1} (see Chapter 2, section 2.4.2) and is affected by the concentration of amino acids, carbohydrates and electrolytes. If quantities of a liquid with a higher osmolality

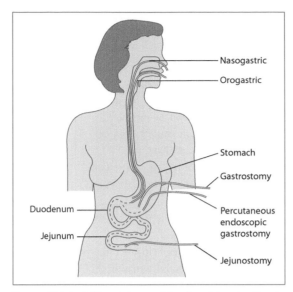

Figure 10.16 Different types of feeding tubes leading to the stomach. Nasoduodenal, nasojejunal and percutaneous jejunostomy tubes extend to the small intestine.

than the gut contents are administered, water is drawn into the intestine; such a process leads to diarrhoea, nausea and distension. The osmolality of normal body

Table 10.1 Some liquid medications that are physically *incompatible* with most enteral fluids
• Brompheniramine (Dimetane Elixir, Wyeth, USA)
• Calcium gluconate (Rugby, USA)
• Ferrous sulfate (Feosol Elixir, GSK, UK)
• Guaifenesin (Robitussin Liquid, Wyeth, USA)
• Lithium citrate (Cibalith-S syrup, CIBA, USA)
• Potassium chloride liquid (Wyeth, USA)
• Pseudoephedrine hydrochloride (Sudafed Syrup, Pfizer, USA)

fluids is 300 mOsm kg^{-1} and isotonic formulations have values close to this. Table 10.2 lists liquid medications that have osmolalities greater than 300 mOsm kg^{-1}. The exact osmolalites will vary with the exact formulations used and will often differ between various brands of a formulation.

The exact osmolalities will vary with the exact formulations used and will often differ between various brands of a formulation.

There are some liquid preparations that are not suitable for administration by enteral feeding tubes. Some may be too viscous and may occlude the tubes.

Table 10.2 Some liquid medications with osmolalities greater than 300 mOsm kg^{-1}

- Acetominophen (paracetamol) elixir, 65 mg mL^{-1}
- Amantadine HCl solution, 10 mg mL^{-1}
- Chloral hydrate syrup, 50 mg mL^{-1}
- Cimetidine solution, 60 mg mL^{-1}
- Docusate sodium syrup, 3.3 mg mL^{-1}
- Lactulose syrup, 0.67 mg mL^{-1}
- Metoclopramide HCl syrup, 1 mg mL^{-1}
- Promethazine HCl syrup, 1.25 mg mL^{-1}

Reproduced with permission from Dickerson RN, Melnik G. Osmolality of oral drug solutions and suspension. *Am J Hosp Pharm* 1988;45:832–834.

Syrups with pH values below 4 often produce incompatibility with the enteral nutrition (EN) formulations, which may result in clumping, increase in viscosity and clogging of the tubes. Not all syrups produce this effect.

Solid conventional-release dose forms can be crushed for administration with EN fluids. The finely ground tablet is added as a suspension in water (15–30 mL). The contents of liquid gelatin capsules are often viscous and it is not easy to remove all of the contents from a single capsule. Delayed-release pancreatic enzyme capsules that contain enteric-coated beads[26] can be mixed with apple sauce or juice for administration via feeding tube. It has been suggested that the soft gelatin capsule can be dissolved in hot water and the whole contents administered. Extended-release tablets and capsules have to be treated as special cases: the contents of capsules containing coated pellets can be mixed with EN fluids, but there can be a tendency for these to clump and block narrow-bore feeding tubes.

Drug interactions with nutrient formulations

Certain drugs have been found to interact with nutrient solutions. It is not surprising, given the nature of these solutions, that drugs may bind to proteins or be affected by electrolytes. Phenytoin, carbamazepine, warfarin and some fluoroquinolones have been reported to have lowered bioavailability because of various interactions. Phenytoin absorption has been reported to be reduced by up to 70% on co-administration with enteral feeds.[27,28]

Summary

This chapter has covered many of the areas in which drug formulation is important clinically for specific age groups. Special formulations for paediatric and geriatric patients form a group of products that are key to optimising therapy in these vulnerable age groups. The fact that both groups are themselves diverse emphasises the importance of the appropriate choice of medication and delivery system and hence the need for closer attention to the individual as a patient. Some wider issues are also discussed, including enteral feeding, interactions of drugs with nutritional fluids and the osmolalities of liquid formulations and there is renewed emphasis to devise and produce new administration systems and formulations to advance personalised medicine through personalised medicines.

References

1. Johnson TN. The development of drug metabolising enzymes and their influence on the susceptibility to adverse drug reactions in children. *Toxicology* 2003;192:37–48.
2. Strassburg CP *et al*. Developmental aspects of human hepatic drug glucoronidation in young children and adults. *Gut* 2002;50:259–265.
3. Ernest TB *et al*. Developing paediatric medicines: identifying the needs and recognizing the challenges. *J Pharm Pharmacol* 2007;59:1043–1055.
4. Lowey AR, Jackson MN. A survey of extemporaneous preparation in NHS trusts in Yorkshire, the North East and London. *Hosp Pharm* 2008;15:217–219.
5. Berger-Gryllaki M *et al*. The development of a stable oral solution of captopril for paediatric patients. *Eur J Hosp Pharm Sci* 2007;13:67–72.
6. Mulla H *et al*. Variations in captopril formulations used to treat children with heart failure: a survey in the United Kingdom. *Arch Dis Child* 2007;92:409–411.
7. Thompson JE, Davidson LW. Vehicles for oral delivery. In: *A Practical Guide to Contemporary Pharmacy Practice*, 3rd edn. Philadelphia, PA: Wolter-Kluwer.
8. American Academy of Pediatrics. Ethanol in liquid preparations intended for children. *Pediatrics* 1984; 73:405–407.
9. Casella SJ *et al*. Accuracy and precision of low-dose insulin administration. *Pediatrics* 1993;91:1155–1157.
10. Gnanalingham MG *et al*. Accuracy and reproducibility of low dose insulin administration using pen-injectors and syringes. *Arch Dis Child* 1998;79:59–62.
11. Thomson SA *et al*. Minitablets: new modality to deliver medicines to preschool-aged children. *Pediatrics* 2009;123: e235–e238.

12. Barennes H *et al*. Sublingual sugar administration as an alternative to intravenous dextrose administration to correct hypoglycemia among children in the tropics. *Pediatrics* 2005;116:e648–e653.

13. Harris DI *et al*. Dextrose gel for neonatal hypoglycaemia (the Sugar Babies study): a randomised, double-blind, placebo-controlled trial. *Lancet* 2013;382:2077–2083.

14. Marran K, Segal D. SKINNY – Skin thickness and Needles in the Young. *South Afr J Child Health* 2014;8:92–95.

15. Delgado-Charroe MB, Guy RH. Effective use of transdermal drug delivery in children. *Adv Drug Del Rev* 2014;73:63–82.

16. Coulter RA. Pediatric use of topical ophthalmic drugs. *Optometry* 2004;75:419–429.

17. Wildhaber JH *et al*. Inhalation therapy in asthma: nebulizer or pressurized metered-dose inhaler with holding chamber? In vivo comparison of lung deposition in children. *J Pediatr* 1999;135:28–33.

18. Wooten JM. Pharmacotherapy considerations in elderly adults. *South Med J* 2012;105:437–445.

19. Gidal BE. Drug absorption in the elderly: biopharmaceutical considerations for the antiepileptic drugs. *Epilepsy Res* 2006;68S:S65–S69.

20. Perkins AC *et al*. The use of scintigraphy to demonstrate the rapid esophageal transit of the oval film-coated placebo risedronate tablet compared to a round uncoated placebo tablet when administered with minimal volumes of water. *Int J Pharm* 2001;222:295–239.

21. Schindler JS, Kelly JH. Swallowing disorders in the elderly. *Laryngoscope* 2002;112:589–602.

22. Wahlich J *et al*. Medicines for older adults. Learning from practice to develop patient centric drug products. *Int J Pharm* 2013;456:252–257.

23. Kaestli L-Z *et al*. The use of transdermal formulations in the elderly. *Drugs Ageing* 2008;25:269–280.

24. Russell TL *et al*. Upper gastrointestinal pH in seventy-nine healthy, elderly, North American men and women. *Pharm Res* 1993;10:187–196.

25. Williams NT. Medication administration through enteral feeding tubes. *Am J Health-Syst Pharm* 2009;65:2347–2357.

26. Ferrone M *et al*. Pancreatic enzyme pharmacotherapy. *Pharmacotherapy* 2007;27:910–922.

27. Gilbert S *et al*. How to minimise interaction between phenytoin and enteral feedings. Two approaches. *Nutr Clin Pract* 1996;11:28–31.

28. Doak KK *et al*. Bioavailability of phenytoin acid and phenytoin sodium with enteral feedings. *Pharmacotherapy* 1998;18:637–6645.

11

Physicochemical interactions and incompatibilities

This chapter deals with some practical consequences of the physical chemistry of drugs, especially their interactions with each other, with solvents and with excipients in formulations. Sometimes the interaction is beneficial and sometimes not. In this chapter you will appreciate that there are several physicochemical causes of interactions. These include:

- pH effects – changes in pH that may lead to precipitation of the drug
- change of solvent characteristics on dilution, which may also cause precipitation
- cation–anion interactions in which complexes are formed
- salting out and salting in – the influence of salts in decreasing or increasing solubility, respectively
- chelation – in which a chelator molecule binds with a metal ion to form a complex
- ion-exchange interactions – in which ionised drugs interact with oppositely charged resins
- adsorption to excipients and containers – causing loss of drug
- interactions with plastics – another source of loss of material
- protein binding – through which the free concentration of drugs *in vivo* is reduced by binding to plasma proteins.

The chapter discusses the topic of drug interactions from a physicochemical rather than a pharmacological or pharmacodynamic viewpoint. Many drug interactions *in vitro* are, not surprisingly, readily explained by resorting to the physical chemistry discussed in earlier chapters of this book. There is no reason why the same forces and phenomena that operate *in vitro* cannot explain many of the observed interactions that occur in the body, although of course the interplay of physicochemical forces and physiological conditions makes a fascinating exercise. Interactions such as protein binding, adsorption of drugs on to surfaces, chelation and complexation all occur in physiological conditions and are predictable to a large degree. We can also observe drug–drug and drug–excipient interactions.

Drug–drug or drug–excipient interactions can take place before administration of a drug. These may result in precipitation of the drug(s) from solution, loss of potency or chemical instability. Under some circumstances they can occur even in the solid state. With the decline in traditional forms of extemporaneous dispensing, this aspect of pharmaceutical incompatibility may seem to have decreased somewhat in importance. However, extemporaneous preparation still is important, for example, in the form of addition of drugs to intravenous (IV) fluids where interactions can be critical, and which should be carried out with pharmaceutical oversight, particularly with new drugs and new formulations and especially during clinical trials.

An *incompatibility* occurs when one drug is mixed with other drugs or agents and produces a product unsuitable for administration either because of some modification of the effect of the active drug, such as increase in toxicity, or because of some physical change, such as decrease in solubility or stability. Some drugs designed to be administered by the IV route cannot safely be mixed with all available IV fluids. If, as discussed in Chapter 4, the solubility of a drug in a particular infusion fluid is low, crystallisation may occur sometimes very slowly when the drug and fluid are mixed. Microcrystals may be formed that are not immediately visible. When infused, these have potentially serious effects. The mechanism of crystallisation from solution will often involve a change in pH; the problem is a real one because the pH of commercially available infusion fluids can vary within a pH range of perhaps 1–2 units. Therefore, a drug may be compatible with one batch of fluid and not another. The proper application of the equations relating pH and pK_a and solubility discussed in section 4.2.4 should allow additions of drugs to be made safely or to be avoided.

We now discuss, in turn, some of the potential interactions that can occur. Not all interactions between drugs or between drugs and excipients are detrimental to therapeutic effects; one example discussed in the chapter is the interaction used to limit the duration of action of general anaesthetics such as rocuronium by the infusion of a cyclodextrin derivative sugammadex, which binds and inactivates the anaesthetic, thus causing the desired reversal of action.

11.1 pH effects *in vitro* and *in vivo*

The pH of a medium, whether in a formulation or in the body, can be a primary determinant of drug behaviour. For convenience we here discuss separately pH effects in the laboratory and in the body.

11.1.1 *In vitro* pH effects

Chemical, as well as physical, instability may result from changes in pH, buffering capacity, salt formation or complexation. Chemical instability may give rise to the formation of inactive or toxic products. Although infusion times are generally not greater than 2 hours, chemical changes following a change in pH may occur rapidly. pH changes often follow from the addition of a drug substance or solution to an infusion fluid, as

shown in Table 11.1. This increase or decrease in pH may then produce physical or chemical changes in the system.

The titratable acidity or alkalinity of a system may be more important than pH itself in determining compatibility and stability. For example, an autoclaved solution of dextrose may have a pH as low as 4.0, but the titratable acidity in such an unbuffered solution is low, and thus the addition of a drug such as benzylpenicillin sodium, or the soluble form of an acidic drug whose solubility will be reduced at low pH, may not be contraindicated. As seen from Table 11.1, the additive may itself change the pH of the solution or solvent to which it is added. As little as 500 mg of ampicillin sodium can raise the pH of 500 cm^3 of some fluids to over 8, and carbenicillin or benzylpenicillin may raise the pH of 5% dextrose or dextrose saline to 5.6 or even

Table 11.1 Changes in pH of 5% dextrose (1000 cm³) following addition of three drugs

Drug	Quantity	ΔpH	Final pH
Aminophylline	250 mg	+4.2	8.5
	500 mg	+4.2	8.5
Cefalothin sodium	1 g	+0.1	4.2
	2 g	+0.2	4.3
Oxytetracycline hydrochloride	500 mg	−1.25	2.9
	1 g	−1.45	2.7

Reproduced with permission from Edwards M. pH – an important factor in the compatibility of additives in intravenous therapy. *Am J Hosp Pharm* 1967;24:440.

higher. Both drugs are, however, stable in these conditions.

The solubility of calcium and phosphate in total parenteral nutrition (TPN) solutions is dependent on the pH of the solution. TPN solutions are, of course, clinically acceptable only when precipitation can be guaranteed not to occur. Dibasic calcium phosphate, for example, is soluble only to the extent of 0.3 g dm⁻³, whereas monobasic calcium phosphate has a solubility of 18 g dm⁻³. At low pH the monobasic form predominates, while at higher pH values the dibasic form becomes available to bind with calcium and precipitates tend to form.

Calcium solubility curves for TPN solutions containing 1.5% (w/v) amino acid and 10% (w/v) dextrose at pH 5.5 are shown in Fig. 11.1. The broken straight lines show the calcium and phosphate concentrations at 3 : 1 and 2 : 1 ratios. The dotted curve for Aminosyn solutions shows the concentrations at which precipitation occurs after 18 hours at 25°C followed by 30 minutes in a water bath at 37°C. The full curve is for TrophAmine solutions, and represents calcium or phosphate concentrations at which visual or microscopic precipitation or crystallisation occurs. Compositions to the left of the curves represent physically compatible solutions. The compatibility and stability of additives in parenteral nutrition mixtures are discussed in a review by Allwood and Kearney.[1]

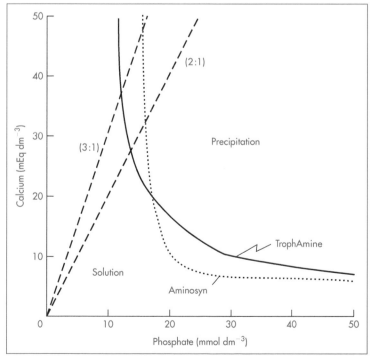

Figure 11.1 Solubility curves for total parenteral nutrition solutions containing amino acid (15 g dm⁻³) and 10% dextrose at pH 5.5. Dotted line: Aminosyn. Solid line: TrophAmine. Dashed lines: relative calcium-to-phosphate ratios.

Modified with permission from Fitzgerald KA, MacKay MW. Calcium and phosphate solubility in neonatal parenteral nutrient solutions containing TrophAmine. *Am J Hosp Pharm* 1986;43:88–93.

11.1.2 *In vivo* pH effects

The sensitivity of the properties of most drugs to changes in the pH of their environment means that the hydrogen-ion concentration will be an important determinant of solubility, crystallisation and partitioning. Gastric pH is 1–3 in normal subjects, but the measured range of pH values in the human stomach is wide, as can be seen in Fig. 11.2. Remembering that pH is a logarithmic scale, the order of the change in the gut and its effect on aqueous and lipid solubility in particular can be appreciated. Changes in the acid–base balance therefore have a marked influence on the absorption and thus on the activity of drugs.

Ingestion of antacids, food and weak electrolytes will all change the pH of the stomach. Weakly acidic drugs, being un-ionised in the stomach, will be absorbed from the stomach by passive diffusion. One might expect, therefore, that concomitant antacid therapy would delay or partially prevent absorption of certain acidic drugs. The main mechanism would be an increase in pH of the stomach, increasing ionisation of the drug and reducing absorption. A problem in generalisations of this kind is that the acid-neutralising capacity of antacids is very variable, as the results quoted in Table 11.2 show. Some acidic drugs, listed in Table 11.3, are also known to be absorbed in the intestine, in which case the co-administration of an antacid is not necessarily prohibited, as its effects may be transitory.

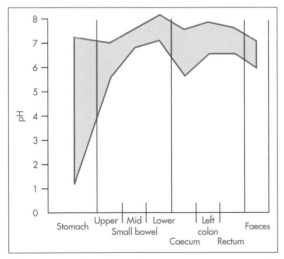

Figure 11.2 pH profile in the gut as measured by radio-telemetric capsule; the shaded area represents extremes of values observed in 9 subjects.

Reproduced with permission from Watson BW *et al.* pH profile of gut as measured by radiotelemetry capsule. *Br Med J* 1972;2:104.

Clinical point

The effects of antacids are not always clear-cut, as pointed out at the beginning of this chapter. There are contradictory reports of the effect of antacids on the absorption of levodopa, as one example. Levodopa is metabolised within the gastrointestinal tract and more rapidly degraded in the stomach than in the intestine, so the rate at which the drug is emptied from the stomach can affect its availability. It has been suggested that, when an antacid is administered prior to the drug, serum levodopa concentration is increased because it is transferred to the intestine more rapidly.

The use of ranitidine, nizatidine, famotidine and other H_2-antagonists has given rise to the possibility of a drug interaction involving the subsequent increase in gastric pH, as these drugs inhibit gastric acid secretion. A few subjects have transient achlorhydria after oral cimetidine, so increased absorption of acid-labile drugs is a predictable side-effect, as breakdown is reduced.

Sodium bicarbonate (sodium hydrogen carbonate) is one of the most effective antacids in terms of neutralising capacity. It can greatly depress the absorption of tetracycline – the mean amount of drug appearing in the urine of patients receiving only drug was 114 mg at 48 hours and was 53 mg for those also given sodium bicarbonate. Chelation (see section 11.5) is not possible with the monovalent Na^+ ion as it is with the multivalent components of other antacids, nor does adsorption occur. If the drug is dissolved prior to administration, the antacid does not affect the excretion of the antibiotic, suggesting that in normal dosage forms it is the rate of dissolution of the drug that is affected by the antacid, as explained below in the case of tetracycline.

The aqueous solubility of tetracycline at pH 1–3 is 100-fold greater than at pH 5–6. Consequently, its rate of solution, dc/dt, at this lower pH is greatly reduced as, according to equation (11.1),

$$\frac{\mathrm{d}c}{\mathrm{d}t} = kc_\mathrm{s} \qquad (11.1)$$

where c_s is the solubility. A 2 g dose of $NaHCO_3$ will increase the intragastric pH above 4 for a period of

Table 11.2 Amounts of various antacids required to neutralise 50 mEq HCl

Antacid	Neutralising capacity of 1 g or 1 cm³		Dose required to neutralise 50 mEq	Weight of tablet (g)	No. of tablets
	cm³ 0.1 mol dm⁻³ HCl	mEq HCl			
Powders					
NaHCO₃	115	11.5	4.4 g		
MgO	85	8.5	5.9 g		
CaCO₃	110	11.0	4.5 g		
Magnesium trisilicate	10	1.0	50 g		
MgCO₃	8	0.8	63 g		
Suspensions					
Al(OH)₃ gel	0.7	0.07	715 cm³		
Milk of Magnesia	27.7	2.8	17.8 cm³		
Titralac	24	2.4	20.6 cm³		
Aludrox	1.7	0.17	294 cm³		
Oxaine	2.4	0.24	208 cm³		
Mucaine	1.7	0.17	294 cm³		
Kolantyl gel	3.4	0.34	147 cm³		
Tablets					
Gastrogel	5.0	0.5	100 g	1.08	93
Gastrobrom	15.0	1.5	33.3 g	1.48	23
Glyzinal	2.5	0.25	200 g	0.72	278
Actal	7.7	0.77	65 g	0.60	109
Amphotab	2.5	0.25	200 g	1.04	192
Gelusil	2.5	0.25	200 g	1.36	147
Nulacin	10.0	1.0	50 g	3.12	17
Kolantyl wafer	5.0	0.50	100 g	1.64	61
Titralac	42.5	4.25	11.8 g	0.65	18
Almacarb	3.0	0.3	167 g	1.28	130
Dijex	4.6	0.46	109 g	1.65	66

Reproduced from Piper DW, Fenton BH. Antacid therapy of peptic ulcer. II. An evaluation of antacids in vitro. *Gut* 1964;5:585, copyright 1964, with permission from BMJ Publishing Group Ltd.
Note that proprietary preparations available in different countries may not have the same formulation.

20–30 minutes, sufficient time for 20–50% of the undissolved tetracycline particles to be emptied into the duodenum, where the pH (at 5–6) is even less favourable for solution to occur. The fraction of drug absorbed is therefore decreased.

Effects of antacids other than directly on pH

The effect of antacids on gastric-emptying rate is a factor that makes difficult a direct physicochemical analysis of the problem. The difficulty in predicting the effect of antacids is clearly shown by studies with naproxen, a weakly acidic non-steroidal

Table 11.3 Drugs whose absorption may be affected by antacid administration

Drug whose activity would be reduced	Drug whose activity would be potentiated
Tetracyclines	Theophylline
Nalidixic acid	Chloroquine
Nitrofurantoin	Mecamylamine
Benzylpenicillin	Amfetamine
Sulfonamides	Levodopa

anti-inflammatory with a pK_a of 4.2. Several textbooks of drug interactions state that antacids decrease the absorption of acidic drugs such as nalidixic acid, nitrofurantoin and benxylpenicillin (as indicated in Table 11.3), but antacids both increase and decrease the absorption of naproxen. Magnesium carbonate, magnesium oxide and aluminium hydroxide decrease absorption and, as these are insoluble agents, adsorption effects that reduce the quantity of free drug in solution are suspected (Fig. 11.3). On the other hand intake of Maalox, which contains magnesium and aluminium hydroxides, slightly increased the area under the curve. The extent to which Al^{3+} and Mg^{2+} ions chelate with nalidixic acid is not clear, but the structure of the drug suggests it has chelating potential (see section 11.5).

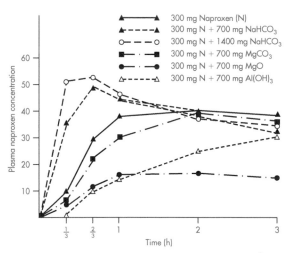

Figure 11.3 Mean plasma concentrations ($\mu g\ cm^{-3}$) of naproxen in 14 male volunteers with and without intake of sodium bicarbonate, magnesium oxide or aluminium hydroxide.

Modified with permission from Segre EJ *et al.* Letter: Effects of antacids on naproxen absorption. *N Engl J Med* 1974;291:582.

Clinical point

Even though gastric emptying tends to become more rapid as the gastric pH is raised, antacid preparations containing aluminium or calcium are prone to retard emptying, and magnesium preparations to promote it. The caution about the co-administration of antacids containing divalent or trivalent metals and tetracyclines should be extended to antacids containing sodium bicarbonate or any substance capable of increasing intragastric pH.

Similar principles can be applied to intestinal absorption, although here the pH gradients between the contents of the intestinal lumen and capillary blood are smaller. Sudden changes in the acid–base balance may, none the less, change the concentration of drugs able to enter cells, providing that the pH change does not alter binding of the drug to protein, or drug excretion, which of course it invariably does. Accurate prediction of the effect of a change in the acid–base balance on the activity of any drug requires a knowledge of its site of action and the potential effect of pH

Clinical point

Ingestion of some antacids over a period of 24 hours will increase urinary pH and hence affect renal resorption and handling of some drugs. For example, administration of sodium bicarbonate with aspirin reduces blood salicylate levels by about 50%, probably owing to its increased excretion in the urine. Although high doses of alkalising agents that raise the pH of the urine will increase the renal excretion of free salicylate and result in lowering of plasma salicylate levels, in some commercial buffered aspirin tablets (such as Bufferin) there is insufficient antacid to cause a change in the pH of the gastric fluids. The small amount of antacid is sufficient, however, to aid the dissolution of the acetylsalicylic acid and this leads to more favourable absorption rates.

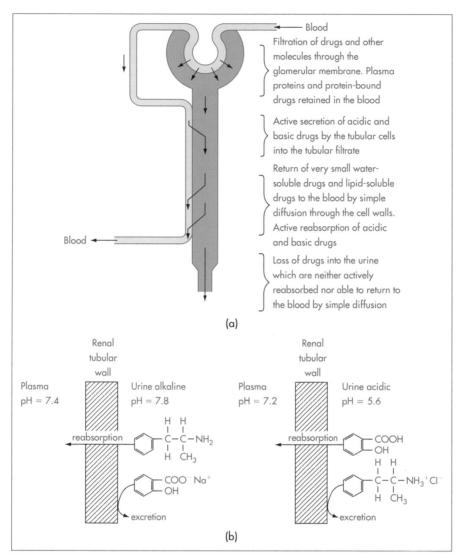

Figure 11.4 (a) A highly simplified diagram of a kidney tubule to illustrate the filtration and secretion of drugs from the blood into the tubular filtrate, and their subsequent reabsorption or loss in the urine. (b) Schematic representation of the influence of urinary pH on the passive reabsorption of a weak acid and a weak base from the urine in the renal tubules; at a high pH the passive reabsorption of the weak base and the excretion of the weak acid are enhanced, while at a low pH value the reabsorption of the weak acid and the excretion of the weak base are enhanced.

changes on its excretion and biotransformation, and requires knowledge of the extent of pH changes throughout the body.

The importance of urinary pH

Change in the pH of urine will change the rate of urinary excretion of many drugs (as represented in Fig. 11.4). When a drug is in its un-ionised form it will more readily diffuse from the urine to the blood. In an acidic urine, acidic drugs will diffuse back into the blood from the urine. Acidic compounds such as nitrofurantoin are excreted faster when the urinary pH is alkaline. Amfetamine, imipramine and amitriptyline are excreted more rapidly in acidic urine. The control of urinary pH in studies of pharmacokinetics is thus vital. It is difficult, however, to find compounds to use by the oral route for deliberate adjustment of urinary pH. Sodium bicarbonate and ammonium chloride may be used but are unpalatable. IV administration of acidifying salt solutions presents one approach, especially for the forced diuresis of basic drugs in cases of poisoning.

Clinical point

Urinary pH can be important in determining drug toxicity more directly. A preparation containing the urinary antiseptic methenamine mandelate and sulfamethizole caused turbidity in the urine of 9 out of 32 patients. The turbidity was higher in acidic urine, and was caused by precipitation of an amorphous sulfonamide derivative containing 63% sulfamethizole. The efficacy of both agents is reduced by precipitation and the danger of renal blockade is, of course, increased.[2]

Precipitation of drugs in vivo

Pain on injection may be the result of precipitation of a drug at the site of injection brought about either by solvent dilution or by alteration in pH. Precipitation of drugs from formulations used intravenously can, of course, lead to thromboembolism. The kinetics of precipitation under realistic conditions must be appreciated, since a sufficiently slow rate of infusion may obviate problems from this source as the drug precipitates and then redissolves. A simple but important equation[3] yields the flow rate (Q) of blood or normal saline required to maintain a drug in solution during its addition to an IV fluid:

$$Q = \frac{R}{S_m} \qquad (11.2)$$

where R is the rate of injection of drug in mg min^{-1} and S_m is the drug's apparent maximum solubility in

Clinical point

Too rapid injection of the diazepam preparation directly into the venous supply might result in precipitation; slow venous blood flow would contribute to the effect. This would perhaps explain a finding that thrombophlebitis occurs less frequently when smaller veins are avoided and when injection of diazepam is followed by rigorous flushing of the infusion system with normal saline.[4]

the system (mg cm^{-3}). Using diazepam and normal saline as an example, if R is 5 mg min^{-1}, S_m is approximately 0.3 mg cm^{-3}, so Q would have to exceed 17 cm^3 min^{-1} to prevent observable precipitation. As this is a high rate of infusion, it is evident that the administration of diazepam through the tubing of an IV drip is likely to result in precipitate formation.

11.2 Dilution of mixed-solvent systems

In several cases the special nature of a formulation will preclude dilution by an aqueous infusion fluid. Injectable products containing phenytoin, digoxin and diazepam may come into this category if they are formulated in a non-aqueous but water-miscible solvent (such as an alcohol–water mixture) or as a solubilised (e.g. micellar) preparation. Addition of the formulation to water may result in precipitation of the drug, depending on the final concentration of the drug and solvent. It has been suggested that precipitation of the relatively insoluble diazepam may account for the high (3.5%) incidence of thrombophlebitis that occurs when diazepam is given intravenously.

Other additives in formulations may give rise to subtle problems that are not immediately obvious. One diazepam injection contains 40% propylene glycol and 10% ethanol; it is buffered with sodium benzoate and benzoic acid and preserved with benzyl alcohol. Addition of this formulation to normal saline results in the formation of a precipitate; a precipitate also forms on addition of the diazepam solution to human plasma.

A graphical technique has been described to predict whether a solubilised drug system will become supersaturated and thus have the potential to precipitate. When a drug dissolved in a cosolvent system is diluted with water, both drug and cosolvent are diluted. The logarithm of the solubility of a drug in a cosolvent system generally increases linearly with the percentage of cosolvent present (Fig. 11.5a). On dilution, the drug concentration falls linearly with a fall in the percentage of cosolvent. The aim of the graphical method is to plot dilution curves and solubility curves on the same graph. This is achieved in Fig. 11.5b, where the dilution curves have been plotted semilogarithmically for three systems containing initially 1, 2 and 3 mg cm^{-3} of drug substance (plots I, II and III, respectively).

With solution III, dilution below about 30% cosolvent causes the system to be supersaturated; with solution II, below 20% cosolvent the solubility line and the dilution line touch. Only solutions containing 1 mg cm^{-3} can be diluted without precipitation.

11.3 Cation–anion interactions

The interaction between a large organic anion and an organic cation may result in the formation of a relatively insoluble precipitate. Complexation, precipitation or phase separation can occur in these circumstances, the product being affected by changes in ionic strength, temperature and pH. Examples of cation–anion interactions include those between procainamide and phenytoin sodium, procaine and thiopental sodium, and hydroxyzine hydrochloride and benzylpenicillin (Scheme 11.1). The nature of many of these interactions has not been studied in detail. In the absence of this it is necessary to predict possible incompatibilities from a knowledge of the physical properties of the drug and other components in the formulation. Sometimes, as when chlorpromazine and morphine injections are mixed, the incompatibility is

not due to an interaction between the two drugs but to drug–bactericide interaction; the chlorocresol contained in the morphine injection precipitates with the chlorpromazine, possibly by an anion–cation interaction. Nitrofurantoin sodium must be diluted prior to use with 5% dextrose or with sterile water for injection; alkyl *p*-hydroxybenzoates (parabens), phenol or cresol, all of which tend to precipitate the nitrofurantoin, must be absent.

Phase diagrams such as that shown in Fig. 11.6 are useful in determining regions of incompatibility and compatibility in cation–anion mixtures because admixture is not always contraindicated. The example shown here is for mixtures of disodium cromoglicate (DSCG, sodium cromoglicate) which is a di-anionic drug with a cationic surfactant, tetradecyldimethylammonium bromide (C$_{14}$BDAC). As can be seen, the interaction is strongly concentration-dependent. In some regions, below the line AB, the two ions coexist. Ion pairs (see below) form in the shaded region below AB. Above this solubility product line, turbidity occurs in the hatched region. On increasing the concentration of surfactant, the complex is solubilised so that the interaction is masked.

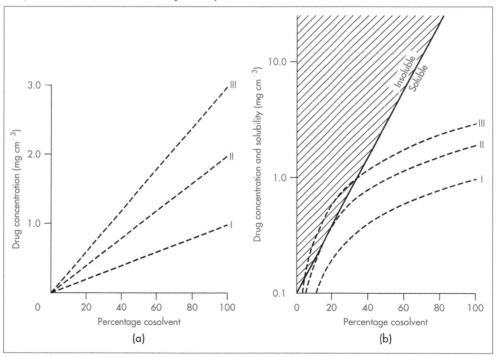

Figure 11.5 (a) Dilution profiles for three solutions (I, II and III) in pure cosolvent containing 1, 2 and 3 mg cm^{-3} drug, respectively. (b) Curves from (a) plotted on semilog scale along with typical solubility line.

Reproduced with permission from Yalkowsky SH, Valvani S. Precipitation of solubilized drugs due to injection or dilution. *Drug Intell Clin Pharm* 1977;11:417.

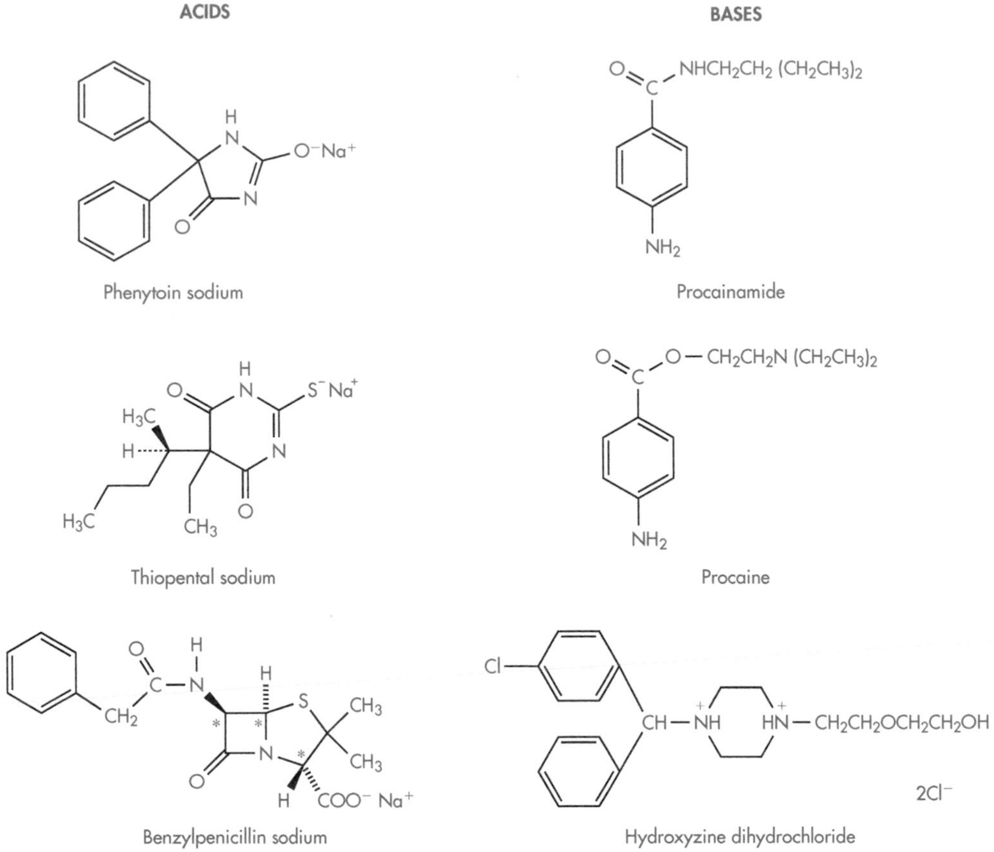

ACIDS
BASES
Phenytoin sodium
Procainamide
Thiopental sodium
Procaine
Benzylpenicillin sodium
Hydroxyzine dihydrochloride

Scheme 11.1

A
B
Solubilisation
Free ions
DSCG (mol dm⁻³)
C14BDAC (mol dm⁻³)

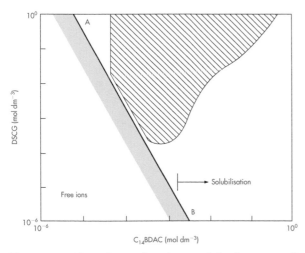

Figure 11.6 Phase diagram for mixtures of disodium cromoglicate (DSCG, sodium cromoglicate) and tetradecyldimethylammonium bromide ($C_{14}BDAC$).

Reproduced with permission from Tomlinson E. *Pharm Int* 1980;1:156–158.

The incompatibility of organic iodide contrast media and antihistaminic drugs (added to reduce anaphylactic reactions) is due to the acidity of the antihistamine solutions, resulting in the precipitation of the organic iodide.[5] One of the antihistamines, promethazine, reacted strongly with all the contrast media, probably because its solution had the lowest pH of the drugs studied. It is not only with IV fluids that such interactions may occur. Examples have been quoted of the inadvisable mixture of syrups; for example, immediate precipitation in a prescribed mixture of a syrup containing cloxacillin sodium and a syrup containing the bases codeine and promethazine. Precipitation was followed by a 20% loss in antibiotic activity in 5 hours and 99% loss in 5 days. The double-decomposition reactions involved are likely to be those shown in Fig. 11.7.

Complexes that form are not always fully active. A well-known example is the complex between neomycin sulfate and sodium lauryl sulfate that will form when Aqueous Cream BP is used as a vehicle for neomycin sulfate. Aqueous cream comprises 30% emulsifying ointment, which itself is a mixture of emulsifying wax

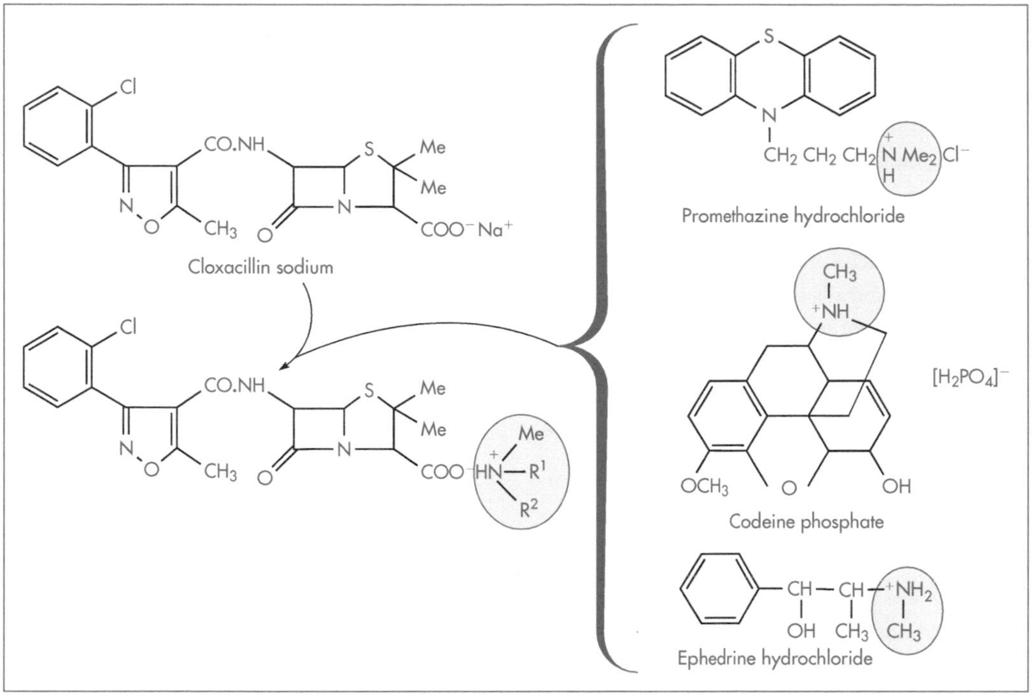

Figure 11.7 The interaction of cloxacillin sodium with promethazine hydrochloride, codeine phosphate and ephedrine hydrochloride.

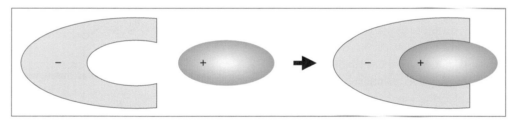

Figure 11.8 Representation of an organic ion-pair – the anion is shown here interacting with a cationic molecule of complementary shape (purely schematic), thus masking the exposure of the charge to the aqueous environment.

that contains 10% of sodium lauryl sulfate or a similar anionic surfactant.

Interactions are also not always visible. The formation of visible precipitates depends to a large extent on the insolubility of the two combining species in the particular mixture and the size to which the precipitated particles grow.

Interactions between drugs and ionic macromolecules are another potential source of problems. Heparin sodium and erythromycin lactobionate are contraindicated in admixture, as are heparin sodium and chlorpromazine hydrochloride or gentamicin sulfate. Tables of incompatibilities abound with such examples. Interference with the sulfate groups reduces the anticoagulant activity of heparin.

Ion-pair formation

Ion-pair formation may be responsible for the absorption of highly charged drugs such as the quaternary ammonium salts and sulfonic acid derivatives, the absorption of which is not explained by the pH-partition hypothesis. Ion pairs may be defined as neutral species formed by electrostatic attraction between oppositely charged ions in solution, which are often sufficiently lipophilic to dissolve in non-aqueous solvents. The formation of an ion pair (Fig. 11.8) results in the 'burying' of charges and alteration to the physical properties of the drug. Interactions between charged drug species and appropriate lipophilic ions of opposite charge may constitute a drug interaction and may occur *in vitro* or *in vivo*.

11.4 Polyions and drug solutions

The extensive clinical use of polyionic solutions for IV therapy means that drugs are frequently added to systems of a complex ionic nature. Reduction in the solubility of both weak electrolytes and non-electrolytes can occur through salting out, a phenomenon discussed in section 4.2.3.

Most physicochemically based drug interactions can take place in the body, or outside it, or during concomitant drug administration, so it is probably not profitable to consider them separately. Some interactions, such as complexation, which are probably more important *in vivo* than *in vitro,* are discussed below.

Clinical point

Sodium sulfadiazine and sulfafurazole diolamine in therapeutic doses (1 mg) added to 5% dextrose and 5% dextrose and saline solution have been found to be compatible, yet when added to commercial polyionic solutions (such as Abbott Ionosol B, Baxter electrolyte No. 2), both rapidly form heavy precipitates. pH and temperature are two vital parameters, but the pH effect is not simply a solubility-related phenomenon. Polyionic solutions of a lower initial pH (4.4–4.6) cause crystallisation of sulfafurazole at room temperature within 2.5 hours, the pH values of the admixtures being 5.65 and 5.75, respectively.

Other solutions with slightly higher initial pH levels (6.1–6.6) formed crystals only after preliminary cooling to 20°C at pH values from 4.25 to 4.90. If the temperature remains constant, the intensity of precipitation varies with the composition and initial pH of the solution used as a vehicle.[6]

11.5 Chelation

The term chelation (derived from the Greek *chele,* meaning lobster's claw) relates to the interaction between a metal atom or ion and another species, known as the *ligand,* by which a heteroatomic ring is formed. Chelation changes the physical and chemical

characteristics of both the metal ion and the ligand. It is simplest to consider the ligand as the electron-pair donor and the metal the electron-pair acceptor, the donation establishing a coordinate bond. Many chelating agents act in the form of anions that coordinate to a metal ion. For chelation to occur there must be at least two donor atoms capable of binding to the same metal ion, and ring formation must be sterically possible. For example, ethylenediamine (1,2-diaminoethane, $NH_2CH_2CH_2NH_2$) has two donor nitrogens and acts as a bidentate (two-toothed) ligand. When a drug forms a metal chelate, the solubility and absorption of both drug and metal ion may be affected, and drug chelation can lead to either increased or decreased absorption. Tetracyclines have similar chelating groups in their structure. Therapeutic chelators are used in syndromes where there is metal ion overload. Deferiprone (**I**) chelates iron. Ethylenediaminetetraacetic acid (EDTA) (**II**) as the monocalcium disodium salt is used in the treatment of lead poisoning.

Structure I Deferiprone, shown as chelate with iron

Structure II Ethylenediaminetetraacetic acid (EDTA)

Tetracyclines

Probably the most widely quoted example of complex formation leading to decreased drug absorption is that of tetracycline chelation with metal ions. Polyvalent cations such as Fe^{2+} and Mg^{2+}, and anions such as trichloracetate or phosphate, interfere with absorption in both model and real systems. Figure 11.9 shows the effect of a dose of 40 mg ferrous ion on serum levels following 300 mg of tetracycline. As can be seen from this figure, the nature of the iron salt ingested is important. Ferrous sulfate has the greatest inhibitory effect on tetracycline absorption, perhaps because it dissolves in water more quickly than organic iron compounds. The ability of the various iron compounds to liberate ferrous or ferric ions in the upper part of the gastrointestinal tract before tetracycline is absorbed would seem to be an essential step in the interaction. The order of activity of the different iron salts in the chelation process *in vivo* turns out to be the same as the order of the intestinal absorption of these iron compounds. All the active tetracyclines form stable chelates with Ca^{2+}, Mg^{2+} and Al^{3+}. The antibacterial action of the tetracyclines depends on their metal-binding activity, as their main site of action is on the ribosomes, which are rich in magnesium.

The tetracyclines have an avidity for divalent metals similar to that of glycine (**III**) but they have a greater affinity for the trivalent metals, with which they form 3 : 1 drug–metal chelates. Therapeutically active tetracyclines form 2 : 1 complexes with cupric, nickel and zinc ions while inactive analogues form only 1 : 1 complexes.

The structures of some tetracyclines are reproduced in Table 11.5, together with their pK_a values; from these data it should be possible to determine something of the relative affinities of the tetracyclines for metal ions. One piece of evidence relating to the site of chelation is that isochlortetracycline, which lacks the C-11, C-12 enolic system, does not chelate with Ca^{2+} ions.

Structure III The 1:1 copper-glycine chelate

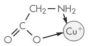

Clinical point

The complexing of tetracyclines with calcium poses a problem in paediatric medicine. Discoloration of teeth results from the formation of a coloured complex with the calcium in the teeth; the deposition of drug in the bones of growing babies can lead to problems in bone formation.[7]

Table 11.4 shows that there is no correlation between the binding capacity of a tetracycline with iron and that with calcium, suggesting different modes of complexation. The *in vitro* data are simpler to interpret: the serum levels are the result of two processes, the chelation of the tetracycline and the partitioning of the chelate. Clinical studies have shown that the absorption of doxycycline is not significantly affected by milk in conditions where the absorption of tetracycline itself is reduced.

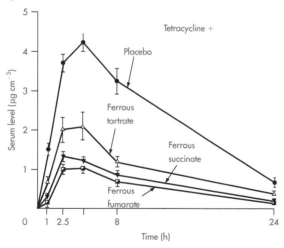

Figure 11.9 The effect of simultaneous ingestion of various iron salts (dose equivalent to 40 mg elemental iron) and tetracycline hydrochloride (500 mg) on serum levels of tetracycline (mean levels in 6 patients).

Reproduced from Neuvonen PJ, Turakka H. Inhibitory effect of various iron salts on the absorption of tetracycline in man. *Eur J Clin Pharmacol* 1974;7:357, with kind permission from Springer Science and Business Media.

Table 11.4 Relative calcium-binding capacities of tetracycline derivatives and decreases in serum levels after 200 mg ferrous sulfate

Tetracycline	Calcium binding[a] (%)	Decrease in serum concentration (%) after 200 mg ferrous sulfate
Demeclocycline	74.5	n.s. [b]
Chlortetracycline	52.7	n.s. [b]
Tetracycline	39.5	40–50
Methacycline	39.5	80–85
Oxytetracycline	36.0	50–60
Doxycycline	19–22	80–90

[a] Percentage of dissolved antibiotic (5 mg/50 cm³ H_2O) bound to calcium phosphate after overnight shaking. Reproduced from Osol A, Pratt R. *The United States Dispensatory*, 27th edn. Philadelphia, PA: Lippincott, p. 1155ff.
[b] n.s. = not studied.

The decreased aqueous solubility of chelates suggests increased lipophilicity but, in the case of the tetracycline chelates, precipitation would decrease the biological activity of the drug as it would be less available for transport across membranes; the larger molecular volume of the chelate would also prevent easy absorption in the intact form.

Complex formation of a coumarin derivative occurs between magnesium ions present in antacid formulations. In this case the formation of a more absorbable species is indicated, since plasma levels of bishydroxycoumarin are elevated in the presence of magnesium hydroxide but are unaffected by aluminium hydroxide; neither antacid influenced warfarin absorption.[8] A magnesium–bishydroxycoumarin chelate having the structure (IV) has been isolated. Adsorption may counteract a chelate-mediated increase in absorption, so the adsorptive properties of aluminium hydroxide may be responsible for the lack of effect of this antacid on the absorption of the

Table 11.5 Structures and pK_a values for some tetracyclines

	R¹	R²	R³	R⁴	pK_{a1}	pK_{a2}	pK_{a3}
Chlortetracycline	Cl	Me	OH	H	3.27	7.43	9.33
Oxytetracycline	H	Me	OH	OH	3.5	7.6	9.2
Tetracycline	H	Me	OH	H	3.33	7.7	9.5
Demeclocycline	Cl	H	OH	H	3.3	7.16	9.25
Doxycycline	H	Me	H	OH	3.4	7.7	9.7

Structure IV   Suggested form of the bishydroxycoumarin-Mg chelate

drug. Results are shown in Fig. 11.10. It has been suggested that the more rapid and complete absorption of warfarin makes it less susceptible to interactions of this type.[8]

Chelation of ciprofloxacin (**V**) by aluminium hydroxide and calcium carbonate reduces bioavailability, as seen in Fig. 11.11. Other quinolones (**VI–IX**) undoubtedly suffer the same fate.

Following treatment of acrodermatitis enteropathica with diiodohydroxyquinolone (**X**), the absorption and retention of dietary zinc and other trace metals have been found to be greater than in subjects not receiving the drug. Chelation of zinc and other trace metals by the drug could have resulted in the increased absorption from the intestinal lumen.

Desferrioxamine (as the mesylate) is used as a drug to sequester iron in iron poisoning or chronic iron overload; penicillamine is similarly used to aid the elimination of copper in Wilson disease. Chelation is also used for the safe delivery of toxic ions such as gadolinium (Gd^{3+}), which is used as a magnetic resonance imaging enhancing agent. One such preparation is gadobenic acid (**XI**), which is a gadolinium–benzyloxypropionic tetraacetate (BOPTA) (**XIa**) octodentate chelate.

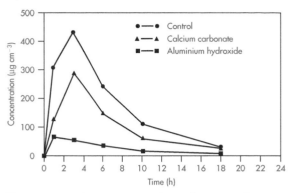

Figure 11.11 Concentrations of ciprofloxacin in the urine following administration of 50 mg to 12 healthy volunteers in a three-way randomised crossover design by RW Frost *et al.* (*Antimicrob Agents Chemother* 1992;36:830), who write: '*The precise conditions required for ciprofloxacin to form chelate complexes with other cations have not been fully elucidated, but the carboxyl group seems to be the most likely site for chelation. Thus, the gastric pH would need to be elevated sufficiently to ionise the carboxyl group. Therefore, the lack of interaction with dairy products might be attributable to a gastric pH that was not elevated sufficiently to ionise the carboxyl group. Alternatively, it could be due to a decrease in the availability of calcium to chelate ciprofloxacin because of a lipid barrier.*'

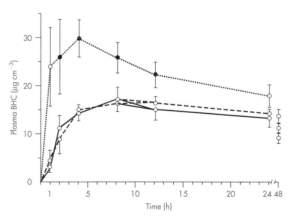

Figure 11.10 Plasma levels of bishydroxycoumarin (BHC), also known as dicoumarol, in 6 subjects after a 300 mg oral dose with water (solid line), magnesium hydroxide (dotted line) or aluminium hydroxide (dashed line). Closed data points represent a significant difference from control.

Reproduced with permission from Ambre JJ, Fischer LF. Effect of coadministration of aluminium and magnesium hydroxides on absorption of anticoagulants in man. *Clin Pharm Ther* 1973;14:231–237.

Structure V Ciprofloxacin

Structure VI Nalidixic acid

Structure VII Ofloxacin

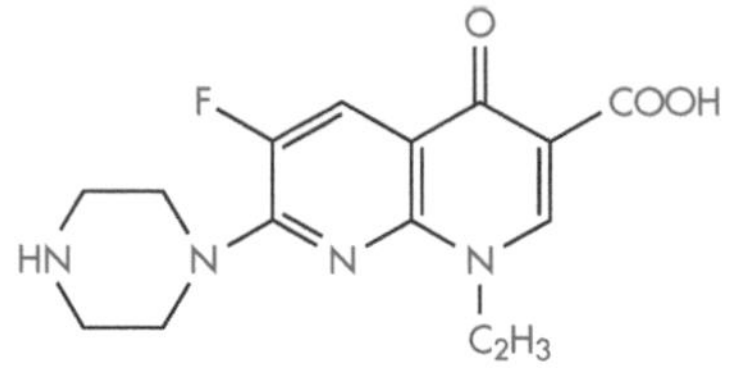

Structure VIII Enoxacin

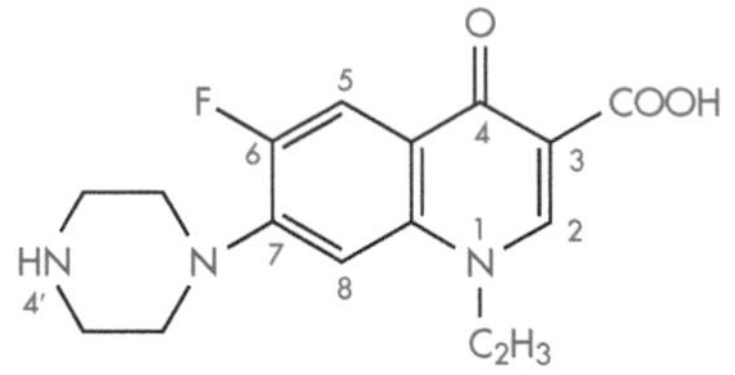

Structure IX Norfloxacin

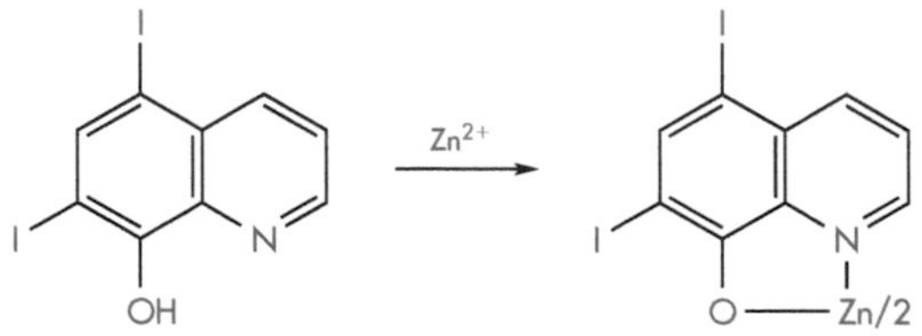

5, 7 - diiodo-8-hydroxyquinoline

Structure X Suggested form of the chelate of zinc-diiodo-hydroxyquinolone

11.6 Other complexes

Molecular complexes of many types may be observed in systems containing two or more drug molecules.

Generally, association follows from attractive interactions (hydrophobic, electrostatic or charge transfer interactions) between two molecules. In the charge transfer system one component is usually an aromatic compound; the second may be a saturated moiety containing an electron lone pair (donor atom) or a weakly acidic hydrogen (acceptor atom). The interaction therefore takes place between electron-rich donors and electron-poor acceptors. Interactions between aromatic rings in which there is a parallel overlap of π-systems fall into this category, as in the following example involving nicotinamide (acceptor) and the indole moiety of tryptophan (donor) (**XII**).

The imidazole moiety (**XIII**) is involved in many interactions; it is regarded as aromatic and the molecule is planar. Not surprisingly, caffeine (**XIV**) and theophylline (**XV**) are frequently implicated in interactions with aromatic species. Caffeine increases the solubility of not only ergotamine but also that of benzoic acid. The marked difference in the solubilising properties of caffeine and dimethyluracil (**XVI**) towards substances such as benzoic acid suggests that the imidazole ring of the xanthine nucleus is the portion involved in the interaction. In the main, 1 : 1 complexes are formed but 2 : 1 drug–caffeine complexes may also be found. Hydrophobic interactions are also implicated in the interaction, since caffeine has a greater solubilising capacity than theophylline, which, as can be seen, lacks the NCH_3 group in the imidazole nucleus.

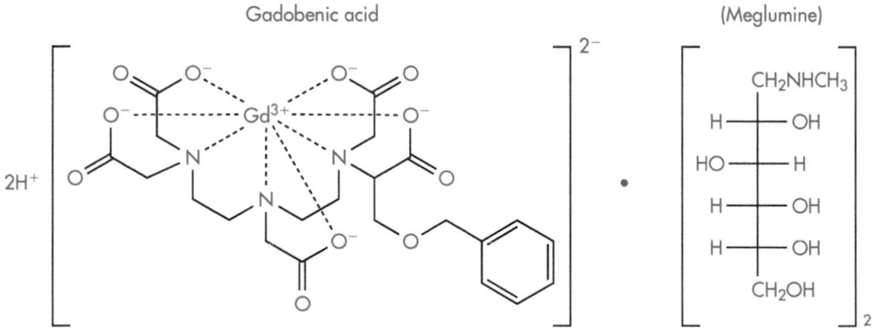

Structure XI Gadobenic acid as the meglumine salt

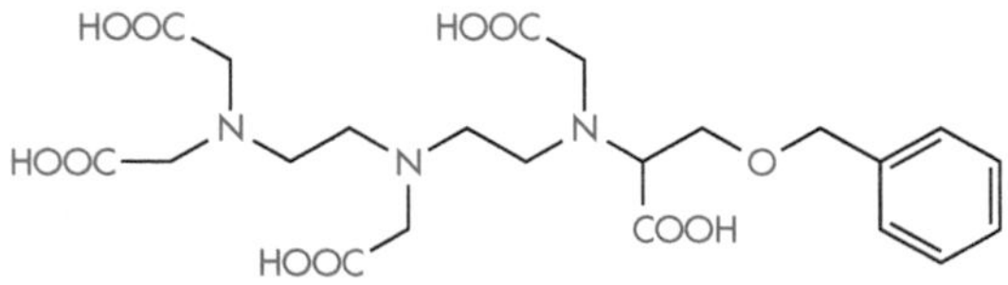

Structure XIa Benzyloxypropionic tetraacetate (BOPTA)

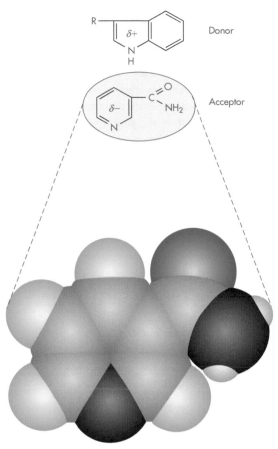

Structure XII Example of donor–acceptor interaction between tryptophan (donor) and nicotinamide

Structure XIII Imidazole

can accept protons (moderately strong base)

can lose proton (weakly acidic)

Structure XIV Caffeine

Structure XV Theophylline

Structure XVI Dimethyluracil

11.6.1 Interaction of drugs with cyclodextrins

Compounds that have interior cavities large enough to incarcerate organic 'guest' molecules have been named molecular container compounds.

Over the last decade there has been growing interest in the interaction of drugs with one group of container compounds, the β-cyclodextrins (cyclic D-glucose oligomers) and their now myriad derivatives. The cyclodextrin molecules have cyclic structures with internal diameters of 0.6–1 nm (see section 4.6). The interior cavity of the cyclodextrin ring is hydrophobic in nature and binds a hydrophobic portion of the 'guest' molecule, usually forming a 1 : 1 complex. The possible structure of β-cyclodextrin complexes of aspirin is shown in Fig. 11.12.

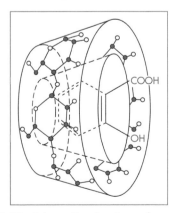

Figure 11.12 Schematic drawing of an aspirin–β-cyclodextrin complex.

Reproduced from Loftsson T, Masson M. Cyclodextrins in topical drug formulations: theory and practice. *Int J Pharm* 2001;225:15–30. Copyright Elsevier 2001.

Inclusion of some drugs (including peptides) into cyclodextrins increases their solubility, chemical stability and absorption. The solubilising effect of β-cyclodextrin on flufenamic acid suggests that a 1 : 1 complex is formed in aqueous solution. A relationship between the oil/water partition coefficient of a drug and its tendency to form inclusion complexes has generally been found.[9] This indicates that the hydrophobic cavity of the cyclodextrin 'eye' is more attractive to lipophilic guest molecules. The formation constants for mefenamic acid were, however, lower than expected from the Me or Cl *ortho* substituent. α-Cyclodextrin showed no appreciable interaction with the anti-inflammatory acids, mefenamic acid and meclofenamic acid, suggesting that its cavity is not large enough to contain the drug molecules.[10]

The altered environment of the drug molecules leads to changes in stability. The cyclodextrins catalyse a number of chemical reactions, such as hydrolysis, oxidation and decarboxylation. Although interactions between drugs and cyclodextrins have been mostly the result of deliberate attempts to modify the behaviour or properties of the drug, they are included here to illustrate an additional mode of interaction with other components that may well occur inside the body as well as in the laboratory.

Sugammadex: a beneficial interaction with anaesthetics

Three of the widely used general anaesthetics, the neuromuscular blocking agents *cis*-atracurium, vecuronium and rocuronium, have durations of action of around 37–81 minutes, 36–137 minutes and 33–119 minutes respectively, according to one survey. Such anaesthetics may require reversal depending on the surgical procedures being undertaken. Atracurium was designed to have a short duration of action, but vecuronium and rocuronium have significantly longer actions. These latter are distinguished from atracurium in having their –N-onium groups separated by a steroidal backbone, as can be seen from their structures, and they interact in the blood with sugammadex when it is administered IV. This complex renders them inactive, thus reversing their action. This is a good example of a beneficial interaction. Sugammadex is a γ-cyclodextrin derivative which effectively acts as an antagonist[11] (Fig. 11.13) and is therefore a modified

excipient used therapeutically. The complex is excreted mainly in the urine.

According to Chemistry Beta (chemistry.stackexchange.com): 'Sugammadex binds rocuronium really tightly. The reason for this is straightforward – lipophilic interactions with the inner cavity of the cyclodextrin, which is the perfect size ... The negatively charged carboxylate groups lock into place with the protonated amine'.

Clearly sugammadex has affinities with other anaesthetic molecules of similar dimensions (Fig. 11.14) such as vecuronium, but the affinity for vecuronium is 2.5 times lower. It does not interact with atracurium which, as can be seen from its structure, has bulky benzyl-isoquinolinium groups that cannot be accommodated in the cavity of this particular cyclodextrin.

Clinical point

Levels of atracurium will not be changed by administration of sugammadex, but vecuronium levels are reduced. Although its affinity for sugammadex is weaker, it is itself seven times more potent than rocuronium, so that fewer molecules are present. Vecuronium blockage can thus be successfully achieved. The possibilities of forming complexes with other steroidal molecules such as aldosterone and glucocorticoids have been found to be insignificant.

11.6.2 Ion-exchange interactions

Ion-exchange resins are now being used medicinally and as systems for modified release of drugs (Fig. 11.15). Colestyramine and colestipol are insoluble quaternary ammonium anion-exchange resins that, when administered orally, bind bile acids and increase their elimination because the high-molecular-weight complex is not absorbed. As bile acids are converted *in vivo* into cholesterol, colestyramine is used as a hypocholesteraemic agent. When given to patients receiving other drugs as well, the resin would conceivably bind anionic compounds and reduce their absorption. Phenylbutazone (**XVII**), warfarin (**XVIII**),

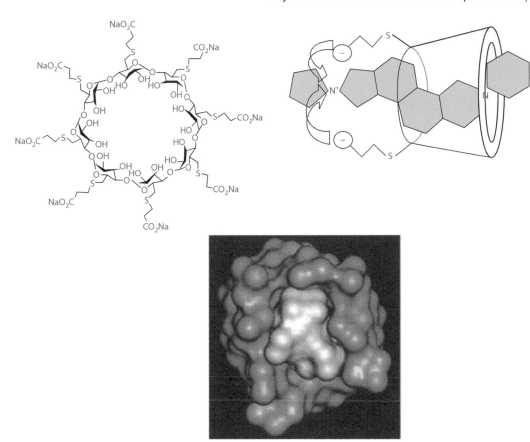

Figure 11.13 (Top left) Sugammadex structure with a cavity of 1.1 nm; (top right) a schematic view of the interaction of sugammadex with the steroidal neuromuscular-blocking agent, rocuronium and (below) a space-filling model of the sugammadex with rocuronium, this being reproduced with permission from Raft J *et al.* 51° *Congrès National d'Anésthesie et de Réanimation*. Elsevier-Masson; 2009.

Structure XVII   Phenylbutazone

Structure XVIII   Warfarin

Structure XIX   Chlorothiazide

chlorothiazide (**XIX**) and hydrochlorothiazide are bound strongly to the resin *in vitro*.

Colestyramine had no effect in animal experiments on the blood levels of these drugs. However, 95% of both warfarin and phenylbutazone were bound and peak blood levels of the latter were halved, although the same total amount was eventually absorbed. A single dose of resin did not significantly reduce the pharmacological effect of warfarin. Nevertheless, it is prudent to administer drugs orally a short time before colestyramine to preclude delay in the action of the

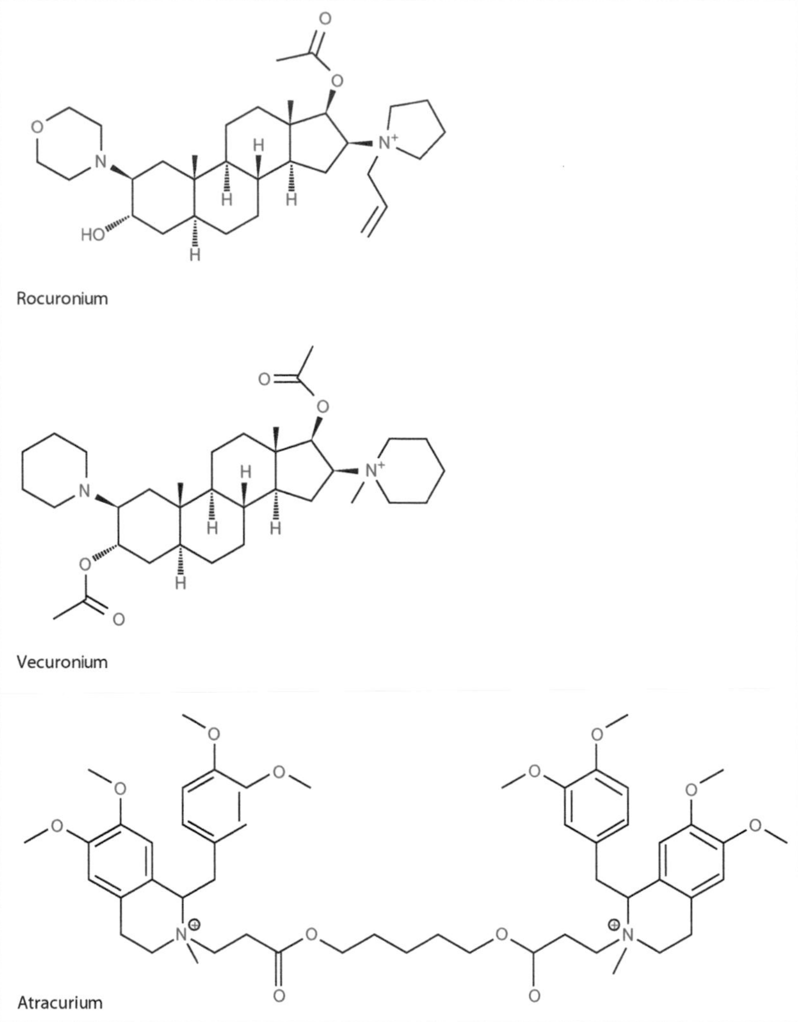

Figure 11.14 Neuromuscular blocking agents: rocuronium, vecuronium and atracurium.

drug through adsorption and slow leaching. Table 11.6 shows the effect of very high resin levels on the serum

Table 11.6 The effect of colestyramine administration on sodium fusidate levels

Resin dose (mg kg^{-1})	Mean serum concentration (µg cm^{-3})
0	3.7
72	2.5
215	1.9
356	0.8

Reproduced from Johns WH, Bates TR. Drug-cholestyramine interactions. II. Influence of cholestyramine on GI absorption of sodium fusidate. *J Pharm Sci* 1972;61:735. Copyright Wiley-VCH Verlag GmbH & Co. KGaA. Reproduced with permission.

concentration of sodium fusidate. Since the binding is pH-dependent (Table 11.7), an ion-exchange resin can bind any drug with an appropriate charge under pH conditions in which both species are ionised. Decreased drug absorption caused by colestyramine or colestipol in the main has been reported with thyroxine, aspirin, phenprocoumon, warfarin, chlorothiazide, cardiac glycosides and ferrous sulfate as a consequence of binding. Absorption of vitamin K and vitamin B$_{12}$ is decreased indirectly by competition of the resin for binding sites on intrinsic factor molecules.[12,13]

The influence of buffer ions on the binding of the drug in Table 11.7 indicates one of the problems of making *in vitro* measurements and attempting to assess the biological significance of the results. Binding

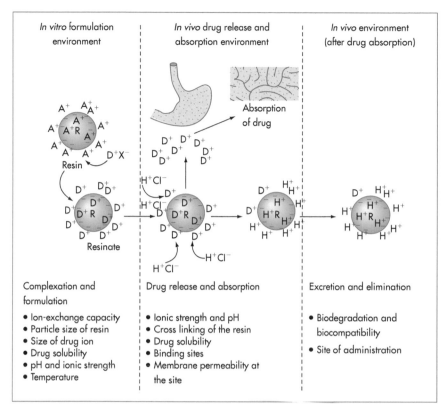

Figure 11.15 The basis of the ion-exchange process in drug delivery with factors affecting the therapeutic efficacy of the system at each stage. R and a blue circle represent resin; a minus sign depicts the integral ion of the resin, and A⁺ is the counterion. D is the drug ion, X⁻ is the ion associated with drug cation and H⁺Cl⁻ is hydrochloric acid. Ions inside and outside the resin indicate ions adsorbed at the surface, as well as in the interior, of the resin structure.

Reproduced from Anand V *et al. Drug Discov Today* 2001;6:905–915.

Table 11.7 Binding of acetylsalicylic acid (aspirin) *in vitro* to colestyramine

	Percentage binding			
	pH 2	pH 3	pH 5	pH 7.5
Buffer	5	–	6	6
Water	51	95	98	97

Reproduced from Halin K-J *et al.* Effect of cholestyramine on the gastrointestinal absorption of phenprocoumon and acetylosalicylic acid in man. *Eur J Clin Pharmacol* 1972;4:142, with kind permission from Springer Science and Business Media.

Structure XX Lincomycin (R = OH) and clindamycin (R = Cl)

of cefalexin, clindamycin (**XX**) and the components of co-trimoxazole to colestyramine has been measured; *in vivo* absorption of these substances in the presence of the resin is delayed and somewhat reduced, but the changed pattern of absorption is unlikely to affect therapeutic efficacy, except perhaps with cefalexin, where it is more pronounced.

Colestilan

A quite recent introduction is the product colestilan, a crosslinked copolymer of 2-methylimidazole and epichlorohydrin (**XXI**) which acts as an anion exchanger resin with an affinity for phosphate. It binds the ions in the gut, removing them from the enterohepatic circulation. Colestilan is not absorbed from the gut. It is used in the treatment of hyperphosphataemia in adult patients with chronic kidney disease receiving haemodialysis or peritoneal dialysis.

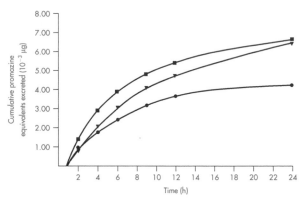

Structure XXI Colestilan

11.7 Adsorption of drugs

The process of adsorption and its medical and pharmaceutical applications have been dealt with in some detail in Chapter 5. The use of adsorbents to remove noxious substances from the lumen of the gut is considered there. Adsorbents generally are nonspecific so will adsorb nutrients, drugs and enzymes when given orally. It is not uncommon for adsorbents to be administered in combination with various drugs and it becomes a matter of practical importance to determine the extent to which adsorbents will interfere with the absorption of the drug substance from the gastrointestinal tract.

Several consequences of adsorption are possible. If the drug remains adsorbed until the preparation reaches the general area of the absorption site, the concentration of the drug presented to the absorbing surfaces will be much reduced. The driving force for absorption would then be reduced, resulting in a slower rate of absorption. During the course of absorption of the drug, it is probable that the adsorbate will dissociate in an attempt to re-establish equilibrium with drug in its immediate environment, particularly if there is competition for absorption sites from other substances in the gastrointestinal tract. As a consequence, the concentration of free drug in solution would be maintained at a low level and the absorption rate would be reduced. Alternatively, the release of drug from the adsorbent might be complete before reaching the absorption site, possibly hastened by the presence of electrolytes in the gastrointestinal tract, in which case absorption rates would be virtually identical to those in the absence of adsorbent. Figure 11.16 shows the reduced amounts of promazine excreted in the urine when the promazine was administered with activated charcoal – evidence of a reduced absorption rate of this drug in this situation.

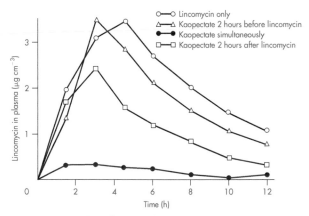

Figure 11.16 Cumulative amounts of promazine equivalents excreted in the urine following administration of various dosage forms to humans: ■, promazine in simple aqueous solution; ▼, promazine plus activated attapulgite; ●, promazine plus activated charcoal.

Reproduced from Sorby DL. Effect of adsorbents on drug absorption. I. Modification of promazine absorption by activated attapulgite and activated charcoal. *J Pharm Sci* 1965;54:677. Copyright Wiley-VCH Verlag GmbH & Co. KGaA. Reproduced with permission.

Figure 11.17 The influence of Kaopectate (kaolin and pectinic acid) on the absorption of lincomycin in humans after oral application; note the decrease in plasma levels caused by the simultaneous administration of the absorbent.

Reproduced with permission from Wagner JG. Design and data analysis of biopharmaceutical studies in man. *Can J Pharm Sci* 1966;1:55.

A further example is the delayed absorption of lincomycin (**XX**) when administered with kaolin and pectinic acid (Kaopectate) (Fig. 11.17). The dramatic effect of several antacids on the adsorption of digoxin from elixirs is shown in Fig. 11.18. In view of the relatively low doses of these glycosides, these adsorption effects are likely to impair digoxin bioavailability.

If the possibility of adsorption on to formulation ingredients is not kept in mind, erroneous conclusions may be drawn from bioavailability studies, as was the case in the suspected *in vivo* interaction between

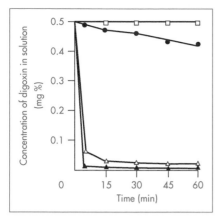

Figure 11.18 Adsorption of digoxin from Lanoxin paediatric elixir at 37 ± 0.1°C by: ●, Aluminium Hydroxide Gel BP (10% v/v); △, Magnesium Trisilicate Mixture BPC (10% v/v); ▲, Gelusil suspension (10% v/v); □, Lanoxin elixir diluted 1 : 10 with water.

Reproduced from Khalil SAH. The uptake of digoxin and digitoxin by some antacids. *J Pharm Pharmacol* 1974;26:961. Copyright Wiley-VCH Verlag GmbH & Co. KGaA. Reproduced with permission.

p-aminosalicylic acid (PAS) and rifampicin. It was thought that PAS impaired the intestinal absorption of rifampicin, reducing its serum levels to about half those occurring when it was administered by itself (Fig. 11.19). It was later found that bentonite, a naturally occurring mineral (montmorillonite), consisting chiefly of hydrated aluminium silicate, present in the PAS granules was adsorbing the antibiotic and delaying its absorption[14] (Fig. 11.19). It can readily be seen how the initial erroneous conclusion was drawn.

Loss of activity of preservatives can arise from adsorption on to solids commonly used as medicaments. Benzoic acid, for example, can be adsorbed to the extent of 94% by sulfadimidine. Adsorption can be suppressed, however, with hydrophilic polymers. In solid-dosage forms, talc, a commonly used tablet lubricant, has been reported to adsorb cyanocobalamin and consequently to interfere with intestinal absorption of this vitamin.

11.7.1 Protein and peptide adsorption

The pharmaceutical properties of peptides and proteins are discussed in Chapter 13. Adsorption can be a problem because of the amphipathic nature of many peptides, and becomes pharmaceutically important when they are present in low concentrations in solution. The adsorption of peptides on to glass has been ascribed to bonding between their amino groups and the silanol groups of the glass. A decapeptide derivative of LHRH, the natural luteinising hormone-releasing hormone, has two basic amino groups posi-

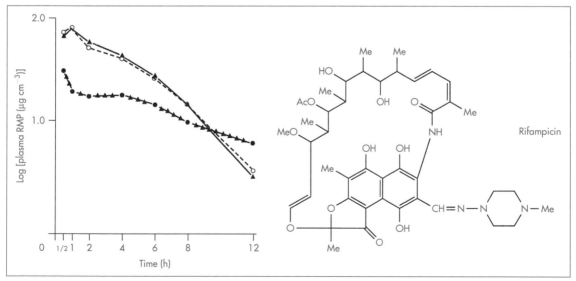

Figure 11.19 Plasma concentrations of rifampicin (RMP) after oral administration in solution (10 mg kg^{-1}) given alone (▲), with *p*-aminosalicyclic acid (PAS) granules (●) or with Na-PAS tablets (○); mean values (*n* = 6 patients) are indicated.

Reproduced from Boman G *et al*. Mechanism of the inhibitory effect of PAS [*p*-aminosalicylic acid] granules on the absorption of rifampicin. Adsorption of rifampicin by an excipient, bentonite. *Eur J Clin Pharm* 1975;8:293–299, with kind permission from Springer Science and Business Media.

tively charged at low pH, providing an opportunity for binding to silanol groups.[15] Siliconisation of the glass did not inhibit adsorption completely, suggesting that ionic binding was not the only mechanism of interaction. Phosphate buffer at 0.1 mol dm^{-3} concentration and acetate ions at 0.16 mol dm^{-3} concentration (both at pH 5) were most effective in preventing adsorption.

11.7.2 Protein aggregation and interactions

As Bee and co-authors discuss,[16] 'proteins can aggregate during processing, shipping, storage and delivery to the patient. Formulation conditions are chosen to maximise protein stability over its shelf-life. However, even thermodynamically and colloidally stable proteins may aggregate after interaction with the container-closure system, container leachates, or particulate contaminants because the stability with respect to surfaces may involve different physical processes than those that determine stability in bulk solution'. We can classify at least some of these adverse events as incompatibilities and interactions. The following are listed by Bee *et al.*[16]:

- nucleation of the aggregation of recombinant human platelet-activating factor acetylhydrolase has been attributed to the presence of silica nanoparticles from glass containers
- Teflon as the cause aggregation of insulin[17]
- silicone rubber delivery tubing decreasing the activity of interleukin-2 by 97%[18]
- silicone oil syringe lubricant inducing aggregation of several model proteins[19]
- leachates from tungsten causing protein precipitation
- stainless-steel particles shed from a filler pump in the laboratory environment caused aggregation of a monoclonal antibody
- Teflon containers fostering aggregation of an IgG$_2$ during freeze thawing.

Protein aggregation in ambulatory pumps can be serious: not only can aggregation reduce the biological activity of macromolecules, but the aggregates can cause blockage of needles. There are several mechanisms of protein aggregation, but the two most relevant to the present chapter are nucleation-controlled aggre-

gation and surface-induced aggregation.[20] In the first, the native monomer interacts with a nucleus and adsorbs on to the nucleus, often with partial unfolding; this can lead to growth and visible precipitation. In the latter mechanism, the native monomer adsorbs on to the surface of containers or closures and partly unfolds; this can trigger growth through aggregation.

11.8 Drug interactions with plastics

In Chapter 7 we discussed the adsorption of insulin on to glass and plastic materials used in syringes and giving sets. The plastic tubes and connections used in IV containers and giving sets can adsorb or absorb a number of drugs (Fig. 11.20), leading to significant losses in some cases. Drugs that show a significant loss when exposed to plastic, in particular poly(vinyl chloride) (PVC), include insulin, glyceryl trinitrate, diazepam, chlormethiazole, vitamin A acetate, isosorbide dinitrate and a miscellaneous group of drugs such as phenothiazines, hydralazine hydrochloride and thiopental sodium.

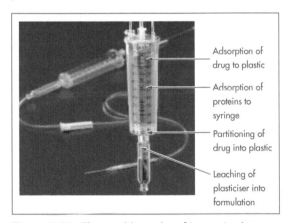

Adsorption of drug to plastic

Adsorption of proteins to syringe

Partitioning of drug into plastic

Leaching of plasticiser into formulation

Figure 11.20 The possible modes of interaction between a drug formulation and the plastic of a giving set.

A theoretical treatment to account for the loss of glyceryl trinitrate from solution to plastic containers has been developed[21] (Derivation Box 11A).

Some idea of the rate and extent of disappearance of warfarin sodium from PVC infusion bags can be gained from Fig. 11.21. The marked effect of pH is seen. Losses can obviously be significant. When medazepam is present at an initial concentration of

40 μg cm^{-3} in 100 cm^3 normal saline stored in similar bags, a 76% loss of the drug occurs in 8 hours at 22°C (Table 11.8).[22]

Preservatives such as the methyl and propyl parabens present in formulations can be sorbed into rubber and plastic membranes and closures, thus leading to

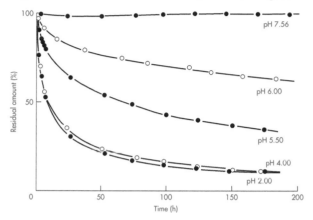

Figure 11.21 Disappearance of warfarin sodium from aqueous buffered solutions stored in 100 cm^{-3} poly(vinyl) chloride infusion bags at room temperature.

Reproduced with permission from Illum L, Bundgaard H. Sorption of drugs by plastic infusion bags. *Int J Pharm* 1982;10:339–351. Copyright Elsevier 1982.

Table 11.8 Loss of drugs from normal saline solutions in poly(vinyl chloride) (PVC) bags stored at 22°C for 8 hours

Drug	Initial solute conc. (μg cm^{-3})	% loss	
		PVC (100 cm^3)	PVC (500 cm^3)
Diazepam	40	60	31
	120	58	31
Medazepam	40	76	–
Oxazepam	40	22	12
Nitrazepam	40	15	10
Warfarin sodium[a]	20	49	–
Warfarin sodium	20	29	–
Glyceryl trinitrate	200	54	–
Thiopental sodium[b]	30	25	–
Pentobarbital sodium	30	0	0
Hydrocortisone acetate	20	0	0

Reproduced from Illum L, Bundgaard H. Sorption of drugs by plastic infusion bags. *Int J Pharm* 1982;10:339–351. Copyright Elsevier 1982.
[a] At pH 2 and pH 4.
[b] At pH 4.0 and pH 7.2.

decreased levels of preservative and, in the extreme, loss of preservative activity.

11.9 Protein binding

This is a topic that requires a chapter to itself for full coverage. Here we have space only for a treatment of mechanisms of protein binding that might enable readers to recognise molecules likely to be protein-bound. High levels of protein binding alter the biological properties of the drug as free drug concentrations are reduced. The bound drug assumes the diffusional and other transport characteristics of the protein molecule. In cases where drug is highly protein-bound (around 90%), small changes in binding lead to drastic changes in the levels of free drug in the body. If a drug is 95% bound, 5% is free. Reduction of binding to 90% by, for example, displacement by a second drug doubles the level of free drug. Such changes are not evident when binding is of a low order.

Most drugs bind to a limited number of sites on the albumin molecule. Binding to plasma albumin is generally easily reversible, so that drug molecules bound to albumin will be released as the level of free drug in the blood declines. Drugs bound to albumin (or other proteins) are attached to a unit too large to be transported across membranes. They are thus prevented from reacting with receptors or from entering the sites of drug metabolism or drug elimination until they dissociate from the protein.

Plasma albumin consists of a single polypeptide chain of molecular weight 67 000 ± 2000 Da. Human albumin contains between 569 and 613 amino acid residues. It is a globular molecule with a diameter of 5.6 nm (calculated assuming the molecule to be an anhydrous sphere). With an isoelectric point of 4.9, albumin has a net negative charge at pH 7.4, but it is amphoteric and capable of binding acidic and basic drugs. Subtle structural changes can occur on the binding of small molecules. Fatty-acid binding produces a volume increase and a decrease in the axial ratio. This is due primarily to non-polar inter-action between the hydrocarbon tail of the fatty-acid molecule and the binding site, and reflects the adaptability of the albumin molecule. When a hydrophobic chain penetrates into the interior of the globular albumin molecule, the helices of the protein separate,

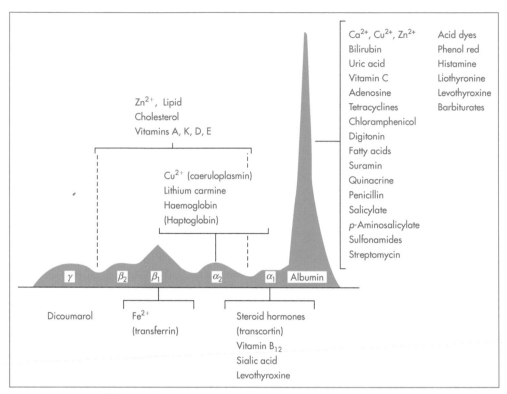

Figure 11.22 Interactions of drugs and chemicals with plasma proteins; plasma proteins are depicted according to their relative amounts.

Modified from Putnam FW. In: Neurath H (ed.) *The Proteins*, 2nd edn, vol. 3. New York: Academic Press; 1965.

producing a small change in the tertiary structure of the protein.

What are the binding sites? Organic anions are thought to bind to a site containing the amino acid sequence Lys-Ala-Try-Ala-Val-Ala-Arg. The five non-polar side-chains of these residues form a hydrophobic 'pool'. A cationic group is present at each end. It has been proposed that the ε-amino group of lysine is the point of attachment for anionic drugs. Albumin is, however, capable of binding molecules that are not ionised at all, such as cortisone or chloramphenicol. Acidic drugs such as phenylbutazone, indometacin and the salicylates may establish primary contact with the albumin by electrostatic interactions, but the bond can be strengthened by hydrophobic interactions. The dual interaction would therefore limit the number of possible binding sites for anionic organic drugs. In spite of electrostatic interactions, a number of drugs bind to albumin according to their degree of lipophilicity. Evidence for the importance of the hydrophobic interaction has been obtained from studies of the binding of phenol derivatives, which depends mainly on the hydrophobic character of the substituent, the phenolic hydroxyl group playing no significant role in the binding process. Similarly, penicillin derivatives and phenothiazines bind in a manner that depends on the hydrophobic characteristics of side-chains. It has been concluded that binding to albumin is a process comparable to partitioning of drug molecules from a water phase to a non-polar phase. The hydrophobic sites are not necessarily 'preformed'. Fatty acids and warfarin are both capable of inducing conformational changes that result in the formation of hydrophobic 'pools' in the protein.

Plasma proteins other than albumin may also be involved in binding; examples of such interactions are shown in Fig. 11.22. Blood plasma normally contains on average about 6.72 g of protein per 100 cm³, the protein comprising 4.0 g of albumin, 2.3 g of globulins and 0.24 g of fibrinogen. Although albumin is the main binding protein, dicoumarol is also bound to β- and γ-globulins, and certain steroid hormones are specifically and preferentially bound to particular globulin fractions.

If protein binding is assumed to be an adsorption process obeying the law of mass action, then the following equations can be derived (Derivation Box 11B) for the number of moles of drug, r, bound to the protein in a system,

$$r = \frac{nKD_f}{1 + KD_f} \tag{11.3}$$

or

$$\frac{1}{r} = \frac{1}{n} + \frac{1}{nKD_f} \tag{11.4}$$

where K is the equilibrium constant, D_f is the molar concentration of unbound drug and n is the number of binding sites per protein molecule.

Protein-binding results are often quoted as the fraction of drug bound, β. This fraction varies generally with the concentration of both drug and protein, as shown in equation (11.5), which relates β with n, K and concentration:

$$\beta = \frac{1}{1 + D_f/(nP_t) + 1/(nKP_t)} \tag{11.5}$$

where P_t is the total molar concentration of protein.

11.9.1 Thermodynamics of protein binding

Estimation of the thermodynamic parameters of binding allows interpretation of the mechanisms of interaction. Table 11.9 gives the thermodynamic parameters of binding of a number of agents to bovine serum albumin. The negative value of ΔG implies that binding is spontaneous. ΔH is negative, signifying an exothermic process and a reduction in the strength of the association as temperature increases. ΔS is positive, most likely signifying loss of structured water on binding. A diagrammatic representation of this last process is shown in Fig. 11.23. This diagram shows the change in the ordered water in the hydrophobic cavity of the albumin and around the non-polar portion of the drug. The loss of the structured water gives rise to the positive entropy change, which contributes to a negative free-energy change.

11.9.2 Lipophilicity and protein binding

Given the data in Table 11.9 it is not surprising to find that the extent of protein binding of many drugs is a linear function of their partition coefficient P (or log P).

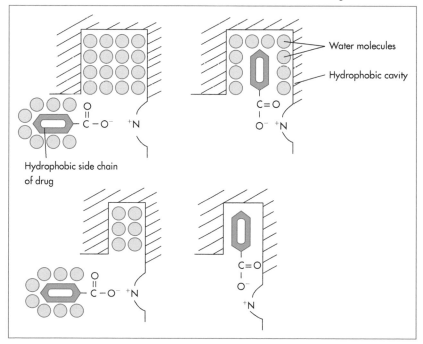

Figure 11.23 Electrostatic contact and hydrophobic binding of a molecular model with anionic and hydrophobic properties.
Reproduced with permission from Hasseblatt A. Interactions of drugs at plasma protein binding sites. *Proc Eur Soc Study Drug Toxic* 1972;13:89.

Table 11.9 Thermodynamic parameters of binding of drugs to bovine serum albumin

Drug	Percentage bound	ΔG (kJ mol^{-1}) at 22 °C	ΔH (kJ mol^{-1})	ΔS (J mol^{-1} K^{-1})
Aminopyrine (aminophenazone)	24.7	−17.7	−5.19	+42.2
Antipyrine (phenazone)	21.4	−17.1	−4.98	+41.0
4-Aminoantipyrine	22.7	−17.4	−5.27	+41.0
Phenylbutazone	84.6	−28.9	−6.1	+77.4
Oxyphenylbutazone	80.3	−27.4	−5.90	+73.2

Reproduced with permission from Ozeki S, Tejima K. Drug interaction II. Binding of some pyrazolidine derivates to bovine serum albumin. *Chem Pharm Bull* 1974;22:1297.

A linear equation of the form log(percentage bound/percentage free) = 0.5 log P − 0.665 has been found to be applicable to serum binding of penicillins. Although there may be an electrostatic component to the interaction, the binding increases with the degree of lipophilicity, suggesting, as is often the case, that more than one binding interaction is in force.

 Clinical point

Binding to protein outside of the plasma may determine the characteristics of drug action or transport. Muscle protein may bind drugs such as digoxin and so act as a depot. Differences in the bioavailability of two antibiotics following intramuscular administration have been ascribed to differences in protein binding. Dicloxacillin, 95% bound to protein, is absorbed more slowly from muscle than ampicillin, which is bound only to the extent of 20%.

Drug binding often changes with drug concentration and with protein concentration. On increasing the drug/protein ratio, saturation of some sites can occur and there may be a decrease in binding (as indicated by total percentage). Hence the importance of determining binding at realistic albumin concentrations (about 40 g dm^{-3}). There may be more than one binding site for a drug.

In determining the pharmacological importance of protein binding, several factors have to be considered. If drug molecules not bound to plasma protein are freely distributed throughout the body, on leaving the blood they enter a volume 13 times as large as the plasma volume. Entry into the cerebrospinal fluid (CSF) depends on the concentration of free, diffusible drug in the plasma. Sulfanilamide enters CSF faster than sulfamethoxypyridazine because less is bound to serum albumin. Such binding factors may override the intrinsic lipophilicities, which in some cases may suggest a different order of penetration from that observed.

When binding occurs with high affinity and the total amount of drug in the body is low, drug will be present almost exclusively in the plasma. Drugs with lower association constants ($K \approx 10^6$ or 10^7) will be distributed more in the body water spaces. When the number of available binding sites is reduced by a second drug, it will appear as if there has been an increase in overall drug concentration.

Although drugs are predominantly bound to albumin, the amount taken up by erythrocytes must not be neglected. More directly, the effect of protein binding on antibiotic action is worth considering.

Comparisons between antibiotics are best made with activity–time plots and not serum concentration profiles, as the free levels often differ from the total antibiotic levels (see, for example, values for cloxacillin and benzylpenicillin in Table 11.10).

The second important consequence of protein binding is related to the fact that only free drug is able to cross the pores of the capillary endothelium. At equilibrium, levels of free drug on both sides of the capillary wall are equal. Albumin levels in most sites are considerably less than those in serum, so there is little bound drug in extravascular regions. There is,

Table 11.10 Protein binding and other characteristics of some penicillins and cephalosporins

Antibiotic	Log P[a]	Serum protein binding (%)	Serum concentration ($\mu g\ cm^{-3}$) during continuous infusion (500 mg h^{-1})		Peak serum levels after 500 mg kg^{-1}	
			Total	Free	Total	Free
Dicloxacillin	3.24	96–98	25	1	15	0.3
Cloxacillin	2.49	94–96	15	0.9	–	–
Oxacillin	2.38	92–94	10	0.8	15	0.8
Nafcillin	–	89–90	9	0.9	6	0.6
Benzylpenicillin	1.72	59–65	16	5.6	4.5	1.6
Methicillin	1.06	37–60			16	10
Ampicillin	–	20–29	29	23.2	12	9
Carbenicillin	–	50	73	36.5	–	–
Ceftriaxone	–	95	–	–	–	–
Cefazolin[b]	–	89	–	–	–	–
Cefditoren	–	88	–	–	–	–
Cefalotin	0.5	65	18	6.3	7.6	2.6
Cefaloridine	–	20	24.7	19.7	18.5	14.8
Cefalexin	0.7	15	27	23	–	–
Cefradine[b]	–1.2	14	–	–	–	–

[a] Log P values from Ryrfeldt A. *J Pharm Pharmacol* 1971;23:463 and Jack DB. *Handbook of Chemical Pharmacokinetic Data*. London: Macmillan; 1992.
[b] Additional values from Singhri SM *et al. Chemotherapy* 1978;24:121.
Reproduced with permission from Lien EJ *et al.* Diffusion of drugs into prostatic fluid and milk. *Drug Intell Clin Pharm* 1974;8:470 (originally published in *Annals of Pharmacotherapy*.

 Clinical point

Penicillins and cephalosporins bind reversibly to albumin. Only the free antibiotic has antibacterial activity. Oxacillin in serum at a concentration of 100 $\mu g\ cm^{-3}$ exhibits an antibacterial effect similar to that of 10 $\mu g\ cm^{-3}$ of the drug in water. A high degree of serum protein binding may nullify the apparent advantage of higher serum levels of some agents (Table 11.10). An increase in the lipophilicity of penicillins results in decreased activity, although one normally expects that this should enhance penetration of bacterial cell walls and also absorption. The hydrophobic binding of penicillins to serum proteins reduces their potency *in vivo* by decreasing their effective concentration.

however, no correlation between the degree of protein binding and peak serum levels of the penicillins and cephalosporins of Table 11.10; other factors such as rates of elimination also determine the peak levels. Protein binding will affect transport into other tissues, however, as the gradient that determines move-

ment is the gradient caused by free drug. Both ampicillin (50 mg kg^{-1} every 2 hours) and oxacillin (50 mg $kg^{-1}\ h^{-1}$) produced similar peak levels in the serum when given as repeated IV boluses. Levels of free drug are markedly different, however, as oxacillin is 75% bound and ampicillin is 17.5% bound in rabbit serum.

11.9.3 Penetration of specialised sites

Muscle, bone and synovial and interstitial fluid are readily accessible to intravascular antibiotics by way of aqueous pores in the capillary supply. The CSF, brain, eye, intestines and prostate gland lack such pores, and entry into these areas is by way of a lipoidal barrier. There is evidence that extensive protein binding may prevent the access of antibiotics into the eye and the inflamed meninges.

The level of free drug in serum is important in determining the amount of drug that reaches tissue spaces.[23] The total concentration of a drug in tissue fluid can be predicted from the serum concentration, the extent of serum protein binding and the protein binding in the tissue fluid. Equation (11.6) has been shown to be highly predictive under equilibrium conditions[23]:

$$C_t = \frac{C_s f_s}{f_t} \tag{11.6}$$

where C_t is the tissue fluid drug concentration, C_s is the serum drug concentration and f_s and f_t are the free fractions of drug in serum and tissue fluid, respectively. If protein binding in the serum and tissue fluid is identical then, provided the same proteins are present in both 'phases', the tissue fluid drug concentration will equal the serum concentration; this is true for both high and low protein-containing extravascular fluid.

Clinical point

In the treatment of bacterial prostatitis; most currently available antibiotics do not readily pass across the prostatic epithelium. The pH of the prostatic fluid is lower than that of plasma, being around 6.6; milk has a pH of 6.8. In passage of drugs both into prostatic fluid and into milk, the degree of dissociation of the drug appears to be the most important factor determining the degree of penetration. The partition coefficient plays a secondary role.

When the prostatic fluid/plasma ratios of sulfonamides were studied it was found that the results could be predicted more closely from the ratio of undissociated/dissociated drug rather than from log P values. It is probable that this is because lipophilic drugs will be highly protein-bound and thus unable to penetrate the boundary membranes.

11.10 Reflections on interactions

The information in this chapter demonstrates the multitude of ways in which drugs can interact with other drugs, with excipients, with the body, with containers. Lists of course can be consulted, but lists (such as the one which closes this chapter) are a starting point to understanding. The subject is undoubtedly complex and to make predictions from the body of knowledge that there is to cases involving new drugs or new formulations and dose regimes requires a high degree of understanding of the possibilities. We have covered many of these in this chapter, and address others in the following chapter on adverse events. But the following is a case history as it were of a search of recent medico-scientific literature on one group of drugs, which begins with the observation of the effects of a group of anticancer drugs and the effect on their absorption of the ingestion of acid-reducing agents, antacids, proton pump inhibitors or buffered medications. It points out that sometimes other factors are involved, not least the bioavailability of the product in question and whether or not it is optimised in a formulation (see the case of vemurafenib below), the dose/solubility ratio and the situation when over-the-counter (OTC) medicines are themselves involved in the picture (see the first clinical point below).

Clinical point[*]: OTC antacid drug combinations and interactions

The availability of OTC medicines as combination formulations of an antacid and an H_2-receptor antagonist can be a concern because these will increase the risk of drug–drug interactions by two mechanisms: a gastric pH-dependent mechanism by the drug itself and a cation-mediated chelation mechanism by antacids.

[*]From Ogawa R, Echizen H. Clinically significant drug interactions with antacids. *Drugs* 2011;71:1839–1864.

11.10.1 A narrative of anticancer drugs and proton pump inhibitors (PPI)*

Clinical point

Many cancer patients frequently take acid-reducing medicines to alleviate symptoms of gastro-oesophageal reflux, thus potentially affecting the absorption of anticancer drugs and possibly jeopardising therapy. Clinical data suggest that the interactions are most relevant for anticancer drugs whose solubility varies over the pH range 1–4, the latter value being the pH of the stomach when the patient has used acid-reducing agents. Figure 11.24 shows the effect on the maximum absorbable dose of such drugs whose solubility is affected by an acid-reducing agent.

Protein kinase inhibitors such as dasatinib, erlotinib, gefitinib (Fig. 11.25) and lapatinib *inter alia* are used in the treatment of non-small-cell lung cancer with activating epidermal growth factor receptor mutations. Their use comes with a long list of potential side-effects, many of which will be determined by their pharmacokinetics. They have a pH-dependent solubil-

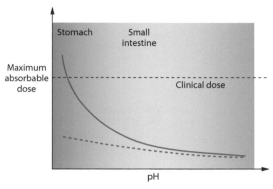

Figure 11.24 Graph showing (solid line) the maximum absorbable dose of drug as a function of pH, the clinical dose and (dashed line) the potential influence of acid-reducing agents in the stomach/small intestine.

ity. Vemurafenib differs in that it has a low solubility over all pH ranges, and has a high dose regimen up to 960 mg. Thus the effect of acid-reducing agents on a drug such as dasatinib will differ from that on vemurafenib (hence the danger of assuming that drugs in a pharmacological class behave identically).

Table 11.11 shows recorded effects of famotidine or omeprazole on dasatinib.

Omeprazole reduces the AUC of erlotinib by 46% and the C_{max} by 61%. These are significant effects.

The effects on absorption of acid-reducing agents on drugs in the four different Biopharmaceutics Classification System and Biopharmaceutical Drug Disposition Classification System classes are summarised in Table 11.12.

Table 11.11 Effect of acid-reducing agents (ARA) on the area under the curve (AUC) and peak plasma concentration (C_{max}) of dasatinib

Drug	ARA	Mean change AUC	C_{max}
Dasatinib[b]	Famotidine 40 mg 10 h ptd[a]	↓61%	↓63%
	Famotidine 40 mg 2 h after dose	NSE[d]	NSE
Dasatinib[b]	Maalox 30 mL 2 h ptd[a]	NSE	↑26%
	Maalox 30 mL coadministered	↓55%	↑58%
Dasatinib[c]	Omeprazole 40 mg daily for 5 days and on day 5 with dose	↓43%	↓42%

[a] ptd = prior to dose.
[b] Eley T *et al. J Clin Pharmacol* 2009;49:700–709.
[c] Clinical study report 2009.
[d] NSE = no significant effect.
Reproduced from Budha NR *et al*. Drug absorption interactions between oral targeted anticancer agents and PPIs: is pH-dependent solubility the Achilles heel of targeted therapy? *Clin Pharmacol Ther* 2012;92:203. Copyright Wiley-VCH Verlag GmbH & Co. KGaA. Reproduced with permission.

*From Budha NR *et al*. Drug absorption interactions between oral targeted anticancer agents and PPIs: is pH-dependent solubility the Achilles heel of targeted therapy? *Clin Pharmacol Ther* 2012;92:203–213.

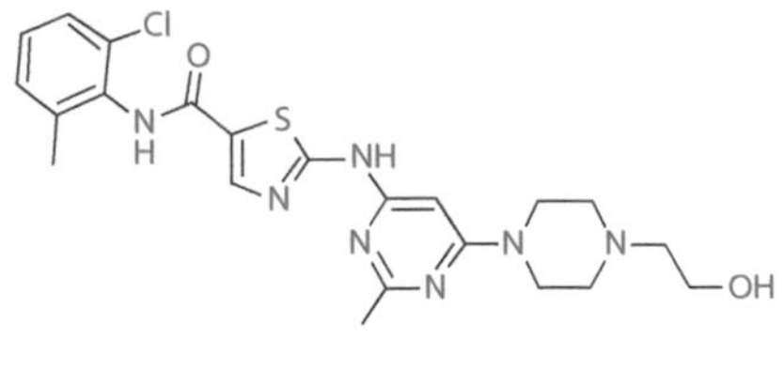

Dasatinib [BCS class II]
Solubility 18 mg ml^{-1} at pH 2.6 to <0.01 mg ml^{-1} at pH 7

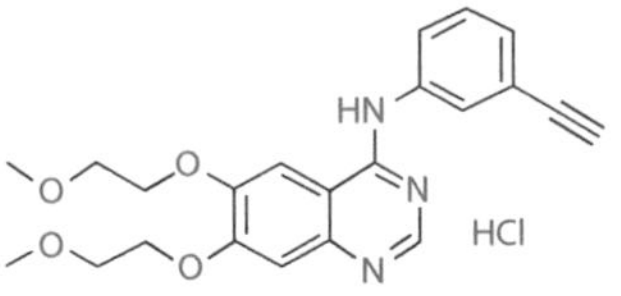

Erlotinib [BCS class II]
Maximum solubility of 0.4 mg ml^{-1} occurs at pH 2

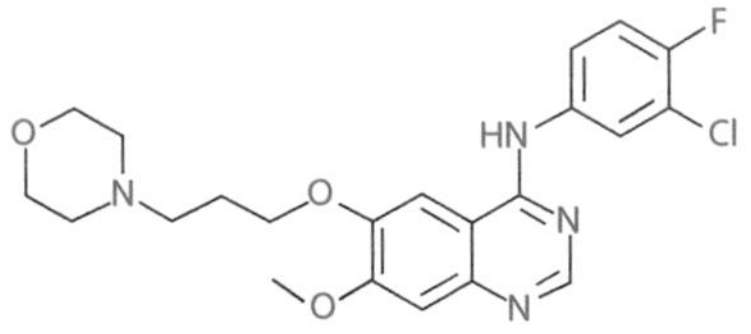

Gefitinib [BCS class II]
Solubility 21 mg at pH 1, decreasing to <0.001 mg ml^{-1} at pH 7,

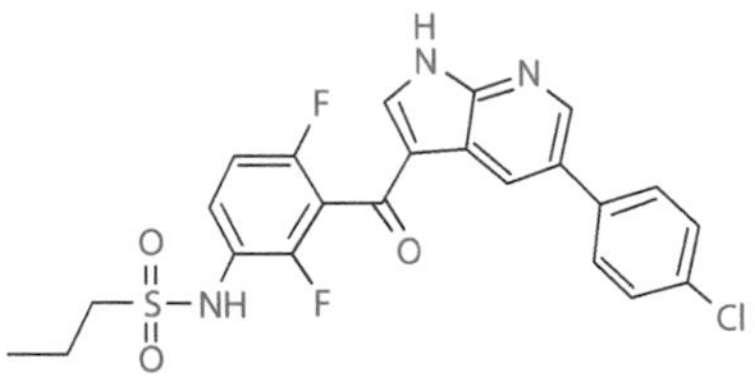

Vemurafenib [BCS class IV/II]
Solubility 0.00026 mg ml^{-1} across pH range

Figure 11.25 The structures, solubilities and Biopharmaceutics Classification System (BCS) class of four anticancer agents of related activity (protein kinase inhibitors). The pKa values of these drugs are: dasatinib: 3.1, 6.8 and 10.8; erlotinib: 5.4; gefitinib: 5.4 and 7.2; vemurafenib: 7.9.

In a comprehensive examination of approved kinase inhibitors,[24] it is emphasised that 'Oral exposure involves interplay of multiple factors, including solubility, dissolution rate, permeability, disposition properties and food effects. Therefore, decent clearance, moderate/high permeability and appropriate formulation vehicles may overcome the effect of low intrinsic solubility, and result in an adequate oral exposure to achieve efficacy.'

Vemurafenib

In examining the data on these kinase inhibitors and the effect of acid-reducing agents, other issues around

bioavailability also appear. This demonstrates the pharmaceutical difficulties encountered in drug development. Vemurafenib is now available as Zelboraf (Roche), formulated as a coprecipitate with hypromellose acetate succinate. The early formulations of a crystalline form demonstrated poor oral bioavailability dosed in capsules which were reported to be 'challenging to manufacture and store', because the crystal form with the highest solubility was unstable. To improve solubility and stability, it was reformulated as a coprecipitate with hypromellose acetate succinate, which resulted in a *sixfold* increase in bioavailability compared to the crystalline formulation.[25] The

Table 11.12 The impact of acid-reducing agents on the absorption of 15 molecular targeted anticancer drugs

Class	BCS description	BDDCS description	Impact on absorption with acid-reducing therapy
I	High solubility High permeability	High solubility Extensive metabolism	Minimal to none
II	Low solubility High permeability	Low solubility Extensive metabolism	Moderate to high
III	High solubility Low permeability	High solubility Poor metabolism	Minimal to none
IV	Low solubility Low permeability	Low solubility Poor metabolism	Moderate to high

Reproduced from Budha NR *et al.* Drug absorption interactions between oral targeted anticancer agents and PPIs: is pH-dependent solubility the Achilles heel of targeted therapy? *Clin Pharmacol Ther* 2012; 92:203. Copyright Wiley-VCH Verlag GmbH & Co. KGaA. Reproduced with permission. BCS = Biopharmaceutics Classification System; BDDCS = Biopharmaceutical Drug Disposition Classification System.

amorphous nature of the coprecipitate aids dissolution (Fig. 11.26).

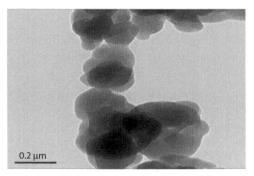

Figure 11.26 Photomicrograph of a coprecipitated bulk powder of a drug prepared with soluble polymers such as hypromellose acetate succinate.

Reproduced from Shah N *et al.* Development of novel microprecipitated bulk powder (MBP) technology for manufacturing stable amorphous formulations of poorly soluble drugs. *Int J Pharm* 2012;438:53–60. Copyright Elsevier 2012.

The effect of acid-reducing agents begs the question of the effect of food. A study in 2014[26] showed that a high-fat/high-calorie meal intake prolonged the T_{max} of vemurafenib from 4 to 8 hours, but increased the AUC threefold.

The work to determine the optimum conditions in which to administer these anticancer agents continues. As the authors Ribas *et al.*[26] state, 'The exact mechanism of how a high-fat meal increased the single-dose exposure of vemurafenib is unknown, but it is likely the result of a combination of factors that influence the *in vivo* dissolution of the tablet and the absorption of vemurafenib. The predominant effect of food after a single oral dose of 960-mg vemurafenib tablets is on the absorption phase, with little or no effect on the terminal drug elimination. The variability associated with PK [pharmacokinetic] parameters seems greater in the fasted condition than in the fed condition.'

Summary

This chapter has dealt with the wide range of physicochemical factors that might cause changes in formulations or drug absorption processes. These have included effects of pH and solvent, interactions between cations and anions, salting in and salting out, ion-exchange reactions, adsorption and interactions with plastics, as well as protein binding, often mediated by hydrophobic interactions. It is, as always, difficult to anticipate the exact quantitative nature of the events that follow from these effects, especially in the body, where there are many compensating and contradictory influences. However, a knowledge of the theoretical possibilities allows us to rationalise what has been observed. By analogy we should therefore be able to predict likely effects with new drugs. One has to be cautious, and aware that what we anticipate theoretically may not take place *in vivo*, where a dynamic situation exists. But the physicochemical basis of interactions and incompatibilities must be appreciated if we are to rationalise interactions.

The Appendix contains tables of drug interactions that could be considered to be physicochemically driven. However, it is important that continuously updated sources are consulted, such as *Stockley's Drug Interactions* (e.g. via Medicines Complete, which is updated frequently online).

Appendix: Drug interactions based on physical mechanisms

The following information was taken originally from a comprehensive listing of drug interactions published by Ruth Ferguson in *Drug Interactions of Clinical Significance* (Auckland: IMS; 1977).

This selection is intended *for illustrative purposes only* and must *not* be used as a definitive source and of course does not contain drugs introduced post-1977. The objective is to illustrate general mechanisms, or the physiochemical principles.

A: Interactions affecting absorption of drugs			
Drugs	**Effect**	**Mechanism/note**	**Recommendation**
Calcium therapy + aluminium hydroxide	Chronic aluminium hydroxide antacid intake (600 cm^3 weekly) can cause osteomalacia	Calcium absorption is prevented	Use alternative antacid. Special care should be taken with people with calcium deficiency
Chlorpromazine + aluminium hydroxide, magnesium oxide, magnesium trisilicate	Reduced blood levels of chlorpromazine, with possible inhibition of therapeutic effect	Possibly due to alteration of gastrointestinal pH by the antacid	Doses should be spaced by 2–3 h
Dicoumarol, warfarin + colestyramine	Anticoagulant absorption is reduced and slowed (25% lower blood levels)	Binding to colestyramine	Space doses by 2–3 h
Dicoumarol, warfarin + laxatives	Chronic laxative administration may cause loss of anticoagulant control	Two possible effects: lubricant oil action may cause decreased absorp- tion of anticoagulant; decreased absorption of vitamin K, particularly with oils and emulsions	Periodic long-term monitoring of prothrombin times in all suspect patients
Dicoumarol + magnesium hydroxide, magnesium oxide	Opposite effects have been reported: (1) Decreased absorption and lower blood levels (up to 75%) of dicoumarol (2) Increased absorption	Possibly adsorption on drug leading to decreased absorption. Chelation might lead to more lipophilic species increased absorption	Space doses by 2–3 h
Digitalis glycosides + docusate sodium (DOSS)	Increased absorption of digitalis to a possibly toxic level	Surface-active properties of DOSS increase wetting and perhaps solubility and absorption of poorly absorbed digitalis	Space doses by 2–3 h
Digoxin, digitoxin + colestyramine	Greatly reduced absorption of digitalis alkaloids with concurrent administration	Binding effect (anionic resin)	Space doses by about 8 h
Digoxin + disodium edetate	Disodium edetate chelates calcium ions, thus antagonising the action of digoxin	Chelation of digoxin in the plasma	May be necessary to monitor blood calcium levels
Digoxin + magnesium trisilicate	Absorption of digoxin reduced by up to 90%	Surface absorption effect	Space doses 2–3 h. Use alternative antacid
Lincomycin + kaolin	Reduced gastrointestinal absorption of lincomycin by up to 90%	Absorption of drug to kaolin	Space doses by 2–3 h
Oxyphenonium bromide + magnesium trisilicate	Reduced blood levels of oxyphenonium with reduced effect	Oxyphenonium adsorbed on to the surface of magnesium trisilicate, reducing availability	Space doses by at least 2–3 h
p-Aminosalicyclic acid (granule formulation) + rifampicin	Reduced blood levels of rifampicin and hence impaired effect	Impaired gastrointestinal absorption rifampicin due to binding to bentonite	Space doses by 8–12 h
Propantheline bromide + magnesium trisilicate	Reduced blood levels (with reduced action) of propantheline		Space doses by 2–3 h

A: Interactions affecting absorption of drugs *(continued)*

Drugs	Effect	Mechanism/note	Recommendation
		Adsorption of propantheline to magnesium trisilicate, reducing availability for absorption	
Salicylates + colestyramine	Greatly decreased absorption of salicylates	Adsorption to ion-exchange resin	Space doses by 4–5 h
Tetracycline + iron preparations	Lower blood levels of tetracycline, possibly below minimal active concentration	Chelation effect	Either space doses at least 2–3 h or alternative antibiotic therapy
Tetracycline + milk products, aluminium, bismuth, calcium and magnesium ions	Gastrointestinal absorption of tetracycline and blood levels of tetracycline greatly reduced	Chelation effect	Space doses by 2–3 h; possible exception minocycline
Tetracycline + sodium bicarbonate (N.B.: Sodium bicarbonate is present in many antacid and effervescent preparations)	Impaired absorption of tetracycline	pH increase in gastrointestinal tract prevents dissolution of complete dose	Space doses by 2–3 h
Thiazide diuretics + colestyramine	Decreased absorption and effect of diuretic	Colestyramine can bind thiazide	Space doses by 2–3 h
Thyroid hormones + colestyramine	Absorption of thyroid hormone prevented	Thyroid hormones become bound to the anionic resin	Space doses by 2–3 h

B: Interactions involving protein binding

Drugs	Effect	Mechanism/note	Recommendation
Chlorpropamide, tolbutamide + sulfonamides	Increased blood level of hypoglycaemic drug. Hypoglycaemic shock reported	Displacement from protein binding and possible metabolic inhibition, competition for excretion	Not reported with sulfadimethoxine, sulfafurazole, sulfamethoxazole. Monitor patient
Chlorpropamide, tolbutamide + salicylates	Introduction of oral salicylate therapy can result in a hypoglycaemic reaction	Displacement from protein binding, salicylates increase tissue glucose uptake	Warn patients against high-dose or chronic salicylate therapy. With long-term salicylate therapy patients should be monitored and restabilised if necessary
Dicoumarol, warfarin + indometacin	Possible elevated blood levels of anticoagulant with risk of haemorrhage. Risk of gastrointestinal bleeding	Displacement from protein	This combination best avoided
Dicoumarol, warfarin + methandienone, norethandrolone, oxymetholone	Increased hypothrombinaemia with several reported cases of haemorrhage	Possibly due to displacement from protein	If combination is definitely indicated, patients should be carefully monitored
Dicoumarol, warfarin + p-aminosalicyclic acid	Increased anticoagulant serum levels with risk of haemorrhage	Displacement from protein	Monitor anticoagulant effect, especially with initiation or cessation of therapy
Dicoumarol, warfarin + paracetamol	With especially large doses, increase in anticoagulant effect	Possibly displacement from protein. Depression of clotting factor synthesis	Use low doses of paracetamol. Probably the safest mild analgesic to use with oral anticoagulants
Dicoumarol, warfarin + sulfadimethoxine, sulfamethoxypyridazine, sulfaphenazole	Increased anticoagulant blood levels with risk of haemorrhage	Displacement from protein by strongly bound sulfonamide	Use alternative chemotherapy. Monitor patient with initiation of cessation of therapy

B: Interactions involving protein binding (continued)

Drugs	Effect	Mechanism/note	Recommendation
Methotrexate + salicylates	Potentiation of methotrexate toxicity	Displacement of methotrexate from protein-binding sites	Owing to severity of methotrexate toxicity, salicylates should not be given to patients receiving methotrexate
Methotrexate + sulfonamides	Potentiation of methotrexate with high risk of toxicity	Displacement from protein binding (sulfafurazole reduces methotrexate binding from 70% to 28%)	Owing to severity of methotrexate toxicity, sulfonamides that are protein-bound should never be administered
Penicillin + probenecid	Threefold increase in serum penicillin level with increase also in spinal fluid levels but decreased brain level	Displacement from protein binding, decreased renal tubule secretion and decreased biliary excretion	Combination can be used when high serum and spinal fluid levels are required
Thyroid hormones, levothyroxine + phenytoin	Rise in thyroxine blood levels with reported tachycardia	Displacement of thyroxine by phenytoin from protein binding	Great care should be taken in administering parenteral phenytoin to people on thyroid therapy
Warfarin + aspirin	Significant increase in anticoagulant effect with possible severe gastrointestinal blood loss	Displacement from protein	Combination should be avoided if possible. Use alternative analgesic such as paracetamol or pentazocine
Warfarin + clofibrate	Higher blood levels of warfarin with risk of haemorrhage	Displacement from protein	Warfarin dose may require a reduction of one-third to one half according to coagulation test
Warfarin + etacrynic acid	Increased blood level of warfarin with haemorrhage risk	Displacement from protein	Monitor patient with initiation and cessation of therapy
Warfarin + mefenamic acid	Enhanced anticoagulant blood levels with risk of haemorrhage and enhanced risk of gastrointestinal bleeding	Displacement from protein	Concurrent administration is best avoided. If necessary, coagulation times should be monitored
Warfarin + nalidixic acid	Possible hypothrombinaemia with associated haemorrhage risk	Displacement from protein (N.B.: In vitro evidence)	Combination administration should be used with care and patient coagulation monitored
Oral anticoagulants + naproxen	Increased anticoagulant effect and risk of gastrointestinal bleeding	Naproxen has ulcerogenic potential. Displacement from protein	Best to avoid concurrent administration. Monitor patient

References

1. Allwood MC, Kearney MCJ. Compatibility and stability of additives in parenteral nutrition admixtures. *Nutrition* 1998;14:697–706.
2. Lipton JH. Incompatibility between sulfamethizole and methenamine mandelate. *N Engl J Med* 1963;268:92–93.
3. Jusko WJ *et al.* Precipitation of diazepam from intravenous preparations. *J Am Med Assoc* 1973;225:176.
4. Langdon DE *et al.* Thrombophlebitis with diazepam used intravenously. *J Am Med Assoc* 1973;223:184–185.
5. Marshall TR *et al.* Pharmacological incompatibility of contrast media with various drugs and agents. *Radiology* 1965;84:536–539.
6. Barbara AC *et al.* Physical incompatibility of sulfonamide compounds and polyionic solutions. *N Engl J Med* 1966;274:1316–1317.
7. Sanchez AR *et al.* Tetracycline and other tetracycline-derivatives staining of the teeth and oral cavity. *Int J Dermatol* 2004;43:709–715.
8. Ambre JJ, Fischer LJ. Effect of coadministration of aluminum and magnesium hydroxides on absorption of anticoagulants in man. *Clin Pharm Ther* 1973;14:231–237.
9. Ikeda K *et al.* Inclusion complexes of β-cyclodextrin with antiinflammatory drugs fenamates in aqueous solution. *Chem Pharm Bull* 1975;23:201–208.
10. Ikeda K *et al.* Circular dichroism study on inclusion complexes of β-cyclodextrin with antiinflammatory fanamates. *J Pharm Sci* 1974;63:1168–1169.

11. Hemmerling TM, Geldner G. Sugammadex: good drugs do not replace good clinical practice. *Anesth Analg* 2007;105:1506.

12. Gross L, Brotman M. Hypoprothrombinemia and hemorrhage associated with colestyramine therapy. *Ann Intern Med* 1970;7295–7296.

13. Coronato A, Glass GBJ. Depression of the intestinal uptake of radio-vitamin B$_{12}$ by colestyramine. *Proc Soc Exp Biol Med* 1973;142:1341–1344.

14. Boman G *et al.* Mechanism of the inhibitory effect of PAS [*p*-aminosalicylic acid] granules on the absorption of rifampicin. Adsorption of rifampicin by an excipient, bentonite. *Eur J Clin Pharm* 1975;8:293–299.

15. Anik ST, Hwang J-Y. Adsorption of D-Nal(2)^{6}LHRH, a decapeptide, onto glass and other surfaces. *Int J Pharm* 1983;16:181–190.

16. Bee JS *et al.* Monoclonal antibody interactions with micro- and nanoparticles: adsorption, aggregation and accelerated stress studies. *J Pharm Sci* 2009;98:3218–3228.

17. Sluzky V *et al.* Mechanism of insulin aggregation and stabilisation in agitated aqueous solutions. *Biotech Adv* 2007;25:318–324.

18. Tzannis ST *et al.* Adsorption of a formulated protein on a drug delivery device surface. *J Colloid Interface Sci* 1997;189:216–228.

19. Jones LS *et al.* Silicone oil induced aggregation of proteins. J Pharm Sci 2005;94:918–927.

20. Philo JS, Arakawa T. Mechanisms of protein aggregation. *Curr Pharm Biotechnol* 2009;10:348–351.

21. Malick AW *et al.* Loss of nitroglycerin from solutions to intravenous plastic containers: a theoretical treatment. *J Pharm Sci* 1981;70:798–801.

22. Illum L, Bundgaard H. Sorption of drugs by plastic infusion bags. *Int J Pharm* 1982;10:339–351.

23. Peterson LR, Gerding DN. Protein binding and antibiotic concentrations. *Lancet* 1978;312:376.

24. O'Brien Z, Moghaddan MF. Small molecule kinase inhibitors approved by the FDA from 2000 to 2011: a systematic review of preclinical ADME data. *Exp Op Drug Metab Toxicol* 2013;9:1597–1612.

25. Shah N *et al.* Improved human bioavailability of vemurafenib, a practically insoluble drug, using an amorphous polymer-stabilized solid dispersion prepared by a solvent-controlled coprecipitation process. *J Pharm Sci* 2013;102:967–981.

26. Ribas A *et al.* The effects of a high-fat meal on single-dose vemurafenib pharmacokinetics. *J Clin Pharmacol* 2014;54:368–374.

Further reading

Baxter K, Preston CL. *Stockley's Drug Interactions*, 10th edn. London: Pharmaceutical Press; 2013 (*Medicines Complete: Stockley's Drug Interactions* http://www.medicines complete.com).

Trissel LA. *Handbook on Injectable Drugs*. Bethesda, MD: American Society of Health-System Pharmacists; 2011.

12

Adverse events: the role of formulations and delivery systems

The main purpose of formulations is to deliver active substances in accurate doses in medicines that are stable and of a high and consistent quality. Drugs are often the smallest proportion of a medicine, and the variety of other ingredients within most dose forms is large. Some of these excipients serve more than one purpose and some have some biological activity. The reason we discuss in this textbook adverse events which may follow from administration of medicines is that some of the problems that arise are the result of excipients interacting physically or chemically with drugs or with themselves, or creating instability or, in some instances, having biological activity of their own. That activity may not be a direct pharmacological or toxicological action, though some agents, such as some non-ionic surfactants, may cause anaphylactic responses or affect drug absorption rates and extent by solubilisation effects or by acting on P-glycoprotein receptors, thus influencing bioavailability. Drug delivery systems have obviously progressed beyond tablets, capsules and injections to a number of devices, such as catheters, drug-eluting stents and implanted devices such as pacemakers. Apart from physical interactions with body tissues, one problem has been bacterial infection associated with the use of some of these. Bacterial interaction with surfaces is very much dependent on physical forces of attachment, the hydrophobicity of the bacteria in question, electrostatic forces and the nature of the adsorbing surface. These and other issues are discussed in this chapter. Of course we do not discuss all adverse drug reactions, as these are contained in more specialised texts.

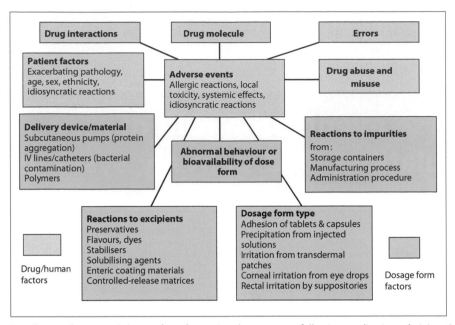

Figure 12.1   Drug/human factors and dosage form factors in adverse events following medication administration.

Modified from Uchegbu IF, Florence AT. Adverse drug events related to dosage forms and delivery systems. *Drug Saf* 1996;14:39–67, with kind permission from Springer Science and Business Media.

12.1 Introduction

It is often assumed when an adverse reaction or adverse event (Box 12.1) occurs that the drug is the causative agent. It is generally the case that the drug itself is the cause of most adverse reactions and effects, but there are instances when formulation factors come into play. Sometimes, as we discuss later in this chapter, excipients may have their own biological effect, and sometimes the way in which the product is constructed and behaves in the body may cause the drug to have enhanced toxicity.*

This chapter summarises the potential for formulations, their form or the ingredients that they contain, to precipitate adverse reactions or events. Figure 12.1 shows both product and patient factors in the causation of adverse events. Errors of choice of product or drug aside, when the correct drug and formulation have been administered, there are still many opportunities for matters to go awry. These include effects which are the result of:

● abnormal bioavailability (both large and small) caused by a product or manufacturing defect or change

Box 12.1 Adverse events and adverse drug reactions

Adverse reactions following administration of a medicine or use of a device can be discussed in terms of *adverse events* (where the causality is not known) or *adverse reactions* (where the causative factor is the drug itself or a specific component of a formulation).

When both drug and formulation are involved, or when an excipient is implicated, the term *adverse event* is possibly the more accurate.

● sensitivities to formulation ingredients (excipients)
● reactions to impurities and breakdown products of either drug or additives, or both
● aggregation of protein and peptide drugs in devices such as pumps
● device failure, for example, with medicated stents or infusion pumps
● the nature of the formulation or dosage form, for example, adhesive tablets lodging in the oesopha-

* There are also psychological factors, outside the scope of this textbook, where, for example, patients receiving placebos in clinical trials report adverse effects, or are influenced by the colour of capsules, tablets or even inhalers.

Table 12.1 Some 'classic' adverse events as a result of use of formulations

Dosage form	Trade name	Adverse event
Indometacin osmotic minipump tablets	Osmosin	Intestinal perforation
Fluspirilene intramuscular injection	Redeptin	Tissue necrosis at site of injection
Epidural injection of prednisolone injection containing benzyl alcohol as preservative	Depo Medrol	Mild paralysis
Inhalation of nebulised ipratropium bromide solution containing benzalkonium chloride as preservative	Atrovent	Paradoxical bronchoconstriction
Povidone-iodine solution for vaginal application		Anaphylactoid reaction
Timolol eye drops	Timoptic	Bronchoconstriction
Fentanyl transdermal patch	Duragesic	Respiratory depression and death

Reproduced from Uchegbu IF, Florence AT. Adverse drug events related to dosage forms and delivery systems. *Drug Saf* 1996;14:39–67, with kind permission from Springer Science and Business Media.

gus or drug precipitating from administered injections.

Figure 12.1 elaborates on the topic, dividing adverse events into those dependent on patient factors and those related to formulations and devices. Adverse events include allergic reactions, local toxicities, systemic effects or idiosyncratic reactions. It is not the place here to recount patient-related factors in detail, although there are of course dosage form–patient interactions that make these of interest. Changed physiology in the postnatal growth period, in childhood and in the elderly can mean that dosage forms may behave differently in certain patient groups (for example with changed gastrointestinal transit times, or patients with underlying pathologies such as dysphagia; see Chapters 8 and 9). Some factors include concomitant pathologies, age, sex and ethnicity. The following sections deal with some product-related adverse effects.

The variety of adverse events that have occurred in the recent past is illustrated in Table 12.1. Historical or 'classic' cases are valuable as they can provide clues to adverse events occurring with new therapeutic agents or delivery systems.

The example of the indometacin osmotic tablets (see Chapter 7, section 7.7) was a case of three factors conspiring to produce the adverse effects: the nature of the drug itself, the osmotic core of potassium chloride and the localised release of the drug from the tablet. The formulation was withdrawn from the market.

12.2 Excipient effects

Excipients, as discussed elsewhere in this text, are components of formulations other than the drug or other active ingredient. Their functions are many, variously to aid processing, to aid dissolution of solid-dose forms or conversely, to retard release of the drug, to stabilise the formulation or to protect the drug from adverse environments both *in vitro* and *in vivo*. Excipients are the dominant material in many tablet and capsule formulations, as sometimes their main role is to provide sufficient bulk for a low-dose drug to be administered safely. This section deals with the potential of excipients to influence outcomes of medication.

Excipients are not always the inert substances that we presume. Some cases and reports of the adverse action of excipients are discussed here. While labelling requirements insist on the listing of ingredients in some products, the plethora of trade names (e.g. for surfactants, polymers, lipids and other excipients) can make accurate identification of materials difficult. The European Commission guidelines require that all excipients must be declared on the labelling if the product is an injectable, or a topical preparation (for skin, for inhalation, delivery to the vaginal, nasal or rectal mucosae) or an eye preparation.

Batch-to-batch variation of many excipient raw materials adds another layer of complexity in tracking down and comparing case histories. One problem faced is that products available in one national market may have different formulations from those marketed in another. The clinical literature does not always detail the formulations or product brands used in clinical studies.

12.2.1 Not always inert

Excipients are intended to be inert, but they are not always so in all patients.[1] Excipients must be of high quality, safe and must have a high degree of functionality, that is, a total fitness for use.

Fitness for use in one application may not mean fitness for use in another, for example, by another route of administration. Even though adverse reactions to additives might be relatively rare, it is for this reason that the possibility that an excipient might be the cause of any adverse event should be kept in mind. Fillers like lactose bulk out a low dose (milligrams or micrograms) so that the resulting tablet or capsule can be manufactured and is of a sufficient size to be handled. Lactose is also used in dry-powder inhaler formulations as a carrier for the drug. There may be lubricants such as magnesium stearate to aid the flow of powders and their subsequent tableting or filling into capsules (see Chapter 1).

Preservatives and dyes used widely in formulation are listed in Tables 12.2 and 12.3, which is the result of surveys of these ingredients and their frequency of use,[2] albeit not in the UK. These figures are used here to give an impression of the excipients most likely to be encountered.

Relatively simple molecules are used as excipients in formulations, from substances such as lactose or magnesium stearate through surfactants, preservatives, colours and flavours to macromolecules. With small molecules, such as the *para*-aminobenzoic acid esters (parabens), it is possible to know whether the compound is pure, and thus exactly what is in the formulation. It is not possible to generalise about the effects of excipients with all their structural diversity and uses. Many polymeric materials are complex (see Chapter 7), not only because of the existence in any one sample of a range of molecular weights, but also because many contain plasticisers to adjust their physical properties or agents to aid production. Plasticisers such as diethyl phthalate leach out from plastic giving sets into infusions, particularly those that have ingredients (such as surfactants) that might

Table 12.2 Preservatives found in liquid pharmaceutical formulations (*n* = 73)

Preservatives	% of formulations
Methylparaben	45.2
Propylparaben	35.6
Sodium benzoate	32.8
Sodium metabisulfite	11
Benzoic acid	8
Hydroxyparabenzoate	4
Potasssium sorbate	2
Hydroxyparabenzoic acid	1
No preservatives	2

Reproduced with permission from Balbani APS *et al.* Pharmaceutical excipients and the information on drug labels. *Rev Bras Otorinolaringol* 2006;72:400–406.

Table 12.3 Dyes found in pharmaceutical formulations (*n* = 73)

Dyes	% of formulations
Dusk Yellow (FD&C #6)	15
Tartrazine Yellow (FD&C #5)	9.5
Erythrosine	6.8
Ponceau 4R Red	5.4
Caramel	4.1
Red #40	4.1
Food Red	4.1
Bordeaux S Red	2.7
Quinoline Yellow	2.7
Yellow #10	2.7
Blue #1	1.3
Red #10	1.3
Iron oxide	1.3

Reproduced with permission from Balbani APS *et al.* Pharmaceutical excipients and the information on drug labels. *Rev Bras Otorinolaringol* 2006;72:400–406.

aid the solubilisation of the phthalate. Dioctyl phthalate and dioctyl adipate have been found in some silicone tubing.

With polymers and other macromolecules one needs to know their molecular weight, or more likely, their molecular weight distribution, and about the presence of impurities, such as catalysts and peroxides, the latter occuring in polysorbate 80 (see Chapter 5). Cremophor EL, a castor oil polyoxyethylene surfactant derivative which is used in paclitaxel formulations, is 'cleaned' rather than pure.

Excipients are rarely produced to the extremely high standards of purity that apply to drug substances. Hence the presence of impurities rather than the material itself might be the cause of any adverse event, perhaps by inducing degradation of the drug. There may be batch differences or brand differences in excipients, which are confusing.

Problems with excipients to which the American Academy of Pediatrics have drawn attention are shown in Table 12.4. Note that the route of administration and sometimes the mode of administration (for example, a particular device such as a nebuliser) and the concentration will affect the appearance or severity of many adverse effects.

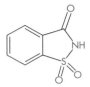

Structure I Saccharin, an *o*-toluene sulfonamide

12.3 E-numbers

From Table 12.4 it is clear that there are many ways of referring to additives. A classification system has been developed that codifies additives both in food and in pharmaceuticals in terms of E-numbers. Box 12.2 gives the general numbering system for several classes of ingredients. It is useful when trying to detect cross-reactivity and sensitivities to know the E-numbers of dyes, preservatives and other ingredients. Each additive has a number within the classifications shown in Box 12.2.

Box 12.2 General system of E-numbers

E100–E199   Colours
E200–E299   Preservatives
E300–E399   Antioxidants, acidity regulators
E400–E499   Thickeners, stabilisers, emulsifiers
E500–E599   Acidity regulators, anti-caking
            agents
E600–E699   Flavour enhancers

Further deconstruction of E-numbers might be useful in identifying possible causes of adverse events.

- E100–109 are yellow dyes; for example, tartrazine (F&DC Yellow 5) is E102.
- E140-149 are green dyes. E430–439 are polyoxyethylene derivatives such as polysorbate 80, which is E433.
- E210–219 are benzoates.
- E230–239 are phenols and methanoates.
- E220–220 are sulfites (e.g. sodium metabisulfite has an E-number of 223).

The structures of some of these dyes are quite complex and, perhaps not surprisingly, some do have pharmacological effects[3], listed in Table 12.5. Another report[4] discussed patients with reactions to E102 (tartrazine: F&DC Yellow 5) in oxytetracycline tablets and to E131 (Patent Blue V) in a doxycycline formulation.

Table 12.4 Excipients that have caused problems in paediatric and adult medicines[a]

Excipient or class	Selected observed reactions
Sulfites	Wheezing, dyspnoea, anaphylactoid reactions
Benzalkonium chloride	Paradoxical bronchoconstriction, reduced forced expiry volume
Aspartame	Headache, hypersensitivity
Saccharin (**I**)	Dermatological reactions; avoid in children with sulfa allergies
Benzyl alcohol	In high concentrations can cause neonatal death
Various dyes	Reactions to tartrazine, similar to aspirin intolerance; patients with the 'classic aspirin triad' reaction (asthma, urticaria, rhinitis) may develop similar reactions from other dyes such as amaranth, erthyrosin, indigo, carmine, Ponceau, Sunset Yellow, Brilliant Blue
Lactose	Problem in lactose-sensitive patients (those with lactase deficiency)
Propylene glycol	Localised contact dermatitis topically; lactic acidosis after absorption

[a]Data from American Academy of Pediatrics. *Pediatrics* 1997; 99:266–278.

Case report[3]

During the 1999/2000 influenza outbreak, a 53-year-old man consulted because of a persistent productive cough that followed flu-like illness. The patient was examined and prescribed erythromycin (Erymax™, Elan). He made it clear that he had a previous history of aspirin allergy and was reassured that there was no known cross-sensitivity between erythromycin and aspirin. Two days later, the patient's wife came into the surgery; she was angry and upset because shortly after taking the erythromycin capsules, her husband had developed some tingling and swelling of his fingers and feet similar to the symptoms he had previously experienced with aspirin. They were both disturbed to find the following warning in the patient information leaflet: '*Capsules contain the colouring agent E110. This can cause allergic-like reactions including asthma. You are more likely to have a reaction if you are also allergic to aspirin*'. This case raised many issues. Was the patient allergic to E110 (Sunset Yellow FCF, Orange Yellow S, FD&C Yellow 6), or was the patient allergic to erythromycin itself? The physician concerned was unaware both of the presence of E110 in the formulation and of the apparent cross-reactivity between aspirin and this colouring agent, there being no mention of either in the physician's BNF [*British National Formulary*] or in the Pharmaceutical Data Sheet Compendium. To be able to foresee such interactions requires that the structures of the molecules concerned be known and this is a tall order. However, understanding after the event is a reasonable goal for avoiding future occurrences.

Taken verbatim from Millar JS. Pitfalls of 'inert' ingredients. *Br J Gen Pract* 2001;51:570.

Table 12.5 Adverse effects of dyes and colouring agents[5]

Compound	Structure	Adverse effects
Sunset Yellow		Urticaria exacerbation
Indigo carmine		Urticaria exacerbation
Tartrazine		Headache, gastrointestinal disturbance, exacerbation of asthma, dangerous in aspirin-intolerant individuals
Amaranth		Potential carcinogenicity (banned)
Brilliant Blue		Hypersensitivity reactions

Reproduced from Pifferi G, Restani P. The safety of pharmaceutical excipients. *Il Farmaco* 2003;58:541–550. Copyright Elsevier 2003.

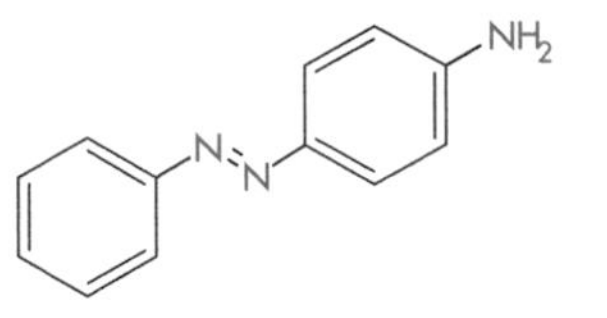

para aminoazobenzene (PAAB)
(II)

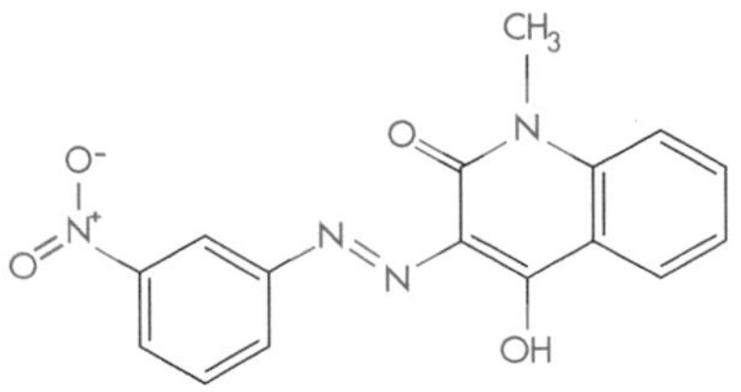

Disperse Yellow 3
(III)

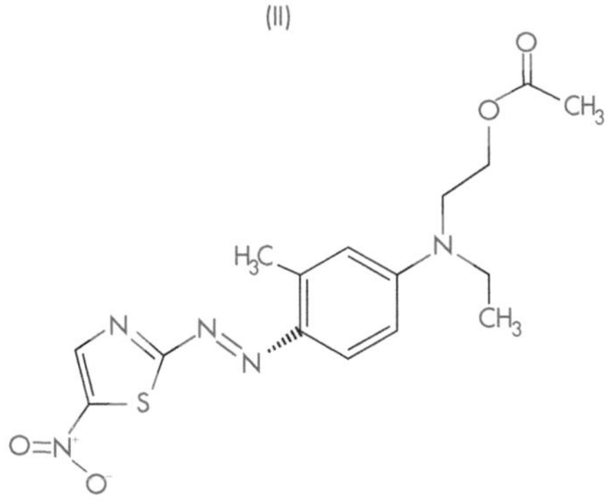

Disperse Blue 124
(IV)

Structures II–IV   Azo compounds used as dyes

Azo dyes (those with the –N=N– linkage) account for 60–70% of dyes used in food and textile manufacture. Their acute toxicity is low but some azo dyes have been banned from foods because of the toxicity of dye breakdown products rather than the dye itself. The mechanism by which tartrazine causes allergic reactions is not fully understood.

12.4 Cross-reactivity of drugs

Cross-reactivity can be defined as:

- a reaction to different compounds which may or may not have some structural similarity. Often the immune system is involved.

Cross-reactions between different azo dyes and *para*-amino compounds have been studied[6] in azo dye-sensitive subjects, in the clinical aspects of azo dye dermatitis, and to attempt to relate the pattern of cross-sensitisations to the chemical structure of the different dyes. Out of 6203 consecutively tested patients, 236 were sensitised to at least one of six azo compounds employed as textile dyes. One hundred and seven subjects reacted to Disperse Orange 3 (DO3), 104 to Disperse Blue 124 (DB124), 76 to *para*-aminoazobenzene (PAAB), 67 to Disperse Red 1 (DR1), 42 to

Disperse Yellow 3 (DY3) and 31 to *p*-dimethylaminoazobenzene (PDAAB). Co-sensitisations to *para*-phenylenediamine were present in most subjects sensitised to DO3 (66%) and PAAB (75%), in 27% and 36% of DR1 and DY3-sensitive subjects, and in only 16% of subjects sensitised to DB124. After the hands and the face, the neck and the axillae were the most frequently involved skin sites. Cross-sensitisations between azo dyes and *para*-amino compounds can partially be explained on the basis of structural similarities, as may be seen from structures **II–IV**.

12.5 Non-ionic surfactants

Non-ionic surfactants are widely used in formulations as wetting agents and solubilising agents. As discussed in Chapter 5, because surfactants are by structure and nature surface-active they will accumulate at interfaces, the air–water interface and the oil–water interface as well as the membrane–water interface. They can influence the fluidity of the membrane, and at higher concentrations, generally above their critical micelle concentration, they will cause membrane damage because they can solubilise structural membrane lipids and phospholipids.

While non-ionic surfactants allow poorly water-soluble drugs to be formulated as injectables, some have side-effects that are by now well known. The two most commonly used, and therefore cited as causing adverse events, are polysorbate 80 (Tween 80; E433) and a polyoxyethylated castor oil (Cremophor EL). Anaphylactic reactions are the most frequently cited, although they occur in a minority of patients. Hence it is essential, if such reactions to injections occur in new or experimental formulations, that their presence be recognised. Some products that contain, or have contained (see key point box below), Cremophor EL include teniposide, ciclosporin and paclitaxel formulations; docetaxel contains polysorbate 80, as does etoposide. The pharmacological effects of formulation vehicles have been discussed in detail elsewhere.[7]

> **Key point**
>
> Different formulations of these drugs exist in different countries under different trade names, hence the true composition of the product in question must be ascertained in assessing outcomes.

12.6 Polyoxyethylene glycols

Polyoxyethylene glycols (PEGs) (macrogols) are not surface-active as they are completely hydrophilic with no hydrophobic domains, but they can exert an adverse effect when used as suppository bases through being hygroscopic. They absorb water from the rectal tissues and thus cause irritation, but this can be minimised by first moistening the PEG base before insertion. This affinity for water is the result of the interaction of water molecules with the oxygen of the repeating – CH_2CH_2O- units; a macrogol of molecular weight 44 500 Da has approximately 1000 such ethylene oxide units, each interacting with up to four H_2O molecules. Macrogols 4000 and 3350 are used to sequester water in the bowels (Idrolax (Ipsen) or Laxido (Galen)).

Note: 'giving fluids with macrogols may reduce the dehydrating effect sometimes seen with osmotic laxatives.' (*British National Formulary* 68).

Its presence in laxative formulations is most likely to aid the penetration of water into the faecal mass. Paediatric powder formulations of PEGs are available for faecal impaction and constipation (Movicol Paediatric, Norgine) with a dose of 6.56 g of Macrogol 3350. Sodium dodecyl (lauryl) sulfate is also an ingredient of an osmotic laxative, Relaxit Micro-enema. Usually it is found as a wetting agent in pharmaceuticals.

12.7 Adjuvants as therapeutic substances

This subsection is appropriate in this chapter as it emphasises again the fact that adjuvants can be biologically active.

12.7.1 Nonoxynol-9

Nonoxynol-9 (**V**) is similar to many non-ionic surfactants used as excipients. It is used as a spermicide because, being membrane-active, it interacts with spermatozoal membranes and reduces sperm mobility. It has also some activity against human immunodeficiency virus (HIV). However, it is also suspected to increase HIV access through the vaginal wall as, like other surfactants, it can damage biomembranes. It also has been shown to increase rectal infection by the herpes simplex virus. The microscopic evidence is clear that the compound damages the epithelial wall, as shown in Fig. 12.2 in the case of rectal tissue.[8]

12.7.2 Poloxamers

Poloxamers are ABA block copolymer surfactants (see Chapter 5, section 5.5.3); in designating them, A is the hydrophilic polyoxyethylene chain and B is the hydrophobic polyoxypropylene chain. The properties of the poloxamers depend on the length of each chain. ABA block copolymer surfactants such as the poloxamers

Structure V Nonoxynol 9

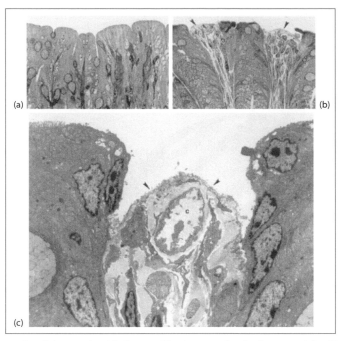

Figure 12.2 Light micrographs of the rectal epithelium and lamina propria of mice treated for 10 minutes with phosphate-buffered saline (PBS) (a) and nonoxynol-9. (b). Control (PBS-treated) tissue is characterised by a continuous epithelium of columnar and goblet cells. In tissue treated with nonoxynol-9, epithelial cells appear necrotic. In some areas the epithelium is missing and connective tissue is directly exposed to the rectal lumen (arrows). In the transmission electron micrograph shown in (c), connective tissue (arrows) appears to be exposed to the rectal lumen. Epithelial cells are missing microvilli. A capillary is shown in (c).

Reproduced from Phillips DM, Zacharopoulous VR. Nonoxynol-9 enhances rectal infection by herpes simplex virus in mice. *Contraception* 1998;57:341–348, with kind permission from Springer Science and Business Media.

have many pharmaceutical uses, as wetting, solubilising and emulsifying agents, but some, like poloxamer 188 (Pluronic F68) have some useful biological activity. It improves microvascular blood flow by reducing blood viscosity, particularly in low-shear conditions. Its mechanism of action is not clear, but it is suggested that the surfactant binds to cells via the hydrophobic B portion, leaving the polyoxyethylene chains to provide a hydrated barrier, reducing cell–cell, cell–protein and protein–protein interactions in the blood.[9]

Poloxamer 188 can have a protective effect on damaged heart muscle cells. Purified poloxamer 188 also has a beneficial effect on the treatment of sickle-cell disease,[10] perhaps because it decreases the adhesion of sickle cells to the microvasculature.

It has been suggested that Poloxamer 188 may also operate as a cell repair agent or membrane sealant,[11] as shown in Fig. 12.3.

12.7.3 Talc as therapeutic agent and excipient

Talc is hydrated magnesium silicate; there are variable amounts of calcium, magnesium and iron present in different samples of talc. Its particle size can vary considerably. Humble talc is used not only in baby care but also as a lubricant in the manufacture of tablets and as a lubricant for surgical gloves.

There is one less well-known use of talc, which is as an active agent rather than as an excipient. This is in the procedure of pleurodesis, when the membranes around the lung adhere. Talc prevents the build-up of fluid between the membranes. An irritant such as bleomycin, tetracycline or talc powder is instilled inside the pleural cavity to instigate an inflammatory response that 'tacks the two pieces together'.[12] Talc is one of the most effective agents to achieve the desired outcome, but there have been concerns about side-effects, especially acute respiratory distress syndrome (ARDS), assumed to be related to both the particle size and

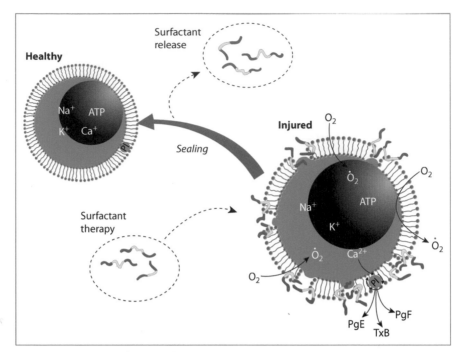

Figure 12.3 Suggested mechanism of action of Poloxamer 188, operating as a cell repair agent or membrane sealant. The surfactant, shown with its hydrophobic portion in light grey and hydrophilic part in blue, interacts with the injured cell, 'sealing' the membrane and returning it to normal. ATP, adenosine triphosphate; PgE, PgF, prostaglandins E and F, respectively; T × B, thromboxane B.

Reproduced with permission from Agarwal J, Walsh AM, Lee RC. *Ann NY Acd Sci* 2005;1006:295–309.

perhaps the shape of the talc particles.[13] Particle size has been found to be key in determining the distribution of talc in the body,[14] suggesting the possibility of migration of talc through the lymphatics.

In the USA, talc used in this procedure has a smaller particle size than in European samples, and it is in the USA that most cases of ARDS seem to occur. It has been shown[15] in comparing two sizes of talc (normal and large) that they both elicit the same benefit in pleurodesis but the smaller sizes have greater pulmonary and systemic deposition of talc particles and cause greater pleural inflammation. This is another example where the physical properties of a material influence its biological effect. Small particles, once they gain entry, can in fact translocate throughout the body, depending on their size and surface properties, an issue discussed in Chapter 14 on pharmaceutical nanotechnology.

The smaller the particles of any substance, the farther they can travel, hence there is real concern about the migration of such particles, whether inhaled, swallowed or inadvertently placed in contact with open wounds, for example. There are similar concerns with cytotoxic drugs in powder form, which can be inhaled or absorbed through the skin (to be discussed).

12.8 Active excipients in multiple therapies

Box 12.3

When an excipient in one formulation affects, say, P-glycoproteins (P-gp), and it is administered along with another product whose absorption is P-gp-dependent, then interpretation of interactions can be obscured if the excipients in both products are not taken into account.

Examples to illustrate the point made in Box 12.3 might include paclitaxel formulations with Cremophor EL and polysorbate 80 when used along with other formulations. Several non-ionic surfactants have been found to inhibit P-gp-mediated transport *in vitro*[16]; in one system the descending order of effect was Toco-pheryl Polyethylene Glycol 1000 Succinate (TPGS) > Pluronic PE8100 > Cremophor EL > Pluronic PE6100 ≈ Tween 80. These surfactants had no effect on multiple drug resistance protein 2 function, suggesting specific action.

The well-known effects of surfactants on absorption enhancement have in the past been thought to be mainly due to direct interactions of the surfactant with biomembranes, at low concentrations causing increased fluidity and transport and at high concentrations causing solubilisation of key membrane components. Sometimes surfactants affect absorption in multiple ways, by interacting with the barrier membrane, by forming a microemulsion and thus aiding dispersal of lipophilic drugs or by affecting intestinal secretory transit.[17]

12.9 Influence of dosage form type

12.9.1 Adhesion of tablets

Oesophageal damage caused by tablets is discussed later, but it is important to consider here the following two case studies.

Case studies

A tablet of pantoprazole (Protonix) was seen 'perched' in the oesophagus of a 57-year-old woman with oesophageal dysmotility; this patient with diffuse bronchiolar disease required hospitalisation.[18] In another patient an enteric-coated aspirin tablet, its coating still intact, was seen in an ulcer in the gastric antrum of another patient.[19] Adhesion or simply entrapment in diverticula may be an issue, In this case, as with others, a combination of pathology and dose form conspired to cause a problem.

Adverse events are rarely simple. The manner in which dose forms behave in the presence of small or larger amounts of aqueous media, which may be found respectively in the oesophagus or later in the stomach, are varied. Simple *in vitro* studies can be illuminating, as Fig. 12.4 illustrates.[20] This shows the unusual disintegration properties of two tablet formulations, the lower example being an extreme case typical of emopronium bromide (**VI**) tablets, once marketed as Cetiprin for the treatment of nocturnal enuresis.

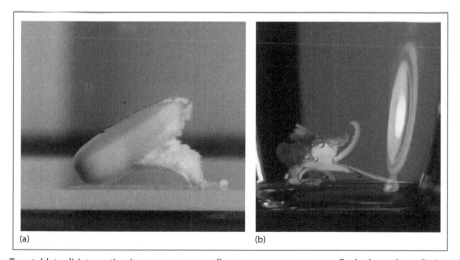

(a) (b)

Figure 12.4 Two tablets disintegrating in an aqueous medium at room temperature. Both show the splitting of the coating layer on the tablets, but (b) shows a now-discontinued tablet of emopronium bromide (Cetiprin) that is unravelling to expose the core of pure drug, irritant to the oesophageal lining.
Reproduced with permission from Florence AT, Salole EG (eds). *Formulation Factors in Adverse Reactions*. London: Wright; 1990.

Structure VI Emopronium bromide, showing its surfactant-like nature

The Cetiprin tablet is seen to break apart, exposing a core of pure drug, which has surfactant properties. If this occurred in the oesophagus, pain and damage would result and this indeed was the case. Given its indication, many patients took the tablets with insufficient water and many cases of dysphagia were reported. The product was subsequently withdrawn from the market.

In this case the combination of adherence and the presence of a potentially irritant drug create the problem. Close connection between epithelia and product leads to high concentrations of drug and to damage. The oesophagus is a primary site for such adverse events, since tablets and capsules will generally not have disintegrated during their oesophageal transit and retain their bulk. Small uncoated tablets may also cause problems in the oesophagus because they can adhere firmly to the mucosal surface. A range of drugs have been reported to cause oesophageal injury, as shown in Table 12.6 and discussed in Box 12.4.

Table 12.6 Some drugs that have caused oesophageal injury

- Alendronate
- Alprenolol
- Aspirin
- Clindamycin
- Doxycycline
- Emopronium bromide
- Ferrous salts
- Indometacin
- Potassium chloride
- Risendronate
- Tetracycline
- Thioridazine

Box 12.4

What, if any, are the common features of the drugs listed in Table 12.6? What might be the main reason or reasons for each to cause injury?

These include the acidity of the concentrated solutions of some of the drugs (aspirin, alendronate and risendronate); the proximity of high concentrations of drugs such as doxycycline which chelate calcium and hence disrupt the epithelial lining; the surface activity of agents such as emopronium bromide; or high electrolyte concentrations from the inorganic drugs.

N.B.: If these agents are in dosage forms that are swallowed with sufficient water and do not lodge in the oesophagus, damage is less likely to be caused.

Dosage forms have other effects and influences in modulating or causing adverse events, apart from the influence they have on pharmacokinetics and bioavailability. Precipitation of drugs from injection solutions is one prime example. Figure 12.1 reminds us of others:

- irritation from the adhesives of transdermal patches
- corneal irritation from eye drops
- rectal irritation from the use of suppository bases (such as PEGs) that, as discussed, extract water from the mucosa.

12.10 Tear films and eye drops

The formation and rupture of tear films were explained over 40 years ago by Holly.[21] Eye drops can disrupt the natural tear film, either by the action of the drugs they contain or through additives such as benzalkonium chloride. The latter is a component of eye drops, but it can be toxic as it is a cationic surfactant. It is not a single compound, but comprises a mixture of alkyl chains[†] (see Chapter 5); the component molecules can adsorb on to the corneal surface in dry-eye syndrome, rendering that surface even more hydrophobic. The

† Benzalkonium chloride (BKC) is a mixture comprising derivatives with different alkyl chain lengths, hence its generic "alkonium" name.

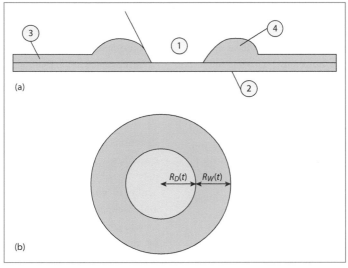

Figure 12.5 (a) Simplified diagram showing a thin liquid film (3) on a surface such as the cornea (2). When the film reaches a critical thickness, instability causes the film to rupture and surface forces pull the film away from that point, leaving an exposed surface (1). The liquid in the film is gathered in a rim (4). The contact angle between the broken film and the corneal surface will be reduced on addition of an agent that lowers surface tension. On the other hand, the adsorption of, say, benzalkonium chloride on the surface, with the onium group towards the negative cells, will render the surface in (1) more hydrophobic, exacerbating the situation. (b) Schematic diagram used to calculate the radial velocity of de-wetting.

Reproduced with permission from Njobuenwu DO. Spreading of trisiloxanes on thin water film: dry spot profile. *Leonardo J Sci* 2007;6:165–178.

film can then de-wet the surface, thereby exposing the corneal epithelial cells to the air. The process may start at a given point on the corneal surface. A critical thickness for stability is breached and the film breaks, as shown in Fig. 12.5.

The film break-up time (Fig. 12.6) is measured in the clinic and is a useful measure to compare artificial tear fluids or severity of the syndrome of dry eye.

Tear film formation may be compromised, but not necessarily cause clinical problems unless the eyes are challenged with smoke or dust or certain drugs.

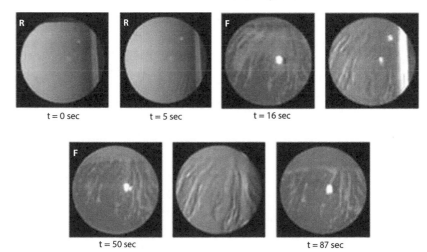

Figure 12.6 Time course and spatial topography of tear film break-up for subject AL obtained during a 90-second period of non-blinking. The time immediately after a blink is $t = 0$ sec. R = retro-illumination image; F = fluorescein image. The lack of a blink allows the drying out of the film, especially when the surface has been made more hydrophobic by adsorption of, say, benzalkonium chloride.

Reproduced with permission from Himebaugh NL *et al.* IUSO Visual Sciences Groups 1999 Indiana University. Available online at: www.opt.Indiana.edu (accessed 25 March 2015).

Contact lenses may also of course affect tear film formation and stability.

As discussed in Chapter 10, neonates have normal tear fluid but low rates of blinking.[23] This incomplete blinking[24] allows time for the film to evaporate, as discussed above, and to cause the dry spots that lead to exposed points on the corneal epithelium. A low rate of tear fluid turnover is also believed to be the cause of reduced barriers to potential pathogens. The tear film in effect has a 'washing function', reducing the likelihood of bacterial adhesion to the corneal surface. This is similar to the case with saliva, which removes bacteria on teeth.

12.10.1 Fluoroquinolone eye drops

How do different fluoroquinolones behave in tears? In one study, three fluoroquinolone solutions were evaluated[25]: ciprofloxacin 0.3% (Ciloxan), norfloxacin (Chibroxin) and ofloxacin 0.3% (Ocuflox). The pH of the tear film for the first 15 minutes after instillation of each of the drugs is determined by the pH of its formulation. Rapid precipitation of ciprofloxacin was seen in a model system 8 minutes after dosing owing to the supersaturation of the drug in tears, while the tear concentration of ofloxacin and norfloxacin remained below saturation solubility at all pH values studied. These findings may explain the reports of precorneal deposits following the use of ciprofloxacin. The reasons for the precipitation of Ciloxan were discussed in Chapter 4 (section 4.2.4) and the relevant figure is shown again here. Figure 12.7 shows the solubility–pH plots for the three drugs, which explain the problem that occurs with Ciloxan in the model tear system when drug tear concentration exceeds solubility. One can see that the solubility line crosses the concentration line in the diagram for Ciloxan (Box 12.5).

Box 12.5

The pH–solubility profiles of the fluoroquinolones up to pH 7.2 are typical of a base. Solubility decreases with increasing pH, with a minimum in solubility around pH 7. If the pH were to increase above 7.5, solubility would increase again as the compound possesses a carboxyl group. The pH of tear fluids is just over 6.8. When the solubility curve falls below the concentration curve, precipitation can be anticipated, a quick way of predicting the occurrence of precipitation.

12.11 Reactions to impurities

Reactions to impurities generally refer to the effect of breakdown products of the active ingredient, which may be initiated by interactions with moisture or acidity or with excipients or materials from containers and packaging. The manufacturing process may contribute some impurities, although these will be limited by the marketing authorisation, but the validity of these requirements and limitations will depend on the same route of synthesis and production being adhered to.

12.11.1 Heparin

 Case study

In January 2008, Baxter Healthcare Corporation withdrew batches of nine lots of heparin sodium in the USA[26] because around 700 acute allergic-type adverse reactions had been reported after their use. The number of deaths was 19. The source of the active ingredient for this product was the Scientific Protein Laboratories (SPL) in Changhzou, China. The US Food and Drug Administration found that the heparin batches associated with the reactions contained 5–20% of a heparin-like compound as a contaminant.

In the case above the contaminant was identified as over-sulfated chondroitin sulfate[27] (Fig. 12.8). More than 80 adverse reactions were also reported in Germany with products where the heparin was also sourced from China, although from another company.

This example illustrates that the final product safety is compromised if the raw material has been sourced from an unreliable supplier. In-house testing of the incoming material should have detected that there

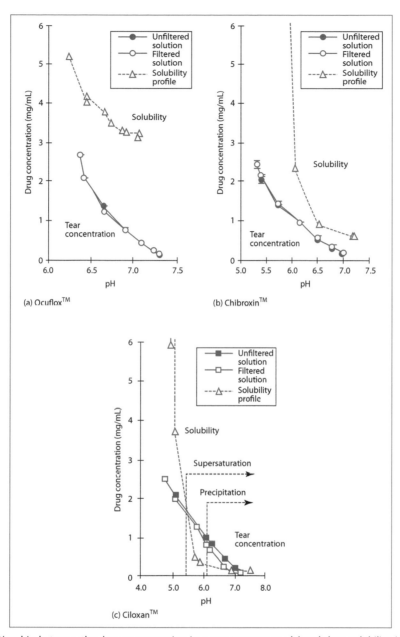

Figure 12.7 Relationship between the drug concentration in a tear turnover model and drug solubility (dashed lines).

Reproduced from Firestone BA *et al*. Solubility characteristics of three fluoroquinolone ophthalmic solutions in an *in vitro* tear model. *Int J Pharm* 1998;164:119–128. Copyright Elsevier 1998.

was a problem, given the high percentage of the impurities, but it is difficult to cater for previously unknown impurities.

12.11.2 Hyaluronic acid

Hyaluronic acid (HA) is used in osteoarthritis as a synovial fluid supplement (see Chapter 7). It is also used in ophthalmic surgery. *In vivo* metabolic degradation of HA by hyaluronidase is one of the determinants of its biological half-life. HA can be sourced from bacteria, from rooster combs or from human umbilical cord, and the resulting HA products will contain different impurities.[28] Several commercially available products in one study did not degrade on digestion with hyaluronidase, clearly indicating that biological

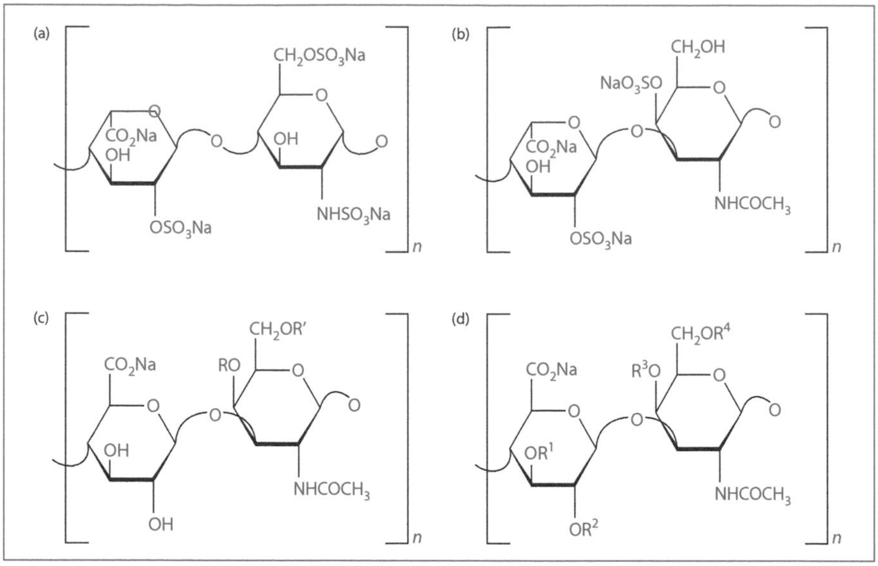

Figure 12.8 Structural formulae of (a) heparin; (b) dermatan sulfate; (c), chondroitin sulfate A and C; and (d) oversulfated chondroitin sulfate (OSCS). For chondroitin sulfate A, group R represents the sulfated moiety, as for chondroitin sulfate C the residual group R' is sulfated. For OSCS, R^1–R^4 label possibly sulfated moieties. The dermatan in heparin preparations is a signal of poor purification methods.

Reproduced from Beyer T *et al.* Quality assessment of unfractionated heparin using ^{1}H nuclear magnetic resonance spectroscopy. *J Pharm Biomed Anal* 2008;48:13–19. Copyright Elsevier 2008.

half-life will not be the same. Vigilance is necessary and, where problems arise, the provenance of biological products must be determined. Sources matter, processing matters, purification matters and, of course, proving quality by the application of the highest-quality analytical technology is essential.

12.11.3 Oligomeric impurities in penicillins

Acute sensitivity to penicillins occurs in a minority of patients, but the reaction is well known in practice. Nevertheless, the source of at least some of the adverse reactions is not always appreciated. Impurities in penicillins have been blamed for sensitivities and allergies to this class of drug. The number of impurities found in samples of amoxicillin (**VII**) is quite remarkable.[29]

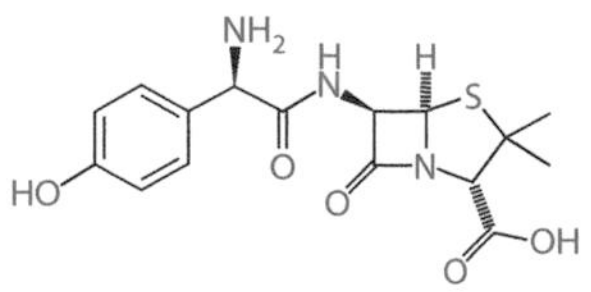

Structure VII Amoxicillin

Such impurities may include 2-hydroxy-3-(4-hydroxyphenyl)pyrazine, 4-hydroxyphenylglycine, 4-hydroxyphenylglyclamoxicillin, 6-aminopenicillanic acid, amoxicilloic acid and seven others, not including the dimer and the trimer (Fig. 12.9). These latter and other oligomers are possibly prime culprits in penicillin allergies as they are formed with peptide bonds and resemble peptides.

12.11.4 Contamination from containers

Sensitisation of the skin to topical products may not always be the result of either the drug or of the excipients. There is the potential for contamination by substances that have leached from the containers. The aluminium tube is still the most widely used container for topical creams and ointments; the tubes are lacquered to prevent direct interaction between product and aluminium. Epoxy resins are used as the protective layer in most cases, particularly bisphenyl A diglycidyl ether (BADGE)-based resins. Leaching of BADGE and its congeners depends to an extent on the formulation and the mechanical stresses applied to the tubes.[30]

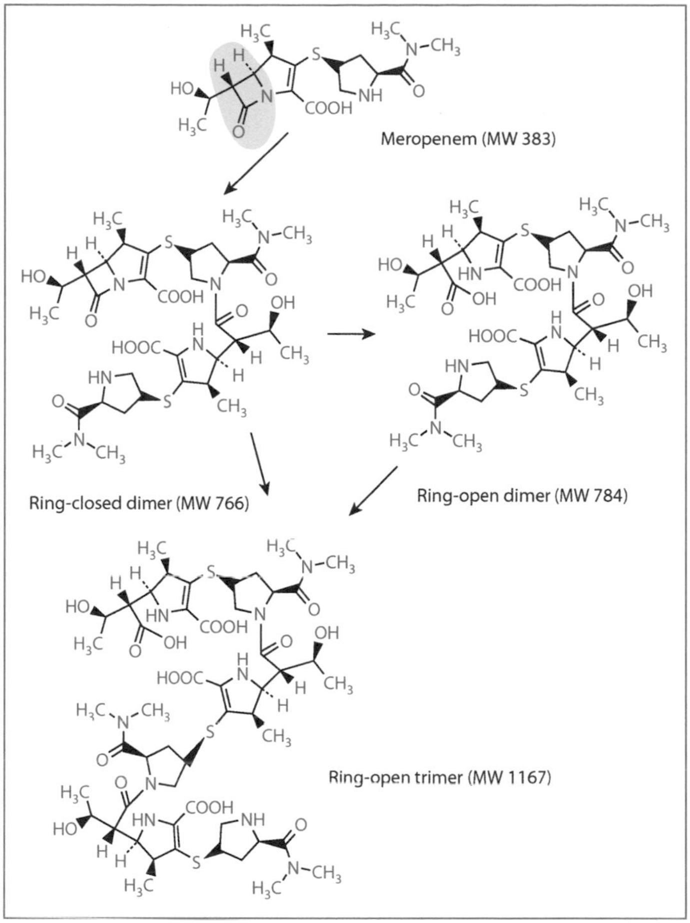

Figure 12.9 Ring-opened and ring-closed dimers and a ring-open trimer. The ring in question, the β-lactam ring, is highlighted.

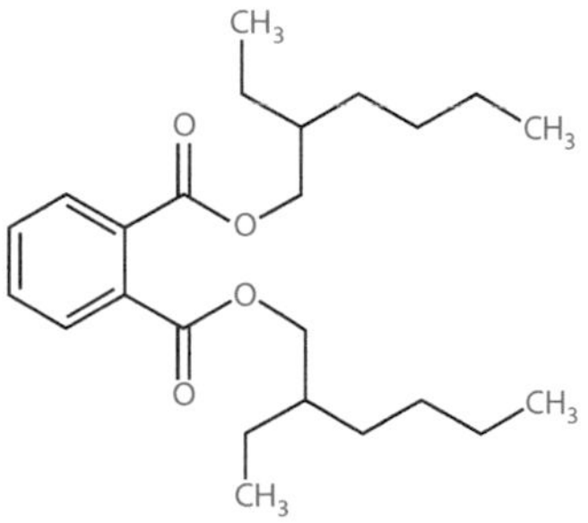

Structure VIII Di(2-ethylhexylphthalate) (DEHP)

Adverse effects due to these leachables have not been assessed but they are a potential cause, for example, of contact dermatitis.

Figure 12.10 shows the time scale of the leaching process from poly(vinyl chloride) bags into intravenous etoposide formulations.

Di(2-ethylhexylphthalate) (DEHP) (**VIII**) has a log P (octanol/water) of 7.5 and an aqueous solubility of 3 µg L^{-1}. Hence lipids and surfactants in formulations will encourage the transfer from the bags to the contents.

12.11.5 Delivery devices and materials

There is an increasing number of devices and bio-materials that are used to deliver drugs, genes and vaccines. Issues can arise with the materials used in such devices, which include syringes and giving sets, or with the manner in which the device as a whole behaves (system plus active material). There might also be technical failure of a pump or reservoir, or conditions in the device that destabilise the drug, especially if it is a protein.

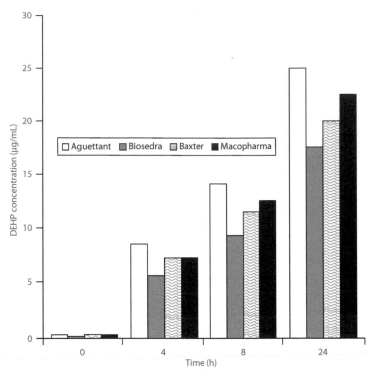

Figure 12.10 Levels of di(2-ethylhexylphthalate) (DEHP) (μg mL^{-1}) leached from bags of intravenous etoposide from different manufacturers, as shown.

Reproduced with permission from *J Clin Hosp Pharm* 2002;27:139–142.

12.11.6 Insulin pumps

One example of problems that arise through system–drug interactions is the phenomenon of protein aggregation in insulin pumps,[31] as aggregation is accompanied by a significant loss of biological activity. Various problems have been encountered with insulin pumps: obstruction in the infusion set or leakage at the infusion set connection or from the infusion site. Insulin aggregation (when insulin fibrils form) can also occur owing to agitation of the pump during wear and to temperature fluctuations. The stability is influenced by the type of insulin, the solvent and concentration.[32] Metal-ion contamination has also been implicated and the use of ethylenediaminetetra-acetic acid has been recommended to sequester ions in formulations.[33] Insulin aggregates will at times block delivery channels.

Figure 12.11 illustrates the different deposition patterns of insulin in solution following administration by pen injector, a jet injector and an external insulin pump. The diffusion of insulin from sites of administration is important for its activity; retention of insulin and its degradation at the site of deposition might reduce biological activity. Pharmacokinetic differences between these modes of administration might also be found.

In one study of bovine zinc-insulin, aggregation occurred only when there was both agitation and hydrophobic surfaces.[34]

Other proteins also degrade physically in pumps: interleukin-2 can lose 90% of its activity over a 24-hour period of infusion. Adsorption, which is a precursor of aggregate formation in some insulin systems, does not occur with interleukin-2, but irreversible structural changes can occur.[35]

Adsorption of proteins on to solid surfaces is a well-known phenomenon. Insulin adsorbs to glass, so that in low concentrations drug can be lost. Figure 12.12 shows the rate at which Asp^{B25} insulin adsorbs on to a silanated silica wafer surface.[36] At the higher concentrations adsorption is rapid, as one might expect from diffusion-controlled kinetics. One technique to avoid loss of insulin by adsorption is to add small amounts of albumin to the infusion as the albumin adsorbs first and inhibits further adsorption of the active.

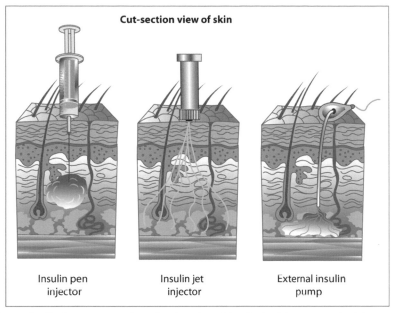

Figure 12.11 Different distribution patterns after administration of insulin by injector pen, jet injector and external insulin pump.

Reproduced from http://adam.about.com/care/diabetes.

12.11.7 Drug-eluting stents

Drug-eluting stents have made an impact in the treatment of restenosis – the proliferation of smooth-muscle cells in response to pressure from foreign objects, such as during balloon angioplasty. So, while the stent opens the artery flow, it simultaneously diminishes the stenosis. Hence, such stents have been considered a breakthrough, acting to reduce the need for repeat revascularisation after bare-metal stenting.[37] The first drug-eluting stents to appear were those with non-biodegradable (or 'durable') polymer coats as the drug reservoir. There has been debate about whether

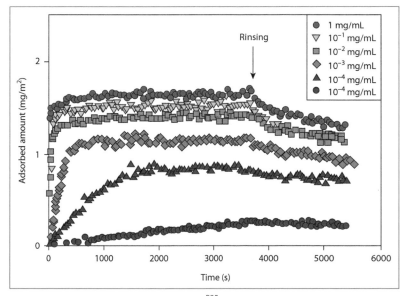

Figure 12.12 Adsorption on to silanised silica surfaces of Asp^{B25} insulin, showing the influence of concentration.

Reproduced from Mollman SH *et al*. Adsorption of human insulin and AspB28 insulin on a PTFE-like surface. *J Colloid Interface Sci* 2005;286:28–35. Copyright Elsevier 2005.

Structure IX Sirolimus

Structure X Zotarolimus

the so-called 'durable' and biodegradable coated stents are equivalent therapeutically, as there have been concerns that the former may induce inflammation. Biodegradable polymers on stents were suggested to be safer because, when degraded, the bare-metal stent is left, reducing any inflammation caused by the polymer.** Of course, some adverse effects might be due to the drug used. Among those incorporated are paclitaxel, and the antiproliferative macrolide lactams sirolimus (**IX**), everolimus and zotarolimus (**X**).

Sirolimus is formulated in a controlled-release polymer coating following coronary intervention. Several large clinical studies have demonstrated lower restenosis rates in patients treated with sirolimus-eluting stents when compared to bare-metal stents, resulting in fewer repeat procedures. A sirolimus-eluting coronary stent has been marketed by Cordis, a division of Johnson & Johnson, under the trade name Cypher. Figure 12.13 shows the proximity of the polymer drug layer on a drug-eluting stent to the tissues being treated, hence the importance of both polymer and drug in beneficial and adverse effects.

Resistance of the stent to withdrawal has been ascribed to the 'stickiness' of the stent, perhaps due to friction between the stent delivery balloon and the drug–polymer coating on the stent. The foregoing emphasises the complex nature of the development of such devices and the need for postmarketing surveillance.

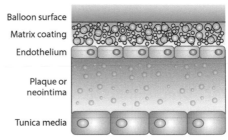

Figure 12.13 Diagram showing the proximity of the polymer drug layer on the stent surface to the endothelial cells, the plaque or neointima.

12.11.8 Catheters and infection

Intravascular catheter-related infections can be an important source of blood stream infections in patients who are critically ill.[38] It is said that more than 250 000 vascular catheter-related bacterial or fungal infections occur each year in the USA alone, with mortalities in critically ill patients of up to 25%. Bacteria can adhere to and form biofilms on catheter surfaces (see Fig. 12.14). Preventive stratagems include cutaneous antisepsis, use of sterile barriers during insertion, application of chlorhexidine-impregnated sponges and the use of antimicrobial, antibiotic-coated or silver-impregnated catheters, which depend generally on antimicrobial polymer coats, both on the external and internal surfaces of the catheters. Antimicrobial polymers are discussed in Chapter 7 and these bear many similarities to polymer therapeutic systems.

** See Chapter 7 for a brief discussion of polymer–biological interfaces.

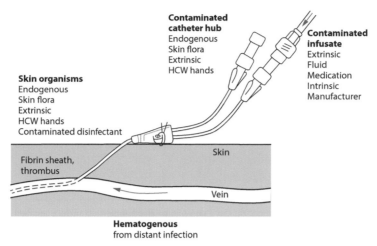

Figure 12.14 Points of entry of bacteria to an indwelling catheter. HCW = health care worker.

Urinary catheters also suffer from bacterial film formation. There are several possible points of entry of bacteria in such systems, as seen in Fig. 12.15. This is clearly an area of great importance, but some of the issues are outside the scope of this book. What is clear is that antibiotic-coated catheters are drug delivery devices and that the bacterial biofilms that form on catheters are the result of bacterial adhesion processes.

Bacterial adhesion

Bacteria adhere to solid surfaces and in so doing cause many problems. Bacterial hydrophobicity can be correlated with the adhesion of bacteria to experimental surfaces such as negatively charged polystyrene. Different bacteria have different hydrophobic properties. Contact angles of water with bacterial surfaces correlate with their hydrophobicity: the higher the contact angle, the higher the hydrophobicity and the greater the potential for adsorption.[39] Different strains of bacteria, e.g. of *Pseudomonas*, behave differently, as can be seen in Table 12.7. However, it is generally unlikely that only one parameter correlates with bacterial adsorption on to a wide range of surfaces, which are not always smooth, as in experimental systems. Nonetheless, knowing the surface properties of bacteria and of the catheter material can be valuable in understanding problems.

Table 12.7 Contact angles of water on different *Pseudomonas* spp.

Strain number and name	Contact angle (°)
Pseudomonas fluorescens	21.2
Pseudomonas aeruginosa	25.7
Pseudomonas putida	38.5
Pseudomonas sp. strain 26-3	20.1
Pseudomonas sp. strain 52	19.0
Pseudomonas sp. strain 80	29.5

Values for other organisms can range up to 60° for an *Arthrobacter* sp. strain 177 and 70° for a *Corynebacter* sp. strain 125.

Cutaneous antisepsis is clearly demanded using povidone-iodine, for example, and by maximising sterile barriers. Several other approaches are in use[38]:

- chlorhexidine-impregnated sponges (placed over site of insertion)

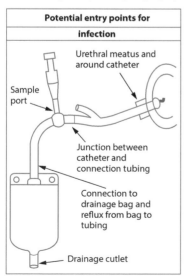

Figure 12.15 Diagram of the arrangement of a urinary catheter, with sources of infection indicated by arrows.

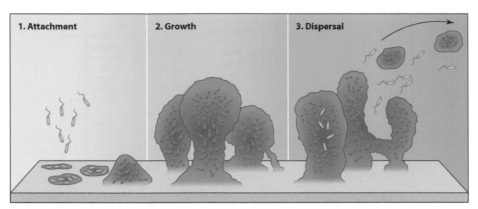

Figure 12.16 The biofilm life cycle. (1) Free-floating bacteria encounter a submerged surface and within minutes can become attached. They produce extracellular polymeric substances (EPS) and colonise surfaces. (2) EPS production allows the emerging biofilm community to develop a complex, three-dimensional structure. Biofilm communities can develop within hours. (3) Biofilms can propagate through detachment of small or large clumps of cells, or by a type of 'seeding dispersal' that releases individual cells.

Reproduced from: http://www.hypertextbookshop.com/biofilmbook/v004/r003/index.html; used with permission from Montana State University Center for Biofilm Engineering.

- antibacterial catheter locks
- antimicrobial catheters:
  - antiseptic catheters
  - antibiotic-coated catheters
  - silver-impregnated catheters.

Biofilms

Biofilms built by accumulation of bacteria are complex structures (Fig. 12.16), which makes access of antimicrobial and antibiotic agents difficult (similar to the difficulties encountered with the hindered delivery of drugs to tumours, discussed in Chapter 14). As with diffusion of solutes into any complex structure, like porous media, the architecture of the structure matters. One of the most important features in the control of access of antibiotics and other solutes is their diffusion into the biofilm, as Stewart[40] emphasised, pointing out that such diffusion can be summarised as follows.

- Diffusion is the predominant solute transport process within cell clusters.
- The time scale for diffusive equilibration of a *non-reacting* solute will range from a fraction of a second to tens of minutes in most biofilm systems.
- Diffusion limitation readily leads to gradients in the concentration of *reacting* solutes and hence to gradients in physiology.

- Water channels can carry solutes into or out of the depths of a biofilm, but they do not guarantee access to the interior of cell clusters.

Studies of the relative diffusion coefficient of small solutes such as sucrose shows that the ratio $D_{\text{biofilm}}/D_{\text{o}}$, (where D_{biofilm} and D_{o} are the diffusion coefficients in the biofilm and in water respectively) falls to around 0.2. The poor penetration and thus the action of several antibiotics are evidenced in the clinical point below.

 Clinical point

'Biofilm-related infections remain a scourge', states Siala and colleagues.[41] In an *in vitro* model of biofilms using *Staphylococcus aureus* reference strains, delafloxacin and daptomycin were found to be the most active among the antibiotics from eight different pharmacological classes.

At clinically meaningful concentrations, delafloxacin, daptomycin and vancomycin caused a ≥25% reduction in viability of the biofilms studied, respectively. The antibiotic penetration within the biofilms ranged from 0.6 to 52% for delafloxacin, 0.2 to 10% for daptomycin and 0.2 to 1% for vancomycin; for delafloxacin, this was inversely related to the polysaccharide proportion in the matrix. Six biofilms were acidic, explaining the high potency of delafloxacin (which has a lower minimum inhibitory concentration at acidic pH).

12.11.9 Transdermal patches as devices

Transdermal patches can be considered to be devices. Problems that have arisen with these include adverse reactions to the adhesive used to adhere the patch to the skin. Allergic contact dermatitis from hydroxymethylcellulose has been reported with an estradiol patch.[42] Mishaps related to use of transdermal patches include many involving patches falling off under a variety of conditions, including subsequent adhesion to another person! Other events include swelling and itching at the application site; too strong adhesion, leading to pain on removal; excessive adhesion of the plastic backing to the adhesive layer, leading to tearing of the patch; inflexible patches that do not flex with the skin; and cases of drug crystals being seen on patches.[43] Cases of burning have been reported when medicated patches containing even small amounts of aluminium are worn during magnetic resonance imaging, as a result of overheating in the area of the patch.[44]

12.12 Crystallisation

Figure 12.17 summarises some of the situations in which the solid state is important clinically. Highlighted are crystalluria, gout, the precipitation of drugs before or after injection, inhalation therapy and understanding the potential toxic effects of particulates.

Case study

A case of crystalluria[45] illustrates one of the propositions put forward in this book. The case concerned a 60-year-old man infected with HIV whose medications included efavirenz, emtricitabine, tenofovir and pravastatin sodium: a heady cocktail. Two hours after he had received aciclovir, his urine became cloudy and white in the proximal part of a Foley catheter. Microscopic analysis showed birefringent needle-like crystals 'consistent with the precipitation of acyclovir [aciclovir]', as shown in Fig. 12.18.

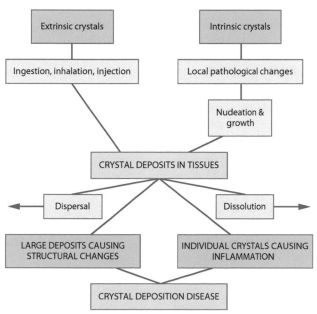

Figure 12.17 Potential clinical issues with crystal forms of drugs.

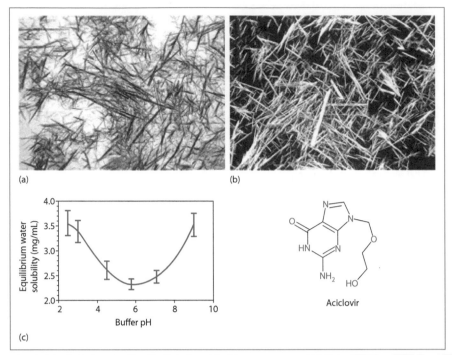

Figure 12.18 (a, b) Photomicrographs of aciclovir crystals harvested from the urine of the patient in question (a), and a pure sample (b). (c) The solubility–pH relationship for aciclovir is shown along with its chemical structure.

(a and b) Reproduced from reference 45.

(c) Reproduced from reference 46.

Additional treatment with intravenous aciclovir did not result in urinary crystallisation of the drug. Aciclovir (pK_a values: 2.27 and 9.25) has a solubility in water at 25°C of > 100 mg mL^{-1}. At physiological pH, aciclovir sodium is un-ionised and has a minimum solubility in water (at 37°C) of 2.5 mg mL^{-1} (Fig. 12.18b).[46] The concentration of aciclovir in human urine after *oral* administration of 200 mg reaches 7.5 μg mL^{-1},[47] clearly not exceeding its aqueous solubility. As urine is concentrated as it passes along nephrons, urine drug concentrations increase. Determination of saturation of drugs in urine is more predictive of problems.

This case illustrates that a knowledge of the solution properties of drugs and the pH at which drugs might precipitate or become saturated in body fluids and compartments is essential if we are to make contributions to patient care using our unique knowledge. Knowledge of the solution properties of drugs is of course applied directly in the formulation and delivery of intravenous mixtures of drugs or when drugs are added to infusion fluids.

Some time ago an editorial in the *Lancet*[48] discussed the topic of crystals in joints. It pointed out that it is not only in gout that crystals (of monosodium urate monohydrate, or of calcium pyrophosphate in pseudo-gout) appear but that calcium hydroxyapatite deposits cause apatite deposition disease. The discussion indicated that synovial fluid may contain pieces of cartilage, strands of fibrin, cholesterol crystals and, in some patients, steroid crystals remaining after intra-articular injection. Biological systems are of course complex. Urine and blood are more complex than water, so simple theories of solution properties cannot be applied directly, especially when we introduce formulations into already multicomponent environments. Nevertheless, theory and equations give clues as to what might be happening *in vivo*. Without them we only guess.

12.13 Abnormal bioavailability and adverse events

Classical examples where the bioavailability has changed after a period when patients have been stabilised and physicians accustomed to responses from a particular dose form or brand include that of digoxin

(Lanoxin). In the 1970s a change in the manufacturing process led to a marked difference in bioavailability through an increase in particle size, resulting from a change in the processing of the drug. Another example was when a change in the main excipient from calcium carbonate to lactose in a brand of phenytoin sodium led to a marked increase in bioavailability and over-dosing. The calcium was clearly forming a poorly soluble calcium salt of the drug, decreasing its intrinsic solubility and its rate of dissolution. Its removal led to faster absorption and toxic effects in titrated patients. Other examples of formulation-related effects are discussed in Chapters 8 and 9.

12.13.1 Testing for adverse effects

How can pharmacists become more involved in searching for the causes of adverse effects and reactions related to dosage forms and devices? This depends on:

- a thorough knowledge of the nature of the ingredients and their purpose in the medication concerned
- understanding the nature of the drug substance and its likely interactions with excipients
- understanding the structure of systems such as controlled-release preparations
- carrying out straightforward tests to investigate potential problems
- improving the scoring of severity and adopting more quantitative approaches to this.

One example derives from work between the University of Strathclyde and the Contact Dermatitis Unit at Belvidere Hospital, Glasgow, some years ago, where modes of quantitative measurement of skin reactions to substances applied to the skin were explored. The aim was to replace more subjective (−, +, ++, +++) clinical scoring of effects. Contact dermatitis is a (skin) reaction resulting from exposure to allergens (allergic contact dermatitis) or irritants (irritant contact dermatitis). Phototoxic dermatitis occurs when the allergen or irritant is activated by sunlight. Contact dermatitis can occur from contact with jewellery but also from drugs and devices (e.g. transdermal patch adhesives).

Contact dermatitis testing

Suspected contact dermatitis is usually tested for by application of a series of patches containing putative causative agents. The formulation of these materials has often been fairly crude (for example, by dispersing nickel sulfate in a paraffin base) and this might affect the outcome. Poor attention to pharmaceutical principles of release, poor choice of vehicle and lack of consideration of particle size all contribute to imprecision.[49] Proprietary patch formulations are available. Test results are often evaluated against a control or controls by clinical scoring of reactions from severe (+++), through (++), (+), 0 and equivocal (<+). Skin reflectance measurements were evaluated as a measure of skin haemoglobin content and correlated well with clinical scoring.[50] The following is an example of a study conducted some time ago.[49]

A group of 43 patients with a clinical history of nickel allergy who exhibited an equivocal or no allergic reaction to a patch test at 48 hours were further challenged using several different formulations of nickel sulfate. This experimental test battery comprised aqueous, dimethyl sulfoxide and propylene glycol solutions of nickel sulfate, and nickel sulfate incorporated into Cetomacrogol cream and yellow soft paraffin (Paraffin Molle Flavum: PMF). Although some of these vehicles were irritant, a formulation-dependent test response was observed, such that in terms of the number of responses per unit weight of nickel sulfate applied to the skin, the vehicles could be ranked: dimethyl sulfoxide > propylene glycol > aqueous solution > Cetomacrogol cream > PMF preparations. This ranking could be correlated with the relative ease with which nickel sulfate could be dialysed from each vehicle *in vitro*. This study demonstrates that, for nickel sulfate, the vehicle can influence the outcome of patch testing, apparently by modifying the quantity of nickel released into the skin for elicitation of the allergic response. (Cetomacrogol is a non-ionic surfactant with a C_{16} hydrocarbon chain and an average 24-unit polyoxyethylene oxide hydrophilic chain.)

Release of nickel sulfate from the test preparations varied considerably, as shown in Fig. 12.19. The correlation between skin blood flow (plotted in Fig. 12.20 as the haemoglobin index) and clinical scoring is good. The response is often a weal which reflects increased blood flow and, of course, heat output. Infrared thermography has also been used.[51] This is a convenient non-invasive technique that employs an infrared camera and can be used to discriminate between irritant and allergic responses and to quantify the latter.

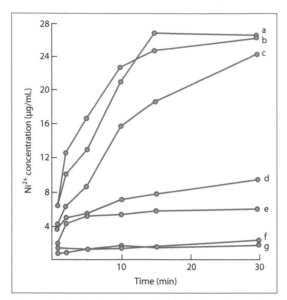

Figure 12.19 *In vitro* release of nickel sulfate from various vehicles at 37°C using a dialysis technique. Curve a, an aqueous solution of nickel sulfate ($NiSO_4$); curve b, propylene glycol solution; curve c, dimethyl sulfoxide (DMSO) solution; curve d, Cetomacrogol cream; curve e, 2.5% $NiSO_4$ in yellow soft paraffin (proprietary formulation); curve f, yellow soft paraffin; curve g, 5% $NiSO_4$ in yellow soft paraffin (proprietary formulation).

Reproduced from Mendelow AY *et al.* Patch testing for nickel allergy. The influence of the vehicle on the response rate to topical nickel sulphate. *Contact Dermatitis* 1985;13:29–33. Copyright Wiley-VCH Verlag GmbH & Co. KGaA. Reproduced with permission.

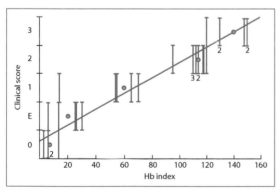

Figure 12.20 Correlation between clinical scores of patient responses to a variety of proprietary test patches and the haemoglobin (Hb) index derived from a skin reflectance technique. The individual test patches contained separately nickel, chromium, colophony fragrances, thiomersal, benzoic acid, parabens, neomycin and a range of other materials implicated in contact dermatitis.

Reproduced from Mendelow AY *et al.* Skin reflectance measurements of patch test responses. *Contact Dermatitis* 1986;15:73–78. Copyright Wiley-VCH Verlag GmbH & Co. KGaA. Reproduced with permission.

Figure 12.21 shows some results after application of the contact dermatitis test patches, both the appearance of the reactions to different formulations and the results when assessed using the infrared camera. The infrared thermograms, which detect the increased blood flow and heat profiles, show not only the intensity but also the spread of the reaction on the skin.

The simple *in vitro* tests for the disintegration behaviour of emopronium bromide tablets discussed earlier in this chapter illustrate clearly that investigation does not necessarily involve expensive equipment. Dissolution testing can also show differences or confirm patients' concerns about generic products, or perhaps detect counterfeit medicines emanating from internet suppliers.

Mechanisms of toxicity of nanosystems are discussed in Chapter 14. Undoubtedly, new adverse effects will arise from the use of nanosytems. Much has still to be learned about the potential downsides of nanomedicines and assurances on the safety of the materials from which they are made are not always sufficient to instill confidence in the complete safety of the nanoparticles. Because of the vast array of possible systems, it is impossible to generalise. Each system will have to be examined and tested on its merits.

The last section deals with light-induced reactions, either following the administration of a drug such as a fluoroquinolone or through photodynamic therapy (PDT). This section has a specific focus on light but it illustrates the multifaceted nature of reactions to drugs and formulations.

12.14 Photochemical reactions and photoinduced reactions

First, it is essential to define a variety of light-induced effects. These include:

- *photoallergy*: an acquired immunological reactivity dependent on antibody- or cell-mediated hypersensitivity
- *photosensitivity*: a broad term used to describe an adverse reaction to light after drug administration, which may be photoallergic or phototoxic in nature
- *phototoxicity*: the conversion of an otherwise nontoxic chemical or drug to one that is toxic to tissues after absorption of electromagnetic radiation

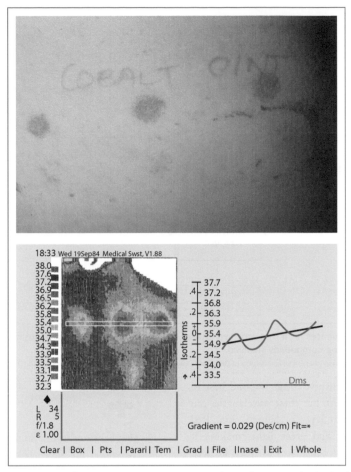

Figure 12.21 (a) Typical appearance of positive reactions to contact with patch tests on the back of a subject. (b) An infrared thermogram of the back of a (different) patient who has been assessed for contact dermatitis to nickel with three formulations of nickel sulfate. The image shows not only differences in intensity but also difference in the spread of the response. These thermograms are more informative than physicians' scoring systems.

- *photodynamic effects*: photoinduced damage requiring the presence of light, photosensitiser and molecular oxygen
- *PDT*: therapy in which photoactive drugs inactive in the unexcited state are administered and activated at particular sites in the body.

Many drugs decompose *in vitro* after exposure to light, but the consequences depend on the nature of the breakdown products (Fig. 12.22). Some derivatives of nifedipine have a very short photochemical half-life, sometimes of the order of a few minutes, while others decompose only after several weeks' exposure. A drug may not decompose after exposure to light, but may be the source of free radicals or of phototoxic metabolites *in vivo*. Adverse reactions occur when the drug or metabolites are exposed to light and the absorption

spectrum of the drug coincides with the wavelength of light to which it is exposed (the wavelengths of ultraviolet-A (UV-A) are 320–400 nm; of UV-B 280–320 nm; and of UV-C 200–290 nm). To behave as a photoallergen, a drug or chemical must be able to absorb light energy present in sunlight and on absorption of the light generate a chemical species capable of binding to proteins in the skin, either directly or after metabolism.[52]

12.14.1 How do photosensitisers work?

In PDT, drugs that can be activated by light are administered intravenously. The drug remains inactive until exposed to light with a wavelength that can penetrate the skin but is not completely attenuated by

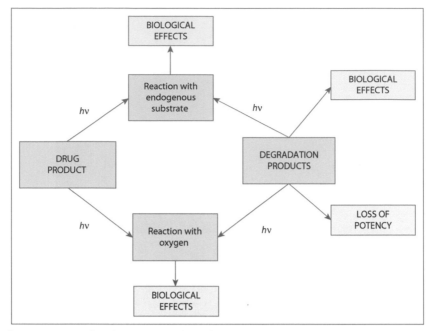

Figure 12.22 The consequences for a light-sensitive drug of interaction with light energy, causing biological effects and loss of potency depending on the compounds involved.
Redrawn with permission from Tønneson HH (ed.). *Photostability of Drugs and Drug Solutions*. London: Taylor and Francis; 1996.

the blood. Most photosensitive drugs respond best to blue or green light *in vitro*, but these wavelengths can pass through only a thin layer of human skin. Red blood cells absorb blue and green light, making it impossible for most photosensitisers to work in deep or bloody places. Texaphyrins, on the other hand, respond best to a specific red light that passes through blood. Light energy is directed to the required site through a fibreoptic device. When activated, the drug – usually a porphyrin derivative – creates oxygen radicals that destroy tissue in its vicinity. Principal side-effects of drugs like Photofrin have a skin sensitivity to light for up to 6 weeks as the drug is available systemically and partitions into lipid layers.

Other drugs cause light sensitivity; these are those that deposit in the skin and either interact with light or degrade to form coloured complexes. Coloration is not always a sign of pathological change.

Temoporfin (**XI**: Foscan) and porfimer sodium (**XII**: Photofrin) are used in PDT of various tumours. Activated by laser light they produce a cytotoxic effect in the tissues in which they accumulate. Temoporfin is licensed in the UK for the therapy of advanced head and neck cancers, while porfimer sodium is used in the PDT of non-small-cell lung cancer and oesophageal cancer.

 Clinical point

The cautions given in the *British National Formulary* for porfimer are to 'avoid exposure of the skin to direct sunlight or bright indoor light for at least 30 days', and for temoporfin 'for at least 15 days', but to avoid prolonged exposure of the injection site to direct sunlight for 6 months after administration.

12.14.2 Chemical photosensitivity

In chemical photosensitivity, patients develop redness, inflammation and sometimes brown or blue discoloration in areas of skin that have been exposed to sunlight for a brief period. This reaction occurs after ingestion of drugs, such as tetracycline, or the application of compounds topically in consumer products such as perfumes or aftershaves. These substances (Table 12.8) may make some skin types more sensitive to the effects of UV light. Some develop hives with itching, which indicates a type of drug allergy triggered by sunlight.

Structures XI and XII Temoporfin and the oligomer (*n* = 0–6) porfimer sodium

Table 12.8 Some substances that sensitise skin to sunlight

Type	Examples
Anxiolytics	Alprazolam, chlordiazepoxide
Antibiotics	Quinolones, sulfonamides, tetracyclines, trimethoprim
Antidepressants	Tricyclics
Antifungals (oral)	Griseofulvin
Antihypertensives	Sulfonylureas
Antimalarials	Chloroquine, quinine
Antipsychotics	Phenothiazines
Diuretics	Furosemide, thiazides
Chemotherapeutics	Dacarbazine, fluorouracil, methotrexate, vinblastine
Antiacne drugs (oral)	Isotretinoin
Cardiovascular drugs	Amiodarone, quinidine
Skin preparations	Chlorhexidine, hexachlorophene, coal tar, fragrances, sunscreens

12.15 Conclusions

Detecting the causes of adverse events is not an easy task, especially when drugs or drug products are novel. It is essential that one looks for analogies, reliable reports on closely chemically and pharmacologically related drugs and similar formulations. This requires a breadth of knowledge of similar events recorded in the literature or from experience. The few examples noted in this chapter may assist in asking the right questions.

C Case study **Burns after photodynamic therapy**

Problems have been reported during a clinical trial with Foscan. This contains temoporfin as its active ingredient. In the trial it was alleged that a high proportion of patients suffered burns.[53] The manufacturer of the product complained that the results were at odds with more extensive trials of the product.[54] It subsequently emerged that in the trials the formulation of the product was different from that of the marketed product. It was claimed that a new solvent had been added so that the drug would be more soluble and less painful to administer. Here was the scenario: trial data are disputed, there is some confusion or inadequate reporting of the formulation used (there are many instances of this, including the problems that arise with the different formulations of amphotericin) and an underlying effect of the active substance, a porphyrin. Later, two of the physicians involved in the trial[55] admitted that there may have been a connection between the leakage and the effect of the solvent as the active agent had spread from the point of administration. The adverse events were not due to extravasation injury itself as they occurred only after photoactivation.[56] This is a good example of the interlocking effects of drug, formulation and the nature of clinical trials, where the influence of the formulation was underestimated or neglected.

The concluding illustration (Fig. 12.23) summarises how one might approach the issues. A fuller record of adverse events and the involvement of delivery systems can be read: the older literature should not be discarded as there may be clues there which might have relevance to new medicines and treatments.

Potential mechanisms should be proposed and the following questions asked:

- Is the event due to the drug?
- Is the event linked to the use of another medication?
- Is it an excipient effect?

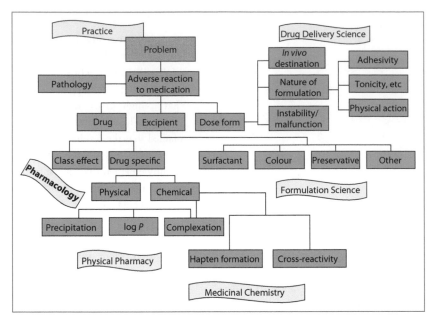

Figure 12.23 Charting the causes of adverse reactions to medications. The many causes are shown in relation to drug, excipient, nature of formulation, the dosage form or device and whether there are physical or chemical causes.

- Is it a vehicle or matrix effect?
- Is it a result of the physical nature of the dosage form?
- Is it the result of concomitant pathologies?
- Is it unrelated to the medication?

The determination or, better, the prediction of potential adverse reactions is an important task. It requires constant attention to the literature, a good knowledge of the chemistry of offending drugs, the influence of the formulation, determining the mechanisms if possible, and certainly looking for trends and patterns. It is a fascinating and vital subject. Nearly all the topics raised here can be the subject of chapters in themselves.

References

1. Uchegbu IF, Florence AT. Adverse drug events related to dosage forms and delivery systems. *Drug Saf* 1996;14:39–67.
2. Balbani APS *et al*. Pharmaceutical excipients and the information on drug labels. *Rev Bras Otorinolaringol* 2006;72:400–406.
3. Millar JS. Pitfalls of 'inert' ingredients. *Br J Gen Pract* 2001;51:570.
4. Cubitt GT. Pitfalls of 'inert' ingredients. *Br J Gen Pract* 2001;51:756.
5. Pifferi G, Restani P. The safety of pharmaceutical excipients. *Il Farmaco* 2003;58:541–550.
6. Seidenari S *et al*. Cross-sensitisations between azo dyes and *para*-amino compound: a study of 236 azo-dye-sensitive subjects. *Contact Dermatitis* 1997;36:91–96.
7. ten Tije AJ *et al*. Pharmacological effects of formulation vehicles: implications in cancer chemotherapy. *Clin Pharmacokinet* 2003;42:665–685.
8. Phillips DM, Zacharopoulous VR. Nonoxynol-9 enhances rectal infection by herpes simplex virus in mice. *Contraception* 1998;57:341–348.
9. Smith CM *et al*. Pluronic F-68 reduces the endothelial adherence and improves the rheology of liganded sickle erythrocytes. *Blood* 1987;69:1631–1636.
10. Orringer EP *et al*. Purified poloxamer 188 for treatment of acute vaso-occlusive crisis of sickle cell disease. *JAMA* 2001;286:2099–2106.
11. Lee R. Pipe dream or paradigm shift? *University of Chicago Magazine* 2006;98(3). Available online at: magazine.uchicago.edu/0602/features (accessed 24 March 2015).
12. Medicine.net.com. *Pleurisy*. Available online at: http://www.medicinenet.com/pleurisy/article.htm (accessed 20 September 2009).
13. Aelony Y. Talc pleurodesis and acute respiratory distress syndrome. *Lancet* 2007;369: 1494–1496.
14. Marchi E *et al*. Talc for pleurodesis. Hero or villain? *Chest* 2003;124:416–417.
15. Ferrar J *et al*. Influence of particle size on extrapleural talc dissemination after talc slurry pleurodesis. *Chest* 2002;1221018–1027.

16. Bogman K *et al.* The role of surfactants in the reversal of active transport mediated by multidrug resistance proteins. *J Pharm Sci* 2003;92:1250–1261.

17. Hu Z *et al.* A novel emulsifier, Labrasol enhances gastrointestinal absorption of gentamicin. *Life Sci* 2001;69:2899–2810.

18. Singh MK *et al.* Another reason to dislike medication. *Lancet* 2008;371:1388.

19. Levy DJ. An aspirin tablet and a gastric ulcer. *N Engl J Med* 2000;343:863.

20. Florence AT, Salole EG (eds). *Formulation Factors in Adverse Reactions.* London: Wright; 1990.

21. Holly FJ. Formation and rupture of the tear film. *Exp Eye Res* 1973;15:515–525.

22. Njobuenwu DO. Spreading of trisiloxanes on thin water film: dry spot profile. *Leonardo J Sci* 2007;6:165–178.

23. Lawrenson JG, Murphy PJ. The neonatal tear film. *Contact Lens Anterior Eye* 2003;26:197–202.

24. McMonnies CW. Incomplete blinking: exposure keratopathy, lid wiper epitheliopathy, dry eye, refractive surgery and dry contact lenses. *Contact Lens Anterior Eye* 2007;30:37–51.

25. Firestone BA *et al.* Solubility characteristics of three fluoroquinolone ophthalmic solutions in an *in vitro* tear model. *Int J Pharm* 1998;164:119–128.

26. *WHO Drug Information* 2008;22:84–85.

27. Beyer T *et al.* Quality assessment of unfractionated heparin using ^{1}H nuclear magnetic resonance spectroscopy. *J Pharm Biomed Anal* 2008;48:13–19.

28. Matsuno Y-K *et al.* Electrophoresis studies on the contaminating glycosaminoglycan in commercially available hyaluronic acid products. *Electrophoresis* 2008;29:3628–3635.

29. Jouyban A, Kenndler E. Impurity analysis of pharmaceuticals using capillary electromigration methods. *Electrophoresis* 2008;9:3531–3551.

30. Haverkamp JB *et al.* Contamination of semi-solid dosage forms by leachables from aluminium tubes. *Eur J Pharm Biopharm* 2008;70:921–928.

31. Guilhem I *et al.* Technical risks with subcutaneous insulin infusion. *Diabetes Metab* 2006;32:279–284.

32. Hirsh IB *et al.* Catheter obstruction with continuous subcutaneous insulin infusion. Effect of insulin concentration. *Diabetes Care* 1992;15:593–594.

33. James DE *et al.* Insulin precipitation in artificial infusion devices. *Diabetologia* 1981;21:554–557.

34. Sluzky V *et al.* Kinetics of insulin aggregation in aqueous solutions upon agitation in the presence of hydrophobic surfaces. *Proc Natl Acad Sci USA* 1991;88:9377–9381.

35. Tzannis ST *et al.* Irreversible inactivation of interleukin 2 in a pump-based delivery environment. *Proc Natl Acad Sci USA* 1996;93:5460–5465.

36. Mollman SH *et al.* Adsorption of human insulin and AspB28 insulin on a PTFE-like surface. *J Colloid Interface Sci* 2005;286:28–35.

37. Waksman R, Maluenda G. Polymer-drug eluting stents: is the future biodegradable? *Lancet* 2013; 378:1900–1902.

38. Raad I *et al.* Intravascular catheter-related infections: advances diagnosis, prevention and management. *Lancet Infect* 2007;7:645–657.

39. van Loosdrecht MCM *et al.* The role of the bacterial cell wall hydrophobicity in adhesion. *Appl Environ Microbiol* 1987;53:1893–1897.

40. Stewart PS. Diffusion in biofilms. *J Bacteriol* 2003;185:1485–1491.

41. Siala W *et al. Antimicrob Ag Chemother* 2014;58:6385–6397.

42. Schwartz BK, Glendinning WE. *Contact Dermatitis* 2006;18:106–107.

43. Wokovich AM *et al.* Transdermal drug delivery systems (TDDS) adhesion as a critical safety, efficacy and quality attribute. *Eur J Pharm Biopharm* 2006;64:1–8.

44. Lowry F. Medicated patch can cause burns during MRI, FDA warns. *Medscape Medical News* 2009. Available online at: www.fda.gov/NewsEvents/Newsroom/PressAnnouncements/ucm149537.htm (accessed 14 May 2009).

45. Mason WJ, Nickols HH. Crystalluria from acyclovir use. *N Engl J Med* 2008;358:e14.

46. Shojaei AH *et al.* Transbuccal delivery of acyclovir: I. In vitro determination of routes of buccal transport. *Pharm Res* 1998;15:1181–1188.

47. Testereci H *et al.* The determination of acyclovir in sheep serum, human serum, saliva and urine by HPLC. *East J Med* 1998;3:62–66.

48. Editorial. Crystals in joints. *Lancet* 1980;1:1006–1007.

49. Mendelow AY *et al.* Patch testing for nickel allergy. The influence of the vehicle on the response rate to topical nickel sulphate. *Contact Dermatitis* 1985;13:29–33.

50. Mendelow AY *et al.* Skin reflectance measurements of patch test responses. *Contact Dermatitis* 1986;15:73–78.

51. Baillie AJ *et al.* Thermographic assessment of patch-test responses. *Br J Dermatol* 1990;122:351–360.

52. Barratt MD. Structure–activity relationships and prediction of the phototoxicity and phototoxic potential of new drugs. *ATLA* 2004;32:511–524.

53. Hettiaratchy S *et al.* Burns after photodynamic therapy. *Br Med J* 2000;320:1245.

54. (a) Bryce R. Burns after photodynamic therapy. *Br Med J* 2000;320:1731. (b) Dow R. *Br Med J* 2000;321:53.

55. Täubel J, Besa C. Burns after photodynamic therapy. *Br Med J* 2000;320:1732.

56. Hettiaratchy S, Clarke J. Burns after photodynamic therapy. *Br Med J* 2000;320:1731.

Further reading

Gonçalo M. Phototoxic and photoallergic reactions. Chapter 18. In Johansen JD *et al.* (eds) *Contact Dermatitis*. Berlin: Springer-Verlag; 2010.

Hatashi N *et al.* New findings on the structure-photosensitivity relationship and photostability of fluoroquinolones with various substituents at position 1. *Antimicrob Agn Chemother* 2004;48:799-803.

McCann MT, Gilmore BF, Gorman SP. *Staphylococcus epidermidis* device-related infections: pathogenesis and clinical management. *J Pharm Pharmacol* 2008;60:1551–1571.

Peptides, proteins and monoclonal antibodies

An increasing number of therapeutic substances are peptides or proteins, whether natural or synthetic in origin or produced by recombinant DNA technology or from transgenic animals. Most peptides and proteins are not absorbed to any significant extent by the oral route because of their degradation in the acidic conditions of the stomach and because of their intrinsic size and charge. Most available formulations of protein pharmaceuticals are therefore parenteral products for injection or inhalation (Table 13.1). DNA, RNA and various oligonucleotides are being used increasingly in gene therapy. These share some of the problems of proteins as therapeutic agents, principally owing to their high molecular weight, relative fragility and ionic nature. Monoclonal antibodies (MAbs) are being increasingly used clinically and the physical and pharmaceutical issues of these products are discussed in the last section of the chapter.

The object of this chapter is to provide some background for the appreciation of the pharmaceutics of proteins, peptide DNA, oligonucleotides and MAbs as therapeutic entities. From an understanding of the nature of amino acids and their physical properties comes an appreciation of the physical nature and properties of peptides, polypeptides and proteins. The solution properties of proteins in simple and complex media have to be understood, together with the factors affecting the stability of proteins in solution. Problems in the formulation and clinical use of proteins to be overcome will then become clearer.

First some definitions:

- *Peptides* have a short chain of residues with a defined amino acid sequence; therapeutic peptides include ciclosporin, octreotide and somatostatin, which are *cyclic peptides*.
- *Polypeptides* have longer amino acid chains, usually of defined sequence and length.
- *Polyamino acids* have random amino acid sequences of varying lengths, generally resulting from

non-specific polymerisation of one or more amino acids. One such is available as a drug for the treatment of multiple sclerosis – glatiramer (Copaxone).

- *Proteins* are those polypeptides that occur naturally and have a definite three-dimensional structure under physiological conditions.
- *Nucleotides* are the building block of nucleic acids, consisting of a five-carbon sugar covalently bonded to a nitrogenous base (adenine, thymine, guanine, cytosine or uracil) and a phosphate group.
- *Oligonucleotides* are short (10–25) sequences of nucleotides.
- *Plasmid DNA* is a circular piece of DNA that exists apart from the chromosome and replicates independently of it.

Other oligomeric substances such as the antisense oligonucleotides and DNA fragments are being used therapeutically and, for these as with proteins, no systematic approaches to their pharmacy have been defined. New modes of delivery of many or all of these agents will need to be developed if they are to be used to their maximal advantage. It is misleading to assume that because many are either natural substances or their close analogues they are safe. Injection of abnormal doses even of endogenous agents at sites where they do not naturally exist can often induce bizarre side-effects. Hence the need for optimised formulations, delivered in appropriate ways to the most appropriate target sites.

Development of improved formulations and delivery systems requires a good understanding of the physical pharmacy of these molecules if we are to avoid typical problems of degradation, unwanted adsorption to glassware and plastics and aggregation in delivery devices such as reservoirs or pumps.

13.1 Structure and solution properties of peptides and proteins

13.1.1 Structure of peptides and proteins

The *primary* structure of a protein is the order in which the individual amino acids are sequenced. This tells us little about the shape that the protein will assume in solution, although the primary structure determines the *secondary*, *tertiary* and even *quaternary* forms. These amino acid building blocks (Table 13.2) give the key to structure and behaviour. The standard three-letter (Glu, Arg, Trp, etc.) and one-letter (G, A, W, etc.) abbreviations for amino acids are also listed: their use makes structural descriptions more accessible.

Secondary structures include the coiled α-helix, and pleated sheets, discussed below and shown in Figs 13.1 and 13.2. Chain folding, arising from cross-linking through hydrogen bonding, the hydrophobic effect and salt bridges, leads to a definition of tertiary structure, and association of these structural units leads to quaternary forms.

Representations in a stylised diagrammatic form of three proteins (interleukin-1β, zinc insulin dimers and the Fc fragment of immunoglobulin) are shown in Fig. 13.3. The nature of the three-dimensional structure shows how difficult it is to define proteins in conventional ways, and how they must be considered in a new light as pharmaceutical entities. They are in many ways fragile molecules. Loss of the unique tertiary or quaternary structure, through denaturation, can occur from a variety of insults that would not affect smaller molecules.

Complex structures are formed in solution because of interactions between the structural amino acids. Unfortunately, knowing the amino acid sequence of a protein is not enough to enable us to predict its physical behaviour. Function is determined by the way the linear chains of amino acids fold in solution to give specific three-dimensional structures comprising the coils, sheets and folds (Figs 13.1 and 13.2). Strides are being made in understanding the 'grammar' of protein folding, through the synthesis of synthetic peptides and sequences and observation of their structures. Some of the primary structures are so complex that it is not possible to predict their physicochemical properties, although modern molecular modelling techniques have made great inroads into understanding tertiary structure and behaviour.

Table 13.1 Some therapeutic proteins and peptides, their molecular weights and actions

Protein/peptide	Size (kDa)	Use/action
Oxytocin	1.0	Uterine contraction
Vasopressin	1.1	Diuresis
Leuprolide acetate	1.3	Prostatic carcinoma therapy
Luteinising hormone-releasing hormone analogues	~1.5	Prostatic carcinoma therapy
Somatostatin	3.1	Growth inhibition
Calcitonin	3.4	Ca^{2+} regulation
Glucagon	3.5	Diabetes therapy
Parathyroid hormone (1–34)	4.3	Ca^{2+} regulation
Insulin	6	Diabetes therapy
Parathyroid hormone (1–84)	9.4	Ca^{2+} regulation
Interferon-gamma	16 (dimer)	Antiviral agent
Tumour necrosis factor-α	17.5 (trimer)	Antitumour agent
Interferon-α$_2$	19	Leukaemia, hepatitis therapy
Interferon-β$_1$	20	Lung cancer therapy
Growth hormone	22	Growth acceleration
DNase	~32	Cystic fibrosis therapy
α$_1$-Antitrypsin	45	Cystic fibrosis therapy
Albumin	68	Plasma volume expander
Bovine IgG	150	Immunisation
Catalase	230	Treatment of wounds and ulcers
Cationic ferritin	400+	Anaemias

Reproduced with permission from Niven RW. Delivery of biotherapeutics by inhalation aerosols. *Pharm Technol* 1993;July: 72.

13.1.2 Hydrophobicity of peptides and proteins

Amino acids have a range of physical properties, each having a greater or lesser degree of hydrophilic or hydrophobic nature. Naturally, if amino acids are spatially arranged in a molecule so that distinct hydrophobic and hydrophilic regions appear, then the polypeptide or protein will have an amphiphilic nature. Table 13.3 lists the relative hydrophobic character of a range of amino acids, where Gly is considered to have a value of zero. The amino acids range from very hydrophobic to very hydrophilic. The side-chains of selected amino acids are shown in the table where their relative hydrophobic properties are shown. Some values of log P (octanol/water) are also given, demonstrating the trend in hydrophobic parameters.

An idea of the overall hydrophobicity of a peptide or protein may be gained from the use of indices of the hydrophobicity of the individual amino acids. Secondary and tertiary structures are important in determining the actual hydrophobic nature of the polypeptide, however, and this complicates the prediction of their physicochemical properties such as solubility and adsorption.

If alternating hydrophilic and hydrophobic amino acid sequences in synthetic peptides are at the right distances in space, the molecule coils with the hydrophobic amino acids on the inside of each coil and the hydrophilic ones to the outside. There are still, however, many structural mysteries: the interior of many protein structures with myriad side-chains, and the way in which metal ions can stabilise three-dimensional structures, have been likened to a *terra incognita*.

13.1.3 Solubility of peptides and proteins

As most proteins are delivered parenterally in solution it is important to understand their properties. In physiological conditions the aqueous solubilities of proteins vary enormously from the very soluble to the virtually insoluble. In section 4.2.4 we discussed the solubility profiles of zwitterions, including tryptophan, which all have biphasic solubility–pH profiles. One would expect proteins with terminal —NH_2 and —COOH groups to behave similarly, although the effect will be complicated by the behaviour of the multitude of the intermediate amino acids, as can be seen from the pH–solubility profile of insulin in Chapter 9, Fig. 9.5. Figure 13.4 shows the general solubility behaviour of a protein (β-lactoglobin) as a function of pH at two ionic strengths.

The solubility of globular proteins increases as the pH of the solution moves away from the isoelectric point, which is the pH at which the molecule has a net

Table 13.2 Nomenclature and structure of the principal amino acids. The common name, the three-letter code and the single-letter code are given

Glycine (Gly) G · Alanine (Ala) A · Valine (Val) V · Serine (Ser) S · Threonine (Thr) T

Methionine (Met) M · Phenylalanine (Phe) F · Tryptophan (Trp) W · Proline (Pro) P · Glutamine (Gln) Q

Leucine (Leu) L · Isoleucine (Ile) I · Cysteine (Cys) C · Tyrosine (Try) Y · Asparagine (Asn) N

Aspartic acid (Asp) D · Glutamic acid (Glu) E · Lysine (Lys) K · Arginine (Arg) R · Histidine (His) H

zero charge and does not migrate in an electric field. Some examples of the isoelectric points of amino acids are shown in Table 13.4. At its isoelectric point a protein has no net charge and has a greater tendency to self-associate. As the net charge increases, the affinity of the protein for the aqueous environment increases and the protein molecules also exert a greater electrostatic repulsion. However, extremes of pH can cause protein unfolding, which not infrequently exposes further non-polar groups.

The relative hydrophilicities of the side-chains of the amino acids correlate well with the hydration of the side-chain; proteins are surrounded by a hydration layer, equivalent to about 0.3 g H_2O per gram of protein, which represents about two water molecules per amino acid residue. Disturbing this layer has an impact on the behaviour of the protein in solution.

The phase behaviour of protein solutions is affected by pH, ionic strength and temperature. Protein–water solutions sometimes exhibit critical

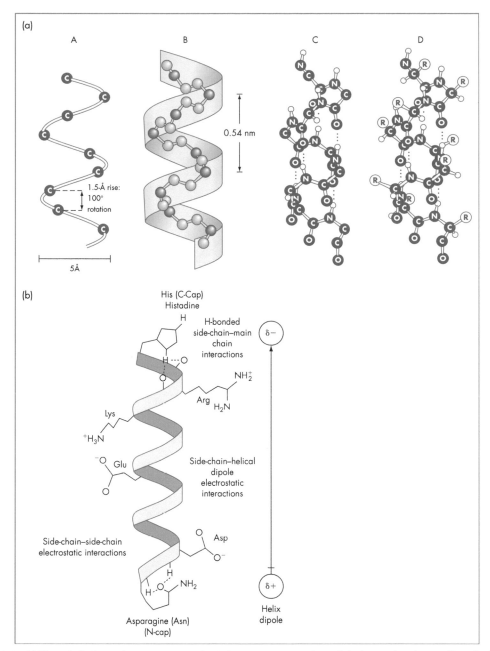

Figure 13.1 (a) The α-helix forms, because —NH and —C=O groups interact through hydrogen bonding, pulling the backbone into a spiral, as shown in this diagram in a 9-amino peptide: in (A) here only the central carbon atoms are shown for clarity; in (B) the nitrogen and carbons of the backbone are shown, and in (C) the oxygen and hydrogen atoms have been added. All the —NH groups point in the same direction 'up' and the —C=O groups point 'down' to allow the formation of —C=O ... H—N— bonds. In (D) the side-chains are added and point outwards from the α-helix. Hydrophobic interactions between some helix-promoting side-chains (the more hydrophobic chains: Table 13.3) help to stabilise the helix. (b) An idealised α-helix, drawn as a ribbon, showing typical stabilising intrahelical interactions. Specific hydrogen-bonded interactions are said to 'cap' the ends of the chain, known specifically as the N-terminal and C-terminal ends of the helix. Free energies (ΔG) of the interactions, compared with the free energy of hydrophobic bonding involving an isobutyl side-chain (-4.18 kJ mol^{-1}), are:
N-cap, 4.2–8.4 kJ mol^{-1}
C-cap, $\sim$2 kJ mol^{-1}
Side-chain–side-chain electrostatic interactions, $\sim$2 kJ mol^{-1}

Reproduced with permission from Bryson JW *et al*. Protein design: a hierarchic approach. *Science* 1995;270:935.

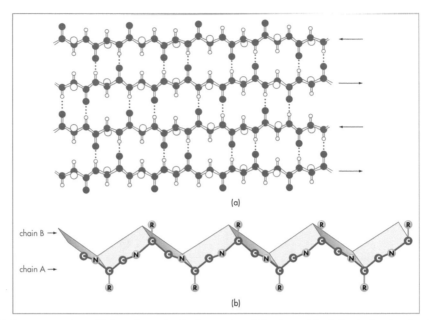

Figure 13.2 (a) A representation of β-sheet formation by four antiparallel polypeptide chains (to be visualised as being in and out of the plane on the paper). The interactions that determine β-sheet stability are more variable than those determining α-helix stability. Different amino acids have different propensities for forming β-sheets. (b) A representation of the concertina shape of a β-sheet showing two antiparallel polypeptide chains, A and B, associated by hydrogen bonding as in (a). Exposed amides at the edge of a β-sheet can hydrogen-bond to other sheets, leading to the formation of insoluble aggregates.

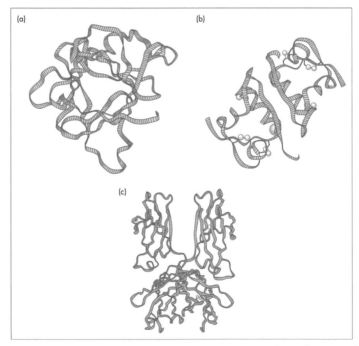

Figure 13.3 Ribbon diagrams of (a) interleukin-1β, (b) zinc–insulin dimer and (c) the Fc fragment of immunoglobulin.
Reproduced from Lesk AM. *Protein Architecture*. Oxford: IRL Press; 1991. Copyright Wiley-VCH Verlag GmbH & Co. KGaA. Reproduced with permission.

Table 13.3 Relative hydrophobic character of amino acid side-chains (Gly = 0)

Side-chain	Amino acid	Hydrophobic character[a]	Log P[b]
(Most hydrophobic)			
$CH_3CH_2CH(CH_3)-$	Isoleucine	1.83	−1.72
$CH_3CH(CH_3)CH_2-$	Leucine	1.80	−1.61
$C_6H_5CH_2-$	Phenylalanine	1.69	
	Tryptophan	1.35	
$CH_3CH(CH_3)-$	Valine	1.32	−2.08
$CH_3-S-CH_2CH_2-$	Methionine	1.10	
	Proline	0.84	
$HSCH_2-$	Cysteine	0.76	
$HOC_6H_5CH_2-$	Tyrosine	0.39	
CH_3-	Alanine	0.35	−2.89
(Standard)	Glycine	0	
$CH_3CH(OH)-$	Threonine	−0.27	
$HOCH_2-$	Serine	−0.63	
	Histidine	−0.65	
$H_2NCOCH_2CH_2-$	Glutamine	−0.93	
H_2NCOCH_2-	Asparagine	−0.99	
$H_2NCH_2CH_2CH_2-$	Ornithine	−1.50	
$H_3N^+-CH_2CH_2CH_2CH_2-$	Lysine	−1.54	−3.31
$HOOCCH_2-$	Aspartic acid	−2.15	−3.38
(Least hydrophobic)			

[a] High positive values indicate very hydrophobic amino acids, and negative values indicate amino acids with hydrophilic character.
[b] From Pliska V *et al. J Chromatogr* 1981;216:79.
Reproduced with permission from Dressler D, Potter H. *Discovering Enzymes.* New York: Scientific American; 1991.

solution temperatures (see Chapter 4 for a discussion of phase separation). Phase transitions are important not only in manufacture and formulation but also because they have some pathophysiological implications. Phase separation of gamma-crystallins causes opacification of the lens of the eye in certain cataracts; Fig. 13.5 shows the phase diagram obtained.

In section 4.2.3 we discussed the effect of salts on the solubility of organic electrolytes. The parabolic effects of salts on protein solubility (Fig. 13.6) might, at first sight, seem unexpected. Data on haemoglobin solubility, produced many decades ago (Fig. 13.6b), show a general increase in solubility with increasing ionic strength of salts such as NaCl, KCl and $(NH_4)_2SO_4$. However, decrease in solubility occurs at

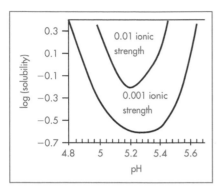

Figure 13.4 A plot of the logarithm of the aqueous stability of β-lactoglobulin versus pH at two different ionic strengths, 0.001 and 0.01 mol kg^{-1}. When the protein is charged at pH values below and above pH 5.3, solubility increases from its lowest point at the isoelectric point. Increased ionic strength shifts the isoelectric point to lower pH values, around 5.2. See also Fig. 13.6.

Table 13.4 Values of pK and isoelectric point (IP) of common L-amino acids

Amino acid	pK$_1$ (COOH)	pK$_2$ (NH$_3$$^+$)	pK$_3$	IP
Alanine	2.34	9.69	–	6.00
Asparagine	2.02	8.80	–	5.41
Aspartic acid	1.88	3.65 (COOH)	9.60 (NH$_3$$^+$)	2.77
Cysteine	1.96	8.18	10.28 (SH)	5.07
Glutamic acid	2.19	4.25 (COOH)	9.67 (NH$_3$$^+$)	3.22
Glutamine	2.17	9.13	–	5.65
Glycine	2.34	9.60	–	5.97
Histidine	1.82	6.00 (imidazole)	9.17 (NH$_3$$^+$)	7.59
Isoleucine	2.36	9.68	–	6.02
Leucine	2.36	9.60	–	5.98
Lysine	2.18	8.95(α)	10.53 (ε-NH$_3$$^+$)	9.74
Methionine	2.28	9.21	–	5.74
Phenylalanine	1.83	9.13	–	5.48
Proline	1.99	10.96	–	6.30
Serine	2.21	9.15	–	5.68
Threonine	2.71	9.62	–	6.16
Tryptophan	2.38	9.39	–	5.89
Tyrosine	2.20	9.11	10.07 (OH)	5.66
Valine	2.32	9.62	–	5.96

higher ionic strengths – a salting-out effect. Several effects are responsible: (1) the preferential interaction of salts with bulk water; and (2) the effect of the salts on the surface tension of water, which is related to the energy of cavity formation. In fact, the degree to which a salt increases the surface tension of water is proportional to its tendency to salt out proteins.

The presence of other polymers in the solution will also tend to reduce protein solubility because of the volume exclusion effect. The addition of a water-soluble polymer (such as polyoxyethylene glycol (PEG)) can lead to the formation of two distinct liquid phases, owing to changes in the energy required to accommodate the protein molecules and to the unfavourable interaction of PEG with charges on the surface of the protein.

PEG molecules grafted to proteins, however, favourably change the properties of therapeutic proteins, as we will discuss later.

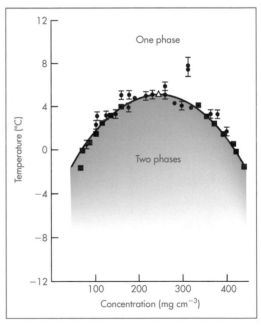

Figure 13.5 The temperature–concentration phase diagram for aqueous gamma-crystallin (mol wt ≈ 20 000 Da) systems (pH = 7, I = 0.24 mol kg^{-1}). ●, cloud point measurements; ■, concentration measurements of separated phases; △, critical point.

Reproduced with permission from Thompson JA *et al.* Binary liquid phase separation and critical phenomena in a protein/water solution. *Proc Natl Acad Sci USA* 1987;84:7079.

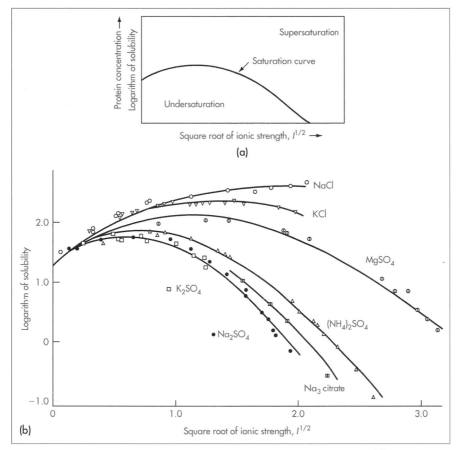

Figure 13.6 (a) A generic plot of log(solubility) as a function of square root of ionic strength ($I^{1/2}$) for proteins. (b) The plot for haemoglobin at 25°C, indicating the influence of the nature of the salt. Solubility is expressed as grams per 1000 grams H_2O. Reproduced from Green AA. *J Biol Chem* 1932;95:47–66.

Key points

- Proteins have, in increasing order of complexity:
  - *primary* structure – the order in which the individual amino acids are arranged
  - *secondary* structures – including coiled α-helix and pleated sheets
  - *tertiary* structure – the three-dimensional arrangement of helices and coils, and sometimes
  - *quaternary* forms, which are the association of ternary forms (e.g. the hexameric form of insulin).
- Proteins have solubilities ranging from very soluble to virtually insoluble. The solubility of globular proteins increases as the pH of the solution moves away from the *isoelectric point*, which is the pH at which the molecule has a net zero charge and a tendency to self-associate.
- Proteins are surrounded by a hydration layer, equivalent to about two water molecules per amino acid residue.
- Aqueous solutions of proteins may exhibit phase transitions. Addition of electrolytes such as NaCl, KCl and $(NH_4)_2SO_4$ decreases solubility and at high ionic strengths proteins precipitate – a *salting-out* effect. Organic solvents tend to decrease the solubility of proteins by lowering solvent dielectric constant.

13.2 The stability of proteins and peptides

In Chapter 3 we examined how the stability of drug formulations may be improved from a knowledge of the principal routes of degradation and the kinetics of breakdown. It has been implicitly assumed that the drugs under discussion were typical low-molecular-weight compounds and it is clear that for this type of drug there is a large body of knowledge relating to all aspects of their stability. The formulation of this important class of peptides and proteins presents more of a challenge.

Protein pharmaceuticals can suffer both physical and chemical instability: the major pathways are summarised in Fig. 13.7. Physical instability refers to changes in the higher-order structure (secondary and above), whereas chemical instability can be thought of as any kind of modification of the protein via bond formation or cleavage, yielding a new chemical entity. For each degradation route we will look at the effect of formulation parameters such as pH and ionic strength on stability and also discuss the application of accelerated stability-testing procedures. We will concentrate on the physical aspects of the problem.

13.2.1 Physical instability

Physical instability is a phenomenon that is rarely encountered with small organic molecules but that arises in peptides and proteins because of the many conditions under which proteins can lose their native three-dimensional structure. Unfolding of stable forms can lead to adsorption, aggregation or further chemical reactivity. Aggregation can lead to precipitation. Loss of the unique biologically active three-dimensional structure (denaturation) can be caused by heating and, conversely, by cooling or freezing, extremes of pH and contact with organic chemicals and denaturants. Most of these act through their influence on solubility or conformation, hence the importance of understanding protein–solvent interactions. It is generally thought that denaturation must first occur before the other processes such as aggregation, adsorption and precipitation can proceed.

Denaturation: reversible and irreversible

Denaturation refers to a disruption of the tertiary and secondary structure of the protein molecule. The denaturation can be *reversible* or *irreversible*. When caused by an increase of temperature, the process is said to be reversible if the native structure is regained on decreasing the temperature. Irreversible denaturation implies that the unfolding process is such that the native structure cannot be regained simply by lowering the temperature. In many cases the protein may become more compact, exposing hydrophobic residues that are normally buried within its core. It is the interaction between these hydrophobic residues in the protein interior that determines the physical stability of the proteins. When they become exposed to the solvent, these residues can interact with other hydro-

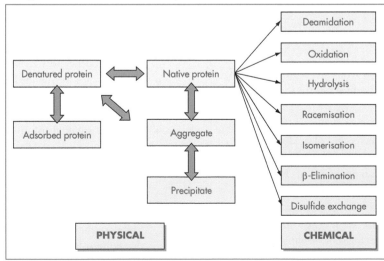

Figure 13.7 Schematic of the major pathways of protein degradation, which may be physical or chemical in origin.

phobic surfaces such as the container walls or the exposed residues of other denatured proteins, leading to the localised accumulation of denatured protein molecules that results in the formation of aggregates. Increase of temperature results in greater flexibility of the proteins and an increased tendency for collision, leading to aggregate formation. An increase of the ionic strength may lead to neutralisation of the surface charge on the protein molecules that is responsible for their mutual repulsion, again resulting in aggregation. Charge neutralisation and subsequent aggregation can also occur when the pH of the solution approaches the isoelectric point of the protein. In both cases, molecules in the aggregated state can undergo denaturation with time as a result of subtle changes in their conformation and the aggregation process becomes irreversible.

Two basic pathways have been observed for proteins during denaturation and folding. The simplest is a two-state model. If we refer to the native state as N and the unfolded, denatured state as D, we can write

$$N \rightleftharpoons D$$

Once critical hydrophobic residues are exposed to solvents they can interact with other surfaces (containers or the air–water interface). The process may involve the formation of intermediate conformations (I) which may be stable and may self-associate during folding. The second general pathway for denaturation includes these stable intermediate species and may be written

$$N \rightleftharpoons I_n \rightleftharpoons \cdots \rightleftharpoons I_2 \rightleftharpoons I_1 \rightleftharpoons D$$

The equation shows the unfolding of a native protein to form an intermediate, I_n, which then unfolds to form other intermediates. If the two-state model is assumed, the concentration of denaturant required to achieve equal concentrations of N and D will give some indication of the process. If the fraction of denatured protein, f_d, is calculated under given conditions (temperature, concentration of additive, etc.) we can write

$$f_d = \frac{[D]}{[N] + [D]} = \frac{K_{ND}}{1 + K_{ND}} \qquad (13.1)$$

where K_{ND} is the equilibrium constant for denaturation $(K_{ND} = [D]/[N])$, related to the free energy of denaturation $\Delta G_{ND}^\ominus$ by

$$K_{ND} = \exp\left(\frac{-\Delta G_{ND}^\ominus}{RT}\right) \qquad (13.2)$$

Hence,

$$\Delta G_{ND}^\ominus = -2.303 RT \log K_{ND} \qquad (13.3)$$

When 50% of the molecules are unfolded $[D] = [N]$ and $K_{ND} = 1$, therefore $\Delta G_{ND}^\ominus = 0$. The temperature at which this occurs is referred to as the melting temperature, T_m. An increase of T_m is indicative of an increase of stability; for example, T_4 lysozyme (lysozyme from bacteriophage T_4) is more stable at pH 6.5 where T_m is 65°C than at pH 2 where T_m is 42°C.

Aggregation/association

Some proteins self-associate in aqueous solution to form oligomers. Insulin, for example, exists in several associated states; the zinc hexamer of insulin is a complex of insulin and zinc that dissolves slowly into dimers and eventually monomers following its subcutaneous administration, so giving it long-acting properties. In most cases, however, it is desirable to prevent association such that only monomeric or dimeric forms are present in the formulations and a more rapid absorption is achieved. Recent studies have been directed towards engineering insulin molecules which are not prone to association,[1,2] or the prevention of association through the addition of surfactants.[3] Protein self-association is a reversible process, i.e. alteration of the solvent properties can lead to the re-formation of the monomeric native protein. There is an important distinction between this association process and the aggregation of proteins, which relates to the usually non-reversible interaction of protein molecules in their denatured state. Aggregation therefore implies that the proteins have undergone some form of denaturation prior to their interaction.

If an intermediate forms that has a solubility less than that of N or D, this can lead to aggregation and eventually to precipitation. For example, the addition of moderate amounts of denaturant to bovine growth hormone can generate a partially unfolded intermediate of low solubility that aggregates. Similarly, γ-interferon is inactivated by acid treatment or by the addition of salt because the dimeric native state is converted into monomers, which are partially denatured. For both proteins the formation of intermediates leads to inactivation.

Surface adsorption and precipitation

The adsorption of proteins such as insulin on surfaces such as glass or plastic in giving sets is important as it can reduce the amount of agent reaching the patient. It can also lead to further denaturation, which can then cause precipitation and the physical blocking of delivery ports in insulin pumps, for example. Insulin adsorption on the surface of the containers and the subsequent 'frosting' effect, due to the presence of a finely divided precipitate on the walls (Fig. 13.8), is accelerated by the presence of a large headspace allowing a greater interaction of the insulin with the air–water interface, which facilitates denaturation.

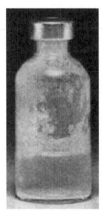

Figure 13.8 A vial of insulin showing the frosted appearance of flocculated and adsorbed protein.
Reproduced from diabetesindogs.com

13.2.2 Formulation and protein stabilisation

There are several possible ways in which the physical stability of the protein can be improved through formulation. We will examine methods for minimising this and chemical degradation in the following sections.

Prevention of adsorption

Some measures can be taken to eliminate, or at least minimise, protein denaturation resulting from surface adsorption. The surface of glass is conducive to adsorption and it is preferable in principle to use more hydrophilic surfaces, although this may not be feasible in practice. Alternatively, when the use of glass cannot be avoided, components may be added to the protein solution to prevent adsorption to the glass surface. These additives can act by coating the surface of glass or by binding to the proteins. For example, serum albumin can be included in the formulation since this will compete with the therapeutic protein for the binding sites on the glass surface and so reduce its adsorption. A similar effect can be achieved by the addition of surfactants such as poloxamers and polysorbates to the protein solution. Consideration must be given, however, to the effects of the surfactants on the pharmacology of the protein and to the toxicological effects of the surfactant itself.

Minimisation of exposure to air

Significant denaturation of proteins can occur when the protein solutions are exposed at the air–solution interface. In this respect the air interface is behaving as a hydrophobic surface and the extent of denaturation is found to be dependent on the time of exposure of the protein at the interface. Agitation of protein solutions in the presence of air or application of other shear forces, such as those that occur when the solutions are filtered or pumped, may also cause denaturation. Again, the inclusion of surfactants can reduce denaturation arising from these processes. Stability testing of protein-containing formulations often involves subjecting the solutions to shaking for several hours and the subsequent assessment of the protein configuration. If the protein has retained its native state and has not aggregated, the formulation is considered to be stable against surface- or shear-induced denaturation.

Addition of cosolvents

Some excipients and buffer components added to the protein solution are able to minimise denaturation through their effects on solvation. These compounds, including polyethylene glycols and glycerol, are referred to as cosolvents. They may act either by causing the preferential hydration of the protein or alternatively by binding to the protein surface. Preferential hydration results from an exclusion of the cosolvent from the protein surface due to steric effects (as in the case of polyethylene glycols); surface tension effects (as with sugars, salts and amino acids) or some

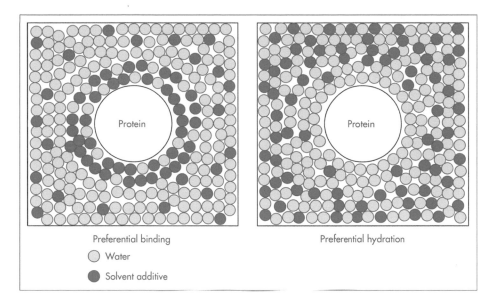

Figure 13.9 Schematic illustration of preferential binding and preferential hydration by solvent additives. In preferential binding the additive occurs in the solvation shell of the protein at a greater local concentration than in the bulk solvent, while preferential hydration results from the exclusion of the additive from the surface of the protein.

Reproduced with permission from Timasheff SN, Arakawa T. In: Creighton TE (ed.) *Protein Structure: A Practical Approach*. Oxford: IRL Press; 1989: 331–345.

form of chemical incompatibility such as charge effects. As a result, more water molecules pack around the protein in order to exclude the additive and the protein becomes fully hydrated and stabilised in a compact form (Fig. 13.9). Alternatively, the cosolvent may stabilise the protein molecule either by binding to it non-specifically or by binding to specific sites on its surface.

Optimisation of pH

In order to avoid stability problems arising from charge neutralisation and to ensure adequate solubility, a pH must be selected that is at least 0.5 pH units above or below the isoelectric point. This is often difficult to achieve, however, since a pH range of 5–7 is usually required to minimise chemical breakdown and this frequently coincides with the isoelectric point.

Characterisation of degradation

If the formulation does not prevent denaturation and aggregation of the protein, then the pharmacology, immunogenicity and toxicology of the denatured or aggregated protein must be studied to determine its safety and efficacy. Several studies must be performed to determine the extent of degradation that is acceptable for administration. If the aggregates are soluble there may be a significant effect on the pharmaco-

kinetics and immunogenicity of the protein. On the other hand, insoluble aggregates are generally unacceptable and instructions are usually given not to administer protein solutions containing precipitates.

 Key points

- *Denaturation* is the disruption of the tertiary and secondary structure of the protein molecule; it can be reversible or irreversible. When caused by an increase of temperature, the process is said to be reversible if the native structure is regained on decreasing the temperature. Irreversible denaturation implies that the unfolding process is such that the native structure cannot be regained simply by lowering the temperature. Hydrophobic residues become exposed to the solvent and can interact with other hydrophobic surfaces (container walls or the exposed residues of other denatured proteins), leading to the localised accumulation of denatured protein molecules and aggregate formation.

- *Aggregation*. Some proteins self-associate in aqueous solution to form oligomers. Although advantageous in some cases (the slow rate of dissolution of the zinc hexamer of insulin into dimers and monomers gives it long-acting properties), self-association is usually prevented, for example, by addition of surfactant. This form of association is reversible, unlike the non-reversible aggregation of protein molecules in their denatured state.

- *Adsorption* of proteins on surfaces such as glass or plastic in giving sets reduces the amount of agent reaching the patient, and can lead to further denaturation and precipitation.

- Formulation procedures to improve the physical stability of the protein include:
  - avoiding contact with glass (if possible) or adding compounds (e.g. serum albumin or surfactants) that coat the glass surface or bind to the proteins, so minimising surface adsorption
  - avoiding exposure at the air–solution interface, agitation of protein solutions in the presence of air or application of other shear forces; inclusion of surfactants can reduce denaturation arising from these processes
  - addition of cosolvents such as polyethylene glycols and glycerol minimises denaturation by causing preferential hydration of the protein or by binding to the protein surface
  - buffering at a pH at least 0.5 pH units above or below the isoelectric point to avoid stability problems arising from charge neutralisation and to ensure adequate solubility.

13.2.3 Chemical instability

Chemical instability can involve one or more of a variety of chemical reactions, including:

- *deamidation*, in which the side-chain linkage in a glutamine (Gln) or asparagine (Asn) residue is hydrolysed to form a carboxylic acid

- *oxidation*: the side-chains of histidine (His), methionine (Met), cysteine (Cys), tryptophan (Trp) and tyrosine (Tyr) residues in proteins are potential oxidation sites
- *racemisation*: all amino acid residues except glycine (Gly) are chiral at the carbon atom bearing the side-chain and are subject to base-catalysed racemisation.
- *proteolysis*, involving the cleavage of peptide (CO-NH) bonds
- *beta elimination*: high-temperature treatment of proteins leads to destruction of disulfide bonds as a result of beta elimination from the cystine residue
- *disulfide formation*: the interchange of disulfide bonds can result in an altered three-dimensional structure.

Table 13.5 lists the amino acids or sequences that are subject to chemical degradation and the formulation approaches used to overcome the problems.

Table 13.5 Amino acids or sequences susceptible to chemical degradation, together with formulation strategies to reduce degradation

Amino acid or sequence	Mechanism of degradation	Formulation strategy
Cysteine–cysteine	Aggregation	Addition of surfactants, polyalcohols and other excipients
Glutamine, asparagine	Deamidation	pH 3–5
Tryptophan, methionine, cysteine, tyrosine, histidine	Oxidation	pH < 7
Methionine	Oxidation	Protect from oxygen
Tryptophan	Photodecomposition	Protect from light
Lysine-threonine	Copper-induced cleavage	Chelating agents
Asparagine-proline, asparagine-tyrosine	Hydrolysis	pH > 7

Reproduced with permission from Parkins DA, Lashmar UT. The formulation of biopharmaceutical products. *Pharm Sci Technol Today* 2000;3:129–137.

13.3 Protein formulation and delivery

It has been said that 'drug delivery represents the potential Achilles' heel of biotechnology's peptide drug industry'. The reasons for this include the range of instabilities discussed above, the inherent low membrane transport by diffusion because of molecular size and hydrophilicity, and often the need for temporal and site control of delivery.

13.3.1 Protein and peptide transport

For a series of 11 model peptides in an *in vitro* intestinal cell monolayer system, a good correlation was found between the permeability coefficient, P, and the log of the partition coefficient of the peptides between heptane and ethylene glycol (rather than octanol and water) (Fig. 13.10), results that also suggest that the principal deterrent to peptide transport is the breaking of hydrogen bonds. Molecular volume (or size) will increasingly be a factor as the molecular weight of the peptide increases.

The diffusion of proteins and peptides in solution is dictated by the same considerations as those discussed in Chapter 2, section 2.6. The rate of translational movement depends on the size of the molecule, its shape and interactions with solvent molecules. The rate of translational movement is often expressed by a frictional coefficient, f, defined in relation to the diffusion coefficient D, by equation (13.4):

$$f = \frac{k_B T}{D} \qquad (13.4)$$

where k_B is the Boltzmann constant and T is the temperature in kelvins. Many proteins are nearly spherical in solution, but if their shape deviates from sphericity this is reflected in a frictional ratio, f/f_0, above unity, where f_0 is the rate of diffusion of a molecule of the same size but of spherical shape. The frictional ratio of lysozyme is 1.24 and that of trypsin is 1.187. Globular proteins have values of f/f_0 in the range 1.05–1.38.

The diffusion coefficients and translational movements of proteins are important in considering the release of proteins from hydrogel matrix devices and other delivery vehicles, and in membrane transport, as far as this can be considered to be a passive diffusion process. Changes in shape during membrane transport in a lipid environment may also have to be considered. Table 13.6 gives some values of the diffusion coefficients of a number of therapeutic peptides and proteins.

13.3.2 Lyophilised proteins

Because of their potential instability in solution, therapeutic proteins are often formulated as lyophilised

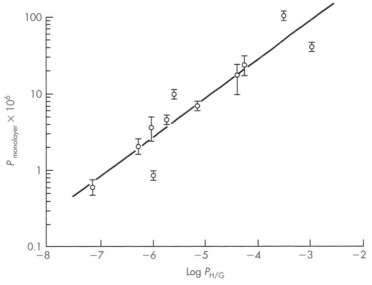

Figure 13.10 A plot of the permeability coefficient P across Caco-2 cell monolayers versus the log P (heptane/glycol) for a series of synthetic peptides to illustrate relationships between lipophilicity and transport.

Reproduced with permission from Paterson DA *et al. Quant Struct–Action Relationships* 1994;13:4–10.

Table 13.6 Diffusion coefficients and molecular weights of peptides and proteins

Compound	Molecular weight (Da)	10^6 D (cm^2 s^{-1})
Oxytocin	1007	4.30
Lys-vasopressin	1056	4.18
Arg-vasopressin	1084	4.27
Somatostatin	1638	3.74
Calcitonin	3418	2.76
Insulin	5807	1.14
Calculated (insulin)		
Monomer	5807	2.03
Hexamer	34 845	0.93

Reproduced from Hosoya O *et al. J Pharm Pharmacol* 2004;56:1501–1507. Copyright Wiley-VCH Verlag GmbH & Co. KGaA. Reproduced with permission.

powders. Even in this state several suffer from moisture-induced aggregation. Proteins such as insulin, tetanus toxoid, somatotropin and human albumin aggregate in the presence of moisture, which can lead to reduced activity, stability and diffusion.

In the presence of water vapour at 37°C, lyophilised recombinant human albumin experiences intermolecular thiol–disulfide interchange and forms high-molecular-weight, water-insoluble aggregates.[4] The use of excipients (e.g. low- and high-molecular-weight sugars, organic acids) to prevent such effects leads to the conclusion that the stabilising effect is correlated with the ability of the additives preferentially to absorb water. Figure 13.11 illustrates the effects on

recombinant human albumin solubility and the influence of sorbitol on the changes in solubility.

13.3.3 Water adsorption

Because of the sensitivity of proteins to moisture, the ability to measure sorption of water is vital in preformulation. Water sorption isotherms from recombinant bovine somatotropin (rbST), a protein with 191 amino acids, molecular weight 22 000 Da, show water content versus the relative vapour pressure (p/p_0) for the sodium salt and the 'internal' salt of rbST (Fig. 13.12). These were fitted to modified BET isotherms which have an additional state of interacting water intermediate to the free water and the strongly bound water states.[5,6] Calculations reveal that a monolayer of water is formed from 88 moles of H_2O per mole of protein for the lyophilised sodium salt of rbST, which is equivalent to about 7.3 g per g of protein. The much higher apparent surface areas obtained using water (as opposed to nitrogen) adsorption isotherms (typically 264 m^2 g^{-1}, compared with 1.3 m^2 g^{-1} with nitrogen) suggest that water penetrates the powder and that the isotherm represents adsorption and absorption. The practical implications of moisture load are seen in Fig. 13.13, which shows the rate of decomposition of rbST (albeit at 47°C) following incubation in sealed vials.

Both solubility and stability have to be addressed, as well as the mode of delivery. The wide range of biodegradable polymers used for the controlled delivery of proteins and peptides includes natural sub-

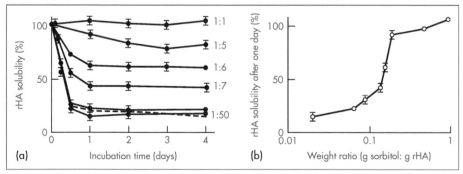

Figure 13.11 Stabilisation of recombinant human albumin (rHA) against aggregation afforded by co-lyophilised sorbitol. (a) The time-dependent change of solubility of rHA co-lyophilised with sorbitol at various sorbitol-to-rHA weight ratios, as indicated (the dashed line depicts the time course of rHA aggregation in the absence of sorbitol). (b) rHA solubility after a 1-day incubation as a function of sorbitol-to-rHA weight ratio, taken from the data in plot (a).

Reproduced with permission from Costantino JR *et al.* Aggregation of a lyophilized pharmaceutical protein, recombinant human albumin: effect of moisture and stabilization by excipients. *Biotechnology* 1995;13:493–496.

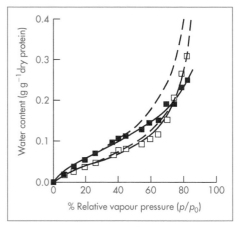

Figure 13.12 Comparison of fits obtained by the Brunauer–Emmett–Teller (BET: dashed lines) and Guggenheim–Anderson–de Boer (GAB: solid lines) models for the sorption isotherms of the sodium (■) and internal (□) salts of bovine somatotropin.

Reproduced with permission from Hageman MJ *et al*. Prediction and characterization of the water sorption isotherm for bovine somatotropin. *J Agric Food Chem* 1992;40:342–347. Copyright 1992 American Chemical Society.

stances, starch, alginates, collagen and a variety of proteins such as crosslinked albumin, a range of synthetic hydrogels, polyanhydrides, polyesters or orthoesters, poly(amino acids) and poly(caprolactones). Poly(lactide-glycolide) (PLGA) is one of the commonest polymers used in microsphere form to deliver, *inter alia*, growth hormone-releasing factor, a somatostatin analogue, ciclosporin and luteinising hormone-releasing hormone antagonists.[7,8]

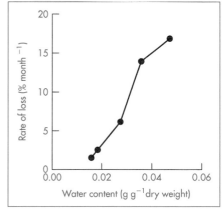

Figure 13.13 The increasing rate of decomposition of a lyophilised recombinant bovine somatotropin formulation with increasing water content following incubation in sealed vials at 47°C.

Reproduced from reference 5.

13.3.4 PEGylation of peptides and proteins

PEG is a versatile molecule. It is used pharmaceutically in molecular weight ranges from 200 to 10 000 Da. The polyoxyethylene chain forms an integral part of many non-ionic surfactants (polysorbate 80, Triton X-100). PEG is used as a vehicle for drug delivery: higher-molecular-weight fractions are used in suppository bases and lower-molecular-weight species (200–300 Da) that are liquid at room temperature are useful drug solvents. The molecule can be coupled in a range of molecular weights and hence lengths to peptides and proteins, enhancing their native properties by creating a hydrophilic 'envelope' around proteins and antibodies (Fig. 13.14). A variety of techniques is also used to modify the properties of liposomes and nanoparticles to reduce their uptake by the reticuloendoethelial system. The PEG chains act to prevent opsonisation and hence reticuloendothelial system scavenging, thus increasing half-life *in vivo*.

Pegylation is the term used to describe this modification of proteins, peptides or, indeed, non-peptide molecules by linking one or more PEG chains to the molecule.[9] PEG is non-toxic, non-immunogenic, non-antigenic and highly soluble in water. The PEG–drug conjugates also have a prolonged circulation time after intravenous administration; they are less susceptible to degradation by metabolic enzymes; and their immunogenicity is reduced. The hydrophilic halo is thus important, sometimes increasing the water solubility of the molecule and potentially its biological activity through modification of interactions with biological target sites. The section on colloid stability should be consulted (Chapter 6, section 6.2) to see how PEG molecules affect the physical stability of emulsions and particles.

Naturally the physical properties of the PEGylated molecules are altered by their acquired hydrophilic chains. Clearly their molecular radius increases: haemoglobin has a molecular weight of 64 kDa and a radius of 3.1 nm. As the molecular weight of the attached PEG chains increases, so too does the radius, more than doubling to 7 nm with large PEG chains of 450 ($-OCH_2CH_2-$) units. The viscosity of solutions increased by nearly fivefold over native haemoglobin solutions. Because of the variety of possible linkages between the PEG molecules and the protein concerned, and because of the choice of PEG molecular size and

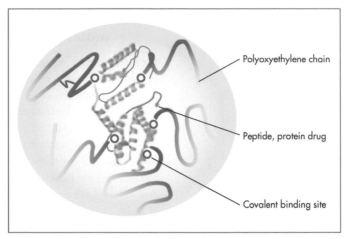

Figure 13.14 A schematic representation of a PEGylated protein, showing the protein surrounded by a polyoxyethylene glycol (PEG) protective sheath.

indeed number of attached molecules, it is vital that the exact structural properties of these modified products are known, especially when generic versions of therapeutic proteins are available. The structure and properties of proteins and MAbs prepared by different methods, and processed in different ways with non-identical excipients, are rarely identical. Thus generic macromolecular products are termed 'bio*similars*' to make this point. Many of the issues surrounding biosimilars are dealt with in Chapter 16.

Pegylated therapeutic proteins

As discussed above proteins have been modified by the covalent addition of PEG chains to their structures. While the intrinsic activity of the protein is generally unaffected, other parameters change so that a pegylated protein must be considered to be a new chemical entity. Pegylation of therapeutic proteins changes their pharmacokinetics and dynamics. It improves the performance of therapeutic proteins, providing them with a longer circulation time *in vivo*, and a reduction in immune responses. There is often also enhanced solubility of the peptide or protein (as might be expected from the addition of these very hydrophilic chains) or improved stability. Increased circulation time decreases the dose of protein necessary for biological action. Reduced antigenicity, immunogenicity and proteolysis are some of the benefits claimed for pegylated over non-pegylated forms of proteins and peptides.

Why is this? The barrier produced by the PEG chains is both a physical and a thermodynamic one. The polyoxyethylene molecules shield the protein,

reducing uptake and loss by the reticuloendothelial system. The resulting larger size of the molecule may, however, confer slower diffusional characteristics on the molecules. The addition of these water-soluble entities not only increases solubility but can also decrease the pH dependency of protein solubility. Above all, the PEG layer shields the protein from opsonisation *in vivo* and thus the molecules are not scavenged by the reticuloendothelial system and hence circulation times are enhanced. As might be anticipated, the length of the PEG chain is important: the longer the chain, the longer the circulation time.

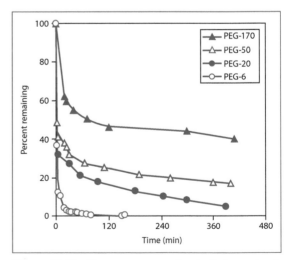

Figure 13.15 The percentage of polyethylene glycols (PEG) remaining in the circulation as a function of their size (molecular weight: 6 = 6 kDa, 20 = 20 kDa etc.).

Reproduced from Mehrar R. Modulation of the pharmacokinetics and pharmacodynamics of proteins by polyoxyethylene glycol conjugation. *J Pharm Pharm Sci* 2000;3:125–136.

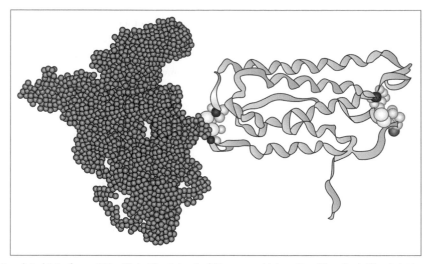

Figure 13.16 Pegylated interferon (Mire Zloh, The School of Pharmacy, University of London). The right-hand portion of the molecule represents the interferon while the left-hand part represents the polyoxyethylene chains.

Figure 13.15 shows the kinetics of free (unattached) PEG molecules as a function of molecular size.[10]

Pegfilgastim is a pegylated recombinant methionyl human granulocyte-stimulating factor indicated in the reduction of the duration of neutropenia and incidence of febrile neutropenia during cancer chemotherapy. It is administered by intramuscular injection, and has a half-life in human subjects of 15–80 hours compared to the 3–4 hours of the parent compound.

PEG-Intron (peginterferon alfa) (Fig. 13.16) is a covalent conjugate of recombinant interferon alfa-2b with monomethoxy polyethylene glycol. Compared to standard interferon alfa, this modified molecule has a longer half-life after injection, allowing once-weekly injections and superior antiviral efficacy in the treat-ment of hepatitis C when used in combination with ribavirin. A case of a local blistering reaction develop-ing in a patient receiving pegylated interferon alfa-2b has been reported.[11] Dalmau *et al.*[12] state that, although injection site pain is infrequent (2–3%), site inflammation and skin reactions (e.g. bruises, itchi-ness, irritation) occur at approximately twice the incidence with pegylated interferon alfa-2b treatment (in up to 75% of patients) compared with ordinary recombinant interferon alfa-2b. Dalmau and co-work-ers suggest that 'because pegylated interferon alfa-2b has almost completely replaced interferon for its most frequent indications, increased awareness of the possi-bility of cutaneous necrosis is necessary for early diagnosis to prevent continuation of pegylated inter-

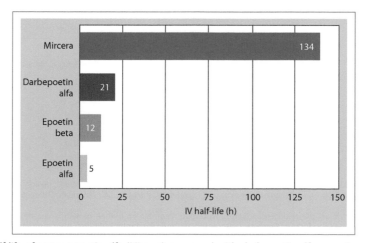

Figure 13.17 The half-life of pegzerepoetin alfa (Mircera) compared with darbepoetin alfa, epoetin alfa and epoetin beta.

feron alfa-2b injections at the involved area'. There are hints that any toxicity at the site of injection might be due to its higher molecular weight and slower diffusion from the site.

Methoxy polyethylene glycol-epoetin beta (pegzerepoetin alfa; Mircera) is given by subcutaneous injection or intravenous infusion. Its half-life is extended over other forms of epoetin alfa or epoetin beta, as shown in Fig. 13.17.

Pegvisomat (Somavert), a pegylated analogue of human growth hormone structurally altered to act as a growth hormone receptor antagonist, comprises 191 amino acids with an average of 4–6 PEG molecules covalently bound to lysine residues and one bound to the terminal phenylalanine. It acts by binding to growth hormone receptors on cell surfaces. The molecular weight of the protein is 21 998 Da and the molecular weight of each PEG chain is 5 000 Da; hence there are three predominant molecular sizes in the product, with molecular weights of 42 000, 47 000 and 52 000 Da.

Thus it is not a homogeneous product, but it should be a *consistent* product in terms of the ratios of the predominant species. Clearly, when generic versions become available, information on the molecular weight of species will be an important parameter. Peak concentrations after subcutaneous administration are achieved 33–77 hours after administration, a result likely to be due to its high molecular weight.

13.3.5 Peptide–albumin complexes

Other strategems to increase the circulation time of peptides include the formation of adducts with serum albumin, an example of which is shown in Fig. 13.18. This is of albuferon, an albumin–interferon-alpha fusion product. While on a molar basis it is less active than the native interferon-alpha, its overall activity is higher, and its half-life is prolonged, which reduces the burden of frequent dosing.

Table 13.7 Routes of delivery for proteins and peptides

Delivery routes	Formulation and device requirements	Commercial products[a]
Invasive		
Direct injection: intravenous, subcutaneous, intramuscular, intracerebral vein	Liquid or reconstituted solid, (syringe)	Activase (alteplase) Nutropin (somatrotropin) RecombiVax (hepatitis B vaccine)
Depot system (subcutaneous or intramuscular)	Biodegradable polymers, liposomes, permeable polymers (not degradable), microspheres, implants	Lupron Depot (leuprolide) Zoladex (goserelin) Decapeptyl (triptorelin)
Non-invasive		
Pulmonary	Liquid or powder formulations, nebulisers, metered-dose inhalers, dry-powder inhalers	Pulmozyme (dornase alfa)
Oral	Solids, emulsions, microparticulates, with or without absorption enhancers	
Nasal	Liquid, usually requires permeation enhancers	Synarel (nafarelin)
Topical	Emulsions, creams or pastes (liposomes)	
Transdermal	Electrophoretic (iontophoresis), electroporation, chemical permeation enhancers, prodrugs, ultrasonics	
Buccal, rectal, vaginal	Gels, suppositories, bioadhesives, particles	

Modified with permission from Cleland JL, Langer R. Formulation and delivery of proteins and peptides: design and development strategies. In: Cleland JL, Langer R (eds) *Formulation and Delivery of Proteins and Peptides*. Washington, DC: American Chemical Society; 1994: 1–19. Copyright 1994 American Chemical Society.
[a]Activase (recombinant human tissue plasminogen activator), Nutropin (recombinant human growth hormone) and Pulmozyme (recombinant human deoxyribonuclease I) are all products of Genentech; RecombiVax (recombinant hepatitis B surface antigen) is produced by Merck; Lupron Depot (leuprolide acetate – poly(lactide-glycolide) (PLGA)) is a product of Takeda Pharmaceuticals; Zoladex (goserelin acetate – PLGA) is produced by AstraZeneca; Decapeptyl is produced by Debiopharm; Synarel (nafarelin acetate) is produced by Roche.

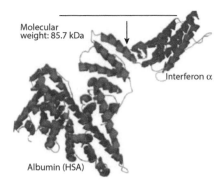

Molecular
weight: 85.7 kDa

Interferon α

Albumin (HSA)

Figure 13.18 An interferon-human serum albumin (HSA) conjugate molecule (Albuferon) combining the activity of interferon-alpha with the longevity in the circulation of albumin.

Reproduced with permission from www.natap.org (2005).

Albumin–drug complexes

To alter the *in vivo* behaviour (such as half-life and stability) of some drugs their conjugates with albumin have been prepared. Hence the albumin with its own circulation and half-life characteristics acts as a carrier for the drug substance. A methotrexate–albumin complex has been studied, as has a doxorubicin conjugate. Another strategy is to create prodrugs with exposed hydrophobic groups which cause the drug to bind to circulating albumin. One such case, the myristic acid derivative of insulin, Levemir, is discussed below in section 13.4.1.

13.3.6 Routes of peptide and protein delivery

Table 13.7 lists the invasive and non-invasive routes of delivery for peptides and proteins, involving direct injection of solutions, depot systems and a variety of oral, nasal, topical and other formulations. Figure 13.19 summarises some of the issues involved in delivery

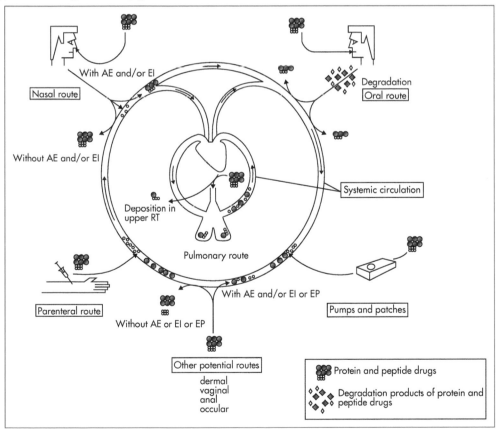

Figure 13.19 A schematic diagram referring to the different routes of administration of protein and peptide drugs, namely the parenteral, nasal, oral and pulmonary routes and by pumps and patches. Of all these, the oral route is the most problematic. Other potential routes, dermal, vaginal, anal and ocular are listed. AE = absorption enhancers; EI = enzyme inhibitors; EP = electroporation or iontophoresis; RT = respiratory tract.

Reproduced with permission from Agu RU *et al*. The lung as a route for systemic delivery of therapeutic proteins and peptides. *Respir Res* 2001;2:198–202.

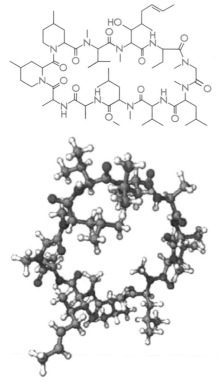

Structure I Ciclosporin in two different modes of representation

of peptides and proteins by different routes. Cyclic peptides such as ciclosporin (**I**) can be absorbed orally; the bioavailability of ciclosporin is of the order of 15%. Such cyclic peptides, although molecularly large, bear a closer resemblance to conventional drugs in many ways, but absorption is quite compound-specific.

Other cyclic peptides include the antibiotics Tyrocidin A and gramicidin S, which are both cyclic decapeptides.

13.4 A therapeutic protein and a peptide

13.4.1 Insulin

It is appropriate that the protein therapeutic substance with the longest pedigree is discussed here. There are three main types of insulin preparations:

- those with a *short* duration of action that have a relatively rapid onset (soluble insulin, insulin lispro, insulin aspart, insulin glulisine)
- those with an *intermediate* duration of action (isophane insulin and insulin zinc suspension)

- those with a slow action, slower in onset and lasting for *long* periods (crystalline insulin zinc suspension; insulin glargine, insulin detemir, insulin degludec).

Some aspects of insulin were dealt with in section 9.2.5. Tables 13.8a and b list some of the insulin formulations designed to produce different durations of onset and action. Insulin is generally self-administered subcutaneously with injection pens, needle-free devices or pumps.

There is discussion of some of the characteristics of these products below. The pharmacokinetics of each formulation may vary greatly among different individuals; in these tables the onset of therapeutic levels of insulin is referred to as the start of the effect, the maximum serum level of insulin is denoted the peak, and the time at which the insulin levels are below therapeutic levels is listed as the end of the therapeutic time course.

Precipitation of insulin and other proteins

Precipitation of insulin in pumps due to the formation of amorphous particles, crystals or fibrils of insulin can lead to changes in release pattern or to blockage that prevents insulin release. 'Amorphous' or 'crystalline' precipitates can be caused by the leaching of divalent metal contaminants or lowering of pH (due to CO_2 diffusion or leaching of acidic substances), but can be prevented. More difficult to solve is the tendency of insulin to form fibrils, as illustrated in Fig. 13.20.

The interactions leading to fibril formation result from the monomeric form, and from changes in the monomer conformation and hydrophilic attraction of the parallel β-sheet forms. Fibril formation is also encouraged by contact of the insulin solution with hydrophobic surfaces.

Propylene glycol, glycerol, non-ionic and ionic surfactants and calcium ions have been used in formulations to achieve greater stability, reducing fibril formation, but the most successful strategy is the addition of calcium ions or zinc, which appear to protect the hexameric form of the insulin (see section 9.2.5).

Recombinant human insulin: insulin lispro and insulin aspart

Insulin lispro and insulin aspart are mentioned in Table 13.8b. Chemical modifications to an endogenous

Table 13.8a Effect of insulin formulation on its pharmacokinetics after subcutaneous injection

Product[a]	Formulation	Pharmacokinetics[b]
Humulin R Novolin R	Zinc-insulin crystalline suspension (acid regular)	Rapid onset, short duration Start, 0.5 h; peak, 2.5–5 h; end, 8 h
Humulin N Novolin N	Isophane suspension protamine, zinc crystalline insulin (buffer water for injection)	Intermediate-acting, slower onset, longer duration than regular insulin
		Start, 1.5 h; peak, 4–12 h; end, up to 24 h
Humulin 70/30[c] Novolin 70/30[c]	70% isophane suspension 30% zinc crystalline	Intermediate-acting, faster onset longer duration
		Start, 0.5 h; peak, 2–12 h; end, up to 24 h
Humulin U	Extended zinc-insulin suspension – all crystalline	Slow-acting, slow onset, longer, less-intense duration than R or N forms
Humulin L Novolin L	70% zinc-insulin crystalline suspension 30% amorphous insulin (cloudy suspension)	Intermediate-acting, slower onset, longer duration Start, 2.5 h; peak, 7–15 h; end, 22 h
Humulin BR	Zinc crystalline insulin dissolved in sodium diphosphate buffer	Rapid onset, short duration; use in pumps only

[a] Humulin products (Eli Lilly & Company) contain recombinant human insulin derived from *Escherichia coli*; Novolin products (Novo Nordisk) are recombinant human insulin derived from *Saccharomyces cerevisiae*; both companies also sell other forms of recombinant human insulin and may have additional forms (formulations or new drugs) in clinical trials.
[b] The pharmacokinetics of each formulation may vary greatly among individuals; the onset of therapeutic levels of insulin is referred to as the start of the effect, the maximum serum levels is the peak, and the time when the levels of insulin are below therapeutic levels is listed as the end of the therapeutic time course.
[c] Solution consists of 70% N form and 30% R form for both products.

Table 13.8b Comparison of the onset peak and duration of action of insulin products

Examples	Products	Onset of action (min)	Peak action	Duration of action (h)
Insulin aspart Insulin lispro Insulin glulisine	Novorapid Humalog Apidra	10–20	30–180 min	2–5
Human sequence soluble insulin	Actrapid, Humulin S	30–90	2–4 h	6–8
Isophane insulin	Insulatard	30–90	6–8 h	11–24
Insulin glargine Insulin detemir Insulin degludec	Lantus Levemir Tresiba	60–120	No peak	20–26

Reproduced with permission from Jacques N, Hackett E. *Clin Pharmacist* 2013;5:75.

protein, however minor, can lead to significant differences in properties and activity. Species differences can also be great. Salmon calcitonin (SCT) is 10 times more potent than human calcitonin (hCT), for example. Recombinant human protein analogues may be subtly different, as in the case of insulin lispro, in which the sequence of proline and lysine at positions 28 and 29 in the B protein chain has been reversed (Fig. 13.21a). This sole difference leads to formation of hexamers, which more rapidly dissociate to monomers on injection, giving a faster onset of action than

human insulin, in which the B28 is proline and B29 is lysine (such as the recombinant product Humulin S, which is injected up to an hour before meals).

Insulin glargine (Lantus, Aventis) has two arginines added to the B30 position (Fig. 13.21b). Its isoelectric point changes from a pH of 5.4 to 6.7, making it a soluble (and thus clear) solution in the acid medium of pH 4 in which it is supplied. When it is injected subcutaneously, however, glargine precipitates at the physiological pH of 7.4, which delays its absorption and prolongs its action. Substituting glycine for aspar-

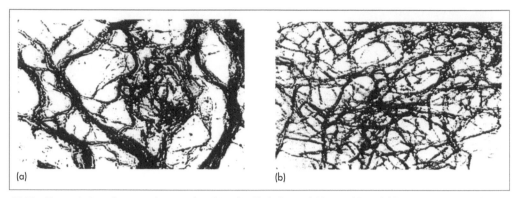

Figure 13.20 Transmission electron micrographs of insulin fibrils formed (a) at 37°C and (b) at 80°C (×100 000).
Reproduced from Brange J. *Galenics of Insulin*. Berlin: Springer; 1987, with kind permission from Springer Science and Business Media.

agine at the A21 position and adding zinc stabilises the hexamer and delays absorption further.

Glargine has a similar insulin receptor affinity to that of NPH (Neutral Protamine Hagedorn, an intermediate-acting insulin that initially achieves slower action through the addition of protamine to short-acting insulin) so that, once absorbed in the circulation, glargine is equipotent to NPH. The result is a relatively constant supply of insulin with an onset of approximately 2 hours and a duration of action of approximately 24 hours.

Insulin detemir (Levemir) is a long-acting human insulin analogue for maintaining the basal level of insulin and is an example of a modified therapeutic agent which allows it to bind to plasma proteins. It is an analogue in which a fatty acid (myristic acid) is bound to the lysine amino acid at position B29. It is quickly absorbed, after which it binds to albumin in the blood through its fatty acid at position B29. It then slowly dissociates from this complex. Figure 13.22 aids the visualisation of the chemistry of this and human and porcine insulin.

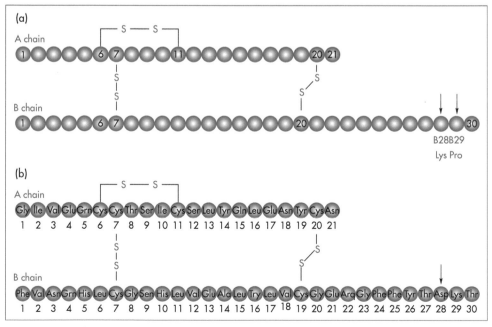

Figure 13.21 (a) Insulin lispro, a product of recombinant DNA technology, is an analogue of human insulin in which the natural sequence of proline and lysine at positions B28 and B29 (arrowed) of human insulin has been reversed. (b) Insulin aspart (Novo Nordisk) has an aspartame at B28 (arrow) replacing the proline of the natural insulin. Insulin glargine has a glycine at position A21 and two arginines at B30.

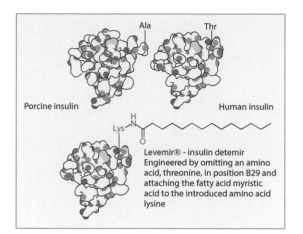

Figure 13.22 The chemical modification by the addition of the hydrophobic myristic acid group to insulin to encourage its binding *in vivo* to albumin and the change in it pharmacokinetics.

Reproduced from Elsadek B, Kratz F. *J Control Release* 2012;157:4–28. Copyright Elsevier 2012.

13.4.2 Calcitonin

Calcitonin, a peptide hormone of 32 amino acids having a regulatory function in calcium and phosphorus metabolism, is used in various bone disorders such as osteoporosis. Salmon, human, pig and eel calcitonin are used therapeutically. hCT has a tendency to associate rapidly in solution and, like insulin, form fibrils, resulting in a viscous solution.[13] The fibrils are 8 nm in diameter and often associate with one another. Heating fibrillated hCT solutions in 50% acetic acid–water converts the system back to soluble monomers. hCT has a pK of 8.7, while sCT has a pK of 10.4. This accounts for the high stability of sCT at pH 7.4, as electrostatic interactions between calcitonin monomers play a role. At pH 7.4, sCT monomers will be charged and will repel each other.

13.5 DNA and oligonucleotides

13.5.1 DNA

DNA of varying molecular weights is used in gene therapy. Figure 13.23 shows the well-known primary structure of DNA and the charge-determining phosphate groups connected to the deoxyribose rings. As DNA is a large hydrophilic, polyanionic and sensitive macromolecule, its successful delivery to target cells

and the nucleus within these cells is an issue. Shearing of high-molecular-weight DNA while stirring in solution can lead to breakage of the molecule. One approach to delivery is to complex the DNA with polymers or particles of opposite charge to produce, by condensation, more compact species. Many studies have been conducted to condense the DNA with cationic polymers (e.g. polylysine and chitosan), cationic liposomes and dendrimers, to produce nanosized complexes that retain an overall positive charge and are able to transfect cells more readily than native or naked DNA. The interaction of DNA with poly-

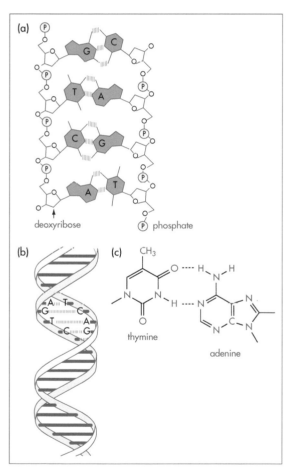

Figure 13.23 (a) Diagrammatic representation of the interactions between two oligonucleotide strands. ////// represents hydrogen-bonding interactions between the base pairs G–C, T–A, C–G, A–T. P represents the phosphate groups, which confer the negative charge on the molecule. (b) Representation of the double helix, again illustrating the hydrogen-bonding interaction that is key to the helical conformation. (c) The detailed primary structure showing the phosphate–deoxyribose–base point sequence for T–A.

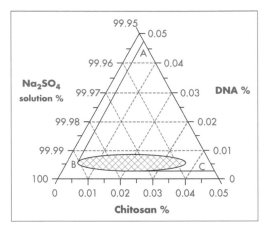

Figure 13.24 Ternary-phase diagram of complex coacervation between a plasmid DNA and chitosan at 55°C in 50 mmol dm^{-3} Na$_2$SO$_4$. Sodium sulfate solution was regarded as one component, since the concentration change in the experiment range was minimal. The region to the right of the line ABC depicts the conditions under which phase separation occurs. The concentration ranges in the small grid area yield distinct particles.

Reproduced from Mao H-Q *et al*. Chitosan-DNA nanoparticles as gene carriers: synthesis, characterisation and transfection efficiency. *J Control Release* 2001;70:399–421. Copyright Elsevier 2001.

cationics like chitosan is akin to a coacervation process[14] (Fig. 13.24).

Through the formation of particulates (Fig. 13.25) cell-uptake characteristics and stability are improved, although transfection inside the cell depends ultimately on the successful release of DNA from the complex and its uptake into the nucleus.

13.5.2 Oligonucleotides

Antisense oligonucleotides (**II**) (used for the sequence-specific inhibition of gene expression) are polyanionic single-strand molecules comprising 10–25 nucleotides. They resemble single-stranded DNA or RNA. They have molecular weights ranging from 3000 to 8000 Da and are hydrophilic, having a log P of approximately −3.5. Like DNA, they clearly do not have the appropriate properties for transfer across biological membranes. They are also sensitive to nucleases and non-specific adsorption to biological surfaces, and hence require to be formulated to achieve delivery and nuclear uptake. Chemical modification of oligonucleotides, which is outside of the scope of this book, can increase the stability and activity of the molecules.

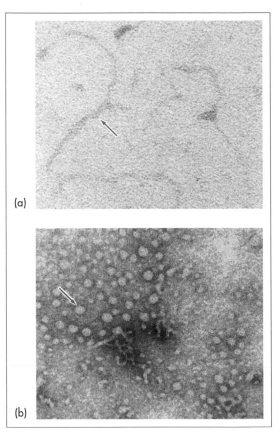

(a)

(b)

Figure 13.25 (a) Electron micrograph of naked plasmid DNA; (b) the same sample after condensation with a cationic partial dendrimer. The size, shape, charge and stability of such complexes depend on the ionic strength of the medium, lipid composition, lipid/DNA ratio and concentration, and even on mixing procedures. Manufacturing issues include those of reproducibility, avoiding aggregation of the resulting colloidal suspension and lyophilisation, as discussed by RI Mahato *et al*. (*Pharm Res* 1997;14:853–859).

Reproduced from Ramaswamy C, Florence AT. Self-assembly of some amphipathic dendrons. *J Drug Del Sci Tech* 2005;15:307–311. Copyright Elsevier 2005.

13.6 Therapeutic monoclonal antibodies

There are growing numbers of MAbs (antibodies produced from a single clone of cells) available for use in the clinic, including MAb–drug conjugates. Typical MAbs include anti-HER2 MAb, trastuzumab (Herceptin, Roche) for breast cancer and rituximab for malignant lymphoma. Although MAbs were first produced in the mid-1970s, there have been several problems with their clinical use, for, in spite of their target specificity,

Structure II An oligonucleotide

their poor distribution and tissue penetration result in the need for high doses. The latter leads to various pharmaceutical issues common to the group. The restricted penetration results from the fact that MAbs are large molecules with molecular weights of the order of 150 kDa, so that they diffuse slowly in tissues, especially in tumours or inflamed sites. Antibodies with a molecular size greater than 150 kDa are prevented from passage through the blood–brain barrier, for example, hence the cerebrospinal fluid level of one MAb, rituximab, is known to be only 0.1% of its serum levels. While there has been evidence suggesting that antibodies against beta-amyloid plaques can reverse cognitive deficits in early Alzheimer disease, promising constructs do not cross the blood–brain barrier. Their physical chemistry can explain in part the properties of MAbs, such as blocking the action of target antigens, their binding to antigens and their diffusion and translocation in tissues.[15]

Many MAbs have doses in the range of mg kg^{-1} when administered by intravenous or subcutaneous routes. Used subcutaneously there is the need to minimise the volume administered, hence the use of concentrated solutions. Such solutions often have an elevated viscosity and the concentrated antibodies tend to be more prone to self-association and aggregation.[16] These large protein molecules have complex structures and complex solution behaviour, as might be expected, often sensitive to impurities or additives: even small amounts of silicone oil used as lubricants for syringes can lead to antibody aggregation,[17] as do some preservatives also. Aggregation generally implies partial loss of activity.

Figure 13.26 shows the simplified structure of a typical MAb with its light and heavy chains. The variable and constant regions of the model structure are also shown. An MAb is represented interacting with a target, and a simplified representation is given of a MAb–drug conjugate (ADC) and a drug conjugate showing the labile disulfide linkage, one of several that can be employed, to control the rate of release of the drug from the conjugate, a key element in its biological activity. See Box 13.1.

> **Box 13.1 Nomenclature of MAbs**
>
> The International Non-proprietary Names of all drugs should convey meaning about the class to which each drug belongs. Trade names do not serve this purpose. All MAbs thus have the -mab suffix in their name. Other elements of the name provide further information. A *source suffix* (before -mab) reveals the cell origin : -u- (human), -o- (mouse), -xi- chimeric, -zu- (humanised), -xi-zu- (hybrid of chimeric and humanised) are examples, as shown in Fig. 13.27. Thus, trastuzumab is a humanised MAb. *Disease targets* can also be included in the name, e.g. -lim- (immune), -les- (infectious diseases), -vir- (viral), -mel- (melanoma), -col- (colon).

13.6.1 Antibody–drug conjugates

Figure 13.28 illustrates many of the vital features of drug conjugates: the antibody itself, the active drug such as a cytotoxic agent attached to the antibody and the linker between antibody and drug. The MAb provides the potential for specific targeting; in other words, it is the vector. The link between drug and MAb can be designed to control payload release. Two examples of ADCs are trastuzumab emtansine (MAb linked to the cytotoxic mertansine) and brentuximab vedotin (MAb linked to monomethyl auristatin E), whose payloads are inactive until binding to their target receptors, the conjugate internalised in lysosomes, linkers cleaved and drug released within the

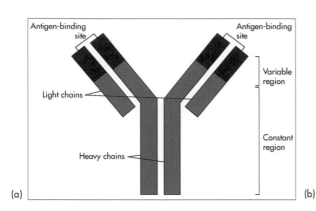

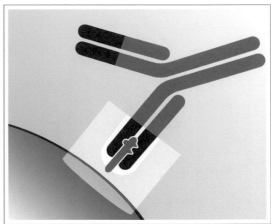

(a)

(b)

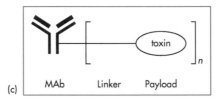

(c)

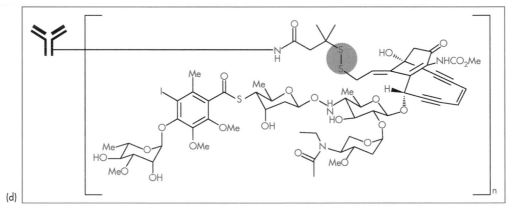

(d)

Figure 13.26 (a) Representation of a typical monoclonal antibody (MAb) showing the light and heavy chains. The variable and constant regions of the model structure are also shown. (b) An MAb interacting with a target. (c) A much simplified representation of an MAb–drug conjugate, the form that many therapeutic approaches now take. (d) (not to scale) A conjugate showing the labile S–S– linkage, one of several that can be employed. The rate of release of the drug from the conjugate can be a key element in its biological activity.

target cells.[*] This is the theory, but there are constraints.

A key point is the ratio of drug to antibody. It is tempting to think that increasing the payload enhances activity, but the attached molecules can begin to interfere sterically with the behaviour of the antibody: increased numbers of drug molecules change the phys-

ical properties of the construct by changing the surface properties, hydrophobicity, charge, shape, and so on. The position of the linker and thus the drug is also important to activity, as are the degradation pathways of the complex. Premature breakdown of the linker will clearly lead to release of drug before the optimal target is reached – a problem discussed in

---

[*] There is also the ingenious use of MAbs for reducing the toxicity of drugs. D Morelli *et al.* (*Cancer Res* 1996:56;2082–2085) report that the murine MAb MAD11 recognises the anthracycline doxorubicin, a drug which can cause gastrointestinal toxicity. Oral administration of MAD11 was found to reduce the drug's toxicity.

Chapter 14 in relation to many drug carriers such as liposomes and nanoparticles.

13.6.2 Aggregation and other forms of instability: the pharmaceutical issues

The antibody constructs can associate in solution, forming dimers, tetramers or larger aggregates. Such changes in the form of the construct can lead to

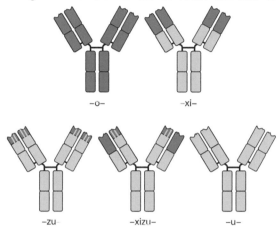

−o− −xi−

−zu− −xizu− −u−

Figure 13.27 Illustrations of mouse (-o-) to human (-u-) monoclonal antibodies with intermediate forms such as chimeric (-xi-), humanised (-zu-) and (-xizu-), a hybrid form derived from chimeric and humanised sources.

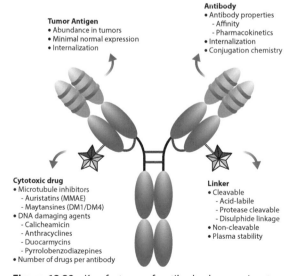

Tumor Antigen
• Abundance in tumors
• Minimal normal expression
• Internalization

Antibody
• Antibody properties
  - Affinity
  - Pharmacokinetics
• Internalization
• Conjugation chemistry

Cytotoxic drug
• Microtubule inhibitors
  - Auristatins (MMAE)
  - Maytansines (DM1/DM4)
• DNA damaging agents
  - Calicheamicin
  - Anthracyclines
  - Duocarmycins
  - Pyrrolobenzodiazepines
• Number of drugs per antibody

Linker
• Cleavable
  - Acid-labile
  - Protease cleavable
  - Disulphide linkage
• Non-cleavable
• Plasma stability

Figure 13.28 Key features of antibody–drug conjugates: the cytotoxic drug, the nature of the link between drug and antibody, the affinity of the antibody to sites of action such as tumour antigen, pharmacokinetics and internalisation.

Reproduced with permission from Panowski S *et al*. Site-specific antibody drug conjugates for cancer therapy. *mAbs* 2014;6:34–45.

decreased therapeutic activity and enhanced immunogenicity and will affect the transport properties of the MAbs or ADCs, as size matters! Figure 13.29 schematically illustrates the potential for change in solution behaviour:

• unfolding of chains
• clustering of unfolded antibodies
• aggregation into soluble clusters
• formation of insoluble particles.

The several processes that contribute to the instability of antibodies are outlined in Figure 13.30, showing chemical instability through oxidation, deamidation, hydrolysis and proteolysis to the physical manifestations of instability, conformational change and aggregation, already discussed.

13.6.3 Rheological changes

Higher concentrations of MAbs increase the viscosity of their solutions, as one would expect from earlier discussions of rheology of colloids (see Chapter 6). But beyond the normal enhanced viscosity due to increased volume fraction, the aggregation of the antibodies has a marked effect on viscosity, as shown in Fig. 13.31, where there is a linear increase in viscosity with the average number of antibodies in each cluster, rising from around 10 cP to more than 400 cP with aggregates containing nine antibodies. This can result in difficulties not only in manufacture and processing but also in the filling of syringes, and their subsequent dispersal from intramuscular and subcutaneous injection sites.

13.6.4 Formulations

As examples we can cite palivizumab (Synagis) or efalizumab (Raptiva) for intramuscular injection, both with a concentration of 100 mg mL^{-1}, while omalizumab (Xolair) for subcutaneous injection exceeds this at 125 mg mL^{-1}. Antibody formulations often contain surfactants such as polysorbate 20 and polysorbate 80 to aid stabilisation of the protein: altering the nature of the solution can influence viscosity also.

13.6.5 Diffusion coefficients and transport

Aggregation may be reversible, as shown in the examples above, by the addition of electrolyte, or

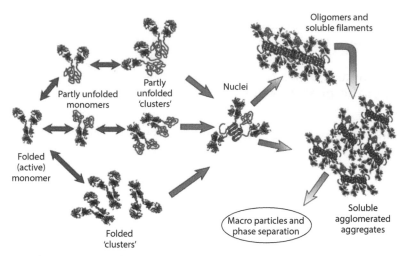

Figure 13.29 A comprehensive survey of the possibilities of the association and aggregation of monoclonal antibodies (MAbs) in solution, starting from the folded active MAb monomers, through partly unfolded, to oligomers and particles. Increasing the net charge on proteins minimises these effects, as does decreasing ionic strength.

Reproduced from Roberts CJ. Therapeutic protein aggregation: mechanisms, design, and control. *Trends Biotechnol* 2014;32:372–380. Copyright Elsevier 2014.

surfactant or other formulation excipients. One consequence of: (1) the size of the MAb and (2) its aggregation is the effect these parameters have on the diffusion coefficient which, as the Stokes–Einstein equation dictates, is a function of the radius of spherical particles, and determines the ability of the molecules or their aggregates to negotiate the body as has been discussed in Chapters 2 and 14.

The aqueous diffusion coefficient of glucose (molecular weight 192 Da) is 6.6×10^{-6} cm^2 s^{-1}; that of insulin (5734 Da) is 2.10×10^{-6} cm^2 s^{-1}, serum albumin (66,500 Da) is 0.6×10^{-6} cm^2 s^{-1} (its

radius is 6 nm) while human IgM (970 000 Da), with a radius of 15 nm, has a diffusion coefficient of 0.32×10^{-6} cm^2 s^{-1}. We know that:

$$t = x^2/2D$$

where t is the diffusion time (the elapsed time after diffusion has begun), D is the diffusion coefficient, x is the mean distance travelled in one axis after time t. Hence the time taken for glucose, insulin and IgM to travel 1 cm is 21 hours, 66 hours and 434 hours respectively. Diffusion in more complex media, e.g. in

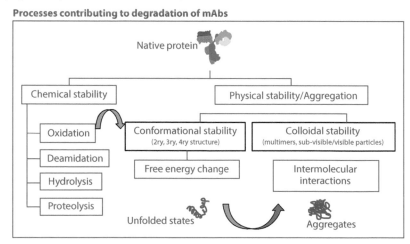

Figure 13.30 The many processes contributing to degradation of monoclonal antibodies (MAbs). Chemical degradation is applied to most actives, coupled with the conformational stability of proteins and macromolecules and physical instability, leading to aggregate formation.

Courtesy of M Connolly, University of Bath.

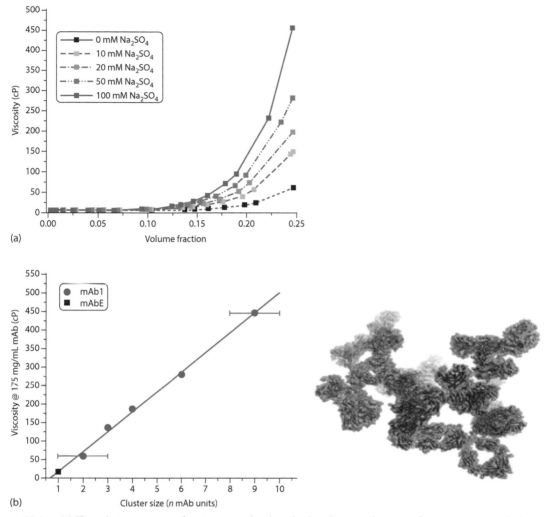

Figure 13.31 (a) The solution viscosity of an Ig_1 monoclonal antibody solution as function of concentration and electrolyte (Na_2SO_4) concentration, showing the sensitivity to both parameters above certain concentrations. (b) The viscosity of 175 mg mL^{-1} solutions as a function of the cluster size determined for each system with a computer model of cluster formation.

Reproduced with permission from Lilyestrom WG *et al.* Monoclonal antibody self-association, cluster formation and rheology at high concentrations. *J Phys Chem B* 2013;117:6373–6384. Copyright 2013 American Chemical Society.

tumours, mucus and tissues, is in general affected also by (1) *binding* of the diffusant to biological molecules and tissues and (2) the *obstruction effect,* where size and surface properties of the molecule and possible *flexibility* come into play as the molecules move through a complex fluid milieu with impenetrable obstacles like fibres and cellular components.

Botulinum toxin diffusion

Botulinum toxins, which can decrease the release of acetylcholine, and thus elicit a neuromuscular blocking effect, are used in many cases to relieve unwanted muscular contractions as occur in strabismus, blephar-

ospasm, hemifacial spasm and spasticity. There are a number of products, processed and purified in different ways, providing a variety of clinical products with different protein content, excipients and so on. As botulinum toxin is obviously a toxic product (in inappropriate concentrations), one characteristic of interest is the diffusion of the toxin molecules,[18] not least when the products are used in cosmetic treatments. Naturally the diffusion, spread and migration of the botulinum toxin A are vital and it is the limited diffusion of the molecule that has allowed this potent molecule to be used safely!

Three of the main products are:

1. Botox/Vistabel (Allergan, NPN onabotulinum-toxinA)
2. Dysport/Azzalure (Ipsen, NPN abobotulinum-toxinA)
3. Xeomin/Bocouture (Merz, NPN incobotulinum-toxinA).

These have markedly different specific activities and cannot be considered to be bio-equivalent. For further discussion of so-called biosimilars, see Chapter 16. A detailed review of the literature is available.[19]

13.7 Vaccine formulation

The field of immunology is complex. Vaccines stimulate production of antibodies and other components of the immune system and comprise four types, which, in the words of the *British National Formulary,* are:

1. *live attenuated* forms of a virus (e.g. measles, mumps and rubella vaccine) or bacteria (e.g. Bacillus Calmette-Guérin (BCG) vaccine)
2. *inactivated* preparations of a virus (c.g. influenza vaccine) or bacteria
3. *detoxified exotoxins* produced by a microorganism (e.g. tetanus vaccine)
4. *extracts of* a microorganism, which may be derived from the organism (e.g. pneumococcal vaccine) or produced by recombinant DNA technology (e.g. hepatitis B vaccine).

 Clinical points

Live attenuated vaccines usually produce a durable immunity, but not always as long-lasting as that resulting from natural infection.
Inactivated vaccines may require a primary series of injections of vaccine to produce an adequate antibody response, and in most cases booster (reinforcing) injections are required; the duration of immunity varies from months to many years. Some inactivated vaccines are adsorbed onto an adjuvant (such as aluminium hydroxide) to enhance the antibody response.
Source: BNF, through Medicines Complete December 2014.

 Clinical point

Vaccines are contraindicated in those who have a confirmed anaphylactic reaction to a preceding dose of a vaccine containing the same antigens or vaccine component (such as antibacterials in viral vaccines). The presence of the following excipients should be noted in some vaccines.

Gelatin	Penicillins
Gentamicin	Polymyxin B
Kanamycin	Streptomycin
Neomycin	Thiomersal

Source: BNF, through Medicines Complete, December 2014.

This short account will discuss some of the issues related to the pharmaceutics of vaccines. There are components and excipients in some vaccines which can cause problems.

The two main areas to be dealt with here are *adjuvants,*† used to boost immune response and delivery options, some of which have already been dealt with earlier in this book. The roles adjuvants play are fascinating, but still offer us some mysteries.

13.7.1 Routes of administration

Most vaccines are given by the intramuscular route, while some are given by the intradermal, deep subcutaneous or oral routes, for example:

- intradermal route – BCG
- deep subcutaneous route – varicella
- oral route – cholera, poliomyelitis, rotavirus and live typhoid vaccines (where the gut-associated lymphoid tissue plays its part in achieving activity).

† Adjuvant derives from the Latin verb *adjuvare,* to help.

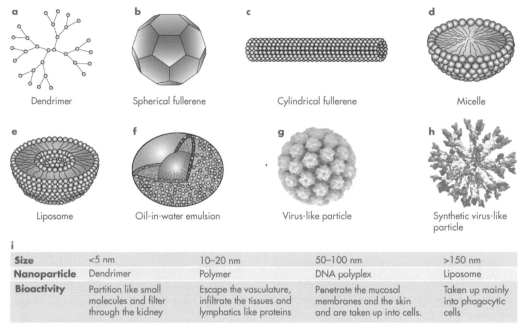

i				
Size	<5 nm	10–20 nm	50–100 nm	>150 nm
Nanoparticle	Dendrimer	Polymer	DNA polyplex	Liposome
Bioactivity	Partition like small molecules and filter through the kidney	Escape the vasculature, infiltrate the tissues and lymphatics like proteins	Penetrate the mucosal membranes and the skin and are taken up into cells.	Taken up mainly into phagocytic cells

Figure 13.32 Representation of types of carriers for vaccines acting (left to right) mainly as depots, or in dual roles as immunostimulants and carriers or as immunomodulators. Immunostimulating complexes (ISCOMs) are relatively stable but non-covalently-bound complexes of the saponin adjuvant Quil-A from *Quillaia saponaria Mollina*, cholesterol and amphipathic Ag in a molar ratio of approximately 1:1:1. ISCOMs have been shown to induce cytotoxic T-lymphocytes.
Reproduced from Smith DM, Simon JK, Baker JR Jr. *Nat Rev Immunol* 2013;13:592–605.

The UK Department of Health has advised against the use of jet guns for vaccination owing to the risk of transmitting blood-borne infections, such as human immunodeficiency virus (HIV), because of the potential for production of sprays through impact on the skin.

13.7.2 Vehicles

Some of the materials used or under study today are represented in Fig. 13.32. These include a number of systems discussed elsewhere in the book: neutral and cationic liposomes, microspheres and nanoparticles (such as PLGA), salts such as alum (aluminium hydroxide), immunostimulating complexes (ISCOMs), water-in-oil and oil-in-water emulsions and saponins.

Alum

Alum (aluminium hydroxide) was first introduced as a vaccine adjuvant in the 1920s and its mode of action in enhancing the action of antigens is still being debated – one of the 'slowest processes in the history of medicine,'** according to De Gregorio *et al.*[20] One hypothesis is that alum, by combining with a soluble

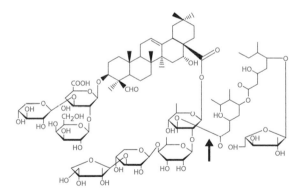

Structure III Quil-A saponin

antigen, forms a precipitate and that slow release of the antigen from the precipitate on injection encourages a prolonged, strong antibody response. However, the desired effects of aluminum-containing adjuvants have also been concluded not to derive from direct antigen adsorption and retention, but rather from other contributions to immunopotentiation.

Since then, a number of adjuvant materials and formulations have been described with different modes of action, but alum is still the only adjuvant licensed in

** The mechanism of action of alum has also been known as the field's 'dirty little secret'.

the USA, while the European authorities have approved two oil-in-water emulsions, MF59 and AS03.

ISCOMs

ISCOMs are relatively stable but non-covalently bound complexes of the saponin adjuvant Quil-A from *Quillaia saponaria Mollina*, cholesterol and amphipathic Ag in a molar ratio of approximately 1:1:1. The adjuvanticity of Quil-A saponin (**III**) depends on its structure; it is composed of hydrophilic sugar sidechains and a hydrophobic aglycone backbone.

Saponins

Saponins derive from many plant sources. Like many adjuvant components they have an amphipathic structure. It is claimed that the overall hydrophile–lipophile balance of the saponins is more important for its adjuvanticity than the structures involved. Being surface active, micelles can be formed by the saponins and these must play a part in the protection and release properties of the adjuvant.

Emulsions

Freund's incomplete adjuvant (Statens Seruminstitut, Copenhagen, Denmark) is a water-in-oil emulsion containing antigen in the aqueous phase, light paraffin oil and an emulsifying agent, mannide monooleate. On injection, this mixture (*Freund's incomplete adjuvant*) induces strong persistent antibody formation. The addition of killed, dried mycobacteria, e.g., *Mycobacterium butyricum,* to the oil phase (*Freund's complete adjuvant*) elicits cell-mediated immunity (delayed hypersensitivity), as well as humoral antibody formation.

MF59 (Novartis) is a squalene (**IV**)-in-water emulsion with a mean globule size of 160 nm, stabilised by sorbitan trioleate and polysorbate. It is used in influenza vaccines. A related product is *AS03* or 'Adjuvant System 03', a squalene-based adjuvant used in various vaccine products by GlaxoSmithKline. A dose of AS03 adjuvant contains 10.69 mg squalene, 11.86 mg DL-α-tocopherol and 4.86 mg polysorbate 80.

Structure IV Squalene

Adjuvant 65 is a marketed water-in-oil emulsion containing antigen in peanut oil with Arlacel A (mannide

monooleate) and aluminum monostearate as the emulsifying agents.

Summary

This chapter has not attempted to provide an overview of proteins and peptides and other complex therapeutics such as DNA, oligonucleotides or MAbs. It has concentrated on giving a flavour of some of the unique physical properties that the substances discussed here have. It has tried to give some feeling for the properties of peptides and proteins and how their physical properties are dictated not only by the properties of their individual amino acids but also by the spatial arrangement of the amino acids in their polypeptide chains, and of course their interaction with water and other ingredients that might be in formulations. Hydrophobic amino acids alternating with hydrophilic, or charged amino acids can produce tertiary and quaternary structures that are quite different from those induced by the spatial separation of hydrophobic and hydrophilic amino acids. The stability of proteins and peptides is of prime pharmaceutical significance. Maintenance of chemical and physical stability is a prerequisite for clinical use. The macromolecular and generally hydrophilic character of all but the smallest peptides makes this class of compound one that is challenging in terms of delivery for therapeutic ends. Some of the issues involved in the formulation of proteins and vaccines, such as botulinum toxin A vaccine, are also discussed.

References

1. Brange J *et al*. Monomeric insulins and their experimental and clinical implications. *Diabetes Care* 1990;13:923–954.
2. Brems DN *et al*. Altering the self-association and stability of insulin by amino acid replacement. In: Cleland J (ed.) *Protein Folding: In Vivo and In Vitro*. ACS Symposium Series 526. Washington, DC: American Chemical Society; 1993: 254–269.
3. Shao Z *et al*. Differential effects of anionic, cationic, nonionic, and physiologic surfactants on the dissociation, alpha-chymotryptic degradation, and enteral absorption of insulin hexamers. *Pharm Res* 1993;102:43–51.
4. Costantino JR *et al*. Aggregation of a lyophilized pharmaceutical protein, recombinant human albumin: effect of moisture and stabilization by excipients. *Biotechnology* 1995;13:493–496.

5. Hageman MJ *et al*. Prediction and characterization of the water sorption isotherm for bovine somatotropin. *J Agric Food Chem* 1992;40:342–347.

6. Zografi G. States of water associated with solids. *Drug Dev Ind Pharm* 1988;14:1905–1906.

7. Cleland JL, Langer R. Formulation and delivery of proteins and peptides: design and development strategies. In: Cleland JL, Langer R (eds) *Formulation and Delivery of Proteins and Peptides*. Washington, DC: American Chemical Society; 1994: 1–19.

8. Ye M *et al*. Issues in long term protein delivery using biodegradable microparticles. *J Control Rel* 2010;146:241–260.

9. Veronese FM, Pasut G. PEGylation, successful approach to drug delivery. *Drug Deliv Today* 2005;10:1451.

10. Mehrar R. Modulation of the pharmacokinetics and pharmacodynamics of proteins by polyoxyethylene glycol conjugation. *J Pharm Pharm Sci* 2000;3:125–136.

11. Gallina K *et al*. Local blistering reaction complicating subcutaneous injection of pegylated interferon in a patient with hepatitis C. *J Drugs Dermatol* 2003;263–67.

12. Dalmau J *et al*. Cutaneous necrosis after injection of polyethylene glycol-modified interferon alfa. *J Am Acad Dermatol* 2005;53:62–66.

13. Arvinte T *et al*. The structure and mechanism of formation of human calcitonin fibrils. *J Biol Chem* 1993;268:6415–6422.

14. Mao HQ *et al*. Chitosan-DNA nanoparticles as gene carriers: synthesis, characterisation and transfection efficiency. *J Control Release* 2001;70:399–421.

15. Breedveld FC. Therapeutic monoclonal antibodies. *Lancet* 2000;355:735–740.

16. Yadav S *et al*. Factors affecting the viscosity of high concentration solutions of different monoclonal antibodies. *J Pharm Sci* 2010;99:4812–4829.

17. Thirumangalathu R *et al*. Silicone oil- and agitation-induced aggregation of a monoclonal antibody in aqueous solution. *J Pharm Sci* 2009;98:3167–3181.

18. Brodksy MA *et al*. Diffusion of botulinium toxins. *Tremor and other hyperkinetic movements*, 2012. Available online at: http://www.tremorjournal.org.

19. Brin MF *et al*. (2014) Botulinum toxin type A products are not interchangeable: a review of the evidence *Biologics: Targets Ther* 2014;8:227–241.

20. De Gregorio E *et al*. Alum adjuvanticity: Unraveling a century old mystery. *Eur J Immunol* 2008;38:2068–2071.

14

Pharmaceutical nanotechnology

This chapter provides an introduction to the characteristics of nanosystems, especially those that are used as carriers for drug delivery and targeting. Wherever possible the preparation, properties and uses of the nanoparticles are related here to issues already discussed in other chapters. Nanoparticles of many types, in view of their size in the range of 1–~200 nm, are colloidal systems, and the laws of colloids (see Chapter 6) apply. The promise of nanosystems which can deliver drugs to specific sites in the body has been partially demonstrated and the reasons for this will be discussed. Not least, physical laws dictate the behaviour of nanosystems *in vivo*. The preparation of nanoparticles often involves processes such as solvent change, supercritical states, emulsion formation and solvent diffusion and evaporation. Many of the biological attributes of nanocarriers depend on their physical chemistry, their surface charge, diameter, hydrophilicity or hydrophobicity, all key attributes. Their movement in cells, tissues and complex media (e.g. mucus) is largely dependent on the laws of diffusion and hence size. We will discuss their diffusion, the adsorption on to their surfaces of proteins (opsonins) and ligands in the blood, and their physical stability. Aggregation and jamming of nanoparticles *in vivo* negate the advantage of their small and controlled size, so this must be controlled, as must the point of release of the drug from any carrier as it traverses the body.

14.1 Introduction

Pharmaceutical nanotechnology deals mainly with particles or constructs that have dimensions ranging from several nanometres to around 250 nm. Natural nanosystems abound (Fig. 14.1) and were known long before the surge in biomedical interest in synthetic versions. Insulin, which can form hexamers (3.5 × 5 nm), and albumin (3 × 3 × 8 nm), which binds and carries drugs, are two examples, while viruses and lipoprotein particles are others. Pharmaceutical nanotechnology encompasses the manipulation and processing of systems, their physicochemical characterisation, their

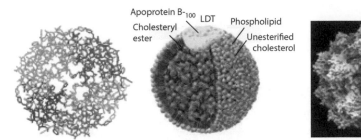

Figure 14.1 Nanosystems that exist in nature (not to scale). Left to right: an insulin hexamer (3.5 × 5 nm), a low-density lipoprotein (LDL) particle (28 nm) and a parvovirus (20–25 nm). LDL with its apolipoprotein ligand is a natural carrier of cholesterol to rapidly dividing cells; viruses are efficient transfection agents.

applications and biological evaluation. The principal pharmaceutical interest in nanoparticles at present is their potential as carriers for drugs and other active entities such as nucleic acids, with the promise of targeting to specific sites in the body, or, a more straightforward goal, to modulate the kinetics of drugs *in vivo*. The active ingredients are encapsulated in, or attached to, the particles and the fate of the nanoparticles determines to a large extent the fate of the drug, which distinguishes nanosystems from the actives themselves. But they have many other potential uses, not least as specialised excipients. There is also the formation of nanoparticles of poorly soluble drugs (as nanocrystals), which is a process that enhances their solubility and bioavailability. Nanoparticles are of course colloidal in nature, hence the topics of colloid science (see Chapter 6) and pharmaceutical nanotechnology overlap considerably.

Although the descriptor *nanotechnology* came to the fore in the late 1980s it has a somewhat longer pedigree in pharmacy, since, in fact, Peter Speiser and his colleagues[1,2] at ETH in Zurich prepared and investigated 'nanoparts' and 'nanocapsules' a decade earlier.[3] Surfactant micelles (see Chapter 5) have diameters of some 1–3 nm and have been studied for more than 70 years as solubilisers of poorly water-soluble drugs. Microemulsions (see section 6.4.5), a name coined in 1959,[4] are more correctly named nanoemulsions and are used in pharmacy, as in the ciclosporin concentrate Neoral, which on dilution forms droplets in the size range 10–100 nm (see section 6.4.6).

Typical nanosized pharmaceutical carrier systems therefore include polymeric or lipidic nanoparticles, nanoemulsions (microemulsions), dendrimers, fullerenes and carbon nanotubes as well as hybrid systems and the smallest liposomes. Some poorly soluble drugs can be prepared as nanosuspensions. Some systems are represented in Fig. 14.2.

Clearly a main focus in pharmaceutical nanotechnology is how to characterise nanosystems. This includes investigation of drug loading capacity, drug release rate and the chemical and physical stability of both drug and carrier (Fig. 14.3). Particle size is of course a key property, and surface charge and character (whether the surface is hydrophilic or hydrophobic) are other defining properties. Shape, flexibility or elasticity of particles can also be factors of importance. Biological evaluation of nanosystems involves knowledge of the absorption, distribution and excretion of both the drug and the carrier along with its load of encapsulated or attached drug. The mode and speed of the biodegradation of the nanoparticle are also required information.

14.2 Rationale for nanoparticles for drug delivery and targeting

The rationale for: (a) the encapsulation of drugs in nanoparticles or (b) in some cases the adsorption of active agents on to the surface of nanoparticles is so that:

1. the active molecules are protected from the external environment until such time as they are released. Once released, any drug will behave as free drug molecules, although being transported by the nanocarriers, the drug may have been deposited in the liver and spleen by the carrier

2. it is the nature, destination and fate of the nanoparticles, rather than the characteristics of the drug, that determine at least the initial fate of the drug because the body 'sees' the carrier rather than the drug

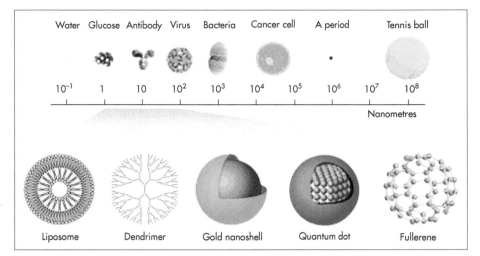

Figure 14.2 Typical nanocarriers and imaging systems in the size range 1–100 nm (not drawn to scale), which will be increasingly used in pharmacy as carriers of drugs and diagnostic agents: shown here in comparison with molecules, viruses, bacteria, cancer cells and a full stop in printing.

Reproduced with permission from McNeil SE. Nanotechnology for the biologist. *J Leukoc Biol* 2005;78:585–593.

3. the pharmacokinetics of the active is modified by its slow release from the carrier and the carrier's trajectory, which may lead to reduction in toxicity.

It is important to distinguish between the *pharmacokinetics* of drug delivered in the carrier and the kinetics of the particles themselves, a subject that is termed *particokinetics.*[5] *Size* is particularly important in determining the ability of nanoparticles to access sites that are out of bounds to larger particles. There is, however, a continuum of diameters and one of the great

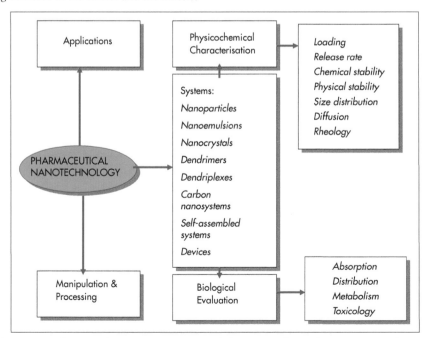

Figure 14.3 Pharmaceutical nanotechnology's main areas of focus, namely, applications, manipulation and processing, physicochemical characterisation and biological evaluation. An understanding of the relevance of the physicochemical properties of these systems and biological barriers and environments they encounter is essential. Absorption, distribution, metabolism and toxicology refer to both the drug once released from the delivery system and the delivery system itself, the two being intertwined.

challenges in drug delivery and targeting is the production of nanosystems with narrow size distributions. Nature achieves this, as we have seen in the case of low-density lipoproteins, which have a mean diameter of 26.7 nm and a size range of 25.8–28.2 nm in young healthy females and 25.5–28.1 nm in males.[6] Small size at the limit where the drug molecules approach the size of the carrier (as with dendrimers in the 2–10 nm range) means a carrier/drug ratio of ≈ 1. Some nanoparticles, such as drug nanocrystals, on the other hand, consist virtually only of drug, as discussed in section 14.6.

One pharmaceutical problem is to design and formulate systems that are stable *in vitro* but can also survive their dilution in blood, and the mixing and shearing forces in flow. There are many changes in the particle environment as it passages through tissues, one of which is a change in surface characteristics brought about by opsonin adsorption, a precursor of uptake by the reticuloendothelial system and hence loss from the circulation.

14.3 Particle structures

To utilise fully the potential of nanotechnology a goal of selective delivery of drugs to cells, organs and tissues

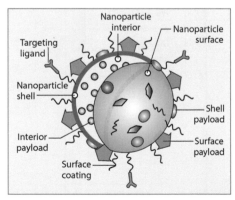

Figure 14.4 General elements of nanoparticles designed for targeting, using targeting ligands to interact with appropriate receptors on target cells or tissues. Surface coatings are used to modify nanoparticle behaviour *in vivo*. Interior, surface or shell-based payloads with the characteristics of the nanoparticle surface and the nature of the particle interior and shell, if present, are other factors in design and characterisation.

Reproduced with permission from Mieszawska AJ *et al.* Multifunctional gold nanoparticles for diagnosis and therapy of disease. *Mol Pharm* 2013;10:831–847.

has been pursued. The general features of targeting systems are drawn in Fig. 14.4, which summarises the complex structural nature of such a nanoparticulate system comprising eight aspects of design:

1. nature of the interior space
2. nature of the shell
3. nature of the surface
4. interior payload levels
5. shell payload level
6. surface payload
7. surface coating
8. targeting ligands.

It may be that the particle is solid, formed from a single polymer without a shell. What is then important is the distribution of the drug throughout the system.

14.4 The primacy of particle size

Nanotechnology is defined to a large extent by the size (or more usually, the size range) of the systems used. Only some systems, such as dendrimers, because they are synthesised as discrete chemical entities, have for any particular type a single size, i.e. they are monodisperse. Many other nanoparticle preparation techniques result in a particle size distribution. It is, however, possible to prepare monodisperse systems as with polystyrene and other commercially available systems which are often used as controls or models in experiments.

Small size brings with it both advantages and disadvantages. Rates of release may be rapid, because of the large surface area per unit particle weight and because diffusional path lengths within the particles are small. Particle size influences many of the properties and behaviour of nanoparticles, as indicated in Fig. 14.5.

 Key question

How can the nanocarriers be designed to release drug only when at a target site? The system could be activated once it had tracked to its destination, for example by elevation of local temperature, making use of enzymatic

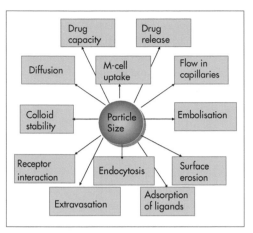

Figure 14.5 Particle size and its bearing either directly or indirectly on the behaviour and fate of nanoparticles. For examples see text.

reactions, or changes in local pH, or by an external stimulus. It should be noted that the circulation times in the body of nanoparticles from a single administration vary depending on the frequency of individual particle uptake into the target. See section on stochatic processes (14.7.4) which discusses the importance of the stochastic nature of extravasation and the consequences for circulation times.

Key parameters

- *Drug release*: the larger surface area per unit weight of nanoparticles leads to potentially high release rates compared to the same weight of larger particles, as solvent penetration will be a function of $n\pi r^2$, where n = number of nanoparticles per unit weight and r is the particle radius.

- *Oral uptake*: although we state in Chapter 8 that drugs must be in their molecular form to be taken up by epithelial cells, there is a mechanism for oral particle uptake. The main site involves the membranous epithelial cells (M cells) of the gut-associated lymphoid tissue. Smaller particles (i.e. those 5–150 nm) with the appropriate surface properties are taken up more readily than the equivalent larger particles (> 300 nm), and above a certain size (around 500 nm) particles will not be absorbed, at least not intact. The oral delivery of large labile molecules such as insulin is being pursued in spite of 90 or more years of failed

experiments, but low uptake of carriers and the sometimes the very low capacity of the carriers for such molecules make this a daunting task if the nanoparticle approach is used for insulin and similar molecules.

- *Flow in capillaries*: once injected, nanoparticles flow in the blood and particle diameter is clearly important. Flow is a complex phenomenon, as discussed in Chapter 6; it depends on the ratio of particle diameter to the diameter of the capillaries, on bifurcations of the capillary network, particle flexibility and particle jamming (see below and Fig. 14.6).

- *Embolisation*: nanoparticles are too small to block blood vessels and capillaries, but if they aggregate then such blockage (embolisation) can occur. The process of particle '*jamming*' can also occur (Fig. 14.6), which hinders free particle movements such as their escape from the circulation and passage though the extracellular matrix or porous media.

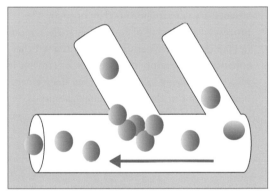

Figure 14.6 A simple illustration of particle jamming at the juncture of two vessels during particle flow. The phenomenon depends on the nature of the particles, their diameter in relation to the diameter of the capillaries and their branches, and the surface properties and flexibility or elasticity under pressure.

- *Surface erosion* is involved in many biodegradation and drug release processes, and will be a function of surface area of the nanoparticles and of course dependent on the nature of the polymer, lipid or other material used to fabricate the system.

- *Adsorption of ligands*: adsorption of proteins, whether derived from the blood or deliberately attached (e.g. polyethylene glycols) to alter the surface properties of nanoparticles. The number of

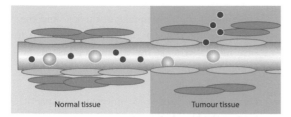

Figure 14.7 Diagrammatic representation of the process of extravasation of nanoparticles in the vicinity of tumours; in normal tissue particle escape is limited.

ligands per particle will depend on the available surface area, and the area/molecule of the adsorbing molecules, the charge and hydrophobicity of the surface.

- *Endocytosis* (uptake of particles by cells) is size-dependent.
- *Extravasation* (escape of particles from the circulation into target cells or tissues) occurs more readily with small particles. Figure 14.7 shows a representation of the escape of nanoparticles from the circulation in the region of tumours where the vasculature is more porous than normal. The process of the potential route of particle tumour uptake by this mechanism has been termed the enhanced permeation and retention effect, but its relevance to many systems has been questioned. Further proof of the range of applicability is required.

- *Physical (colloid) stability* is dependent on radius, the nature of the material, its charge and the presence of any adsorbed molecules whose molecular weight and configuration on the surface are crucial (as discussed in Chapter 6).

 Key question

To what extent can the original properties of a particle designed with surface groups and ligands be retained *in vivo*?

In Fig. 14.8 the dynamic processes that occur at the surface of intravenously administered nanoparticles are illustrated.

- *Diffusion* is vitally important in the translocation of nanoparticles and their transport through mucus and tissues, as well as in tumours and other targets. In a simple fluid medium of viscosity η the influence of particle radius, r, on diffusion coefficient, D, can be recognised from equation (14.1).

$$D = kT/6\pi\eta r \tag{14.1}$$

where k is the Boltzmann constant and T is temperature.

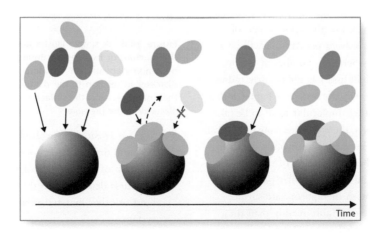

Figure 14.8 Illustration of the dynamics of protein adsorption on to the surface of nanoparticles in the blood. Much depends on the original nature of the particle surface, but a primary corona of biomolecules (light blue) first adsorbs, followed by biomolecules (dark blue and pale blue) with a greater affinity and so on. The surface thus evolves with time.
Reproduced from Monopoli MP *et al. Nature Nanotech* 2012;7:79–786.

Movement in complex media, e.g. cells and gels, will be represented by more complex equations, as given in section 14.7.

As shown in Fig. 14.9:

- The compatibility of drug and carrier system is vital to the even distribution of drug throughout the nanoparticle and to avoid premature release that occurs when the drug migrates to the particle surface.
- The loading of the drug into the particles depends on the nature of the drug and the nature of the carrier material.
- The intravenous route results in mixing of the nanoformulation with blood, perhaps particle adsorption on to erythrocytes,
  opsonisation (which is the adsorption of the proteins or opsonins on to the surface of the nanoparticles which then cause the particles to be recognised as foreign and taken up by the liver and spleen), partial escape from the circulation by extravasation and interaction with the receptor before a cascade of events such as internalisation and diffusion with tissues.

Nanoparticles can be administered by a variety of routes, including the ocular, oral, intravenous, intraperitoneal, intraluminal, subcutaneous, intramuscular, nasal, pulmonary and intratumoral routes. Sometimes nanoparticle-based delivery depends not on any single property. With ocular delivery to the cul-de-sac of the eye, nanoparticles can prolong the action of a drug both by slow-release characteristics and by slowing the loss via the punctae when compared with a solution. The adhesive qualities of some nanosystems can also enhance site-specific activity.[7] Bioadhesive nanoparticles have been advocated to assist adhesion of the carriers to the mucosa and thus increase the probability of arrest, as well as to provide time for the transfer of drug from the carriers or the particles themselves into the gut wall. The importance of the lymphoid tissue in the gut, the gut-associated lymphoid tissue, is crucial to the understanding of some of these possibilities. The M cells and lymphoid tissues of other anatomical regions can be important in particle delivery; for example, the nasal lymphoid tissue, the bronchial tissue and other sites (omentum) provide the possibility of access of particles in small quantities, which may be sufficient for immunisation with vaccines.

14.5 Physicochemical characterisation of nanosystems

The key physicochemical properties of nanoparticles are listed in Table 14.1 under two headings: those of importance in relation to use, and those important in relation to their preparation and properties.

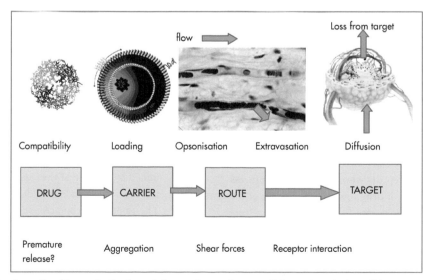

Figure 14.9 A schematic of issues in the formulation and use of nanoparticles as targeted medicines.

Table 14.1 Key physical and chemical properties of nanoparticles as drug carriers

In relation to use
Surface area
Shape
Drug release rate
Biodegradation processes, including rate of degradation
Diffusion (e.g. in tissues and mucus)
Aggregation and flocculation (*in vitro* and *in vivo*)
Adsorption (e.g. to biological and polymer membranes)
Deposition (e.g. on surfaces)
Rheology (e.g. in blood)
Elasticity (to aid progress in capillary networks)
In relation to preparation and properties
Drug–polymer interactions and compatibility (e.g. important in loading drug into systems)
Polymer–polymer interactions (e.g. when two polymers are used to fabricate particles)
Hydrophobicity and hydrophilicity of surfaces
Surface charge
Surface adsorption of macromolecules

To be successful therapeutically, systems must have optimal size and surface characteristics, high loading capacity and loading efficiency, a high degree of chemical and physical stability, as well as appropriate release charactcristics at the target site and be biodegradable and biocompatible.

Not all drug (active)–polymer (carrier) combinations can be readily formulated, sometimes because of the low affinity of the drug for the carrier or indeed incompatibility between drug and carrier. For example, protein drugs do not always mix with polymers without phase separation. (Chapter 7 has a discussion of some of these issues.) Formulations in which drug and carrier material phase-separate (that is, do not produce an isotropic mixture) or whose production process leads to a movement of drug towards the surface of the particles usually demonstrate *burst (initial fast) release* effects. Size polydispersity can also lead to ambiguous results, as it complicates the achievement of targeting because particles of different sizes have different fates.

14.5.1 Hard and soft systems

While size defines all nanosystems, they can differ in their material properties, their chemistry and their physics. It is useful, for reasons that are apparent in relation to movement of nanoparticles *in vivo*, to divide nanosystems into two types, namely 'hard' and 'soft'.

- *Soft systems* include nanoemulsions and polymeric micelles.
- *Hard systems*, which are neither flexible nor elastic, include polymeric nanoparticles, nanosuspensions or nanocrystals, dendrimers and to an extent carbon nanotubes.

Hard systems may block spaces and fenestrae that have the same dimensions as the particles, whereas soft systems can by definition deform and reform (erythrocytes and many liposomes fall into this category). They are thus better able to navigate constricted capillary beds and tissue extracellular spaces.

Key points

- Nanosystems have a size range of several nanometres up to about 150 nm.
- Typical nanosized carrier systems include 'soft systems' such as micelles and nanoemulsions (microemulsions) and 'hard systems' such as polymeric nanoparticles, dendrimers, fullerenes, carbon nanotubes, and polymer nanofibres and nanosuspensions or nanocrystals of drugs themselves.
- The main pharmaceutical interest of nanosystems is as carriers for drugs, which may be encapsulated in or attached to the nanoparticles. This provides two main advantages: the drug is protected from the external environment until it is released, and the fate of the drug *in vivo* is determined by the fate of the carrier rather than the characteristics of the drug itself.
- The important characteristics of nanoparticles are their size and surface characteristics. The size influences a wide range of properties, including drug release, M-cell

uptake, capillary flow, embolisation, surface erosion, adsorption of ligands, endocytosis, extravasation, physical stability and diffusion.

- Their formulation requires an investigation of the drug loading capacity, drug release rate and the chemical and physical stability of both the carrier and encapsulated drug. An important requirement of the formulation is that it should have a narrow size distribution with an even distribution of drug throughout the carrier; it should be stable *in vitro* and be able to survive dilution in blood and the passage through tissues.
- Their biological fate requires knowledge of the absorption, distribution and excretion of both the drug and the carrier.
- Nanoparticles carrying radioactive agents may also be used to aid diagnosis and to locate tumours; some may carry therapeutic agents and are termed 'theranostics'.

14.6 Preparing nanoparticles

There are a large number of methods to prepare nanoparticulate systems, as can be seen from Table 14.2. These depend to a large extent on the material that will form the basis of the carrier, which can include polymers, proteins, metals (gold) or ceramics.

14.6.1 Solvent displacement method

The method of solvent displacement (Fig. 14.10) is perhaps the simplest means of preparing polymeric nanoparticles. The polymer is dissolved along with the drug to be encapsulated in commonly used water-miscible solvents – ethanol, acetone or methanol. The polymer solution is then diluted in the presence of stabilisers such as poly(vinyl alcohol) or polysorbate 80, and forms stabilised nanoparticles with narrow size distributions.

14.6.2 Salting-out method

A variant on the above technique includes a polymer plus a drug dissolved in a water-miscible organic solvent which is added to a stirred aqueous gel containing a salting-out agent and a stabiliser. The polymer–drug combination is salted out as nanoparticles.

Table 14.2 Methods of manufacturing polymeric or protein nanoparticles[a]

Method	Relevant physical events
Solvent displacement	Mixing of solvents to cause the material to come out of solution
Salting out	Reducing solvency: as above, but using another component to salt out the material
Emulsion diffusion	Diffusion of solvent from emulsion droplets, leaving behind the nanoparticle material
Emulsion-solvent evaporation	Evaporation of solvents: Material in the droplets is revealed by removing solvent
Supercritical fluid technology (SCT)	Solvent phase behavior: utilising SCT to produce nanoparticles
Complexation, coacervation	Macromolecular interactions to create a complex mixture of e.g. polymers in the micro or nano size range
Reverse micellar methods	Solubilisation of monomers in inverse micelles and polymerising the monomers by a variety of techniques
In situ polymerisation	Growth of polymers in suspension
Synthesis (e.g. dendrimers)	Covalent growth from a core molecule, by layer addition of linking groups

[a]Some of the above methods are outlined in the text. A fuller account can be found in Florence AT. Pharmaceutical aspects of nanotechnology. In: Florence AT, Siepmann J (eds) *Modern Pharmaceutics*, 5th edn, vol. 2, chapter 12. New York: Informa Healthcare; 2009.

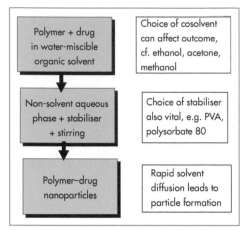

Figure 14.10 A summary of the solvent displacement method. The poly(vinyl alcohol) (PVA) or polysorbate 80 stabilises the particles as they precipitate following the dilution of the non-aqueous solvents. The rapid diffusion of solvent from the polymer phase allows rapid formation and hence a small size distribution.

14.6.3 Emulsion-diffusion method

A different approach is illustrated in Fig. 14.11. A *partly* water-miscible solvent in which the drug and polymer are dissolved forms an emulsion on dilution in an aqueous phase containing a stabiliser. Because of the partial miscibility of the first solvent, it diffuses from the dispersed drops into the bulk to provide polymer nanoparticles containing drug.

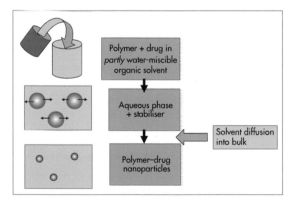

Figure 14.11 Schematic of the emulsion technique wherein the drug and polymer are dissolved in a partly water-miscible solvent. This is then added to an aqueous phase in the presence of surfactant or other stabiliser. Emulsion particles are formed. The solvent, being partly miscible in the water phase, diffuses from the emulsion droplets to form nanoparticles.

14.6.4 Emulsion-solvent evaporation method

Figure 14.12 illustrates a different approach with the emulsion-solvent evaporation technique. It involves the dissolution of the drug–polymer mix in an organic solvent that is immiscible with water, so that on addition to an aqueous phase an emulsion is formed in the presence of emulsifiers. On heating, the internal organic phase can be evaporated in a controlled fashion leaving the polymer–drug nanoparticles, whose size is dependent on the nature of the emulsion.

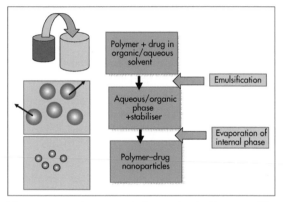

Figure 14.12 A process similar to that in Fig. 14.11. The polymer/drug organic solution is emulsified in water as an oil-in-water system, or the polymer and drug are dissolved in an aqueous phase, which when added to an organic phase forms a water-in-oil emulsion. The internal phase in both cases is evaporated, leaving the polymer–drug particles.

In a variant of this process the drug and the polymer (or protein such as albumin) are dissolved in water, and then added to an organic phase. A water-in-oil emulsion is formed initially, from which the water is removed by evaporation. The oily phase is later 'washed' off.

14.6.5 Using supercritical fluid technology

A supercritical fluid is a substance at a temperature and pressure above its thermodynamic *critical point* (T_c) (Fig. 14.13a). In this state it can diffuse through solids like a gas, and dissolve materials like a liquid. Carbon dioxide and water are the most commonly used supercritical fluids. Supercritical fluid technologies deserve a special mention as they are less commonly applied at a laboratory scale in the preparation of nanoparticles. A drug and polymer are dissolved in an organic solvent or carbon dioxide. Under certain conditions of pressure and temperature (Fig. 14.13(a)) the liquid phase is transformed into the supercritical state, which for CO_2 occurs at pressures > 74 bar (atmospheric pressure $= 1.013$ bar (101.3 kPa)) and temperatures $> 31°$ C (T_c). The rapid expansion of this supercritical solution on exposure to atmospheric pressure causes the formation of microspheres or nanospheres.

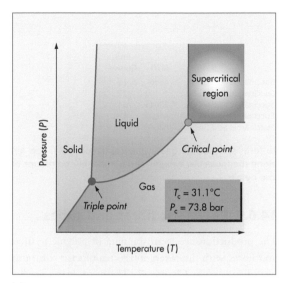

(a)

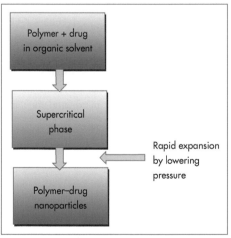

(b)

Figure 14.13 (a) The pressure–temperature phase diagram of CO_2 showing the T_c and P_c at the supercritical region. (b) Schematic of the process of producing nanoparticles using supercritical fluid technology. (See, for example, Byrappa K *et al*. Nanoparticle synthesis using supercritical fluid technology – towards biomedical applications. *Adv Drug Deliv Rev* 2008;60:299–327.)

14.6.6 Coacervation and complexation techniques

A coacervate is a gel-like liquid state of matter that can be treated to produce solid microparticles or nanoparticles. There are several possibilities: one is *complex coacervation*, in which positively charged macromolecules are mixed with negatively charged macromolecules. Under certain conditions of temperature and relative concentration and ionic strength, there will be a phase separation whereby a coacervate forms (Fig. 14.14). In *simple coacervation* with single macromolecules of either charge, solvent change and salting out create the conditions for the formation of coacervate particles.

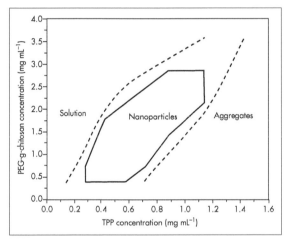

Figure 14.14 A phase diagram of PEGylated chitosan as a function of tripolyphosphate (TPP) concentration showing the region where 'nanogel' coacervate nanoparticles form.

Reproduced with permission from Wu Y. Chitosan nanoparticles as a novel delivery system for ammonium glycyrrhizinate. *Int J Pharm* 2005;295:235–245. Copyright Elsevier 2005.

14.6.7 *In situ* polymerisation

In this mode of synthesis of polymeric nanoparticles (e.g. of polybutylcycanoacrylates), monomeric materials (e.g. butylcyanoacrylate) are dispersed in a suitable solvent and emulsified. An initiator is generally added to the system and the monomers condense to form a polymeric matrix. In the case of the alkyl cyanoacrylates, no initiator is required as the aqueous medium itself acts as the initiator of polymerisation.

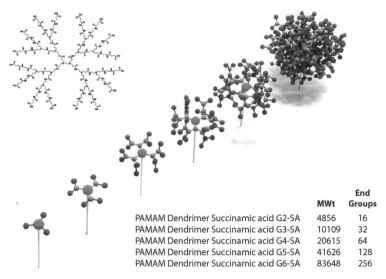

	MWt	End Groups
PAMAM Dendrimer Succinamic acid G2-SA	4856	16
PAMAM Dendrimer Succinamic acid G3-SA	10109	32
PAMAM Dendrimer Succinamic acid G4-SA	20615	64
PAMAM Dendrimer Succinamic acid G5-SA	41626	128
PAMAM Dendrimer Succinamic acid G6-SA	83648	256

Figure 14.15 Scheme of the stepwise synthesis of dendrimers to form spherical or quasi-spherical nanocarriers. Top left: second-generation polyamidoamine (PAMAM) dendrimers; bottom right: the molecular weights and number of end-groups on second- to sixth- generation PAMAM dendrimers. Chapter 7 has more details.

Model, Deutsches Museum, Munich, 2009.

14.6.8 Synthetic and semisynthetic processes: dendrimers and carbon nanotubes

Dendrimers are synthesised 'generation' by 'generation' from a multivalent core molecule, as demonstrated in the model in Fig. 14.15. *Carbon nanotubes* are obtained from soot and processed to form single-walled nanotubes or multiwalled nanotubes, shown in Fig. 14.16.

14.6.9 Polymeric fibres and tubes

The production by electrospinning of polymeric tubes and fibres with diameters in the nanometre size range was discussed in Chapter 7. These are being studied for a variety of delivery challenges.

14.6.10 Drug nanocrystals

Nanocrystals are formed by a variety of techniques, including high-pressure homogenisation, sonochemical processes (e.g. for azithromycin[8]), continuous precipitation techniques, by using microemulsions as tem-

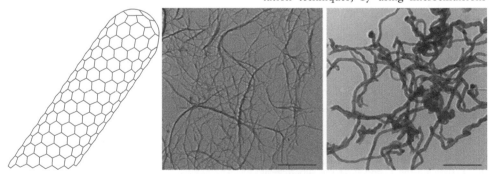

Figure 14.16 Representation of a single-walled carbon nanotube (CNT). In the photomicrograph on the left the native state of carbon nanotubes is seen, and on the right, double-walled nanotubes at the same magnification. The surface of the CNTs can be altered through adsorption of desired molecules or by covalent attachment of molecules for the purpose of stabilisation (for example, to prevent aggregation) or by addition of drug molecules or targeting moieties.

Reproduced with permission from Mérard-Moyen C *et al*. Functionalized carbon nanotubes for probing and modulating molecular functions. *Chem Biol* 2010;17:107–115. Copyright Elsevier 2010.

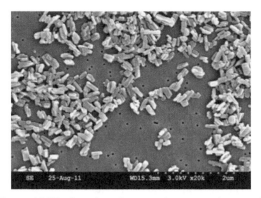

Figure 14.17 Scanning electron microscopy photograph of paclitaxel nanocrystals.

Reproduced from Hollis CP *et al*. www.cntc.uky.edu.

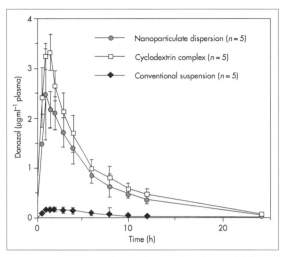

Figure 14.19 Danazol is a drug with a low solubility of *circa* 10 µg mL^{-1}. Here plasma drug levels are plotted as a function of time after administration of three forms of the drug, Including a nanoparticulate dispersion and a hydroxypropyl-β-cyclodextrin complex, using a suspension with a mean particle size of 10 µm as a comparator.

Reproduced from Liversidge GG and Cundy KC. Particle size reduction for improvement of oral bioavailability of hydrophobic drugs: I. Absolute oral bioavailability of nanocrystalline danazol in beagle dogs. *Int J Pharm* 1995; 125: 91–97.

plates (as emulsions can be used to prepare microparticles) or milling in appropriate media. The purpose is to enhance the surface area of poorly soluble drugs with the prospect of enhanced solubility and absorption. Figure 14.17 shows a scanning electron microscopy photograph of paclitaxel nanocrystals, one of many drugs that have been formulated as nanosuspensions.

Nanocrystals of poorly water-soluble drugs are of increasing importance in pharmacy as their greatly reduced particle size increases the surface area per unit weight and hence increases the rate of dissolution of

the drug, all things being equal. The Noyes–Whitney equation (see Chapter 1) relates the change of weight, dw, with time, dt:

$$\mathrm{d}w/\mathrm{d}t = (DA/\delta)(c_\mathrm{s} - c) \qquad (14.2)$$

where A is the surface area of the material, D is the diffusion coefficient, δ is the diffusion layer thickness and c_s is the saturation solubility, c being the concentration of agent in the solution at any given time t. There may be a degree of supersaturation, but the equilibrium solubility is unaffected by particle size until very small particle sizes are reached, as shown in Fig. 14.18. The critical value depends, as can be seen, on the surface energy of the material in question. The combination of increased intrinsic solubility and increased surface area has the potential to change solution, and hence absorption properties dramatically. If the absorption of the drug is dissolution rate-limited this will assist in the extent of absorption; enhanced solubility has the potential to increase concentration gradients across the biological membrane.

Figure 14.19 demonstrates the effect on the plasma level versus time plots of danazol of a nanosized suspension over a conventional suspension. It can be seen that nanocrystal formation leads to results

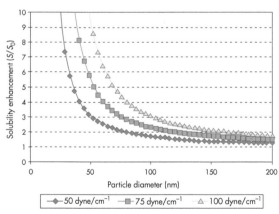

Figure 14.18 The solubility enhancement S/S_0 as a function of particle diameter for three hypothetical compounds with surface energies of 50, 75 and 100 mN m^{-1}. It can be seen that where S_0 is the solubility of a large crystal, and S is the solubility of the crystal of a specific size, the solubility enhancement (S/S_0) does not increase significantly until particle diameters reach below around 75 nm.

Reproduced from Kipp JE. The role of solid nanoparticle technology in the parenteral delivery of poorly water-soluble drugs.*Int J Pharm* 2004;284:109–122. Copyright Elsevier 2004.

equivalent in this case to the effect of solubilisation in a cyclodextrin.

If nanocrystals are used as suspensions clearly as they are colloidal they must be stabilised, for example by surface adsorption of non-ionic surfactants. The ratio of any stabiliser to the drug content must be carefully titrated, as in any stability study. However, nanocrystals can be used not only as suspensions but also as freeze-dried powders for reconstitution; they can be incorporated into liposomes, used as aerosols, incorporated in gels or in microspheres, adsorbed on to microparticles, dispersed in soft gelatin capsules or used as mini-depot tablets.

Key points

- The general approaches to the manufacture of nanoparticles include: comminution, as in the milling of solids or the emulsification of liquids; molecular self-assembly, as in the formation of some dendrimers and polymeric micelles; precipitation from solution; and polymerisation of monomers dissolved in micelles or emulsion droplets. The choice of method is influenced by the nature of the material that forms the basis of the carrier.
- The main methods of manufacture include:
  - solvent displacement
  - salting out
  - emulsion-diffusion
  - emulsion-solvent evaporation
  - use of supercritical fluid technologies
  - coacervation and complexation techniques
  - *in situ* polymerisation
  - nanocrystal formation by a variety of techniques of size reduction.

14.7 Challenges in targeting

There are many potential advantages and exciting opportunities in deploying nanocarriers to achieve end-points that the drugs themselves cannot achieve unaided. This would include enhanced accumulation in particular pathological sites, but one must point out the many challenges that exist in achieving what we might call 'quantitative delivery' of a drug. By and large such efforts have led to 5–10% accumulation of nanoparticles in tumour sites, which translates to a 5–10% drug load only when the nanoparticles are loaded to the highest level. This is a formulation challenge involving the compatibility of drugs, macromolecules and proteins with the materials that make up the nanosystems.

The challenge also partly rests in the changing physical and genetic nature of tumours as they grow and the biological complexities of other targets. That is, the target is a moving target. We will consider some of the factors that fall within the scope of this text.

14.7.1 Complexity of particle flow[9]

Drug targeting using nanoparticulate carriers depends on many factors to achieve quantitative accumulation in target sites. Particles must translocate from the site of injection to distant organs. To an extent, therefore, this depends on the flow patterns of nanoparticles in the blood and in interstitial spaces. The theoretical advantage of nanosystems is that their small size allows freer movement than that of, say, microspheres in the circulation, lymph and tissues. Flow rates are important also in the determination of the possibility and success of interaction of nanoparticles with endothelial receptors prior to internalisation. What is the influence, for example, of nanoparticle *size* on particle flow in the circulation? What is the influence of *shape* on flow and fate? Nanoparticles *in vivo* are driven by the blood flow to distant sites. Particle velocities can be size-dependent because the flow rates across the diameter of the vessels are not constant and hence particle segregation in polydisperse systems might occur, as shown in Fig. 14.20. Flow results in shearing forces at the point of interaction between nanoparticles and the target receptors; smaller particles suffer lower forces likely to dislodge them from receptor surfaces. This is illustrated in Fig. 14.21. Any aggregation of particles, which might even be flow-induced, will alter flow patterns and interactions with receptors.

Larger particles close to the walls of the vessels experience greater shearing forces because of the nature of the flow patterns shown. Adhesion, seen as

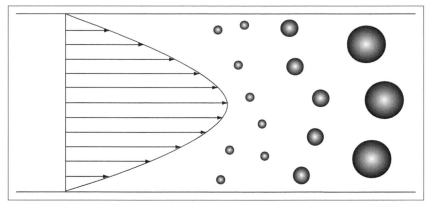

Figure 14.20 Diagram of the velocity pattern in a tube of flowing liquid showing particles of different sizes separating according to their diameter. The large particles, being unable to approach close to the capillary wall, experience the faster fluid streamlines towards the axis and hence move more rapidly.

a prerequisite to cellular uptake from blood and interstitial fluids, is not a foregone conclusion. The determining factors include particle diameter, flow rate, the density of receptors and the force of attraction between particle and receptor.

Figure 14.21 simply reinforces previous points and considers in greater detail the forces involved in nanoparticle interaction with biological surfaces. Particles have to be close to the surface to experience the force of attraction, which allows initial contact with membranes. This diagram again should clearly demonstrate the importance of physical phenomena in the biological environment.

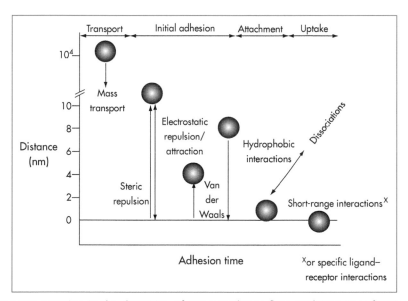

Figure 14.21 Processes occurring in the deposition of nanoparticles in flow conditions as a function of the range of interaction of forces (nanometres) and adhesion times. At the start, mass transport to the surface occurs, initial adhesion occurring through electrostatic attractions and van der Waals forces. Hydrophobic interactions can play their part as well as specific receptor–ligand interactions, which are short-range interactions. Physical adsorption of ligands to the surface of nanoparticles or covalent attachment of ligands changes the nature of the primary surface and may influence each of the forces referred to here.

Drawn with kind permission from Springer Science and Business Media after Vacheethanasee K, Marchant RE. Non-specific *Staphylococcus epidermidis* adhesion: contributions of bacterial hydrophobicity and charge. In: An YH, Friedman RJ (eds) *Handbook of Bacterial Adhesion: Principles, Methods and Applications*. Totowa, NJ: Humana Press; 2000: 73–90.

(a) (b)

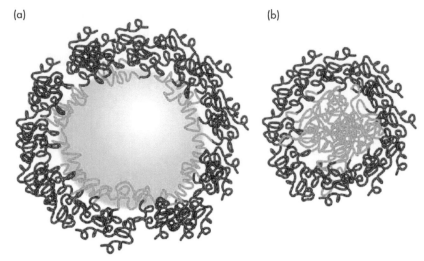

Figure 14.22 A representation of (a) a particle PEGylated with a polyoxyethylene-based block copolymer and (b) a block copolymer micelle with the external hydrophilic chains. The hydrophilic polymer chains on adjacent particles provide both a physical and thermodynamic barrier to aggregation. See also Chapter 6.

14.7.2 Aggregation of particles

Given their large surface to volume/weight ratios, nanoparticles are prone to aggregate. The formulation of a stable nanoparticle suspension in the laboratory is one thing; the maintenance of the monodisperse state *in vivo* is another. Particles will have moved from an aqueous medium (of the formulation) to a more complex situation in blood or tissues. There are biological consequences because opsonins adsorb from the plasma on to the surface of the nanoparticles, which leads to uptake by the reticuloendothelial system. (An opsonin is any molecule that acts as a binding enhancer for the process of phagocytosis, for example, by coating the surface of injected particles and other foreign objects.) In terms of the pharmaceutics of the nanosystems, the potential of the particles to aggregate is critical. Aggregation changes the hydrodynamic size of the particles, decreases their diffusion, restricts extravasation and reduces the effective surface area for interactions with receptors.

PEGylated nanoparticles

PEGylation involves the covalent attachment of poly-oxyethylene glycol (PEG) chains to the surface of the particles. PEGylation (Fig. 14.22) of course creates a hydrated surface on hydrophobic particles, which allows for both steric and enthalpic stabilisation. It also reduces opsonin adsorption, leading to increased circulation times and the enhanced statistical possibil-

ity of nanoparticle uptake after multiple passages through the circulation. PEGylation changes the nature of the surface, turning hydrophobic surfaces into hydrophilic ones. The effect of PEG depends on its chain length.[10] PEG 5000 has a greater effect than PEG 2000 or PEG 750, as predicted by calculations of enthalpic and entropic stabilisation (see Chapter 6).

14.7.3 Nanoparticle diffusion

The Stokes–Einstein equation (see Chapter 2) relates the diffusion coefficient, D, of a molecule or object to the continuous-phase viscosity η and the radius of the diffusing particle, r, as was discussed earlier in the chapter, in the form $D = kT/6\pi\eta r$.

In any one liquid medium, e.g. water, the diffusion coefficient of spherical particles is inversely related to their radius. This alone is important in thinking of the translocation of nanoparticles towards their targets in tissues. Diffusion is important in free solution, in cell culture media, in the gel-like interior of cells, even perhaps in the cell nucleus and in the extracellular matrix. In the brain, for example, diffusion of drugs from nanoparticles or implants is slow and the radius of spread of a drug like paclitaxel after release from implants or nanoparticles is of the order of only millimetres. Gels have been used as models for diffusion of nanoparticles in complex media: the Stokes–Einstein equation applies and the ratio of diffusion in the gel (D) to diffusion in water (D_0) can be calculated.

In gels the viscosity in the equation is not the bulk viscosity but the so-called *microscopic viscosity*,[11] η_0, which is actually close to that of water, as it is the viscosity of the medium in which nanoparticles move between the entangled chains of the macromolecular gels. When the diameter of the particles reaches a critical size in gels, a size approaching the nominal diameter of the pores, diffusion asymptotically approaches zero.

Diffusion within cells is even more complex than within simple gels: first, the cytoplasm is a molecularly crowded zone, a complex gel with structural obstacles such as actin and myosin fibrils and strands. There is the additional tortuosity that occurs in gels as the moving particle avoids the regions of the macromolecular chains and the obstruction effects from the impenetrable regions of the cytoplasm. If we designate by D_e the effective diffusion coefficient and by D_0 the coefficient in water we can write, where τ is the tortuosity factor and ε is the void fraction available to the diffusing solute:

$$\frac{D_e}{D_0} = \frac{\varepsilon}{\tau} \tag{14.3}$$

$\varepsilon = (1 - \phi_p)$ where ϕ_p is the volume fraction of the polymer or other materials that are in the path of the diffusing material. D_G (the diffusion coefficient in the gel) can be written as a ratio with the coefficient in water[12]:

$$\frac{D_G}{D_0} = \frac{(1 - \phi_p)^2}{(1 + \phi_p)^2} \tag{14.4}$$

If $\phi_p = 0.5$, D_G is 0.111 times that in water. When $\phi_p = 0.8$, $D_G \approx 0.012 D_0$. The binding of particles to actin reduces the number of free particles and hence further reduces flux.

Nanoparticle size is important in diffusion in complex media because the diffusional space may be restricted when the diameter of the particle exceeds the 'pore' diameter. The diffusion coefficients of 6 nm dendrimers in the cytoplasm of Caco2 cells and SK/MES-1 cells[13] were determined to be 9.8×10^{-11} cm^2 s^{-1} and $\approx 6 \times 10^{-11}$ cm^2 s^{-1}, respectively, some 1000 times lower than that in water. Adsorption, obstruction and entrapment occur, and at a certain particle radius diffusion virtually ceases.

There are other issues, as shown in Fig. 14.23, where particles of different sizes passing through a gel can be filtered according to their diameters, or two different types of particles can be filtered according to their adhesivity towards the fibres of the gel (or, for example, actin fibres in cells).

14.7.4 Stochastic processes

There can be a tendency to think that events such as ligand–receptor interactions, diffusion of molecules or nanoparticles from A to B, or nanoparticle uptake by specific cells or organs are inevitable. Given time all things might happen. One of the principles of ensuring the long circulation of particles is to enhance their chances of extravasation and interaction with appropriate surfaces. But the movement of molecules free in solution is the result of a number of random walks. This randomness causes events to be referred to as *stochastic*. The chance of an individual nanoparticle extravasating on its passage along a capillary, the chance of a nanoparticle ligand adhering to the appropriate receptor, and so on. Figure 14.24 illustrates Brownian motion of a nanoparticle, motion of particle in confined spaces and a cartoon of the effect of random walks on cell uptake.

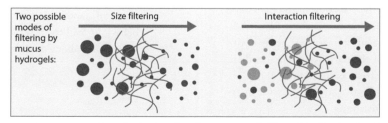

Figure 14.23 Diagrammatic representation of a hydrogel such as mucus: (left) particle filtering by size, the larger particles being held back, and (right) interaction filtering of two particle types, by interaction of one type with the gel strands.
Reproduced from Lieleg O *et al.* Characterization of particle translocation through mucin hydrogels. *Biophys J* 2010;98:1782–1789. Courtesy of Elsevier 2010.

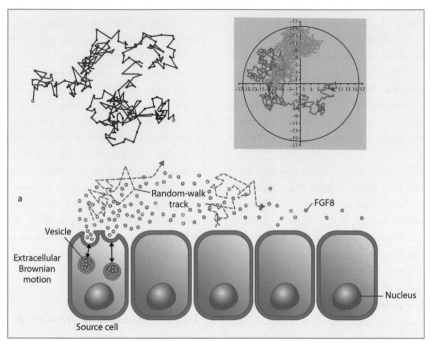

Figure 14.24 Random walks of nanoparticles (top left) of particles in Brownian motion and (top right) in a confined space (such as a cell or large liposome) (Al-Obaidi and Florence). Lower cartoon: the complex track before cell uptake.

 Key points

Physicochemical properties are important in determining the biological fate of nanoparticles:

- The particle size of the nanoparticle influences its flow in blood and interstitial spaces. Polydispersity of size may lead to particle segregation during flow; particle aggregation may be induced by flow, which will alter flow patterns and interaction with receptors. Particle size, flow rate, forces of interaction between particles and receptors, and the density of receptors can all influence the adhesion of the nanoparticles on to receptors.

- Particle aggregation increases the hydrodynamic size of the particles, decreases their diffusion, restricts extravasation and reduces the effective surface area for interaction with receptors.

- Covalent attachment of PEG chains to the nanoparticle surface allows for steric and enthalpic stabilisation and reduces opsonin adsorption.

- The diffusional properties of the nanoparticles are important in their translocation towards their targets in tissues. Diffusion within complex media such as cells is not only determined by the diameter of the nanoparticle but is also strongly influenced by the tortuosity of its path through the cytoplasm, the void volume available for diffusion and any adsorption or entrapment of the particles. Gels have been used as models of diffusion through such complex environments.

- Stochastic processes evident in many stages of nanoparticle movement and behaviour lead to there being a degree of uncertainty about particle destination and fate.

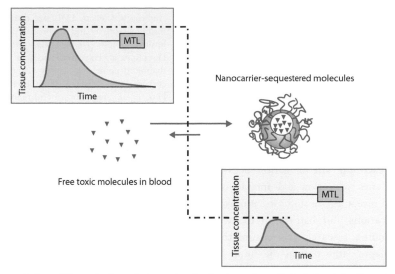

Figure 14.25 Representation of the reduction of plasma levels of a drug above its toxic levels by the administration of empty liposomes. The carrier may contain enzymes to metabolise the absorbed drug where appropriate. MTL, minimum toxic level.

14.8 Detoxification: reducing blood levels

The ingenious converse of drug delivery with carriers such as liposomes is to administer empty carriers which will absorb excess drug in the circulation as a means of detoxification, as demonstrated by Leroux and his colleagues (Fig. 14.25).

14.9 Regulatory challenges: characterisation

Regulatory challenges generally have evolved for good reasons to ensure reproducibility and quality *in vitro* and *in vivo*. Parameters that must be closely defined for nanosystems include those in Table 14.3.

Table 14.3 Parameters and questions that must be addressed before clinical use of nanosystems
• Particle size determination is key: is there a standardised procedure for measuring mean particle diameter and size distribution?
• Is there assurance of stability of size *in vitro*, that is, lack of aggregation/flocculation?
• Standardisation of surface characteristics: what specific methodology is used (zeta potential measurements may be non-specific)?
• The distribution on surfaces and properties of ligands on the surfaces of targeted systems.
• Determination or prediction of stability *in vivo* (especially of particle diameter)
• Measurement and validation of the release rate of active from the systems and the choice of suitable experimental media
• Biocompatibility: is the system compatible with blood?
• Biodegradability: is there evidence of biodegradation of the system to non-toxic products?
• Toxicity of nanosystems: what are reasonable predictive animal or tissue culture tests?
N.B.: Targeted systems congregate in specific organs, and hence can alter the toxicological balance.

Summary

This chapter covers some of the physicochemical principles of the preparation and the use of nanoparticles as drug delivery vectors. It should be clear from this chapter that physical and chemical properties of nanoparticles are crucial in determining their biological fate and success. In targeting it should be remembered that even decorated particles with specific ligands may not reach the site of action because transport to most sites of action and interactions between ligands and receptors are stochastic processes with many complications and barriers in the way. Nonetheless, continuing research will ensure that nanosystems will play a large part in the future of pharmaceuticals – as therapeutic carriers, as carriers of imaging agents or as excipients that are more precise than those that exist today.

References

1. Kreuter J. Nanoparticles and nanocapsules – new dosage forms in the nanometer size range. *Pharm Acta Helv* 1978;533:3–29.
2. Couvreur P *et al*. Nanocapsules: a new type of lysosomotropic carrier. *FEBS Lett* 1977;84:323–326.
3. Kreuter J. Nanoparticles – a historical perspective. *Int J Pharm* 2007;331:1–10.
4. Schulman JH *et al*. Mechanism of formation and structure of microemulsions by electron microscopy. *J Phys Chem* 1959;63:1677–1680.
5. Teeguarden JG *et al*. Particokinetics in vitro: dosimetry considerations for in vitro nanoparticle toxicity assessments. *Toxicol Sci* 2007;95:300–312.
6. Ambrosch A *et al*. LDL size distribution in relation to insulin sensitivity and lipoprotein patterning in young and healthy subjects. *Diabetes Care* 1998;21:2077–2084.
7. De TK *et al*. Polycarboxylic acid nanoparticles for ophthalmic drug delivery: an ex vivo evaluation with human cornea. *J Microencapul* 2004;21:841–855.
8. Pi Z *et al*. Preparation of ultrafine particles of azithromycin by sonochemical method. *Nanomedicine* 2007;3:86–88.
9. Florence AT. Nanoparticle flow: implications for drug delivery. In: Torchilin VP (ed.) *Nanoparticulates as Drug Carriers*. London: Imperial College Press; 2006: 9–27.
10. Mori A *et al*. Influence of the steric barrier of amphipathic poly(ethyleneglycol) and ganglioside GM1 on the circulation time of liposomes and on the target binding of immunoliposomes in vivo. *FEBS Lett* 1991;284:263–266.
11. Ruenraroengsak P, Florence AT. The diffusion of latex nanospheres and the effective (microscopic) viscosity of HPMC gels. *Int J Pharm* 2005;298:361–366.
12. Mackie JS, Meares P. The diffusion of electrolytes in a cationic membrane. I. Theoretical. *Proc Roy Soc Lond A Math Phys Sci* 1955;232:498–509.
13. Ruenraroengsak P *et al*. Cell uptake, cytoplasmic diffusion and nuclear access of a 6.5 nm diameter dendrimer. *Int J Pharm* 2007;331:215–219.

Further reading

Florence AT. 'Targeting' nanoparticles. The constraints of physical laws and physical barriers. *J Control Rel* 2012;164:115–124.

Crommelin DJA, Florence AT. Towards more effective advanced drug delivery systems. *Int J Pharm* 2013;454:496–511.

Date AA, Patravale VB. Current strategies for engineering drug nanoparticles. *Curr Opinion Colloid Interface Sci* 2004;9:222–235.

15

Physical assessment of dosage forms

It is important to have means of studying the key characteristics of quality of formulations during development and for quality control purposes during production and testing. Obviously performance in patients is a product's ultimate test. However, laboratory tests to measure physical properties *in vitro* can give insights into the quality of the product to be used by patients. Formulations are, after all, physical constructs and various aspects of their physical chemistry can inform us about differences between batches of products, and can sometimes explain their behaviour, aberrant or otherwise.

This chapter presents the basics of some *in vitro* tests that can be applied to pharmaceutical products, using the background physical chemistry discussed in earlier chapters. In particular, we will examine how we can measure the influence on drug release rates or product performance using some of the key parameters of pharmaceutical systems, such as aerosol particle size, viscosity of topical products, adhesion of films and patches and tablet hardness, *inter alia*. It is necessary to appreciate the importance of *in vitro* testing in formulation development and in batch-to-batch control of uniformity but also in assessing product defects. *In vitro* tests might be preferred to *in vivo* measures when there is a good correlation between the two, but it should be appreciated that such correlations and physiological verisimilitude are not essential for validity in quality control, where reproducibility of product characteristics is itself a goal.

It is hoped that this brief account of quantitative tests – some simple, some complex – will stimulate thought on how in practice we can assess the products we handle.

15.1 Introduction

One of the key roles of pharmacy in all its dimensions is to ensure the highest quality of drugs and medicines. This is normally achieved in industrial quality control laboratories, but with extemporaneous preparations in hospital or other locations (such as compounding pharmacies in the USA) tests may have to be improvised. Sadly there is another element that in the last few years has clouded the scene, which is the infiltration of counterfeit medicines in the pharmaceutical supply chain. How can we use the resources we have to judge the quality of what we manufacture, prepare and dispense?

With the advent of new technologies, the range of tests which can be applied in the laboratory to dosage forms and their components is growing in number and precision. This account begins with a discussion of methods of evaluating the release rate of drugs from oral dose forms crucial to subsequent pharmacokinetics and pharmacodynamics. Until the 1970s friability and disintegration measurements were the only significant tests applied to solid oral dosage forms but the advent of the serious problems and some deaths with Lanoxin digoxin (see Chapter 12) caused by a change in manufacturing procedure led the (then)

UK Committee on Safety of Medicines to introduce the first dissolution tests for digoxin tablets. The problem arose when a milling procedure was changed, increasing particle size and reducing bioavailability. Patients treated during the period with reduced particle size were in danger when prescribed the same dose after the original milling process was changed. On a more mundane note, Figure 15.1 illustrates today how the poor quality of a product can be evident to a patient simply when a foil pack is opened.

As can be seen in this chapter, *in vitro* tests have evolved and are still evolving with the increased complexity of many formulations. Scheme 15.1 summarises the range of tests that can be applied to a variety of dose forms. What we discuss is not comprehensive but they represent exemplars.

15.2 Dissolution testing of solid oral dosage forms

One of the commonest tests applied to solid oral dosage form is to measure the rate of release of the drug using a dissolution test.

Equations such as the Noyes–Whitney equation cannot readily be applied to deal with the situation of tablet and capsule dissolution because of the constantly changing surface area of the disintegrated tablet components. The presence of additives such as wetting agents, which may alter solubility as well as wettability and the tablet matrix or coating, will also determine release rates. However, the rate of solution of a solid drug substance from a granule or a tablet is dependent to a large extent on its solubility in the solvent phase and its concentration in that phase. Test conditions should provide a reasonable and realistic challenge to the dosage form in terms of degree of agitation, temperature, volume and pH of the dissolution medium. *In vitro* tests thus will provide the opportunity to make precise and reproducible release measurements to distinguish between different formulations of a drug or the effect of ageing, processing or production changes (batch-to-batch variation). The tests do not replace the need for clinical evaluation, but they can pinpoint factors of importance in determining drug release.

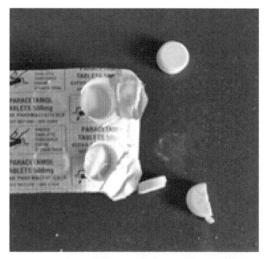

Figure 15.1 Paracetamol tablets, one of which has not survived its removal by the patient (one of the authors). The pieces of the broken tablet were largely recuperated from the clean kitchen surface, but this hardly represented the acme of pharmaceutical expertise. Paracetamol powder can be seen on the black surface.

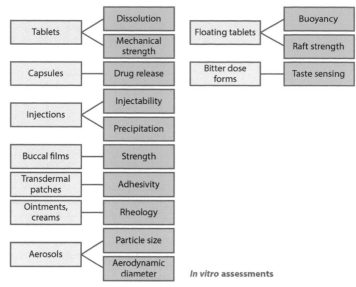

Scheme 15.1 Examples of physicochemical tests applied to formulations and their components. Not discussed in this text are tests for gelatin capsule brittleness (Kontny MJ, Mulski CA *Int J Pharm* 1989;54:79–85), taste sensing with 'electronic tongues' (as described by Woertz K *et al. Int J Pharm* 2011;417:256–271) or measurement of 'dustiness', for example, of cytotoxic drugs (Ohta T *et al. Int J Pharm* 2014;472:251–256).

Dissolution testing, whether routine or during development, is necessary when:

- The drug has low aqueous solubility.
- Dissolution is poor or variable when tested by an official compendial test procedure (British Pharmacopoeia (BP) or United States Pharmacopeia (USP)).
- There is evidence that particle size may affect bioavailability.
- The physical forms of drug – polymorphs, solvates or complexes – have varying solubility and hence likely dissolution characteristics.
- Specific excipients alter dissolution or absorption.
- There is evidence that tablet or capsule coating may interfere with disintegration or dissolution.

The above list refers to solubility, dissolution rate, particle size, polymorphism, excipient interactions and film coating, some of the complexities of formulation.

15.2.1 Methods

In vitro dissolution test methods may be divided into two main types, involving either *natural convection* or *forced convection*. Most practical methods fall into the latter category, as there is a degree of agitation *in vivo*. In natural-convection methods in which, for example, a pellet of material is suspended from a balance arm in the dissolution medium, the conditions are unnatural. In forced-convection methods, a degree of agitation is introduced. These can, in turn, be divided into those that employ non-sink conditions and those that achieve sink conditions in the dissolution medium.

Sink conditions exist when the concentration of solute in the solvent is low and does not affect the dissolution process. In the opposite case of non-sink conditions, the concentration of solute is significant and slows down the dissolution process.

15.2.2 Pharmacopoeial and compendial dissolution tests

The dissolution test method now widely used and described in the British Pharmacopoeia is a variant of the rotating-basket method, shown in Fig. 15.2a. Figure 15.2b shows the alternative rotating-paddle system. The specification of precise dimensions shown in the diagram emphasises the importance of standardisation of equipment to ensure consistency between laboratories.[1]

Tablets or capsules are placed in a basket of wire mesh, the mesh being small enough to retain broken pieces of tablet but large enough to allow entry of solvent without wetting problems. The basket may be rotated at any suitable speed, but most monographs specify 50, 100 or 1500 rpm. The effect of rotation

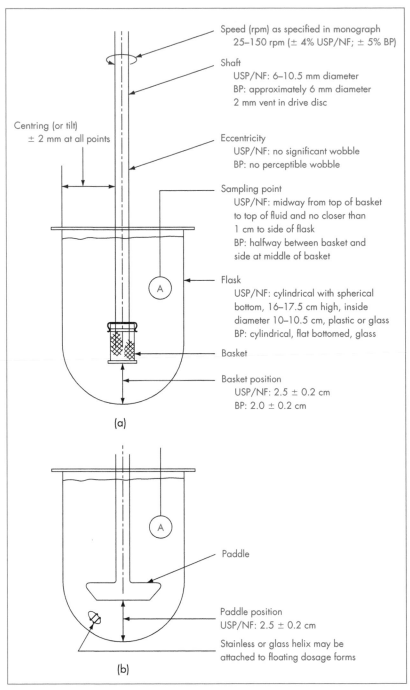

Figure 15.2 The rotating-basket and rotating-paddle versions of the official method for dissolution testing of solid oral dosage forms. (a) The rotating basket – method 1, United States Pharmacopeia and the National Formulary (USP/NF). This method is official for USP/NF and BP. Current specifications describing the geometry and positions for each compendium are shown. (b) The rotating paddle – method 2, USP/NF.

Reproduced with permission from Hanson W. *Handbook of Dissolution Testing*, 2nd edn. Eugene, OR: Aster Publishing; 1991.

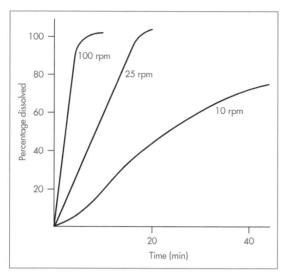

Figure 15.3 Single-tablet dissolution profiles for a sulfamethizole formulation in dilute HCl with USP XVIII method at three stirring rates.

Reproduced from Mattock GL, McGilveray IJ. Comparison of bioavailabilities and dissolution characteristics of commercial tablet formulations of sulfamethizole. *J Pharm Sci* 1972;61:746–749. Copyright Wiley-VCH Verlag GmbH & Co. KGaA. Reproduced with permission.

speed on the dissolution profile of a sulfamethizole formulation is shown in Fig. 15.3, an effect that would be predicted from our understanding of particle dissolution.[2] In all the methods the appropriate pH for the dissolution medium must be chosen, not one that maximises dissolution but one that is physiologically reasonable.

With drugs of very low solubility it is sometimes necessary to consider the use of *in vitro* tests that allow sink conditions to be maintained. This generally involves the use of a lipid phase into which the drug can partition; alternatively, it may involve dialysis or physical replacement of the solvent phase. Mixed-solvent systems such as ethanol–water or surfactant systems may be used to enhance the solubility of sparingly soluble drugs, but some prefer the use of flow-through systems in these cases. Both human and simulated gastric fluids have been used in dissolution tests.[3]

15.2.3 Flow-through systems

A variant on the dissolution methods discussed uses neither basket nor paddle; convection is achieved by solvent flow through a chamber such as that in Fig. 15.4. Dissolution data obtained from this type of system, where continuous monitoring of drug concen-

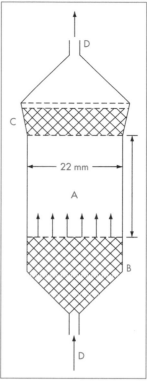

Figure 15.4 A recommended standard design for a flow-through cell: the cell is cylindrical in shape and constructed of glass or other suitable material. A, an internal volume not exceeding 20 cm³ between barrier and filter. B, a bottom barrier of either a porous glass plate or a bed of 1 mm diameter glass beads designed to disperse flow and provide uniform distribution over the dosage chamber A. C, a suitable filter of approximately 25 mm diameter. D, fluid flow from bottom to top.

tration is achieved, must be interpreted with care as the concentration–time profile will be dependent on the volume of solvent, its flow rate and the distance of the detection device from the flow cell, or rather the void volume of solvent.

Clearly there is no absolute method of dissolution testing. Whatever form of test is adopted, results are of most use on a comparative basis, where batches of a product are compared or where a branded product, say, is compared with a generic, and so on.

Factors affecting the release of drugs from other dosage forms can usefully be examined. These include suppositories, topical ointment and cream preparations, and transdermal devices. It is of course always useful to have good *in vitro–in vivo* correlations.

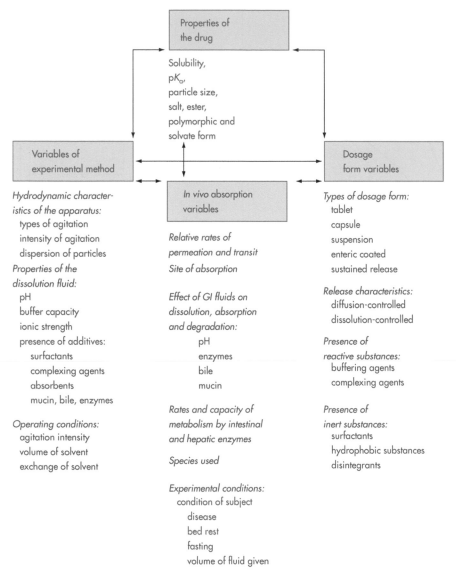

Scheme 15.2 Some interacting variables that influence the sensitivity and degree of *in vivo* correlation of *in vitro* methods for measuring drug release and dissolution.
Modified from Barr WH. *Pharmacology* 1972;8:55.

15.2.4 *In vitro–in vivo* correlations

Some factors that influence the sensitivity and degree of *in vitro–in vivo* correlations are shown in Scheme 15.2. Some relate to the dissolution method, some to the dosage form and some, of course, to *in vivo* behaviour.

15.3 Drug release from parenteral preparations

15.3.1 Suppository formulations

Suppositories are probably more difficult to study than many other dosage forms because it is not a simple matter to simulate conditions in the rectal cavity. In one system,[4] shown in Fig. 15.5, a suppository is placed in a pH 7.8 buffer in a dialysis bag. This bag is placed in a second dialysis bag filled with octanol, and the whole is suspended in a flow system at 37°C.

The amount of drug released into the outer liquid is monitored. The results must be interpreted with care as it is possible for substances that complex with the drug to reduce transport across the dialysis membrane, something that may or may not happen in the body.

A variant on this arrangement was used[5] to obtain the data in Fig. 15.6, which shows the value of such tests, in this case illustrating the reduction in aminophylline release from a Witepsol H15 base as a function of product age.

15.3.2 *In vitro* release from topical products and transdermal systems

Ointments and transdermal systems encounter little water in use but, in the spirit of using release tests to compare basically similar products, useful data can be obtained by measuring release into aqueous media.

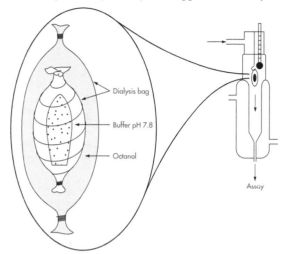

Figure 15.5 An *in vitro* system for studying drug release from suppositories. The suppository is placed in a buffer with a dialysis bag that itself resides in a dialysis bag containing octanol to simulate partitioning into tissue. The amount of drug eluted into a flowing aqueous phase is then measured.

Modified with permission from Ritschel WA, Banarer M. Correlation between *in vitro* release of proxyphylline from suppositories and *in vivo* data obtained from cumulative urinary excretion studies. *Arzneim Forsch* 1973;23:1031–1035.

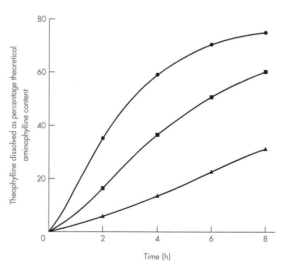

Figure 15.6 Dissolution profiles for aminophylline (theophylline and ethylenediamine mixture) suppositories stored at 35°C: ●, 2 months old; ■, 8 months old; ▲, 12 months old.

Reproduced with permission from Taylor JB, Simpkins DE. Aminophylline suppositories: *in vitro* dissolution and bioavailability in man. *Pharm J* 1981;227:601–603.

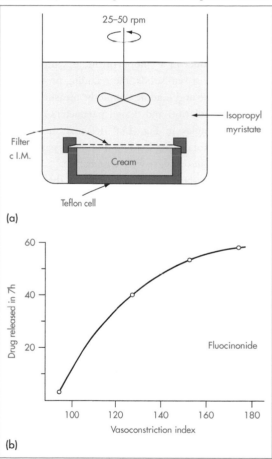

Figure 15.7 (a) An apparatus for the examination of the release of a steroid from a cream formulation: the cream is placed in a Teflon receptacle and covered with a membrane impregnated with isopropyl myristate, and the concentration of fluocinonide is monitored in the bulk isopropyl myristate layer. (b) Release *in vitro* compared with results of vasoconstrictor tests on four formulations.

Modified with permission from Ostrenga JA *et al*. Vehicle design for a topical steroid, fluocinolide. *J Invest Dermatol* 1971;56:392–399.

This information can be predictive of *in vivo* performance. Sometimes an attempt can be made to simulate a lipid biophase to mimic the skin. Some topical products can be tested simply in volunteers. Steroid formulations, for example, can be tested using the vasoconstrictor activity of the steroid to quantitate the results. An *in vitro* system[6] using isopropyl myristate as the 'solvent phase' or 'biophase' is shown in Fig. 15.7. The amount of drug released in 7 hours correlates with the vasoconstriction index for four formulations of fluocinonide. Vasoconstriction evidenced by skin blanching correlates with steroid potency in topical preparations.

A variant of this simple apparatus is that shown in Fig. 15.8, based on the Franz diffusion cell, which has been used to measure the release rate of tacrolimus from an ointment.[7] When a membrane has to be employed to keep the product in a compartment, as with suppositories and most semisolids, the retarding properties of the membrane and loading should be measured before the key formulation and design parameters are determined. Examples in Fig. 15.9 demonstrate how the influence of total drug loading and mean particle size may be seen, in this case with terconazole.[8]

A rotating-bottle apparatus allows the study of the release of glyceryl trinitrate from Deponit transdermal patches (Fig. 15.10).[9] The influence of temperature and pH on release can be examined with this apparatus, confirming that release is essentially determined by the diffusion of drug in the adhesive layer of the product (see section 9.3 in Chapter 9) but is clearly proportional to surface area, as expected.

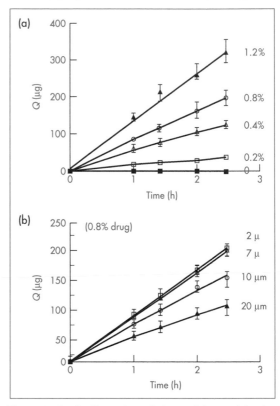

Figure 15.9 An illustration of the usefulness of *in vitro* tests in drug formulation development: the effect on terconazole release rate *in vitro* of (a) drug loading and (b) particle size.

Reproduced with permission from Corbo M *et al*. Development and validation of *in vitro* release testing methods for semi-solid formulations. *Pharm Tech Int* 1993;17:112–118.

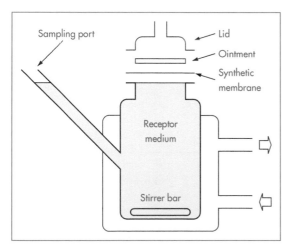

Figure 15.8 A system to measure the release of drug from an ointment via a synthetic membrane into a temperature-controlled and stirred receptor medium.

Reproduced from Yoshida H *et al*. *In vitro* release of tacrolimus from tacrolimus ointment and its speculated mechanism. *Int J Pharm* 2004;270:55–64. Copyright Elsevier 2004.

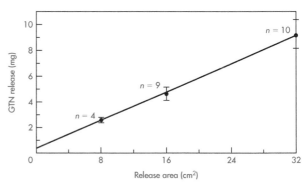

Figure 15.10 *In vitro* glyceryl trinitrate (GTN) release (24 h) into 80 cm³ isotonic NaCl versus release area of Deponit TTS.

Reproduced with permission from Wolff M *et al*. *In vitro* and *in vivo*-release of nitroglycerin from a new transdermal therapeutic system. *Pharm Res* 1985;123–129.

Release increases as temperature increases; between 32°C and 37°C an increase in release rate of between 1 and 2 µg cm^{-2} h^{-1} is detected. The BP specifies a distribution (release) test for transdermal patches based on the paddle apparatus for tablet and capsules.

15.4 Mechanical strength of tablets

There are pharmacopoeial requirements to ensure that tablets possess a suitable mechanical strength to avoid 'crumbling or breaking on subsequent processing, e.g. coating, storage and distribution'. Tablets require strength also to resist the pressures of their extraction by patients from blister packs (see e.g. Fig. 15.1). The examination of the mechanical strength of tablets may sound relatively straightforward, but there are many techniques that can be used; much too is dependent on the shape of tablets (round, flat or capsule-shaped), whether or not they are coated, with or without break lines or are double-layered systems, for example. The mathematics becomes complex too depending on the nature of the test and the nature of the dose form. For a full account the reader should access the excellent review by Podczeck.[10]

Two failure test configurations are shown in Fig. 15.11.

In the diametral test the failure stress (ρ_d) is related to the applied force, F (Newtons), tablet diameter, D (mm) and h, the height of the tablet (mm).

$$\rho_d = 2F/\pi Dh \tag{15.1}$$

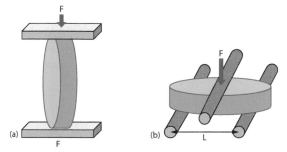

Figure 15.11 Two test configurations for tablets: (a) a diametral test, where stress (F: 0–500 N)) is applied by a flat plate at a constant velocity; and (b) a three-point flexure test, using the same rig and speed and force range.

Reproduced from Mazel V *et al.* Comparison of different failure tests for pharmaceutical tablets: applicability of the Drucker-Prager failure criterion. *Int J Pharm* 2014;470:63–69. Copyright Elsevier 2014.

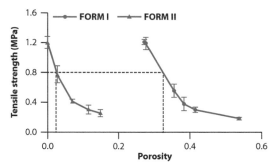

Figure 15.12 Plots of the 'compactability' of ranitidine HCl polymorphs, where the dotted lines show the porosity at which a tensile strength of 0.8 mPa is achieved.

Reproduced from Upadhyay P *et al.* Relationship between crystal structure and mechanical properties of ranitidine hydrochloride polymorphs. *Cryst Eng Comm* 2013;15:3959–3964, with permission of The Royal Society of Chemistry.

In the three-point flexure case, the failure stress (ρ_{3P}) is given by

$$\rho_{3P} = 3FL/2h^2D \tag{15.2}$$

where L is the distance between the supports (mm) (Fig. 15.11). The results from this test are two to three times higher than for the diametral test results; different tests will of course give different results, but within each test system, the value of tensile fracture stress (MPa) is related to the density of the tablet. During compression the porosity is reduced but differences between formulations can be influenced not only by the excipients used but also by polymorphism in the drug substance (Fig. 15.12). Hardness testing is also important and sometimes correlates with differences in dissolution behaviour. Quantitative values obtained from such tests ensure that materials are not over-compressed, as when this occurs the tablets can expand and 'cap' when the stress is relaxed, as shown in Fig. 1.38 of Chapter 1.

15.4.1 Indentation tests

Other tests of hardness include so-called indentation tests, where a sphere or another probe is dropped with a force F on to the surface of a tablet using a variety of commercial apparatus. One example of the configuration is shown in Fig. 15.13, where the hardness is related to the diameter of the sphere, D, and to the diameter d of the impression to produce the Brinell value, HB.

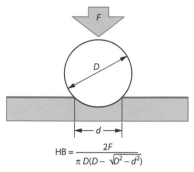

$$HB = \frac{2F}{\pi D(D - \sqrt{D^2 - d^2})}$$

Figure 15.13 One type of indentation test and the equation providing a measure of tablet hardness (HB), where D = ball diameter, d = impression diameter, F = load and HB = Brinell result.

15.5 Rheological characteristics of formulations

The rheological behaviour of liquids and semisolids has been described in other chapters (e.g. Chapter 6). Viscosity monitoring can be used as a quality control procedure, and some practical rheological tests are valuable in optimising product characteristics, as discussed here.

15.5.1 Injectability and flow

The *injectability* of non-aqueous injections and other formulations, which may be viscous and thus difficult to inject, can be assessed by a test for *syringeability*, the ability of a solution or suspension to pass through a hypodermic needle during the transfer of product from a vial to a hypodermic syringe prior to injection. Figure 15.14 shows the microsyringe part of a commercial viscometer which may be used to assess injection force. Table 15.1 shows the relationship between this force and qualitative notions of ease of injection.

Table 15.1 *In vitro* and *in vivo* correlation of injection force (N)

Injection force (*in vitro*)	Injectability (*in vivo*)
0–10	Very easy to inject, further reduction in needle size is possible
11–25	Easy to inject
26–50	Injectable
51–100	Injectable with some difficulty
101–130	Difficult to inject, larger needle size is recommended
> 130	Very difficult to inject, larger needle size is required

The factors which determine injectability include the:

- viscosity of the vehicle
- density of the vehicle
- size of suspended particulate matter
- concentration of suspended drug.

Sesame oil, for example, has a viscosity of 56 cP (56 mPa s^{-1}), but added drugs and adjuvants can increase its viscosity.[11] Injectability is an issue with concentrated protein solutions, as discussed in Chapter 13.

15.5.2 Topical product rheology

The desired physical properties of various topical preparations are listed in Table 15.2. The terms 'soft and unctuous' and 'hard and stiff' are difficult to quantify, but it is useful at least to consider the variety of descriptions that may be applied in a consistency profile of an external pharmaceutical product. Scheme 15.3 lists these comprehensively as primary, secondary and tertiary characteristics. The tertiary properties are probably the most elusive.

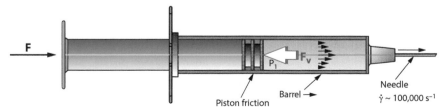

Figure 15.14 The m-VROC microsyringe part of the Rheosense automated viscometer to detect the rheological properties of liquids. It can operate on samples of 20 μL.

Table 15.2 Properties of some topical preparations

Class	Nature	Required physical properties
1	Ophthalmic ointments	Softest type of ointment
2	Other commonly used ointments	Soft and unctuous, but stiff enough to remain in place when applied
3	Protective ointments, e.g. zinc oxide paste	Hard and stiff; remain in place when applied to moist ulcerated areas

Reproduced from Sherman P. *Rheol Acta* 1971;10:121.

15.6 Adhesivity of dosage forms: desired and undesired

A study of the adhesion of dosage forms to epithelial surfaces is important because of the possibility of enhancing contact between oral dosage forms and the gut wall to slow the rate of transit down the gastro-intestinal tract; it is also important in assessing the adhesion of buccal films and tablets. Investigation of adhesion of erythrocytes and bacterial cells to polymer surfaces is also important for an understanding of the blood compatibility of polymers and bacterial infection mediated by catheters.

15.6.1 Undesirable adhesion

- Tablets or capsules to the oesophagus
- bacteria to catheters, skin and medical instruments
- nanoparticles to erythrocytes.

15.6.2 Desirable adhesion

- dosage forms to desired sections of the gastro-intestinal tract
- buccal films and tablets to oral mucosa
- transdermal patches to the skin
- stoma products
- tablet coating materials to tablet surfaces.

Some examples of solid–solid adhesion evaluation processes are shown in Fig. 15.15. Peeling tests for film coats (the separation diagrams in the figure demonstrate the geometry of such tests) are a part of

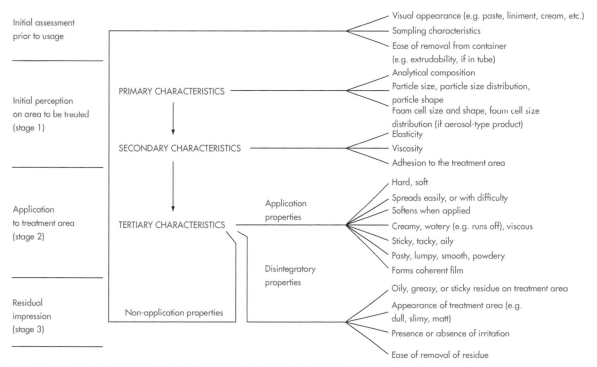

Scheme 15.3 Consistency profile for pharmaceuticals employed externally.

Reproduced from Sherman P. Consistency profiling, and evaluation of pharmaceutical products. *Rheol Acta* 1971;10:121, with kind permission from Springer Science and Business Media.

Common adhesive testing methods

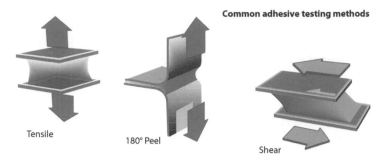

Tensile

180° Peel

Shear

Figure 15.15 Representation of the different stresses to which adhesive bonds are subject: tensile, peeling and shear, which are thus reflected in various tests.

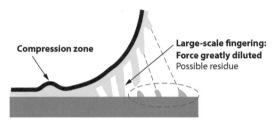

Compression zone

Large-scale fingering: Force greatly diluted Possible residue

Figure 15.16 Diagram illustrating the complexity of the process of separation of a film from a substrate in certain circumstances, showing 'fingering' patterns of polymer as a force is applied to raise the film, and a compression zone on the film.

pharmaceutical development and similar tests for the adhesion of transdermal particles to skin have been used. The measurement of film coat adhesion is discussed in Chapter 7.

The complex nature of the separation of two surfaces separated by an adhesive layer is made clear in Fig. 15.16, emphasising how each test must be considered to be separate but complementary, but most importantly, to be appropriate to the process that occurs in real life.

Several methods of testing oral dosage forms for adhesivity are in use. One involves the raising of the dosage form through an excised porcine oesophagus[12] (Fig. 15.17). Another assesses the adhesion of a moistened capsule or tablet to a tissue surface using a strain gauge[13] (Fig. 15.18).

The effects of polymer concentration and composition and of additives on the adhesivity of film coating materials can be studied using this apparatus, and the force, f, required to separate tablet from substrate can be measured. The force per unit area required to separate two circular plates of radius r initially in

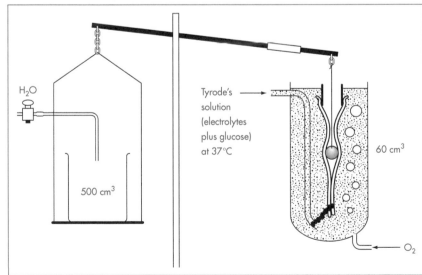

H$_2$O

500 cm^3

Tyrode's solution (electrolytes plus glucose) at 37°C

60 cm^3

O$_2$

Figure 15.17 A system for measurement of the force required to detach a solid-dosage form from an isolated porcine oesophagus.

Reproduced from Marvola M *et al*. Development of a method for study of the tendency of drug products to adhere to the esophagus. *J Pharm Sci* 1982;71:975–977. Copyright Wiley-VCH Verlag GmbH & Co. KGaA. Reproduced with permission.

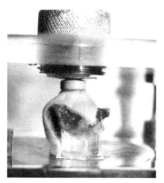

Figure 15.18 A device to measure the force of detachment of tablets or capsules from porcine oesophageal tissue, used to determine the values given in Fig. 15.19.

contact through a liquid layer of thickness h and viscosity η over time t is

$$f - \frac{3k'}{4t} \left[\frac{r^2\eta}{h^2} \right] \tag{15.3}$$

where k', is a constant. This equation applies only when the surfaces are pulled apart slowly.

Clearly the viscosity of the liquid (η) is a key determinant of the force of separation. The 'tackiness' of a system is not, however, simply related to viscosity.[14] High-molecular-weight materials must be present in aqueous solutions, for example, to provide an elastic element to the viscous flow. Rubbery polymers that have partly liquid and partly elastic characteristics are employed as adhesives in surgical dressings and adhesive tapes. It is still unclear what factors influence the adhesivity of high-molecular-weight soluble polymers such as hydroxypropylmethylcellulose (HPMC). HPMC is a component of film coating materials. Figure 15.19 shows the detachment force required to separate tablets from a glass surface when coated with HPMC-606 from a 4% solution, shown here as a function of the thickness of the film coat.[15] The effect of the presence of high concentrations of polyoxyethylene glycol 6000 is to reduce adhesivity, presumably because the glycol solution is less tacky.

The variables likely to affect the process of adhesion of coated tablets to mucosal surfaces are shown in diagrammatic form in Fig. 15.20: film coat thickness, the nature of the film coat, its rate of solution or hydration, the rheology of the solution formed, its surface tension and its elongational characteristics. Eight stages have been identified. Stage I (before contact occurs) defines the system and the variables of film

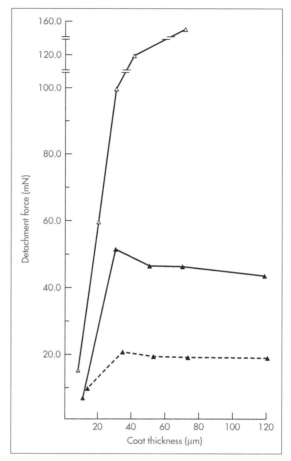

Figure 15.19 The effect of film thickness on the adhesiveness of tablets coated with hydroxypropylmethylcellulose (HPMC)-606 from a 4% solution ($\triangle$) and in the presence of 4% polyoxyethylene glycol (PEG) 6000 (—▲—) and 6% PEG 6000 (··· ▲ ···), i.e. 1: 1 and 1: 1.5 ratios of HPMC to PEG respectively.

Reproduced from Al-Dujaili H *et al*. The adhesiveness of proprietary tablets and capsules to porcine oesophageal tissue. *Int J Pharm* 1986;34:75–79 with permission. Copyright Elsevier 1986.

coating thickness, the nature of the coating and the nature of the tissue surface. In stage II the presence of moisture or water is postulated, and here the wetting characteristics of the film will be important. In stage III the film coat begins to dissolve and we assume that contact is made, or is about to be made, with the tissue; the forces bringing the tablet and the tissue together are not controllable because contact is made by collision and is dependent to some extent on the ratio of tablet size to oesophageal diameter. Stage IV represents contact, when the angle of approach, together with the tablet size and shape, will determine the opportunity for adhesion. Stages V–VIII represent

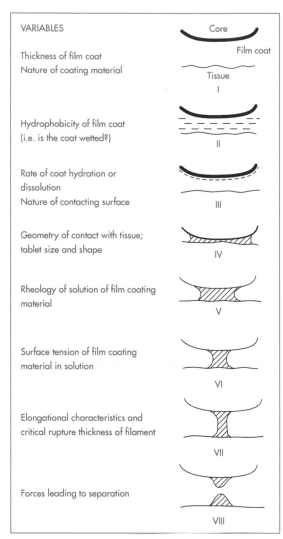

VARIABLES

Thickness of film coat
Nature of coating material

Hydrophobicity of film coat
(i.e. is the coat wetted?)

Rate of coat hydration or
dissolution
Nature of contacting surface

Geometry of contact with tissue;
tablet size and shape

Rheology of solution of film coating
material

Surface tension of film coating
material in solution

Elongational characteristics and
critical rupture thickness of filament

Forces leading to separation

Figure 15.20 Diagrammatic representation of the possible sequence of events in the adhesion of a tablet to a mucosal surface and its subsequent separation, with a partial listing of the many variables in the process.

Reproduced with permission from Florence AT, Salole EG. *Formulation Factors in Adverse Reactions*. London: Wright; 1990.

the detachment process initiated, for example, by swallowing food or water or dry swallowing; here the rheological and elongational characteristics of the adhesive material are important.

15.7 Mechanical strength of buccal films

Buccal delivery can be achieved using orodispersible or buccal films. These have to have a certain strength to withstand application. Thus strength tests have been devised, such as the one shown diagrammatically in Fig. 15.21. It measures the elongation of the film to its break point.

15.8 Gastro-retentive systems: buoyancy tests

Often in practice one seeks to find out differences between branded and generic products. There are now several gastro-retentive systems that rely for their function on their buoyancy in the stomach and hence their retention for reasonable lengths of time. In the words of Timmermans and Moës,[16] 'how well do floating systems float?' It seems that the bulk density is not the most appropriate measure of flotation, but apparent density, which is a function of the porosity of the system, is.[17] The greater the porosity, the lower the apparent density. Simple *in vitro* buoyancy tests are easy to design and perform.

15.8.1 Raft-forming dosage forms

Gaviscon and related products, Algicon, Gastrocote, Gaviscon Advance, Mylanta, Peptac and Rennie Duo, are antacid formulations used in the treatment of gastric oesophageal reflux disease. The formulations have the ability to form a buoyant alginate raft to prevent oesophageal reflux of acidic gut contents. A variety of techniques, including gamma-scintigraphy, radiography and magnetic resonance imaging scanning, have shown that alginates do form physical rafts on the

Table 15.3 Alginate raft resilience measurements

Product	Raft resilience (range) (min)
Algicon	0–0
Gastrocote	2–10
Gaviscon Advance	60–60
Gaviscon Liquid	10–30
Gaviscon Regular Strength[a]	0–0
Gaviscon Extra Strength[a]	0–0
Mylanta Heartburn Relief	2–5
Peptac	2–10
Rennie Duo	0–2

[a] US products.

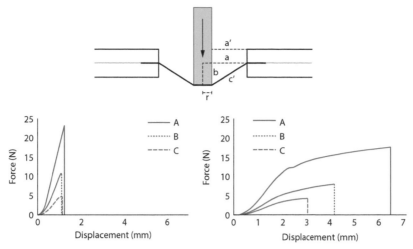

Figure 15.21 top Measurement of elongation to break point of a polymer film. *r* is the radius of the probe, *a* the initial radius of the film, *b* is the probe displacement, *a'* = [*a* −*r*], *c'* is the length of the film after displacement. The force–displacement plots differ according to the materials tested (see lower figures). The energy to puncture a film is related to the area under the curve. Left, paper, and right, polyethylene terephthalate foil using three different probes, A, B and C.

Reproduced from Preis M *et al*. Mechanical strength test for orodispersible and buccal films. *Int J Pharm* 2014;461:22–29. Copyright Elsevier 2014.

stomach contents after ingestion. Techniques have been developed to measure raft strength,[18] including their 'resilience', a measure used to compare a variety of raft-forming products in terms of speed of raft formation, flotation potential and coherence. Figure 15.22 shows the apparatus devised by Hampson *et al*.[18]

Table 15.3 shows some of the resilience data. The higher the value, the stronger the raft.

15.9 Evaluation of aerosols

Analysis of the particle size distribution of aerosol formulations during formulation, development and clinical trial or after storage is of obvious clinical relevance. Aerosols are not easy to size, primarily because in use they are dynamic and inherently unstable systems, as propellants and drug solvents evaporate.

The most widely used instrument in categorising airborne particles is the cascade impactor. It attempts to mimic the obstructions and changes of direction that aerosols experience in the body, albeit in a crude way. Large particles leave the airstream and impinge on baffles or on glass microscope slides. The airstream is then accelerated at a nozzle, providing a second range of smaller-sized particles on the next baffle, and so on (Fig. 15.23). Progressively finer particles are collected at the successive stages of impingement owing to jet velocity and decreasing jet dimension. For more routine examination of medicinal aerosols, 'artificial

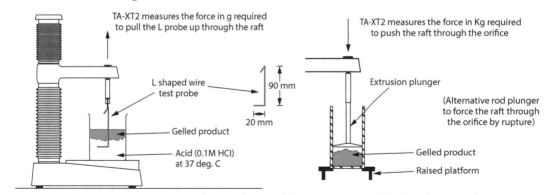

Figure 15.22 Systems to measure the strength or 'resilience' of alginate rafts formed by formulations such as Gaviscon used to prevent gastric acid reflux.

Reproduced from reference 18.

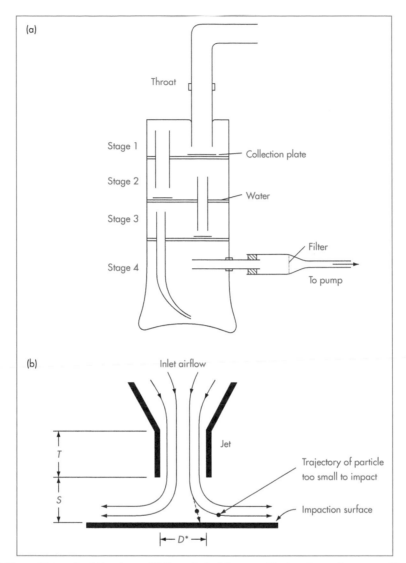

Figure 15.23 (a) The multistage liquid impinger. (b) The principal features affecting the performance of inertial impactors: air flow, the dimensions S and T, the diameter of the jet, D^*, the density, ρ, and the diameter of the particles, d. The trajectory of particles that are too small to deposit is shown.

Reproduced from Hallworth GW. In: Ganderton D, Jones T (eds) *Drug Delivery to the Respiratory Tract*. Chichester: Ellis Horwood; 1987. Copyright Wiley-VCH Verlag GmbH & Co. KGaA. Reproduced with permission.

throat' devices are useful. With these, comparative studies of the behaviour of aerosols can be carried out. In such devices the particles are segregated according to size. Analysis of the collecting layers at the several levels of the device allows the monitoring of changes in released particle size. In devices with an artificial mouth, this can be washed to reveal the extent of fall-out of large particles. The smallest particles of all reach the collecting solvent.

Because of the need for standardisation of test equipment, the BP and other compendia have adopted detailed specifications for impinger devices. Two impinger devices have been adopted by the BP. Apparatus 'A' is shown in Fig. 15.24. All these operate by dividing the dose emitted from an inhaler into the respirable and non-respirable fractions. The device in Fig. 15.24 employs the principle of liquid impingement and has a solvent in both chambers to collect the aerosol. Air is drawn through the system at 60 dm^3 min^{-1} and the inhaler is fired several times into the device. There are several impaction surfaces at the back of the glass throat about 10 cm away from the activator (similar to human dimensions). The upper impinger has a cut-off at a particle size of around 6.4 μm, with the first impact surface known as stage 1 and the last impact surface being in the lower impinger (stage 2), which is considered to be the respirable fraction.

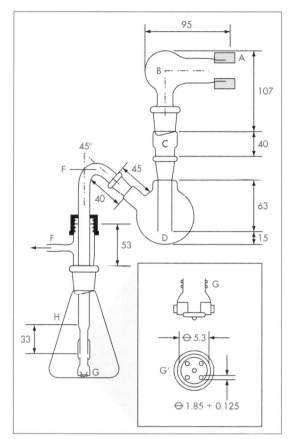

Figure 15.24 Impinger apparatus A, showing dimensions (mm) in order to ensure indenticality between equipment used in quality control.

Source: *British Pharmacopoeia*. London: HMSO, with permission.

Apparatus B (not illustrated) is made of metal and can be engineered to finer tolerances than the glass apparatus A; it is considered to be a superior apparatus for quality control testing and product release.

Typical of the result achieved with Apparatus B are those for two formulations, 1 and 5. Product 1 delivers 1 mg and Product 5 delivers 5 mg per shot. *In vitro*, the respirable fraction was found to be 25% and 20% respectively, while estimates of the percentage of the dose reaching the lung were 12.0% and 8.8% respectively. Some equipment, such as multistage impingers for aerosols, can be predictive of *in vivo* behaviour, or can at least give an assurance of consistency of effect.

An interesting test system for evaluating inhaled nasal delivery systems (Fig. 15.25) combines a physical device with cells in culture so that the interaction of microparticles with living cells can be studied directly. As new delivery systems appear, new tests will be required – as will ingenuity.

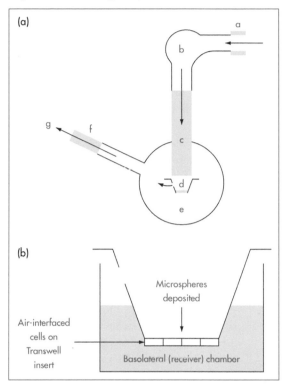

Figure 15.25 An *in vitro* technique for evaluating inhaled nasal delivery systems in which particles/microspheres are deposited on a cell monolayer. Drug that is absorbed through the monolayer can be measured in the basolateral chamber.

Reproduced with permission from Forbes B *et al*. An in vitro technique for evaluating inhaled nasal delivery systems. *STP Pharma Sci* 2002;12:75–79.

Key points

- A selection of tests can be conducted to measure the key parameters of a variety of formulations.
- Tests are not necessarily predictive of performance *in vivo*, but can be used for example to ensure batch-to-batch consistency.
- When good *in vitro–in vivo* correlations have been established, laboratory-based

- tests can be predictive of clinical performance.
- Tests can be applied to rectal and transdermal products by adapting methods used for oral products, altering the receptor phase to mimic the medium to that which the formulation will experience *in vivo*.
- Key parameters are different for different routes of delivery and different formulations: particle size is a key factor in inhalation products and in topical preparations where the drug is dispersed rather than dissolved in the vehicle.
- Adhesivity of oral dosage forms may be a factor in determining their efficacy (as in buccal treatments and delivery) or in causing adverse events (as in oesophageal injury); adhesion of transdermal patches to the skin is clearly important.
- The rheological properties of topical preparations and formulations for nasal administration are important, and a key factor is the syringeability of injectables.
- Each claimed special feature of a product should be the subject of testing in the laboratory from the adhesiveness of transdermal patches or tablets designed to adhere to colonic tissue, to the strength of rafts formed, to the buoyancy of floating oral systems. It is a field which is restricted only by ingenuity.

Summary

In vitro tests are sometimes designed to predict potential behaviour of dosage forms in use or in the body. But not all are. Some tests, for example, that of the hardness of tablets, are simply in place to ensure the survival of tablets throughout their journey from manufacturing plan to patient. Figure 15.1 showed how products can fail at the last hurdle. No laboratory test can mimic the complexity of the biological environment and the dynamic factors involved in drug absorption in patients, but well-designed laboratory experiments can elucidate whether different formulations are comparable in terms of their key features. At best, *in vitro* tests are predictors of quality of performance in the patient; at the least they can ensure consistency of response. For example, where assays of drug content in generic products may give identical results, release studies may show differences due to drug–excipient and other interactions that may be of significance. We should always be on the alert for novel ways of assessing dosage forms before they are used in the clinic. Sometimes simple tests can reveal much. Complex equipment is not always required, but there is now a large array of new techniques which can be brought to bear on the issues of product quality, an understanding of their behaviour *in vivo*, and how they work.

References

1. Hanson R, Gray V. *Handbook of Dissolution Testing*, 3rd edn. Hokessin, DE: DissolutionTechnologies; 2004.
2. Mattock GL, McGilveray IJ. Comparison of bioavailabilities and dissolution characteristics of commercial tablet formulations of sulfamethizole. *J Pharm Sci* 1972;61:746–749.
3. Pedersen BI *et al*. A comparison of solubility of danazol in human and simulated gastro-intestinal fluids. *Pharm Res* 2000;17:891–894.
4. Ritschel WA, Banarer M. Correlation between *in vitro* release of proxyphylline from suppositories and *in vivo* data obtained from cumulative urinary excretion studies. *Arzneim Forsch* 1973;23:1031–1035.
5. Taylor JB, Simpkins DE. Aminophylline suppositories: *in vitro* dissolution and bioavailability in man. *Pharm J* 1981;227:601–603.
6. Ostrenga JA *et al*. Vehicle design for a topical steroid, fluocinolide. *J Invest Dermatol* 1971;56:392–399.
7. Yoshida H *et al*. In vitro release of tacrolimus from tacrolimus ointment and its speculated mechanism. *Int J Pharm* 2004;270:55–64.
8. Corbo M *et al*. Development and validation of *in vitro* release testing methods for semi-solid formulations. *Pharm Tech Int* 1993;17:112–118.
9. Wolff M *et al*. In vitro and in vivo-release of nitroglycerin from a new transdermal therapeutic system. *Pharm Res* 1985;123–129.
10. Podczeck F. Methods for the practical development of the mechanical strength test of tablets – from empiricism to science. *Int J Pharm* 2012;436:214–232.
11. Allahham A *et al*. Flow and injection characteristics of pharmaceutical parenteral formulations using a microcapillary rheometer *Int J Pharm* 2004;270:139–148.
12. Marvola M *et al*. Development of a method for study of the tendency of drug products to adhere to the esophagus. *J Pharm Sci* 1982;71:975–977.
13. Al-Dujaili H *et al*. In vitro assessment of the adhesiveness of film-coated tablets. *Int J Pharm* 1986;34:67–74.

14. Marvola M *et al*. Effect of dosage form and formulation factors on the adherence of drugs to the esophagus. *J Pharm Sci* 1983;72:1034–1036.

15. Al-Dujaili H *et al*. The adhesiveness of proprietary tablets and capsules to porcine oesophageal tissue. *Int J Pharm* 1986;34:75–79.

16. Timmermans J, Moës AJ. How well do floating dosage forms float? *Int J Pharm* 1990;62:201–216.

17. Sauzet C *et al*. An innovative floating gastro-retentive dosage system: formulation and *in vitro* evaluation. *Int J Pharm* 2009;378:23–29.

18. Hampson FC *et al*. Alginate rafts and their characterisation. *Int J Pharm* 2005;294:137–147.

Further reading

Perrie Y *et al*. (eds) Special issue: Advanced characterisation techniques. *Int J Pharm* 2011;417:1 *et seq*.

16

Generic medicines and biosimilars

In this chapter we define and describe generic medicines and biosimilars. The former are products marketed after the expiration of patents on the brand leader. These generally contain conventional drugs, in contrast to biosimilars, which are macromolecular or protein-based drugs whose production processes cannot always be identical to that of the brand leader, hence they are 'similar' and not 'equivalent'. We discuss both chemical equivalence and therapeutic (or bio-)equivalence. Bioequivalence of conventional medicines is measured in volunteers or patients by determination of pharmacokinetic parameters (area under the curve, C_{max}, t_{max}): there is rarely 100% equivalence, hence the licensing authorities allow ranges. When there are several generic products there can be more divergence between products which may or may not be clinically significant. We discuss possible variables between the originator branded product and the one or several generic products. Issues might arise from different excipients, differences in the behaviour of different formulations, different polymorphs of the drug or the use of different salts, and in some cases different routes of synthesis of the drug molecule, leading to different impurities. Generic medicines are not inferior to branded products, but where there are critical issues with treatment, many advise against changing the source of medication.

With biological molecules such as proteins there are the possibilities of differences in the active molecule which could have occured through differences in their often lengthy and complex modes of production, or because of different animal, cell or other sources, hence the term used for post-originator biological products is 'biosimilar'. In both conventional drugs and biological drugs, questions of chemistry, quality and standards come to the fore.

Note that some of the examples of problems here may be historic but which provide instructive lessons when novel drugs are being assessed. One must assume that generic medicines available in pharmacies are approved and therefore bioequivalent, but not necessarily identical. Sustained-release products require special attention when switching products, as it is difficult to define sustained as opposed to normal release, the latter defined by the drug, the former generally by formulation.

16.1 Introduction

The World Health Organization* defines a generic product as 'a pharmaceutical product, usually intended to be interchangeable with an innovator product, that is manufactured without a licence from the innovator company and marketed after the expiry date of the patent or other exclusive rights'. Generic forms of conventional (i.e. small-molecule) medicines contain the same drug as the original product (although the molecule may have been prepared by a different route), and the formulation may differ. The issue of generic equivalence and performance thus certainly lies within the domain of pharmaceutics. It is too simple to say that, as the drug is the same, only the formulation may differ, because, as we will discuss in this chapter, there can be differences in the purity of a drug even when it is within pharmacopoeial limits. The formulation and manufacturing process may indeed influence the stability of the drug and perhaps its physical form. Generic drugs are subject to strict guidelines for licensing so that, within the limits possible with modern analytical techniques and the variability of subjects, they will be bioequivalent, again with certain limits. Equivalence is not identicality. This statement is particularly relevant when one deals with sustained-release or extended-release dosage forms: what is sustained or extended? An additional problem is that a generic product will be tested against the brand leader and there is no requirement to test generic versus generic. This is where these problems can arise, as we will see, and it is this that leads to concerns when the formulations are used in cases where brand changes through generic prescribing and dispensing may be a real or imagined issue.

We distinguish here between so-called conventional, small-molecule drugs and those proteins and other macromolecules that are more complex. Generic forms of biologicals, especially of recombinant proteins, present other issues as the active molecule may contain, say, subtle differences in amino acid sequence due to often inevitable differences in the mode of production and processing. As we discuss below, the manufacture and processing of many biologically active macromolecules can lead to differences in their physical state as well as their composition or conformation. The term 'biosimilars' has evolved for generic forms of such biologicals; alternative terms include follow-on biologics or biogenerics.

We deal first with small-molecule chemical medicines and issues related to branded and generic versions of a medicine. It should be noted that many generic products carry brand names, so in fact the discussion is centred around the orginator's branded product and those products that follow from expiry of patents, and the issue of substitution of a generic for a branded product or one generic for another.

A 2007 survey of recent (Australian) pharmacy graduates' knowledge of generic medicines[1] found that more than 80% believed generic medicines to be inferior, to be less effective and to produce more side-effects when compared with branded medicines. When one considers that many generic medicines are manufactured by companies such as Pfizer, Sandoz, GSK and Merck, whose primary occupation is the development of branded innovative products, one wonders where this perception comes from. There are of course differences in formulation between many generics and their branded equivalents and sometimes these differences can be important for patients, but for the majority of conventional (normal)-release products of most drugs there are few problems. There are some therapeutic categories where one might choose to continue with a product on which the patient has been stabilised, as with antiepileptic drugs (AEDs); clearly, this is where professional intelligence has to be applied.

 Key point

The search for true bioequivalence is important. Given the variability of human drug response, to which we have referred several times, it is even more important that the product which enters the body is as standardised as possible. The combination of human variability and product variability is unthinkable.

---

* www.who.int/trade/glossary

16.2 Regulatory statements on generic products

A generic drug should be identical or bioequivalent to a brand-name drug in dosage form, safety, strength, route of administration, quality, performance characteristics and intended use. The US and European authorities adopt similar approaches.[2] To gain approval, a generic drug must:

- contain the same active ingredients as the innovator drug (inactive ingredients may vary)
- be identical in strength, dosage form and route of administration
- have the same use indications
- be bioequivalent
- meet the same batch requirements for identity, strength, purity and quality
- be manufactured under the same strict standards of good manufacturing practice regulations required for innovator products.

The question of bioavailability has to be looked at in several ways (Fig. 16.1). Products can be bioequivalent yet not therapeutically equivalent, perhaps because the rate of absorption of the drug differs in the first 30 minutes or so. If bioavailability is measured by the area under the plasma concentration–time curve (AUC) over 24 or 48 hours, then these measures of bioavailability might not show up subtle differences.

16.2.1 Generics: a question of quality

Equivalence between medicinal products can be thought of at two levels:

1. *chemical equivalence*, which refers to dosage forms containing the same amount of the same drug in similar dose forms

2. *therapeutic equivalence*, which refers to medicines having not only the same bioavailability (as measured by the AUC), but the same clinical effects.

Figures 16.2 and 16.3 demonstrate the limits of bioequivalence and non-bioequivalence. Figure 16.3 shows how, while two generic products may be equivalent to the first brand product, the two generics may not be equivalent to each other, which may pose problems in practice.

Essential similarity of dose forms of the same drug focuses on the essential similarity of purity of the drug substance as well as similarity of release rates. Chemical equivalence is ensured by pharmaceutical processes and quality assurance and is one prerequisite for therapeutic equivalence. Limits are set for drug substance; for example, tetracycline hydrochloride contains not less than 96% and not more than 102% of the drug. As far as therapeutic equivalence is concerned, the product should have essentially the same safety profile as the comparator product. Regulations do not speak of *identicality* between products, but *essential similarity.* One reason is that drug substances

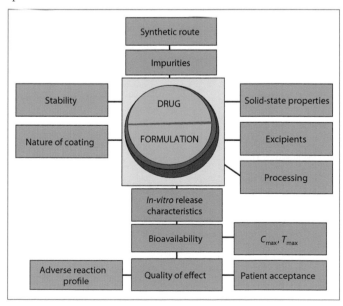

Figure 16.1 The range of issues in determining the equivalence or essential similarity of formulations.

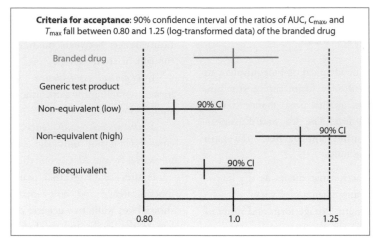

Figure 16.2 The issue of variability in branded and generic products with their 90% confidence limits and the definition of non-equivalence and equivalence in visual form.
Reproduced from Medscape.

can vary in purity within pharmacopoeial guidelines, and there are variations in the amount of drug within each unit of product, again within limits. On top of this there are interpatient and intrapatient variability. This does not excuse differences and indeed sometimes exacerbates differences. Many drugs are absorbed readily and raise no concerns when generic versions become available. It is with drugs that have proven bioavailability problems or that require special formulation techniques that the issue of similarity becomes real. Drugs with a narrow therapeutic index have to be considered with care. On the other hand, solutions and syrups do not need such scrutiny. Simple formulations of soluble drugs for injection are unlikely to cause concern. The only concern might be with drug purity.

Pharmacopoeias of course provide limits on undesirable impurities in the drug substance. Toxic 4-epianhydrotetracycline is limited in tetracycline products. Even if the limit is very low (say 0.005%), there may be three products (or the same product in different batches) with levels of such an impurity at 0.0048%, 0.004% and 0.002%. Are these identical? Much depends on the nature and activity of the impurity.

For conventional tablets, solutions, simple injections and suspensions, generic versions can be used generally without qualms. However, once we enter the field of formulation modification, as with sustained-release products, the picture becomes more complex. One knows that towards the end of the patent life of conventional products, modified-release forms (or

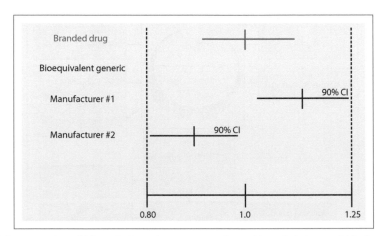

Figure 16.3 Visual demonstration of bioequivalence between generics and branded drugs, which demonstrates clearly, that while generic 1 can be equivalent to the brand, generic 2 may not be equivalent to generic 1. From Medscape.

sometimes new polymorphs of the drug substance) are introduced to delay the introduction of generics and to retain brand loyalty. The relative potentials of oral dosage forms to exhibit bioavailability problems are listed in Table 16.1. It is obvious that the more complex formulations can rarely be identical in originators and branded preparations. Among the 'complex' formulations, one might include liposomes and microparticle and nanoparticulate systems.

Table 16.1 Relative potential of oral medicines to display bioavailability problems

High	Intermediate	Low
Enteric-coated tablets	Suspensions	Solutions
Sustained-release tablets	Chewable tablets	
Complex formulations	Capsules	
Slowly disintegrating tablets		

There are generic versions of some sustained-release formulations, but within a given class of sustained-release product of a given drug, such as theophylline, there will be a spectrum of release rates. The proliferation of sustained- and modified-release forms of branded products at the end of the patent life of a product results not necessarily from the prospect of improved clinical outcomes but for the very reason that generic versions are difficult to produce. Generic modified-release products themselves are therefore usually branded. Having said this, the benefit of having a range of formulations is recognised.[3]

16.2.2 Specific medical conditions and the use of generics

There is just the chance that in the treatment of some conditions differences in the performance of products are relevant. There are also some medical conditions where particular care has to be taken in titrating patients and maintaining therapeutic levels closely throughout treatment. Such is the case with antiepileptic drugs (AEDs). While generic medicines have been an issue at least since the 1970s, problems with AEDs are still current,[4,5] as we discuss below. There are reports on the re-emergence of psychotic symptoms after conversion (a study with $n = 7$) from a brand-name clozapine to a generic formulation.[6] However, the problem with such reports is that they are often specific

to a country; the results will depend on which brand and which generic are being studied. Papers do not always give full pharmaceutical information and hence their value is diminished.

The difficulty in extrapolating results across borders is exhibited by clozapine. It has been found that generic preparations of the drug licensed in the UK are bioequivalent with the branded Clozaril: as the author[7] states: 'There was no evidence of clinical deterioration or the need to use higher doses. Generic clozapine is not inferior to Clozaril.' Some US reports suggest that there are problems in substituting the originators' product with a generic. But another study in the USA of a generic clozapine (Mylan) and Clozaril (Novartis)[8] concluded that they were therapeutically equivalent. Generic bupropion (**I**) extended-release (Budeprion, Impax Labs) was withdrawn for lack of bioequivalence with Wellbutrin XL, the branded product (Fig. 16.4) used for the treatment of depression.

Structure I Bupropion

16.2.3 Antiepileptic drugs: clinical experience and the literature

There is, however, a relative shortage of literature comparing generic substitutions for AEDs. Most of the case reports, letters to the editor and some papers deal with three drugs, carbamazepine, phenytoin and valproate. These reports document breakthrough seizures or adverse events when switching from a branded AED to a generic version. Of around 300 US neurologists, 56% reported adverse events, and 68% reported breakthrough seizures in at least *one* patient when medication was switched from a branded to a generic AED. Burkhardt *et al.*[9] identified eight adult patients whose seizures worsened after switching from branded phenytoin to generic phenytoin. The few blinded, controlled studies reported in the literature have evaluated relative pharmacokinetics of a brand versus generic formulations. Sometimes only one generic version was studied (note Fig. 16.2). No controlled studies have mirrored practice by evaluating safety, efficacy and

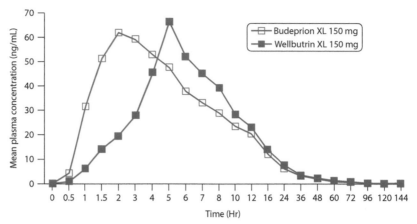

Figure 16.4 Mean plasma concentration of bupropion (Budeprion XL and Wellbutrin XL) as a function of time in 24 fasting healthy volunteers.

See details in Woodcock MD *et al.* Withdrawal of generic budeprion for nonbioequivalence. *N Engl J Med* 2012;367:2463–2465.

compliance with the therapeutic regimen when multiple generic versions are used in succession.

The American Academy of Neurology has produced a number of recommendations regarding generic substitution for AEDs[10,11]:

- Such substitutions can be approved only if the safety and efficacy of treatment are not compromised.
- Specific pharmacokinetic information about each AED generic should be made available to physicians, who should avoid switching between formulations of AEDs.
- Labelling should identify specific manufacturers.
- Pharmacists should be required to inform patients and physicians when switching a product between manufacturers.
- Organisations that encourage or mandate substitution of AEDs should evaluate their responsibility for any problems arising from their policies.

Because changing from one formulation of an AED to another can usually be accomplished, and risks minimised, if physicians and patients monitor blood levels, seizures and toxicity, it is maintained in the USA that the individual and physician should be notified and should give their consent before a switch in medications is made, whether it involves either generic substitution for brand-name products, or generic-to-generic substitutions.

16.3 Reading and deconstructing the literature on bioequivalence

If pharmacokinetic data are available, one needs to ask whether the analytical methodology was up to the task. Was the study sound? The literature can be biased because studies supported by manufacturers of products under study (both generic and branded)[8] might not be published if the results, say, show inequivalence in the former case or equivalence in the latter. In one case, with levothyroxine, it was estimated that analytical techniques commonly used were not sufficiently precise to ascertain equivalence. Figure 16.5 shows data on the levels of thyroxine in plasma after administration of doses from 400 to 600 μg, without taking into account baseline thyroxine concentrations.[12] Such a method would not be able to distinguish between generics if it cannot distinguish between the doses over the range given. Figure 16.5b shows the data taking baseline levels into account. The latter method would be adequate.

The other issue is whether active and active metabolites are being measured, as with risperidone, whose active metabolite, 9-hydroxy-risperidone has a much longer half-life than the parent drug.

16.3.1 Antiretroviral drugs

It is always difficult to generalise from single studies on generic equivalence or non-equivalence. In comparisons of generic and branded anti-human immuno-

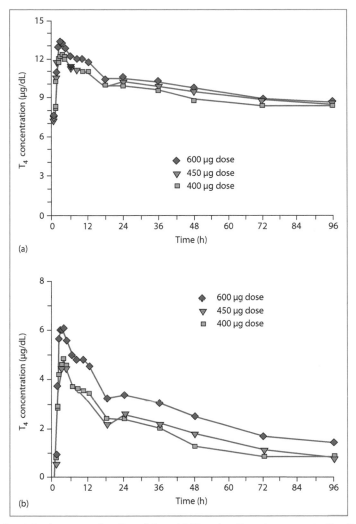

Figure 16.5 Thyroxine levels in plasma as a function of time. (a) Mean levothyroxine concentration time profiles on study day 1 following a single-dose administration of levothyroxine sodium, uncorrected for baseline levothyroxine concentrations. (b) Figures corrected for baseline levothyroxine concentrations.

Reproduced from Blakesley VA. Current methodology to assess bioequivalence of levothyroxine sodium products are inadequate. *AAPS J* 2005;7:E42–E46, with kind permission from Springer Science and Business Media.

deficiency virus (HIV) products containing the three drugs stavudine, lamivudine and nevirapine made in HIV-infected adults,[13] stavudine levels were found to be significantly lower using a generic formulation. A similar but larger study, also in infected adults, found that generic fixed-dose combinations of these drugs were efficacious and safe.[14] Two generic fixed-dose combinations of these drugs for children (Pedimune Baby and Pedimune Junior, Cipla Pharmaceuticals) have been found to be similar to the branded products when tested in healthy adults.[15] As with many products, the true measure of quality is not minor differences in peak plasma levels or AUCs but therapeutic

outcome. Never more so than in developing countries. The stark facts are that, after the introduction of cheaper antiretroviral therapies in Southern India, the numbers using these products increased and death rates decreased from 25 to 5 deaths per 100 persons between 1997 and 2003.[16]

16.3.2 Bioequivalence of ophthalmic products

It is difficult to assess the bioequivalence of ophthalmic products. There have been issues, however,[17] one being high rates of precipitation in a generic prednisone

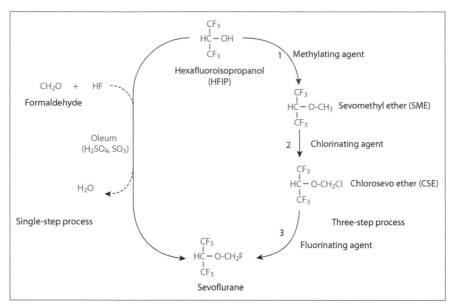

Figure 16.6 Pathways for the single-step and three-step syntheses of sevoflurane from the starting compound hexafluoroisopropanol. The potential impurity from the single-step method is formaldehyde, and from the three-step process is sevomethyl ether (SME) and chlorosevo ether (CSE).

Reproduced with permission from Reference 18.

formulation when administered to the eye. Some products will employ different excipients, which might lead to subtle differences in behaviour of the preparation; a generic timolol gel-forming product possessed a different 'feel' from the branded product. This also apparently gave the impression to the patient that the generic formulation was less efficacious.

16.3.3 The case of sevoflurane

The apparent simplicity of the anaesthetic molecule sevoflurane (II) masks differences in synthetic methods and degradation that may be significant in deciding between products.

Structure II Sevoflurane

Sevoflurane is available in the USA from two manufacturers as Ultane (Abbott) and as a generic product, sevoflurane inhalation anaesthetic (Sevoness) (Baxter Healthcare Corp.). These products are rated therapeutically equivalent by the US Food and Drug Administration, but there are some differences. Ultane is made in a single-step synthetic process, whereas generic

sevoflurane is manufactured using a three-step process, as described by Baker.[18] In the UK sevoflurane is a non-proprietary product. As there is only one UK product, the question of differences will arise only if there are several manufacturers. In the USA, as Baker points out, Ultane contains > 300 ppm water and generic sevoflurane contains ≤ 130 ppm water. Ultane is supplied in a plastic poly(ethylene naphthalate) polymer bottle, while generic sevoflurane is supplied in lacquer-lined aluminium bottles. Here then is an example that typifies some generic issues. The products have different manufacturing processes (Fig. 16.6) and hence different impurities, have different containers, and have potential differences in the rate or extent of sevoflurane degradation.

The significance of the containers has been discussed[18] and relates to the discovery that sevoflurane can be unstable in glass bottles in which the anaesthetic was originally supplied. Reports of a cloudy product with a strong odour appeared. Such batches were found to contain hydrofluoric acid in concentrations up to 863 ppm, as well as a pH below unity. This was linked to Lewis-acid defluorination of the drug. (Lewis acids are usually metal-containing compounds that accept electrons from Lewis bases and result in Lewis base degradation. There are many Lewis acids, such as metal halides and metal oxides, including aluminium oxide (Al_2O_3)). The Lewis acid in this case was identified as rust (iron oxide) on a valve on a bulk shipping container. The drug is especially susceptible to degradation because of the mono-fluoroalkyl ether group. The whole story can be read in Baker's paper.[18]

The base-catalysed conversion of sevoflurane to 'compound A' is as shown in Fig. 16.7. Figure 16.8 shows a range of degradation pathways for the anaesthetic.[19]

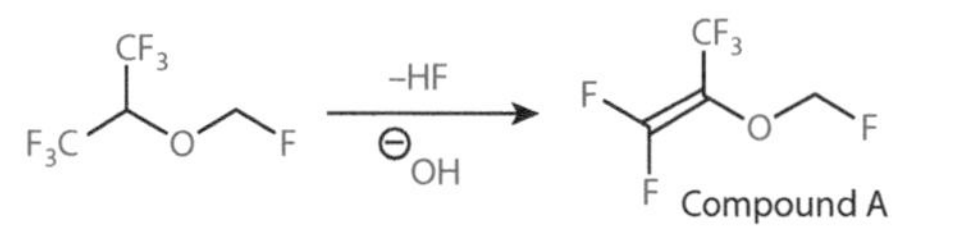

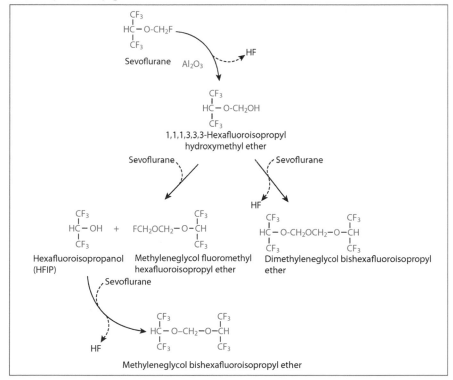

Figure 16.7 Base-catalysed conversion of sevoflurane to so-called compound A.

Carbon dioxide absorption enables the use of low-flow anaesthesia, and a decreased consumption of medical gases and halogenated anaesthetics, as well as reduced pollution. Chemical absorbents (soda lime and barium hydroxide lime (Baralyme)) may produce toxic com-

pounds: carbon monoxide with all halogenated anaesthetics and 'compound A' with sevoflurane (Fig. 16.9). Simple measures against desiccation of the lime prevent carbon monoxide production. The toxicity of compound A, shown in the rat, has not been demonstrated in clinical anaesthesia. Recent improvements in manufacturing processes have decreased the powdering of lime. Moreover, filters inserted between the anaesthesia circuit and the patient abolish the risk for powder inhalation.

A Japanese product is marketed as Sevofrane (Maruishi Pharmaceutical Co., Osaka, Japan)[20] and is available there along with Sevoness. Both products studied contain over 99.998% sevoflurane and fluoride concentrations were the same, at around 0.43 ppm.

The formation and toxicity of anaesthetic degradation products can be an issue.[21] Soon after its introduction in 1935 there were reports of neuropathies following trichloroethylene anaesthesia. These were attributable to the formation of dichloroacetylene through base-catalysed elimination of HCl from the compound. The common cause of their formation is

Figure 16.8 Potential pathways of degradation and the products of degradation of sevoflurane on reaction with alumina (Al_2O_3). The degradation products are detected at very low concentrations in low-flow, long-duration anaesthesia.

Reproduced from Bito H, Ikeda K. Long-duration, low-flow sevoflurane anesthesia using two carbon dioxide absorbents. Quantification of degradation products in the circuit. *Anesthesiology* 1994;81:340–345.

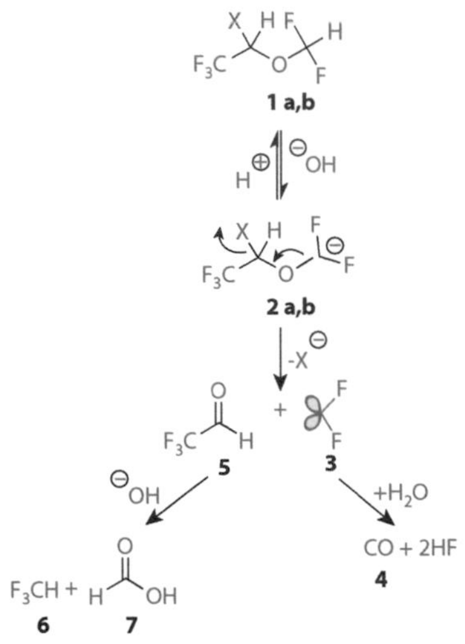

Figure 16.9 Base-catalysed conversion of desflurane and isoflurane (**1a** and **1b**) to CO (**4**). Note also trifluroacetaldehyde (**5**) and trifluoromethane (**6**) and formic acid (**7**).

the reaction of the anaesthetic with the bases in adsorbents in the circuit. (These include sodium hydroxide (soda lime), barium hydroxide lime, potassium hydroxide (KOH)-free soda lime, calcium hydroxide and non-caustic lime. These have different reactivities: sodium hydroxide > soda lime > KOH-free soda lime > calcium hydroxide.) Understanding the nature of these reactions that affect trichloroethylene, desflurane (Fig. 16.9), norflurane and enflurane has helped towards the safe use of these agents.

Although these examples are of a specialised use of these agents, nevertheless the potential formation of very low concentrations of degradants by whatever means can lead to adverse events or certainly to differences in the behaviour of products.

16.4 Biosimilars: protein drugs, monoclonal antibodies

The complexity of proteins as drugs is well known. Peptides and proteins are subject to a variety of chemical and physical instabilities in aqueous solution and at interfaces, and can also suffer during the stresses of some manufacturing processes.

16.4.1 Issues with biomolecular generics

Now that the protein therapeutic market has matured, generic versions of biologicals are becoming available. The source and mode of production of the protein therapeutic are important issues. With the so-called 'follow-on' protein drugs,[22] compound or product identicality cannot always be demonstrated as it can with conventional molecules. Even with the latter there are often small regulated amounts of impurities, such as dimers, breakdown products and products of side-reactions. The impurities in proteins are often very similar to the parent compound and, although present in low concentrations, may be pharmacologically or immunologically active. Small changes in manufacturing processes may lead to final products that are not identical to the originator's product. Aggregation, protein folding and glycosylation may be affected, any of which can lead to differences in pharmacokinetics, immunogenicity or, indeed, efficacy. The formulation may or may not influence outcomes. One example has been seen with recombinant human erythropoietin (Eprex). A change of stabiliser from albumin to polysorbate 80 has been thought to be the cause of the formation of anti-erythropoietin antibodies revealed in pure red cell aplasia,[**] but the issue is complex, as explained in reference 23.

16.4.2 Aggregation of biologicals

The processing of many biological agents is complex. Aggregation of monoclonal antibodies during manufacturing processes is a key problem because, if the correct form of the monoclonal antibodyis not retained, then biological activity will be compromised.[24]

Aggregation during processing includes the events in the following steps:

- cell culture
- purification
- agitation
- ultrafiltration
- pumping at higher shear rates
- buffering procedures
- exposure to pH values close to isoelectric points

[**] Pure red cell aplasia is a rare and serious haematological disorder characterised by loss of erythroid progenitors from bone marrow, severe reticulocytopenia and rapid onset of transfusion-dependent anaemia.

- freezing and thawing
- final filling.

PEGylation of some proteins has been shown to reduce the extent of adsorption and surface-induced aggregation and to increase the reversibility of adsorption compared to native protein. Aspects of PEGylation are discussed in Chapter 13.

16.4.3 Generic biologicals (biosimilars)

A generic is, as stated above, a product that has been shown to be 'essentially similar' to the originator's product. However, biological products (biologics, biologicals, biopharmaceuticals) are more complex than drugs that are small or relatively small organic molecules. Because of their labile nature and the fact that the products may be dependent on the mode of manufacture, it is important to remember that it is has been stated that a process 'cannot be exactly duplicated by another manufacturer'.[25]

Why do these products have such specific problems? The molecules are large and often prepared in cell-based systems; they have complex tertiary and quaternary structures related to their activity; and they may be glycosylated. They are very sensitive to stresses such as temperature and even to shear forces that might be used in their production. DNA, for example, suffers from degradation due to shear forces. A practical pharmacy aspect is the use of International Non-proprietary Names (INNs) for such products. With conventional drugs an identical INN means a bioequivalent product and the same drug substance within pharmacopoeial or other limits. There are dangers if INNs are used for biogenerics that are subtly different.

Methods used to show that small-molecule therapeutics are nearly identical to each other are clearly not sufficient for biologicals. Bioequivalence is usually defined in terms of AUCs, but this is only part of the story with biological products. The nature of impurities is different. These impurities might indeed be analogues with a single amino acid difference, and be potent. If this is the case, this can lead to clinical problems. Impurities might be more difficult to detect in biological products if they are analogues of the main agent, so there is the risk of immunological and other side-effects. It is also possible that the formulation may be the cause of differences in protein products, as discussed above, as with recombinant human erythropoietin (Eprex).

Figure 16.10 summarises the issues that must be considered when dealing with biological generics.[26] The most appropriate description for generic biologicals is that they are 'biosimilar'.

The European Medicines Agency (EMA) has stated that the generic route is not appropriate for biologics, and the US Food and Drug Administration (FDA) stated in September 2006 that it 'has not determined how interchangeability can be established for complex proteins'. Note, however, that for biologics such as insulin, the transfer of patients from one product to another of the same insulin type is commonplace, though carried out with circumspection.

16.4.4 Regulatory views on biosimilar biologicals

The FDA acknowledges that 'biosimilars have not been demonstrated to be interchangeable through any scientific process'. A different naming scheme for these products might involve utilising a different level of granularity, which may be more detailed or less detailed. If the outcome of assigning the same INN to two products with highly similar ingredient(s) creates the implication that the two products are pharmacologically interchangeable *and* there were no scientific data to support that finding, then the FDA would have serious concerns about such an outcome, especially with more complicated proteins. At present, the FDA has not determined how interchangeability can be established for complex proteins.

This initiative reinforces the EMA communication on biosimilar medicines[27] and recognises the uniqueness of these products. It states that they cannot be classified as 'generics' in the same way that chemical compounds may be, owing to the differences stemming from the variability of the active biotechnological substances and manufacturing processes. Further, the EMA document clarifies that 'since biosimilar and biological reference medicines are similar but not identical, the decision to treat a patient with a reference or a biosimilar medicine should be taken following the opinion of a qualified healthcare professional'. This is effective advice against automatic substitution of one biological medicine over another that is ostensibly the same.

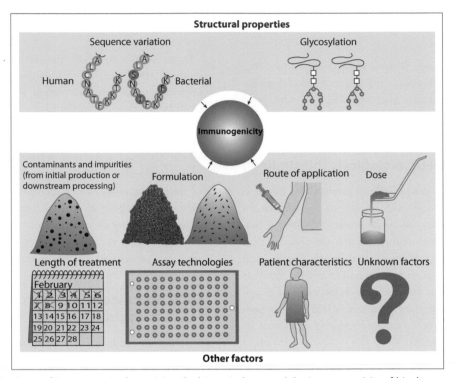

Figure 16.10   Areas of importance in determining the bioequivalence and the immunogenicity of biopharmaceuticals.

Reprinted by permission from Macmillan Publishers Ltd: Schellekens H. Bioequivalence and the immunogenicity of biopharmaceuticals. *Nat Rev Drug Discov* 2002;1:457–462. Copyright 2002.

16.4.5 PEGylated proteins

Some PEGylated proteins are discussed in Chapter 13. Attachment of long-chain polyoxyethylene glycols (PEGs) to proteins is the basis of PEGylation. This can increase the circulation time of proteins with short half-lives and can reduce immunogenicity; however, there are cases[28] where the process can reduce the functional activity of the protein by blocking access to receptors. These modified proteins are clearly not biosimilar to the parent proteins and are essentially new molecules.

16.5 Conclusions

For many medicinal products the initial brand and the subsequent generic products are therapeutically equivalent. There are of course effects of differences, such as the colour of capsules and tablets or the appearance of liquids, which can prejudice patients. There are drugs that have a narrow therapeutic index and that are

perhaps poorly soluble, which perhaps suggests that they might not be used interchangeably, but these are few in number; experts are not agreed even with drugs such as the antiepileptic agents. There is a greater practical problem in that biostudies might have shown both generic 1 and generic 2 to be bioequivalent to the brand leader, but this does not necessarily mean that generic 1 is equivalent to generic 2. Pharmacists have thus to be aware of the source of generics.

With generic versions of biologicals or biosimilars the issues are somewhat more complex. Development in analytical methods and other tests might assist in elucidating the similarity or otherwise of this growing array of drugs in the future. With both conventional drugs and biological drugs, wherever a formulation has been devised to alter the rate of release or delivery of the active agent, it is not automatic that generic versions will produce identical results. To be able to make informed decisions, pharmacists and drugs and therapeutics committees need access to the facts about such products and in particular their biopharmaceutical profiles in patients or volunteers.

References

1. Hassali MA *et al*. Knowledge and perceptions of recent pharmacy graduates about generic medicines. *Pharm Ed* 2007;7;89–95.
2. US Food and Drug Administration, Centre for Drug Evaluation and Research, Office for Generic Drugs. Available online at: http://www.fda.gov/Drugs/ResourcesFor-You/Consumers/BuyingUsingMedicineSafely/Understan-dingGenericDrugs/ucm144456.htm (updated 2009; accessed 23 September 2009).
3. Frijlink HW. Benefits of different drug formulations in psychopharmacology. *Eur Neuropsychopharmacol* 2003;13:S77–S84.
4. Wilner AN. Therapeutic equivalence of generic antiepileptic drugs: results of a survey. *Epilepsy Behav* 2004;5:995–998.
5. Crawford P *et al*. Are there potential problems with generic substitution of antiepileptic drugs? A review of issues. *Seizure* 2006;15:165–176.
6. Mofsen R, Balter J. Case reports of the re-emergence of psychotic symptoms after conversion from brand name clozapine to a generic formulation. *Clin Ther* 2001;23:1720–1731.
7. Paton C. Generic clozapine: outcomes after switching formulations. *Br J Psychiatry* 2006;189:184–185.
8. Healy DJ *et al*. Clinical equivalence of generic clozapine. *Commun Ment Health J* 2005;41:393–398.
9. Burkhardt RT *et al*. Lower phenytoin serum levels in persons switched from brand to generic phenytoin. *Neurology* 2004;63:1494–1496.
10. Assessment: generic substitution for antiepileptic medication. Report of the Therapeutics and Technology Assessment Sub-committee of the American Academy of Neurology. *Neurology* 1990;40:1641–1643.
11. Liouw K *et al*. Position statement on the coverage of anticonvulsant drugs for the treatment of epilepsy. *Neurology* 2007;68:1249–1250.
12. Blakesley VA. Current methodology to assess bioequivalence of levothyroxine sodium products are inadequate. *AAPS J* 2005;7:E42–E46.
13. Byakika-Kibwika P *et al*. Steady-state pharmacokinetic comparison of generic and branded formulations of stavudine, lamivudine and nevirapine in HIV-infected Ugandan adults. *J Antimicrob Chemother* 2008;62:1113–1117.
14. Laurent C *et al*. Effectiveness and safety of a generic fixed dose combination of neviparine, stavudine and lamivudine in HIV-1 infected adults in Cameroon: open label multicentre trial. *Lancet* 2004;364:29–34.
15. L'homme RFA *et al*. Pharmacokinetics of two generic fixed dose combinations for HIV infected children (Pedimune Baby and Pedimune Junior) are similar to the branded products in healthy adults. *J Antimicrob Chemother* 2007;59:92–96.
16. Kumarasamy N *et al*. The changing natural history of HIV disease: before and after the introduction of generic antiretroviral therapy in Southern India. *Clin Infect Dis* 2005;41:1525–1528.
17. Cantor LB. Generic ophthalmic medications: as good as Xerox? *Medscape Ophthalmol* 2008; 26 Nov. Available online at: http://cme.medscape.com/viewarticle/583866 (accessed 23 September 2009).
18. Baker MT. Sevoflurane: are there differences in products. *Anesth Analg* 2007;104:1447–1451.
19. Bito H, Ikeda K. Long-duration, low-flow sevoflurane anesthesia using two carbon dioxide absorbents. Quantification of degradation products in the circuit. *Anesthesiology* 1994;81:340–345.
20. Yamakage M *et al*. Analysis of the composition or 'original' and generic sevoflurane in routine use. *Br J Anaesth* 2007;99:819–823.
21. Anders MW. Formation and toxicity of anesthetic degradation products. *Annu Rev Pharmacol Toxicol* 2005;45:147–176.
22. US Food and Drug Administration. *Follow On Protein Products: Regulatory and Scientific Issues Related to Developing*. Available online at: http://www.fda.gov/Drugs/ScienceResearch/ResearchAreas/ucm085854.htm (accessed 9 January 2015).
23. Locatelli F *et al*. Pure red-cell aplasia 'epidemic' – mystery completely revealed? *Peritoneal Dialysis Int* 2007;27:S303–S307.
24. Vazques-Rey M, Lang DA. Aggregates in monoclonal antibody manufacturing processes. *Biotechnol Bioeng* 2011;108:1494–1508.
25. Bio (Biotechnology Industry Organization). See www.bio.org for various statements on biosimilars; 2015.
26. Schellekens H. Bioequivalence and the immunogenicity of biopharmaceuticals. *Nat Rev Drug Discov* 2002;1:457–462.
27. European Medicines Agency. Committee for Medicinal Products for Human Use (CHMP) *Guideline on Similar Biological Medicinal Products* (CHMP/437/04). 2015. www.ema.europa.eu (accessed 6 April 2015).
28. Kubetzko S *et al*. Protein PEGylation decreases observed target association rates via a dual blocking mechanism. *Mol Pharmacol* 2005;68:1439–1454.

Further reading

Johnston A *et al*. Effectiveness, safety and cost of drug substitution in hypertension. *Br J Clin Pharmacol* 2010;70:320–344. N.B. Although the emphasis in this paper is on hypertension treatment, the review deals with wider therapeutic categories and many of the challenging aspects of the problem of substituting generic products for originator brand products.

Derivations

Chapter 1

Box 1A The Clausius–Clapeyron equation

The Clausius–Clapeyron, which concerns the variation of vapour pressure with temperature, is usually derived from a consideration of the equilibrium between vapour and liquid phases, although in its generalised form it is equally applicable to solid–liquid equilibria. The increased motion of the molecules of the liquid following an increase of temperature leads to a greater tendency for escape of molecules into the vapour phase, with a consequent increase of vapour pressure. The variation of vapour pressure with temperature may be expressed in terms of the molar enthalpy of vaporisation of the liquid, ΔH_{vap}, using the Clapeyron equation:

$$\frac{dP}{dT} = \frac{\Delta H_{vap}}{T\Delta V} \tag{1A.1}$$

In this equation ΔV is the difference in molar volumes of the two phases. Since the molar volume of the vapour, V_v, is very much larger than that of the liquid, ΔV may be approximately equated with V_v. If it is also assumed that the vapour obeys the ideal gas equation, so that V_v may be replaced by RT/P, equation (1A.1) reduces to

$$\frac{dP}{dT} = \frac{P\Delta H_{vap}}{RT^2}$$

or

$$\frac{d\ln P}{dT} = \frac{\Delta H_{vap}}{RT^2} \tag{1A.2}$$

Equation (1A.2) is the Clausius–Clapeyron equation. General integration, assuming ΔH_{vap} to be constant, gives

$$\log P = \frac{-\Delta H_{vap}}{2.303RT} + \text{constant} \tag{1A.3}$$

A plot of log vapour pressure versus reciprocal temperature should be linear with a slope of $-\Delta H_{vap}/2.303R$, from which values of enthalpy of vaporisation may be determined.

Chapter 2

Box 2A Relationship between free energy change and the equilibrium constant

Consider the following reversible reaction taking place in the gaseous phase:

$$aA + bB \rightleftharpoons cC + dD$$

According to the law of mass action, the equilibrium constant, K, can be expressed as

$$K = \frac{(p'_C)^c (p'_D)^d}{(p'_A)^a (p'_B)^b} \tag{2A.1}$$

where p' represents the partial pressures of the components of the reaction at equilibrium.

The relationship between the free energy of a perfect gas and its partial pressure is given by

$$\Delta G = G - G^\ominus = RT \ln p \tag{2A.2}$$

where $G^\ominus$ is the free energy of 1 mole of gas at a pressure of 1 bar.

Applying equation (2A.2) to each component of the reaction gives

$$aG_A = a(G_A^\ominus + RT \ln p_A)$$
$$bG_B = b(G_B^\ominus + RT \ln p_B)$$

etc.

As

$$\Delta G = \sum G_{prod} - \sum G_{react}$$

so

$$\Delta G = \Delta G^\ominus + RT \ln \frac{(p_C)^c (p_D)^d}{(p_A)^a (p_B)^b} \tag{2A.3}$$

$\Delta G^\ominus$ is the standard free energy change of the reaction, given by

$$\Delta G^\ominus = cG_C^\ominus + dG_D^\ominus - aG_A^\ominus - bG_B^\ominus$$

As we have noted previously, the free energy change for systems at equilibrium is zero, and hence equation (2A.3) becomes

$$\Delta G^\ominus = -RT \ln \frac{(p'_C)^c (p'_D)^d}{(p'_A)^a (p'_B)^b} \tag{2A.4}$$

Substituting from equation (2A.1) gives

$$\Delta G^\ominus = -RT \ln K \tag{2A.5}$$

Substituting equation (2A.5) into equation (2A.3) gives

$$\Delta G = -RT \ln K + RT \ln \frac{(p_C)^c (p_D)^d}{(p_A)^a (p_B)^b} \qquad (2A.6)$$

Equation (2A.6) gives the change in free energy when a moles of A at a partial pressure p_A and b moles of B at a partial pressure p_B react together to yield c moles of C at a partial pressure p_C and d moles of D at a partial pressure p_D. For such a reaction to occur spontaneously, the free energy change must be negative, and hence equation (2A.6) provides a means of predicting the ease of reaction for selected partial pressures (or concentrations) of the reactants.

Box 2B Derivation of the van't Hoff equation

From equation (2.15),

$$-\Delta G^{\ominus}/RT = \ln K$$

Since

$$\Delta G^{\ominus} = \Delta H^{\ominus} - T\Delta S^{\ominus}$$

then at a temperature T_1

$$\begin{aligned} \ln K_1 &= -\Delta G^{\ominus}/RT_1 \\ &= -\Delta H^{\ominus}/RT_1 + \Delta S^{\ominus}/R \end{aligned} \qquad (2B.1)$$

and at temperature T_2

$$\begin{aligned} \ln K_2 &= -\Delta G^{\ominus}/RT_2 \\ &= -\Delta H^{\ominus}/RT_2 + \Delta S^{\ominus}/R \end{aligned} \qquad (2B.2)$$

If we assume that the standard enthalpy change $\Delta H^{\ominus}$ and the standard entropy change $\Delta S^{\ominus}$ are independent of temperature, then subtracting equation (2B.1) from equation (2B.2) gives

$$\ln K_2 - \ln K_1 = -\frac{\Delta H^{\ominus}}{R} \left(\frac{1}{T_2} - \frac{1}{T_1} \right)$$

or

$$\log \frac{K_2}{K_1} = \frac{\Delta H^{\ominus}}{2.303R} \frac{(T_2 - T_1)}{T_1 T_2} \qquad (2B.3)$$

Equation (2B.3), which is often referred to as the *van't Hoff equation*, is useful for the prediction of the equilibrium constant K_2 at a temperature T_2 from its value K_1 at a second temperature T_1.

Box 2C Mean ionic parameters

In general, we will consider a strong electrolyte that dissociates according to

$$C_{v+}A_{v-} \rightarrow v_+ C^{z+} + v_- A^{z-}$$

where v_+ is the number of cations, C^{z+}, of valence z_+, and v_- is the number of anions, A^{z-}, of valence z_-.
The activity, a, of the electrolyte is then

$$a = a_+^{v+} a_-^{v-} = a_{\pm}^{v} \tag{2C.1}$$

where $v = v_+ + v_-$

In the simple case of a solution of the 1 : 1 electrolyte sodium chloride, the activity will be

$$a = a_{Na^+} \times a_{Cl^-} = a_{\pm}^2$$

whereas, for morphine sulfate, which is a 1 : 2 electrolyte,

$$a = a_{morph^+}^2 \times a_{SO_4^{2-}} = a_{\pm}^3$$

Similarly, we may also define a *mean ion activity coefficient*, $\gamma_{\pm}$, in terms of the individual ionic activity coefficients γ_+ and γ_-:

$$\gamma_{\pm}^{v} = \gamma_+^{v+} \gamma_-^{v-} \tag{2C.2}$$

or

$$\gamma_{\pm} = (\gamma_+^{v+} \gamma_-^{v-})^{1/v} \tag{2C.3}$$

For a 1 : 1 electrolyte equation (2C.3) reduces to

$$\gamma_{\pm} = (\gamma_+ \gamma_-)^{1/2} \tag{2C.4}$$

Finally, we define a *mean ionic molality*, $m_{\pm}$, as

$$m_{\pm}^{v} = m_+^{v+} m_-^{v-} \tag{2C.5}$$

or

$$m_{\pm} = (m_+^{v+} m_-^{v-})^{1/v} \tag{2C.6}$$

For a 1 : 1 electrolyte, equation (2C.6) reduces to

$$m_{\pm} = (m_+ m_-)^{1/2} = m \tag{2C.7}$$

that is, mean ionic molality may be equated with the molality of the solution.
The activity of each ion is the product of its activity coefficient and its concentration:

$$a_+ = \gamma_+ m_+ \quad \text{and} \quad a_- = \gamma_- m_-$$

so that

$$\gamma_+ = a_+/m_+ \quad \text{and} \quad \gamma_- = a_-/m_-$$

Expressed as the mean ionic parameters, we have

$$\gamma_\pm = a_\pm / m_\pm \tag{2C.8}$$

Substituting for $m_\pm$ from equation (2C.6) gives

$$\gamma_\pm = a_\pm / (m_+^{v+} m_-^{v-})^{1/v} \tag{2C.9}$$

This equation applies in any solution, whether the ions are added together as a single salt or separately as a mixture of salts. For a solution of a single salt of molality, m:

$$m_+ = v_+ m \quad \text{and} \quad m_- = v_- m$$

Equation (2C.9) reduces to

$$\gamma_\pm = \frac{a_\pm}{m(v_+^{v+} v_-^{v-})^{1/v}} \tag{2C.10}$$

For example, for morphine sulfate, $v_+ = 2$, $v_- = 1$, and thus

$$\gamma_\pm = \frac{a_\pm}{(2^2 \times 1)^{1/3} m} = \frac{a_\pm}{4^{1/3} m}$$

Box 2D Chemical potential in two-phase systems

Consider a system of two phases, a and b, in equilibrium at constant temperature and pressure. If a small quantity of substance is transferred from phase a to phase b, then, because the overall free energy change is zero, we have

$$dG_a + dG_b = 0 \tag{2D.1}$$

where dG_a and dG_b are the free energy changes accompanying the transference of material for each phase.
From equation (2.26),

$$dG_a = \mu_a \, dn_a \quad \text{and} \quad dG_b = \mu_b \, dn_b$$

and thus

$$\mu_a \, dn_a + \mu_b \, dn_b = 0 \tag{2D.2}$$

A decrease of dn moles of component in phase a leads to an increase of exactly dn moles of this component in phase b; that is,

$$dn_a = -dn_b \tag{2D.3}$$

Substitution of equation (2D.3) into equation (2D.2) leads to the result

$$\mu_a = \mu_b \tag{2D.4}$$

In general, the chemical potential of a component is identical in all the phases of a system at equilibrium at a fixed temperature and pressure.

Box 2E Chemical potential of a component in solution

Non-electrolytes

In dilute solutions of non-volatile solutes the chemical potential of the solute is given by equation (2E.1):

$$\mu_2 = \mu_2^\ominus + RT \ln x_2 \tag{2E.1}$$

It is usually more convenient to express solute concentration as molality, m, rather than mole fraction using

$$x_2 = mM_1/1000$$

where M_1 = molecular weight of the solvent. Thus

$$\mu_2 = \mu^\ominus + RT \ln m \tag{2E.2}$$

where

$$\mu^\ominus = \mu_2^\ominus + RT \ln M_1 - RT \ln 1000 \tag{2E.2}$$

At higher concentrations, the solution generally exhibits significant deviations from ideality and mole fraction must be replaced by activity

$$\mu_2 = \mu_2^\ominus + RT \ln a_2 \tag{2E.3}$$

or

$$\mu_2 = \mu_2^\ominus + RT \ln \gamma_2 + RT \ln x_2 \tag{2E.4}$$

Electrolytes

The chemical potential of a strong electrolyte, which may be assumed to be completely dissociated in solution, is equal to the sum of the chemical potentials of each of the component ions. Thus

$$\mu_+ = \mu_+^\ominus + RT \ln a_+ \tag{2E.5}$$

and

$$\mu_- = \mu_-^\ominus + RT \ln a_- \tag{2E.6}$$

and therefore

$$\mu_2 = \mu_2^\ominus + RT \ln a \tag{2E.7}$$

where $\mu_2^\ominus$ is the sum of the chemical potentials of the ions, each in their respective standard state, i.e.

$$\mu_2^\ominus = v_+\mu_+^\ominus + v_-\mu_-^\ominus$$

where v_+ and v_- are the number of cations and anions, respectively, and a is the activity of the electrolyte as given in section 2.3.2.

For example, for a 1 : 1 electrolyte, from equation (2C.1) $a = a_\pm^2$. Therefore,

$$\mu_2 = \mu_2^\ominus + 2RT \ln a_\pm$$

From equation (2C.8), $a_\pm = m\,\gamma_\pm$. Therefore,

$$\mu_2 = \mu_2^\ominus + 2RT \ln m\gamma_\pm$$

Box 2F The degree of ionisation of weak acids and bases

Weak acids

Taking logarithms of the expression for the dissociation constant of a weak acid (equation 2.38),

$$-\log K_a = -\log[H_3O^+] - \log\frac{[A^-]}{[HA]}$$

which can be rearranged to

$$pH = pK_a + \log\frac{[A^-]}{[HA]} \tag{2F.1}$$

Equation (2F.1) may itself be rearranged to facilitate the direct determination of the molar percentage ionisation as follows:

$$[HA] = [A^-]\ \text{antilog}\ (pK_a - pH)$$

Therefore,

$$\text{percentage ionisation} = \frac{[A^-]}{[HA] + [A^-]} \times 100$$

$$= \frac{100}{1 + \text{antilog}\ (pK_a - pH)} \tag{2F.2}$$

Weak bases

An analogous series of equations for the percentage ionisation of a weak base may be derived as follows. Taking logarithms of equation (2.40) and rearranging gives

$$-\log K_b = -\log[OH^-] - \log\frac{[BH^+]}{[B]}$$

Therefore,

$$pH = pK_w - pK_b - \log\frac{[BH^+]}{[B]} \tag{2F.3}$$

Rearranging to facilitate calculation of the percentage ionisation leads to

$$\text{percentage ionisation} = \frac{100}{1 + \text{antilog}\ (pH - pK_w + pK_b)} \tag{2F.4}$$

Box 2G Derivation of an expression for the pH of a solution of a weakly acidic drug

We saw above that the dissociation of these types of drugs may be represented by equation (2.38). We can now express the concentrations of each of the species in terms of the degree of dissociation, α, which is a number with a value between 0 (no dissociation) and 1 (complete dissociation):

$$HA + H_2O \rightleftharpoons A^- + H_3O^+$$
$$(1-\alpha)c \qquad \alpha c \qquad \alpha c$$

where c is the initial concentration of the weakly acidic drug in mol dm^{-3}.

Because the drugs are weak acids, α will be very small and hence the term $(1-\alpha)$ can be approximated to 1. We may therefore write

$$K_a = \frac{\alpha^2 c^2}{(1-\alpha)c} \approx \alpha^2 c \tag{2G.1}$$

Therefore,

$$\alpha^2 = \left(\frac{K_a}{c}\right)^{1/2}$$

To introduce pH into the discussion we note that

$$\alpha c = [H_3O^+] = [H^+]$$
$$\therefore [H^+] = (K_a c)^{\frac{1}{2}}$$
$$\therefore -\log[H^+] = -\frac{1}{2}\log K_a - \frac{1}{2}\log c$$
$$pH = \frac{1}{2}\,pK_a - \frac{1}{2}\log c \tag{2G.2}$$

We now have an expression that enables us to calculate the pH of any concentration of the weakly acidic drug provided that its pK_a value is known.

Box 2H Derivation of an equation for buffer capacity

Equation (2.45) may be rewritten in the form

$$pH = pK_a + \frac{1}{2.303}\ln\left[\frac{c}{c_0 - c}\right] \tag{2H.1}$$

where c_0 is the total initial buffer concentration and c is the amount of alkali added. Rearrangement and subsequent differentiation yields

$$c = \frac{c_0}{1 + \exp[-2.303(pH - pK_a)]} \tag{2H.2}$$

Therefore,

$$\beta = \frac{dc}{d(pH)}$$

$$= \frac{2.303c_0 \exp[2.303(pH - pK_a)]}{1 + \exp[2.303 \exp(pH - pK_a)]^2} \tag{2H.3}$$

$$\beta = \frac{2.303c_0 K_a [H_3O^+]}{([H_3O^+] + K_a)^2} \tag{2H.4}$$

Chapter 3

Box 3A A Derivations of rate equations for zero-, first- and second-order reactions

Zero-order reactions
The rate equation is

$$dx/dt = k_0$$

Integration, noting that $x = 0$ at $t = 0$, gives

$$\int_0^x dx = k_0 \int_0^t dt \tag{3A.1}$$

i.e.

$$x = k_0 t \tag{3A.2}$$

First-order reactions
The rate equation is

$$dx/dt = k_1(a - x)$$

Since $x = 0$ at the start of the measurements (that is, when $t = 0$),

$$\int_0^x \frac{dx}{(a - x)} = k_1 \int_0^t dt \tag{3A.3}$$

$$k_1 = \frac{2.303}{t} \log \frac{a}{a - x} \tag{3A.4}$$

Or, rearranging into a linear form,

$$t = \frac{2.303}{k_1} \log a - \frac{2.303}{k_1} \log(a - x) \tag{3A.5}$$

An expression for the half-life $t_{0.5}$ may be derived from equation (3A.4), noting that when $t = t_{0.5}$, $x = a/2$:

$$t_{0.5} = \frac{2.303}{k_1} \log \frac{a}{a/2} \tag{3A.6}$$

Thus,

$$t_{0.5} = \frac{2.303}{k_1} \log 2 = \frac{0.693}{k_1} \tag{3A.7}$$

Second-order reactions

The rate equation is

$$dx/dt = k_2[A][B] \tag{3A.8}$$

If the initial concentrations of reactants A and B are a and b, respectively, equation (3A.8) may be written

$$dx/dt = k_2(a - x)(b - x) \tag{3A.9}$$

where x is the amount of A and B decomposed in time t. Integration of equation (3A.9) by the method of partial fractions yields

$$k_2 = \frac{2.303}{t(a - b)} \log \frac{b(a - x)}{a(b - x)} \tag{3A.10}$$

Rearranging into a linear form suitable for plotting gives

$$t = \frac{2.303}{k_2(a - b)} \log \frac{b}{a} + \frac{2.303}{k_2(a - b)} \log \frac{(a - x)}{(b - x)} \tag{3A.11}$$

For reactions in which both concentration terms refer to the same reactant we may write

$$-d[A]/dt = k_2[A]^2 \tag{3A.12}$$

and

$$dx/dt = k_2(a - x)^2 \tag{3A.13}$$

A similar equation applies to second-order reactions in which the initial concentrations of the two reactants are the same.

Integration of equation (3A.13) between the limits of t from 0 to t and of x from 0 to x yields

$$t = \frac{1}{k_2} \left[\frac{1}{a - x} - \frac{1}{a} \right] = \frac{x}{k_2 a(a - x)} \tag{3A.14}$$

Box 3B Derivations of equations for complex reactions

Reversible reactions

The rate of decomposition of reactant is given by

$$-d[A]/dt = k_f[A] - k_r[B] \tag{3B.1}$$

Equation (3B.1) may be integrated noting that $[A_0] - [A] = [B]$ and introducing the equilibrium condition $k_f[A]_{eq} = k_r[B]_{eq}$ to yield

$$t = \frac{2.303}{(k_f + k_r)} \log \frac{[A]_0 - [A]_{eq}}{[A] - [A]_{eq}} \tag{3B.2}$$

where $[A]_0$, $[A]$ and $[A]_{eq}$ represent the initial concentration, the concentration at time t and the equilibrium concentration of reactant A, respectively. Equation (3B.2) indicates that a plot of t (as ordinate) against log $[([A]_0 - [A]_{eq})/([A] - [A]_{eq})]$ should be linear with a gradient of $2.303/(k_f + k_r)$. k_f and k_r may be calculated separately if the equilibrium constant K is also determined, since

$$K = \frac{[B]_{eq}}{[A]_{eq}} = \frac{1 - [A]_{eq}}{[A]_{eq}} = \frac{k_f}{k_r} \tag{3B.3}$$

where $[B]_{eq}$ is the equilibrium concentration of product B.

Parallel reactions

The rate equation is

$$-d[X]/dt = (k_A + k_B)[X] = k_{exp}[X] \tag{3B.4}$$

where k_A and k_B are the rate constants for the formation of A and B, respectively, and k_{exp} is the experimentally determined rate constant.

Values of the rate constants k_A and k_B may be evaluated separately if it is possible to monitor the concentration of drug X and those of the breakdown products A and B as a function of time. The rate of formation of A can be expressed as

$$\frac{d[A]}{dt} = k_A[X] = k_A[X]_0 e^{-k_{exp}t} \tag{3B.5}$$

where $[A]$ is the concentration of the product A at time t, and $[X]_0$ is the initial concentration of the drug. It is reasonable to assume that the initial concentration of product A is zero and therefore integration of equation (3B.5) gives

$$[A] = \frac{k_A}{k_{exp}}[X]_0(1 - e^{-k_{exp}t}) \tag{3B.6}$$

Similarly, for product B,

$$[B] = \frac{k_B}{k_{exp}}[X]_0(1 - e^{-k_{exp}t}) \tag{3B.7}$$

Plots of $[A]$ or $[B]$ against $(1 - e^{-k_{exp}t})$ should be linear with gradients $k_A[X]_0/k_{exp}$ and $k_B[X]_0/k_{exp}$ respectively, from which values of the rate constants k_A and k_B may be determined. Alternatively, values of the rate constants k_A and k_B may be evaluated from the ratio R of the concentration of products formed by each reaction at equilibrium. From equations (3B.6) and (3B.7)

$$R = \frac{[A]_{eq}}{[B]_{eq}} = \frac{k_A}{k_B} \tag{3B.8}$$

Since

$$k_{exp} = k_A + k_B \tag{3B.9}$$

$$k_{exp} = k_A + k_A/R \tag{3B.10}$$

Solving for k_A gives

$$k_A = k_{exp} \frac{R}{(R+1)} \tag{3B.11}$$

Similarly,

$$k_B = \frac{k_{exp}}{(R+1)} \tag{3B.12}$$

Consecutive reactions

The rate of decomposition of A is

$$- d[A]/dt = k_A[A] \tag{3B.13}$$

The rate of change of concentration of B is

$$d[B]/dt = k_A[A] - k_B[B] \tag{3B.14}$$

and that of C is

$$d[C]/dt = k_B[B] \tag{3B.15}$$

Integration of the rate equation (equation 3B.13) yields

$$[A] = [A]_0 e^{-k_A t} \tag{3B.16}$$

Substitution of equation (3B.16) into equation (3B.14) gives

$$d[B]/dt = k_A[A]_0 e^{-k_A t} - k_B[B] \tag{3B.17}$$

which upon integration gives

$$[B] = \frac{k_A[A_0]}{(k_B - k_A)} [e^{-k_A t} - e^{-k_B t}] \tag{3B.18}$$

At any time,

$$[A]_0 = [A] + [B] + [C] \tag{3B.19}$$

so that

$$[C] = [A]_0 - [A] - [B]$$
$$= [A]_0 \left[1 + \frac{1}{k_A - k_B} (k_B e^{-k_A t} - k_A e^{-k_B t}) \right] \tag{3B.20}$$

Box 3C Non-isothermal methods for determination of drug stability

In the method proposed by Rogers[31] the rise of temperature was programmed so that the reciprocal of the temperature varied logarithmically with time according to

$$(1/T_0) - (1/T_t) = 2.303\, b \log(1+t) \tag{3C.1}$$

where T_0 and T_t are the temperatures at zero time and at time t, respectively, and b is any suitable proportionality constant. Applying the Arrhenius equation at both temperatures and subtracting gives

$$\log k_t = \log k_0 + \frac{E_a}{2.303R}\left(\frac{1}{T_0} - \frac{1}{T_t}\right) \tag{3C.2}$$

Substituting equation (3C.1) into equation (3C.2) gives

$$\log k_t = \log k_0 + \frac{E_a b}{R}\log(1+t) \tag{3C.3}$$

Therefore,

$$k_t = k_0(1+t)^{E_a b/R} \tag{3C.4}$$

For first-order reactions $-\mathrm{d}c/\mathrm{d}t = kc$, where c is concentration. Substituting for k from equation (3C.4) and integrating gives

$$-\int_{c_0}^{c_t}\frac{\mathrm{d}c}{c} = k_0\int_0^t (1+t)^{E_a b/R}\mathrm{d}t \tag{3C.5}$$

where c_0 and c_t are the concentrations at zero time and at time t, respectively. Therefore,

$$\log \mathrm{f}(c) = \log k_0 - \log\left(1 + \frac{E_a b}{R}\right) + \left(1 + \frac{E_a b}{R}\right)\log(1+t) + \log\left[1 - \left(\frac{k_0}{k_t}\right)^{1+R/E_a b}\right] \tag{3C.6}$$

where

$$\mathrm{f}(c) = 2.303\log(c_0/c_t) \tag{3C.7}$$

A similar equation applies to second-order reactions with

$$\log \mathrm{f}(c) = \frac{2.303}{a_0 - b_0}\log\frac{a_t}{b_t} + \frac{2.303}{a_0 - b_0}\log\frac{b_0}{a_0} \tag{3C.8}$$

where a_0 and b_0 are the concentrations of the reactants at the beginning of the experiment, and a_t and b_t their concentrations at time t. The value of the final term of equation (3C.6) rapidly tends to zero as k_t becomes greater than k_0. Thus a graph of $\log \mathrm{f}(c)$ against $\log(1+t)$ will be linear from that time after which k_0 is negligible in comparison with k_t. The gradient of the line is $(1 + E_a b/R)$, enabling E_a to be determined. The rate constant k_0 may then be calculated from the intercept when $\log(1+t) = 0$, which is equal to $\log k_0 - \log(1 + E_a b/R)$. The rate constant at any other temperature may be calculated from k_0 and E_a.

Chapter 4

Box 4A Derivation of an equation for the solubility of an acidic drug as a function of pH

If we represent the drug as HA and the total saturation solubility of the drug as S, and if S_0 is the solubility of the undissociated drug, it is clear that the total solubility is the sum of the solubility of the un-ionised and ionised species, that is

$$S = S_0 + (\text{concentration of ionised species})$$

The dissociation of the acid in water can be written

$$HA + H_2O \rightleftharpoons H_3O^+ + A^- \tag{4A.1}$$

and the dissociation constant K_a is given by

$$K_a = \frac{[H_3O^+][A^-]}{[HA]} \tag{4A.2}$$

Rearranging and substituting S_0 for [HA] gives

$$\frac{K_a}{[H_3O^+]} = \frac{[A^-]}{S_0} \tag{4A.3}$$

but as $[A^-] = S - S_0$,

$$\frac{K_a}{[H_3O^+]} = \frac{S - S_0}{S_0} \tag{4A.4}$$

Taking logarithms,

$$pH - pK_a = \log\left(\frac{S - S_0}{S_0}\right) \tag{4A.5}$$

Hence the solubility of the drug at any pH can be calculated provided pK_a and S_0 are known.

Box 4B Derivation of equations for solubility of basic drugs as a function of pH

The dissociation of the base in water can be written:

$$RNH_2 + H_2O \rightleftharpoons RNH_3^+ + OH^- \tag{4B.1}$$

Therefore,

$$K_b = \frac{[RNH_3^+][OH^-]}{[RNH_2]} \tag{4B.2}$$

That is

$$\frac{K_b}{[OH^-]} = \frac{[H^+]}{K_a} = \frac{S - S_0}{S_0} \tag{4B.3}$$

Taking logarithms,

$$pK_a - pH = \log\left(\frac{S - S_0}{S_0}\right) \qquad (4B.4)$$

or

$$pH - pK_a = \log\left(\frac{S_0}{S - S_0}\right) \qquad (4B.5)$$

Box 4C Derivation of equations for solubility of amphoteric drugs as a function of pH

The equilibria between the species can be written as

The two dissociation constants can be defined in the normal way as

$$K_{a_1} = \frac{[HA^{\pm}][H^+]}{[HAH^+]} \qquad (4C.1)$$

and

$$K_{a_2} = \frac{[A^-][H^+]}{[HA^{\pm}]} \qquad (4C.2)$$

That is

$$\frac{K_{a_1}}{[H^+]} = \frac{[HA^{\pm}]}{[HAH^+]} \qquad (4C.3)$$

and

$$\frac{K_{a_2}}{[H^+]} = \frac{[A^-]}{[HA^{\pm}]} \qquad (4C.4)$$

It is observed that the zwitterion has the lowest solubility (Fig. 4.3 and Table 4.8), which we take to be S_0.

$$\frac{K_{a_1}}{[H^+]} = \frac{S_0}{S - S_0} \qquad (4C.5)$$

and

$$\frac{K_{a_2}}{[H^+]} = \frac{S - S_0}{S_0} \qquad (4C.6)$$

Therefore,

$$pH - pK_a = \log\left(\frac{S_0}{S - S_0}\right) \tag{4C.7}$$

at pH values below the isoelectric point, and

$$pH - pK_a = \log\left(\frac{S - S_0}{S_0}\right) \tag{4C.8}$$

at pH values above the isoelectric point.

Box 4D Partitioning of aggregating and ionising species

Aggregating species

If the solute forms aggregates or otherwise self-associates, the simple expression for partition coefficient given in equation (4.19) no longer applies. For example, the following equilibrium between the two phases 1 and 2 occurs when dimerisation occurs in phase 2:

$$\underset{\text{phase 1}}{2A} \rightleftharpoons \underset{\text{phase 2}}{A \cdot A}$$

$$K = \frac{[A]_{\text{phase2}}}{[A]_{\text{phase1}}^2}$$

Hence

$$K' = \frac{\sqrt{C_2}}{C_1} \tag{4D.1}$$

K' is a constant combining the partition coefficient and the association constant.

Ionisable species

We will consider the distribution of *weakly acidic drugs* between organic and aqueous phases. If we express the dissociation of a weak acid as

$$HA \rightleftharpoons H^+ + A^-$$

the dissociation constant in the aqueous phase, K_a will be given by

$$K_a = \frac{[H^+][A^-]}{[HA]} \tag{4D.2}$$

The true partition coefficient is the ratio of the concentrations of the un-ionised species in organic and aqueous phases, i.e.

$$P = \frac{[HA]_o}{[HA]_w} \tag{4D.3}$$

whereas the apparent partition coefficient is the ratio of the concentration of the un-ionised species in organic phase to the sum of the un-ionised and ionised species in the aqueous phase, i.e.

$$P_{app} = \frac{[HA]_o}{[HA]_w + [A^-]_w} \tag{4D.4}$$

Substituting for $[A^-]_w$ from equation (4D.2) and rearranging using the expression for P from equation (4D.3) gives

$$P_{app} = \frac{[H^+][HA]_o}{[HA]_w\{[H^+]+K_a\}} = \frac{P[H^+]}{[H^+] + K_a} \tag{4D.5}$$

Therefore,

$$\frac{P}{P_{app}} = 1 + \frac{K_a}{[H^+]} \tag{4D.6}$$

Taking logarithms and rearranging gives

$$\log P = \log P_{app} - \log\left[\frac{1}{1 + \frac{K_a}{[H^+]}}\right] \tag{4D.7}$$

Substituting from equation (4D.2),

$$\log P = \log P_{app} - \log\left[\frac{1}{1 + \frac{A^-}{[HA]}}\right] \tag{4D.8}$$

Since, from equation (2.44),

$$pH - pK_a = \log\frac{[A^-]}{[HA]}$$

and therefore,

$$\frac{[A^-]}{[HA]} = 10^{pH-pK_a} \tag{4D.9}$$

Substituting into equation (4D.8) gives

$$\log P = \log P_{app} - \log\left(\frac{1}{1 + 10^{pH-pK_a}}\right) \tag{4D.10}$$

The equivalent expression for the relationship between true and apparent partition coefficients for weakly basic drugs, which may be derived in a similar manner, is

$$\log P = \log P_{app} - \log\left(\frac{1}{1 + 10^{pK_a-pH}}\right) \tag{4D.11}$$

Chapter 5

Box 5A The Gibbs equation

We can treat the thermodynamics of the surface layer in a similar way to the bulk of the solution. The energy change, dU, accompanying an infinitesimal, reversible change in the system is given by

$$dU = dq_{rev} - dw$$

or

$$dU = TdS - dw \tag{5A.1}$$

where dq_{rev} and dw are, respectively, the heat absorbed and the work done during the reversible change (see section 2.2.1).

For an open system (one in which there is a transfer of material between phases) equation (5A.1) must be written

$$dU = TdS - dw + \Sigma \mu_i dn_i \tag{5A.2}$$

where μ_i and n_i are the chemical potential and number of moles of the ith component, respectively.

When applying equation (5A.2) to the surface layer, the work is that required to increase the area of the surface by an infinitesimal amount, dA, at constant T, P and n. This work is done against the surface tension and is given by equation (5.1) as $dw = \gamma \, dA$.

Thus, equation (5A.2) becomes

$$dU^s = TdS^s + \gamma dA + \Sigma \mu_i dn_i^s \tag{5A.3}$$

where the superscript, s, denotes the surface layer.

If the energy, entropy and number of moles of component are allowed to increase from zero to some finite value, equation (5A.3) becomes

$$U^s = TS^s + \gamma A + \Sigma \mu_i n_i^s \tag{5A.4}$$

General differentiation of equation (5A.4) gives

$$\begin{aligned} dU^s = &TdS^s + S^s dT + \gamma dA \\ &+ Ad\gamma + \Sigma \mu_i dn_i^s + \Sigma n_i^s d\mu_i \end{aligned} \tag{5A.5}$$

Comparison with equation (5A.3) gives

$$0 = S^s dT + \Sigma n_i^s d\mu_i + Ad\gamma \tag{5A.6}$$

At constant temperature, equation (5A.6) becomes

$$d\gamma = -\Sigma \Gamma_i d\mu_i \tag{5A.7}$$

where $\Gamma_i = n_i^s / A$ and is termed the *surface excess concentration*. Γ_i is the amount of the ith component in the surface phase s, in excess of that which there would have been had the bulk phases a and b extended to the dividing surface without change in composition.

For a two-component system at constant temperature, equation (5A.7) reduces to

$$dy = -\Gamma_1 d\mu_i - \Gamma_2 d\mu_2 \qquad (5A.8)$$

where subscripts 1 and 2 denote solvent and solute, respectively. The surface excess concentrations are defined relative to an arbitrarily chosen dividing surface. A convenient choice of location of this surface is that at which the surface excess concentration of the solvent, Γ_1, is zero. Indeed, this is the most realistic position since we are now considering the surface layer of adsorbed solute. Equation (5A.8) then becomes

$$dy = -\Gamma_2 d\mu_2 \qquad (5A.9)$$

The chemical potential of the solute is given by equation (2.30) as

$$\mu_2 = \mu_2^\ominus + RT \ln a_2$$
$$d\mu_2 = RT d(\ln a_2)$$

Substituting in equation (5A.9) gives the Gibbs equation:

$$\Gamma_2 = -\frac{1}{RT}\frac{dy}{d(\ln a_2)} = -\frac{a_2}{RT}\frac{dy}{da_2} \qquad (5A.10)$$

Chapter 9

Box 9A Derivation of equation (9.3)

Fick's law of diffusion shows that (for a given vehicle)

$$J \propto \Delta C_v$$

A proportionality constant κ_p may be added. Thus

$$J = \kappa_p \Delta C_v$$

where κ_p is the permeability constant, which provides a means of expressing absorption measurements for comparing different vehicles and conditions. The units of a permeability constant are m s^{-1}, the concentration term being mol m^{-3}, so that J has the correct units of mol m^{-2} s^{-1}. It has been shown that

$$\kappa_p = \frac{PD}{\delta}$$

so that equation (9.3) is readily obtained.

Chapter 11

Box 11A Adsorption of glyceryl trinitrate on to plastic containers

Consider a two-stage loss of drug:

$$A \underset{k_2}{\overset{k_1}{\rightleftharpoons}} B \overset{k_3}{\longrightarrow} C$$

where

    A = glyceryl trinitrate in aqueous solution

    B = adsorbed glyceryl trinitrate

    C = glyceryl trinitrate dissolved in the matrix

Then,

$$\frac{dA}{dt} = -k_1 A + k_2 B \tag{11A.1}$$

$$\frac{dB}{dt} = k_1 A - k_2 B - k_3 B \tag{11A.2}$$

and

$$\frac{dC}{dt} = k_3 B \tag{11A.3}$$

It is found that $dB/dt \gg dC/dt$. At steady state, $dB/dt = 0$, and at $t = 0$, $A = A_0$, $B = 0$ and $C = 0$. Rate constant k_1 is a function of the amount of drug in solution, the surface area available for adsorption and the nature of the plastic, and k_3 is a function of the volume of the plastic matrix and the solubility of the glyceryl trinitrate in the plastic matrix. The ratio k_3/k_2 describes the partitioning of the drug between the plastic and the aqueous phase. So, if P is the partition coefficient,

$$\frac{k_3}{k_2} = aP \tag{11A.4}$$

a being a proportionality constant related to the mass of the plastic, the volume of the solution and other parameters. The ratio k_1/k_2 can be related to a Langmuir type of adsorption constant. The final form of the equation accurately predicts the amount (A) of glyceryl trinitrate remaining in solution:

$$A = 8.957e^{-0.028t} + 14.943e^{-0.235t} \tag{11.A5}$$

Box 11B Estimation of the degree of protein binding

Protein binding can be considered to be an adsorption process obeying the law of mass action. If D represents drug and P the protein we can write

$$D + P \rightleftharpoons (DP) \quad \text{(protein – drug complex)}$$

At equilibrium,

$$D_f + (P_t - D_b) \rightleftharpoons D_b \tag{11B.1}$$

where D_f is the molar concentration of unbound drug, P_t is the total molar concentration of protein, and D_b is the molar concentration of bound drug (= molar concentration of complex). If one assumes one binding site per molecule, the equilibrium constant, K, is given by

$$K = \frac{k_1}{k_{-1}} = \frac{\text{rate constant for association}}{\text{rate constant for dissociation}} \tag{11B.2}$$

From equation (11B.1)

$$K = \frac{D_b}{D_f(P_t - D_b)} \tag{11B.3}$$

It is obvious that $k_1 > k_{-1}$. The rate constant for dissociation, k_{-1}, is the rate-limiting step in the exchange of drug between free and bound forms. From equation (11B.3) we obtain

$$KD_fP_t - KD_fD_b = D_b \tag{11B.4}$$

That is,

$$KD_fP_t = D_b + KD_fD_b = D_b(1 + KD_f) \tag{11B.5}$$

Therefore,

$$\frac{KD_fP_t}{1 + KD_f} = D_b \tag{11B.6}$$

or

$$\frac{D_b}{P_t} = r = \frac{KD_f}{1 + KD_f} \tag{11B.7}$$

where r is the number of moles of drug bound to total protein in the system. If there are not one, but n, binding sites per protein molecule, then

$$r = \frac{nKD_f}{1 + KD_f} \tag{11B.8}$$

or

$$\frac{1}{r} = \frac{1}{n} + \frac{1}{nKD_f} \tag{11B.9}$$

Protein-binding results are often quoted as the fraction of drug bound, β. This fraction varies generally with the concentration of both drug and protein, as shown in equation (11B.10), which relates β with n, K and concentration:

$$\beta = \frac{1}{1 + D_f/(nP_t) + 1/(nKP_t)} \tag{11B.10}$$

Index